Auditory Processing Deficits

Assessment and Intervention

Vishakha Waman Rawool, PhD, CCC-A, FAA
Professor of Audiology
Department of Communication Sciences & Disorders
West Virginia University
Morgantown, West Virginia

Thieme
New York • Stuttgart • Delhi • Rio de Janeiro

Editorial Director, Educational Products: Anne M. Sydor
Managing Editor: Elizabeth Palumbo
Director, Editorial Services: Mary Jo Casey
International Production Director: Andreas Schabert
Vice President, Editorial and E-Product Development:
    Vera Spillner
International Marketing Director: Fiona Henderson
International Sales Director: Louisa Turrell
Director of Sales, North America: Mike Roseman
Senior Vice President and Chief Operating Officer:
    Sarah Vanderbilt
President: Brian D. Scanlan

Library of Congress Cataloging-in-Publication Data

Rawool, Vishakha Waman, author.
Auditory processing deficits : assessment and intervention /
    Vishakha Rawool.
p. ; cm.
Includes bibliographical references and index.
ISBN 978-1-60406-838-2 (softcover) – ISBN 978-1-60406-
837-5 (eISBN)
I. Title.
[DNLM: 1. Auditory Perceptual Disorders–diagnosis.
    2. Auditory Perceptual Disorders–therapy. 3. Auditory
    Cortex–physiopathology. WV 270]
RF290
617.8–dc23   2014032047

© 2016 Thieme Medical Publishers, Inc.

Thieme Publishers New York
333 Seventh Avenue, New York, NY 10001 USA
+1 800 782 3488, customerservice@thieme.com

Thieme Publishers Stuttgart
Rüdigerstrasse 14, 70469 Stuttgart, Germany
+49 [0]711 8931 421, customerservice@thieme.de

Thieme Publishers Delhi
A-12, Second Floor, Sector-2, Noida-201301
Uttar Pradesh, India
+91 120 45 566 00, customerservice@thieme.in

Thieme Publishers Rio de Janeiro, Thieme Publicações Ltda.
Edifício Rodolpho de Paoli, 25º andar
Av. Nilo Peçanha, 50 – Sala 2508
Rio de Janeiro 20020-906 Brasil
+55 21 3172-2297 / +55 21 3172-1896

Cover design: Thieme Publishing Group
Typesetting by DiTech Process Solutions

Printed in China by Everbest Printing Co.   5 4 3 2 1

ISBN 978-1-60406-838-2

Also available as an e-book:
eISBN 978-1-60406-837-5

Important note: Medicine is an ever-changing science undergoing continual development. Research and clinical experience are continually expanding our knowledge, in particular our knowledge of proper treatment and drug therapy. Insofar as this book mentions any dosage or application, readers may rest assured that the authors, editors, and publishers have made every effort to ensure that such references are in accordance with **the state of knowledge at the time of production of the book.**

Nevertheless, this does not involve, imply, or express any guarantee or responsibility on the part of the publishers in respect to any dosage instructions and forms of applications stated in the book. **Every user is requested to examine carefully** the manufacturers' leaflets accompanying each drug and to check, if necessary in consultation with a physician or specialist, whether the dosage schedules mentioned therein or the contraindications stated by the manufacturers differ from the statements made in the present book. Such examination is particularly important with drugs that are either rarely used or have been newly released on the market. Every dosage schedule or every form of application used is entirely at the user's own risk and responsibility. The authors and publishers request every user to report to the publishers any discrepancies or inaccuracies noticed. If errors in this work are found after publication, errata will be posted at www.thieme.com on the product description page.

Some of the product names, patents, and registered designs referred to in this book are in fact registered trademarks or proprietary names even though specific reference to this fact is not always made in the text. Therefore, the appearance of a name without designation as proprietary is not to be construed as a representation by the publisher that it is in the public domain.

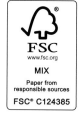

To my parents and Dr. David Goldstein

Contents

Acknowledgments

This book is dedicated to my parents and Dr. David Goldstein. My parents did their best in ensuring a great educational foundation. My father, Waman, ensured a multilingual vocabulary to enhance the ability to gain knowledge from several resources, and my mother, Shobha, encouraged me to write and publish at a very young age. Both of them emphasized self-discipline, which has been very valuable in completing this book and other similar projects. Dr. David Goldstein, who is one of my mentors from Purdue University, was highly instrumental in my acquisition of the PhD degree and was influential in ensuring a path of clinical research to guarantee high quality audiology services.

I would like to acknowledge Topiwala National Medical College and B. Y. L. Nair Charitable Hospital at Bombay (now Mumbai) University, Mumbai, India, for providing me with exceptional clinical knowledge and skills in the areas of audiology and speech and language pathology at the undergraduate level. I was fortunate in being selected for a special training program in oral education of deaf children at the same institute. I benefited from the extensive clinical experience that I gained by working at the same institute in providing speech, hearing, and language services for various populations, including children with hearing loss.

Additionally, I would like to acknowledge the Speech-Language Pathology Department at the University of Texas at El Paso for providing extensive training and clinical experience in speech-language pathology at the graduate level. My undergraduate training in speech language pathology and audiology, my diploma in educating the deaf from Bombay University, my master's training in speech-language pathology from the University of Texas at El Paso, my doctoral education in audiology at Purdue University, and my post-doctoral training at Johns Hopkins University was very helpful in writing this book. During my doctoral course work, I greatly benefited from a doctoral level seminar in language impairment taught by Dr. Laurence B. Leonard.

Chapter 1

Introduction

1 Introduction

To gain a complete understanding of auditory processing deficits (APDs), a detailed understanding of the central auditory system is necessary. Such details can be found in general anatomy and physiology textbooks. A brief review of the anatomy and physiology of the auditory system is included in this chapter with reference to such deficits.

1.1 Auditory Nervous System

The auditory nervous system is fairly complex with several redundant ascending and descending projections. Auditory evoked potentials, including the auditory brainstem response, middle latency response, and late cortical potentials (see Chapter 4), are useful in evaluating the functional status of the auditory system. A brief review of the auditory system is provided below. The system can be broadly divided into the afferent (▶ Fig. 1.1) and efferent systems.

1.1.1 Afferent Auditory Pathways

Auditory Nerve Fibers

Each hair cell in the cochlea has several afferent auditory nerve fibers at the base. Most of the afferent nerve endings are at the base of inner hair cells, although a few also arise from the outer hair cells (▶ Fig. 1.2). The nerve fibers maintain the tonotopic organization within the cochlea. The fibers that are located at the base of the cochlea are arranged toward the outside of the auditory nerve tract, and those that are located at the apex are arranged centrally. The fibers are tuned to specific frequencies depending on their attachments to the hair cells. In other words, they are most sensitive to particular frequencies and are not so sensitive to the surrounding frequencies.

Auditory neurons usually fire at a baseline rate without any auditory stimuli. This is referred to as the *spontaneous firing rate.* Following auditory stimuli, the firing rate of the neuron increases above the spontaneous rate. The rate increases further with the increase in the loudness of the stimuli. In response to tone bursts, a peak is apparent at the onset of the stimulus in the firing rate pattern. With continuation of the tone burst, there is a gradual decrease in the firing rate, and the discharge rate stabilizes. When the stimulus is turned off, the discharge activity drops sharply below the spontaneous rate, then gradually rises up to the baseline spontaneous rate. This type of response pattern is referred to as the *primary-like response pattern* given that the auditory nerve fibers leaving the cochlea are considered the primary neural units within the auditory pathway.

Damage to the outer portion of the auditory nerve results in a high-frequency hearing loss because the fibers tuned to higher frequencies are located toward the outer portion of the auditory nerve. Besides a perceptual deficit, other deficits can occur within the auditory nerve fibers. For example, under certain circumstances, such as an auditory nerve tumor, the fibers may fire continuously without auditory input, giving rise to the perception of tinnitus. In other circumstances, the firing may show excessive adaptation. In this case, even in the presence of a continuous loud tone, the patient may hear the sound at the beginning but may cease to perceive it within a few seconds.

Cochlear Nucleus

After leaving the inner ear through the internal auditory canal, the auditory nerve enters the brainstem, and the neurons of the nerve synapse with cell bodies within the cochlear nucleus. After entering the cochlear nucleus, each nerve fiber distributes branches to the various sections of the cochlear nucleus. The cochlear nucleus can be divided into three regions: the anteroventral cochlear nucleus (AVCN), the posteroventral cochlear nucleus (PVCN), and the dorsal cochlear nucleus (DCN).

The ventral cochlear nucleus (VCN) has different types of units that can be classified based on their response properties as primary-like, chopper, build-up, onset, and pausers. The primary-like units show discharge patterns similar to those of the auditory nerve fibers. The chopper units show response patterns that look as if segments have been chopped out of the pattern. The chopping probably occurs due to regularly spaced, preferred discharge times. Build-up units show a response pattern that shows a gradual increase in the discharge rate following stimulus onset until it becomes stable. Pausers show an initial large discharge peak or spike rate that is followed by a pause in response, which in turn is followed by a

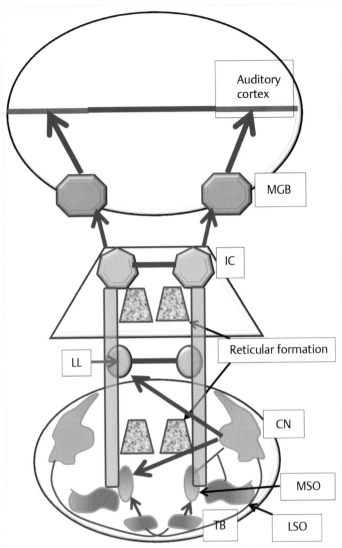

Fig. 1.1 Schematic of the afferent auditory pathway. CN, cochlear nucleus; IC, inferior colliculus; LL, lateral lemniscus; LSO, lateral superior olive; MGB, medial geniculate body; MSO, medial superior olive; TB, trapezoid body.

lower rate of response that lasts until the stimulus is turned off. Onset units respond only at the onset of the stimulus.

The tonotopic organization of the cochlea and the auditory nerve is maintained in the cochlear nucleus and at all higher levels in the auditory pathway. For example, neurons arriving from the basal portion of the cochlea synapse mainly with cell bodies in the dorsal portion of the dorsal cochlear nucleus.

Trapezoid Body

The neural fibers arising from the VCN or ventral acoustic stria form the trapezoid body. The fibers of the trapezoid body cross to the opposite side and synapse with the cell bodies of the contralateral superior olivary complex (SOC) or form connections with the contralateral lateral lemniscus. Other fibers from the trapezoid bodies connect with the ipsilateral SOC.

Superior Olivary Complex (SOC)

The SOC consists of a medial accessory nucleus and a lateral principle nucleus. Fibers from the left and right VCN mainly synapse with the medial accessory nucleus. Thus, the SOC receives input from both ears.

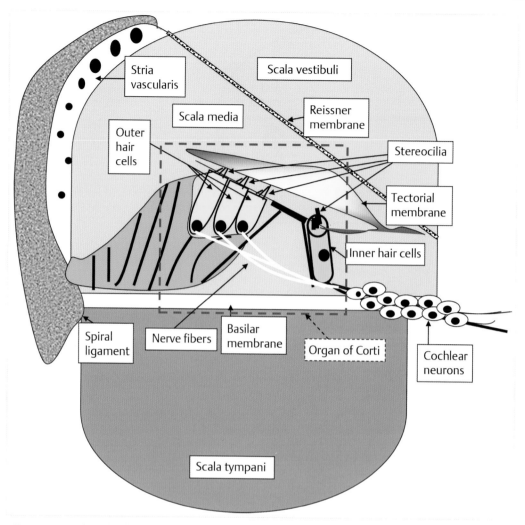

Fig. 1.2 Origin of auditory nerve fibers within the cochlea.

Lateral Lemniscus

Fibers from the medial accessory nucleus of the SOC travel up through the lateral lemniscus on the same side. Besides fibers from the SOC, the lateral lemniscus includes fibers from the trapezoid body and the acoustic stria, as mentioned previously. Some fibers from the cochlear nuclei form direct connections to the contralateral lateral lemniscus. This ensures at least partial travel of neural impulses within the ascending pathway in the presence of dysfunction within the trapezoid bodies or at the SOC level. In addition, there are fibers called the commissural fibers of Probst that connect the lateral lemnisci on the left and the right side.

Inferior Colliculus

The inferior colliculus is considered an important obligatory relay station in the midbrain that integrates information from all lower streams (Winer & Schreiner, 2005). Ascending neural fibers, including those arising from the lateral lemnisci, synapse with inferior colliculi within the midbrain. The left and right inferior colliculi are connected through the commissure of the inferior colliculus. The tonotopic organization apparent in the lower auditory pathways is maintained in the inferior colliculus but is characterized as being heterogeneous and patchy (Ress & Chandrasekaran, 2013).

Medial Geniculate Body (MGB)

The MGB has three divisions: the ventral, medial, and dorsal. The fibers from the inferior colliculus and other ascending fibers that bypass the inferior colliculi synapse with the neurons in the MGB.

1.1.2 Auditory Cortex

The auditory (geniculotemporal) radiations from the MGB project to the transverse temporal gyrus, or Heschl gyrus, in the temporal cortex on the same side. This cortical area is numbered as 41 and 42 within Brodmann's (2006) classification system. Area 41 is referred to as the primary auditory cortex and includes the middle portion of the anterior and part of the posterior temporal gyri. Area 42 is referred to as the auditory association cortex and includes parts of the posterior transverse and superior temporal gyri. The primary and associated auditory cortices connect with each other through neural fibers. The auditory cortices on the left and the right side are connected via the corpus callosum. The auditory association area is connected with several other areas in the brain.

The degree of activation of the primary auditory cortex varies depending on the frequency, intensity, and complexity of auditory stimuli. For example, larger areas are activated in response to a 1000 Hz tone compared to a 4000 Hz tone. Louder tones increase the degree of activation compared to softer tones. Listening to a spoken message leads to greater activation compared to tones (Strainer et al., 1997). Mental auditory imagery for familiar melodies can also lead to significant activation of the auditory cortices (Oh, Kwon, Yang, & Jeong, 2013).

Auditory cortical response patterns can be modified by auditory attention to specific frequencies in a dual-stream listening task. As an example of this task, listeners are presented with a low-frequency tone of 250 Hz and a high-frequency tone of 4000 Hz simultaneously. They are instructed to focus attention on one stream and are asked to switch attention from one frequency to the other every 30 seconds. Attention to low-frequency tone enhances neural responses within low-frequency areas relative to high, and a reversed pattern is apparent when the attention is focused on the high-frequency tones. This shows that the auditory cortex can switch activation on demand and tune in to attended stimuli (Da Costa, van der Zwaag, Miller, Clarke, & Saenz, 2013). Such findings suggest that the auditory cortex probably plays an

important role in fusion or segregation of auditory streams to allow perception of auditory objects through analyses of pitch and other temporal properties, spectral properties, spatial location, or phonemic identity.

1.1.3 Amygdala

The amygdala is located just beneath the surface of the front, medial part of the temporal lobe. It is composed of several nuclei, including the accessory basal, basal, central, lateral, medial, and cortical nuclei (LeDoux, 2007).

Projections are sent from the auditory and other sensory cortices and the thalamus to the lateral nucleus of the amygdala (Romanski, Clugnet, Bordi, & LeDoux, 1993). Information from the lateral nucleus is then transferred to several other cortical and subcortical areas through the central nucleus.

The amygdala appears to play an important role in mediating responses to auditory stimuli with affective significance (LeDoux, 2007). Auditory stimuli can activate the caudate in addition to the auditory cortex and thalamus during the nonrapid eye movement (NREM) sleep cycle and while being awake. In addition, during NREM sleep, the activation of the left amygdala and the left prefrontal cortex is greater for auditory stimuli with affective significance (e.g., a name) when compared to activation for neutral (tones) stimuli (Portas et al., 2000).

Although acoustic features activate the amygdala through the auditory cortex, stimulus valence (aversiveness in sounds, e.g., a squeal of chalk on a blackboard) may modulate the auditory cortex activation through the amygdala, suggesting complex interactive connections between the two structures (Kumar, von Kriegstein, Friston, & Griffiths, 2013). Pathologic processes (e.g., tumors) affecting the amygdala and hippocampus during early developmental periods can lead to pervasive developmental disorders, such as autism, which is characterized by abnormalities in social interaction, affective expression, and communication (Hoon & Reiss, 1992).

1.1.4 Efferent Auditory Pathways

The efferent auditory pathways play an important role in shaping the sensory input through both inhibitory and excitatory influences. From the cortex efferent connections are made to the inferior colliculi and the medial geniculate bodies. These are referred to as *corticofugal pathways.* Several other efferent tracts arise from anatomical structures higher in the brainstem, including the medial geniculate bodies, inferior colliculus, nuclei of the lateral lemniscus, and cerebellum.

Olivocochlear Bundle (OCB)

There are efferent fibers that arrive from the medial and lateral superior olivary bodies and enter the cochlea to form direct connections at the bottom of the outer hair cells and indirect connections to the inner hair cells via synapses on their afferent nerve fibers. These descending efferent fibers are referred to as the olivocochlear bundle (OCB). This efferent pathway was originally described by Rasmussen and thus is sometimes referred to as the Rasmussen bundle. The OCB can be classified as crossed and uncrossed.

Crossed Olivocochlear Bundle (COCB)

The crossed olivocochlear bundle (COCB) has mostly myelinated neurons with relatively large diameters that originate from the vicinity of the medial superior olive. These fibers cross to the opposite side of the brainstem and form direct connections on the outer hair cells. The crossed pathway also includes a few unmyelinated fibers from the lateral superior olive, making indirect connections with contralateral inner hair cells. The effect of the action of the COCB can be clinically evaluated by recording otoacoustic emissions with and without application of noise to the contralateral ear. In the presence of normal function of the COCB, the amplitude of the otoacoustic emissions is reduced following application of noise.

Uncrossed Olivocochlear Bundle (UOCB)

The uncrossed olivocochlear bundle (UOCB) consists of fibers that do not cross to the opposite side but instead make connection with the hair cells in the cochlea on the same side. Most of these fibers arrive from the lateral superior olive, are unmyelinated, have relatively small diameters, and synapse with the afferents of the inner hair cells. In addition, a few myelinated fibers from the medial superior olive make connections with the outer hair cells on the same side.

Efferent Middle Ear Reflex Pathway

This path consists of an efferent connection from the SOC or trapezoid body to the stapedial motor nuclei and projections from the stapedial motor nuclei to the stapedius muscle in the middle ear. The efferent action occurs in the presence of relatively loud stimuli and results in contraction of the stapedius muscle, leading to reduction of low-frequency input to the cochlea. The function of this efferent path can be evaluated by recording the middle ear acoustic reflex. The middle ear reflex is absent or elevated in the presence of damage to the afferent portion of the reflex pathway, including the auditory nerve, cochlear nucleus, trapezoid bodies, and superior olivary complex, and to the efferent portion of the pathway (▶ Fig. 1.3).

1.2 Auditory Processing

The normal auditory system has a capability to perceive auditory stimuli varying from simple (tones) to complex (music or degraded speech) in quiet and noisy surroundings. Humans can perceive and process various stimuli in the environment simultaneously. The key dimensions of auditory stimuli are temporal, spatial, spectral, and intensity, which are discussed throughout this book in various contexts. Introduction to the dimension of stimulus intensity and the related loudness perception is provided below.

1.2.1 Loudness Perception

Loudness perception can be assessed using various techniques. Stimuli of varying intensity can be presented to the listener, and the listener can be asked to judge the loudness of the stimulus, as shown in ▶ Fig. 1.4. In ▶ Fig. 1.4 stimuli between 40 and 60 dB HL (hearing level) are judged as being comfortably loud at 500 Hz. For the 4000 Hz tone, stimuli between 45 and 65 dB HL are judged as being comfortably loud. The maximum level at which the sounds are judged as being comfortable can be referred to as the maximum comfortable loudness levels (MaxCLs). In the case shown in ▶ Fig. 1.4, MaxCLs are 60 dB HL at 500 Hz and 65 dB HL at 4000 Hz. The uncomfortable loudness level in this case is above 90 dB HL, which will be judged as being uncomfortably loud.

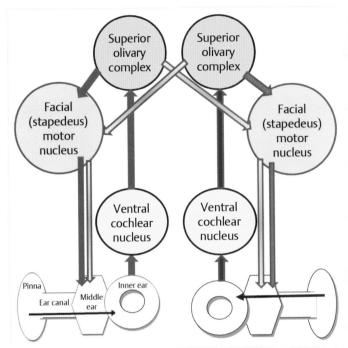

Fig. 1.3 Schematic of the acoustic reflex pathway. Right ipsilateral pathway (*red arrows*); left ipsilateral pathway (*blue arrows*). Crossed pathways are represented by lighter arrows.

Effect of Hearing Loss on Loudness Perception

Hearing loss can change loudness perception (Rawool, 1998a), as shown in ▶ Fig. 1.5. The data for listeners with hearing impairment and normal listener in this figure are obtained by averaging the presentation levels judged in a particular loudness category. For example, as shown in ▶ Fig. 1.4, the normal listener judged two presentation levels of 70 and 75 dB HL as being very loud at 4000 Hz. The average presentation level in this case that was perceived as being loud is 72.5 dB HL and is shown in ▶ Fig. 1.5. As shown in ▶ Fig. 1.5, listener HI (hearing impaired) 3 has the same threshold of 70 dB HL as the two other listeners but has a very narrow dynamic range of 15 dB (93–78 dB) with sounds presented at 78 dB being perceived as very soft and those presented at 93 dB being perceived as loud. Using a similar procedure, the dynamic range for the normal-hearing listener is 47.5 dB. ▶ Fig. 1.5 also shows variation in the loudness growth function across the three listeners with hearing impairment. Therefore, the loudness growth function of each listener should be considered in fitting hearing aids.

There is a significant correlation between the maximum comfortable loudness levels at 1 kHz and acoustic reflex thresholds obtained with a probe frequency of 678 Hz in individuals with hearing loss. A similar correlation exists between maximum comfortable loudness levels at 2 kHz and acoustic reflex thresholds obtained with a probe frequency of 1000 Hz (Rawool, 2001). Thus, for older adults with cognitive deficits, acoustic reflex measures can be used to predict maximum comfortable loudness levels for fitting hearing aids.

Effect of Aging on Loudness Perception

▶ Fig. 1.6 shows a comparison between the loudness judgment obtained in a younger adult and an older adult. Loudness perception tends to be more variable in older adults above the age of 80 years compared to younger adults probably due to higher internal noise level and greater variability in internal noise (Rawool, 1998b). Such variability can lead to constant fiddling with the television (TV) remote or volume controls on hearing aids.

Effect of Temporal Lobe Pathology on Loudness Perception

In a different task involving loudness perception, participants can be asked to balance the loudness between the two ears. This task has been referred

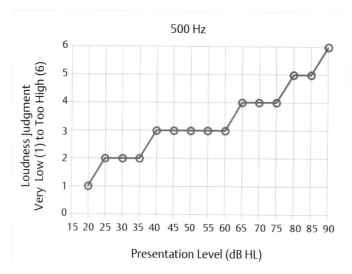

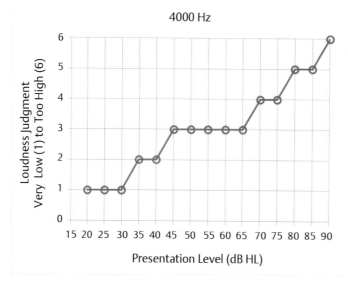

Fig. 1.4 Loudness judgment for 500- and 4000-Hz tones in the right ear for a 21-year-old listener with normal hearing. 1, very low or too soft; 2, low or soft; 3, comfortable; 4, high or loud; 5, very high or very loud; 6, too high or too loud.

to as the alternate binaural loudness balance (ABLB, Fowler, 1936) technique. In one ear a reference tone is presented at a set level, and the listener is asked to adjust the level of the tone in the other ear until the loudness in both ears is judged as being equal. In normal cases, approximately equal sensation levels are necessary to judge the loudness as being equal, as shown in the left panel of ▶ Fig. 1.7.

In some cases with temporal lobe pathology, the ear opposite the site of pathology needs higher sensation levels than the normal ear to judge the loudness as being equal in both ears (Jerger, 1960), as shown in the right panel of ▶ Fig. 1.7. This phenomenon has been referred to as loudness decruitment (Davis & Goodman, 1966). The abnormal performance on this task may not be related to abnormal growth of loudness, as during monaural tasks, patients show normal loudness growth in each ear. The phenomenon is most likely related to difficulty in judging the loudness of stimuli that are presented simultaneously to both ears (Mencher, Clack, & Rupp, 1973).

1.2.2 Auditory Scene Analyses

The term *auditory scene analyses* (Bregman, 1990) refers to the process by which the auditory system uses various properties of auditory stimuli, including temporal, spectral, spatial, and intensity, to group certain sounds together to recognize the source of that sound (e.g., a movie from TV) and to segregate sounds from different sources (e.g., a movie from TV, birds singing outside the window, a plane flying above the house). Auditory scene analyses can involve the use of various cues or auditory processing skills, as discussed in Chapters 5, 6, and 7. As an introduction to these chapters, the following section includes two specific examples of tasks related to auditory scene analysis.

Stream Segregation

Stream segregation (see Chapter 5) can be evaluated in various ways. In one test procedure, two

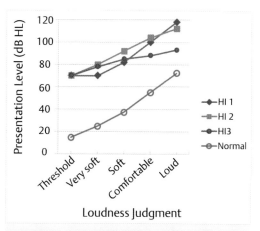

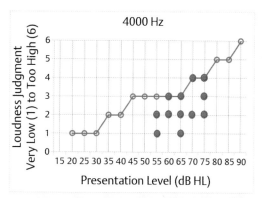

Fig. 1.5 Loudness growth at 4000 Hz as a function of presentation level (dB HL) in three individuals with hearing impairment (HI) and a threshold of 70 dB HL and for the normal listener shown in ▶ Fig. 1.4 with a threshold of 15 dB HL. Note that the dynamic range (DR) for the normal listener from very soft (25) to loud (72.5) is 47.5 dB. The DR for HI 1 is 48 dB, which is very similar to that of the normal listener. The dynamic range for HI 2 is 32 dB, which is less than that for the normal listener. The range for HI 3 is only 15 dB, showing a very narrow dynamic range.

Fig. 1.6 Effect of aging on loudness perception. Loudness judgments of an 80-year-old listener with hearing loss (*filled circles*) are shown, along with data from a young normal-hearing adult (*open circles*). Note the variability in perception. For example, the presentation level of 75 dB HL is judged as being soft, comfortable, or loud during various trials by the older listener.

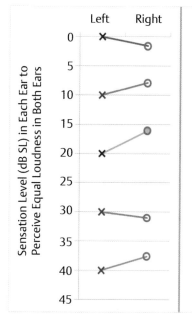

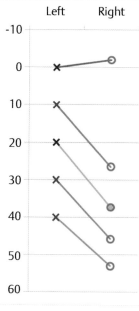

Fig. 1.7 Loudness balance obtained by presenting a reference tone in the left ear and asking the listener to adjust the tone in the right ear until tones in both ears sound equally loud. The left panel shows results from a normal-hearing listener, and the right panel shows the results from an individual with temporal lobe pathology (based on Mencher, Clack, & Rupp, 1973).

tones of different frequencies are presented simultaneously to the listener. The listener is asked to report if he or she perceives two distinct sound streams or just one fused sound. The difference in the two frequencies is slowly changed. At some critical difference in frequency of the two tones, the perception changes from hearing one stream to two. When the two tones are perceived as one stream, a distinct beating sound is heard by listeners. This perception is also influenced by other factors, such as rate of stimulus presentation and previous experience with the specific sounds being segregated (e.g., picking a particular instrument from a piece of complex music).

Auditory Perceptual Restoration or Continuity Illusion

Another example of auditory scene analyses is the perception of interrupted speech (see Chapter 5). When tiny segments are removed temporally from ongoing speech, the speech still remains intelligible. The intelligibility continues when the removed segments are replaced by broadband noise. This has been referred to as the *continuity illusion* or *auditory perceptual restoration* and can be demonstrated by presenting tonal stimuli that are masked occasionally by brief noise bursts. Listeners report the perception of a continuous tone through the periods of noise. The illusion can continue after switching the tone off during the periods of noise bursts. The responses of the auditory system during the auditory perceptual restoration period tend to mimic the responses that would have occurred if the sound was in fact continuous and not masked (Petkov & Sutter, 2011).

1.3 Auditory Processing without Active Attention

The auditory system can continue to process stimuli without active attention. Examples of such processing include auditory processing during sedation or sleep.

1.3.1 Auditory Processing During Sedation

Several evoked potentials can be recorded in response to auditory stimuli. These include the auditory brainstem response (ABR), Mismatch Negativity (MMN), and the P300a or P300b responses. ABRs can be recorded during sedation,

suggesting that processing of stimuli in the brainstem occurs in the absence of active attention. MMN can also be recorded, although it is strongly reduced, during deep sedation. In addition, the P300a component is visible during deep sedation (Koelsch, Heinke, Sammler, & Olthoff, 2006).

1.3.2 Auditory Processing During Sleep

ABRs, MMN, and even P300 (see Chapter 4) can be recorded during sleep. In addition, as previously mentioned, there are differences in the response patterns to simple stimuli, such as beeps, and complex emotionally relevant stimuli, such as the person's own name (Portas et al., 2000). Enhanced P300 response patterns are not observed to any other people's names during sleep (Perrin, Garcia-Larrea, Mauguiere, & Bastuji, 1999). Overall these findings suggest that processing of auditory stimuli and detection of meaningful events can occur during sleep (Portas et al., 2000) or without active attention.

Functional magnetic resonance imaging (fMRI) shows similarity in activation of the thalamus, auditory cortex, and caudate during NREM sleep and wakefulness (Portas et al., 2000). Even P300b can be recorded in sleep stage 2, suggesting active processing of deviant tones (Ruby, Caclin, Boulet, Delpuech, & Morlet, 2008). Such processing has functional significance and may allow protection from dangerous events. For example, young mothers usually are able to hear their own infants' cries during deep sleep.

1.4 Auditory Processing in the Damaged Auditory System

In the presence of damage to the auditory system, some processing can continue partially due to the several redundancies in the central nervous system and neural plasticity.

1.4.1 Auditory Processing in the Damaged Auditory Cortex

In the presence of extensive bilateral destruction of the auditory cortices, including primary auditory fields, the patient may lack conscious awareness of sounds when not attending to auditory stimuli; this phenomenon has been referred to as deaf hearing, auditory agnosia, or cortical deafness. However, effortful or selective attention can allow conscious perception of the onset and offset of sounds even in the presence of such extensive damage; such perception is accompanied by an increase in the blood flow in the prefrontal cortices, the spared middle temporal cortices, and the cerebellar hemisphere. Selective attention may be insufficient for performing complex auditory tasks such as localization, identification of sounds or words, and discrimination of simple and complex patterns in the presence of such extensive damage (Engelien et al., 2000). However, some patients may be able to discriminate loudness of pure tones and some environmental sounds, and their auditory awareness can be enhanced by lipreading (Kaga, Shindo, & Tanaka, 1997).

1.4.2 Auditory Processing During the Persistent Vegetative State

A persistent vegetative state (PVS), or coma, is a profound or deep state of unconsciousness. Bilateral activation of Brodmann areas 41 and 42 has been demonstrated using O-radiolabeled positron emission tomography (PET) in patients in a coma, suggesting neural encoding of basic sound attributes (Boly et al., 2004).

In a subpopulation of patients with PVS with preserved thalamocortical feedback connection and background electroencephalographic (EEG) activity greater than 4 Hz, cortical information processing is apparent using various evoked potentials. This includes undifferentiated processing suggested by the N1–P2 complex; preattentive, cortical orientation documented by mismatch negativity; deep cortical analysis of physical stimuli, as shown by P300; and analyses of semantic stimuli documented by evoked responses to semantic oddball tasks (e.g., counting animal names and ignoring all other words), including P600 (Kotchoubey et al., 2005).

1.4.3 Auditory Processing During the Minimally Conscious State

A minimally conscious state (MCS) is a condition in which minimal but definite evidence of self- or environmental awareness is apparent, although the patient cannot communicate. Acoustic clicks can activate the superior temporal gyri (Brodmann areas 41, 42, and 22) in patients in an MCS, and such patients show some functional connectivity between the secondary auditory cortex and temporal and prefrontal association cortices,

suggesting the potential or prognosis for gaining conscious auditory perception (Boly et al., 2004). This view is further supported by the fact that MCS patients show greater activation in the temporal, parietal, and frontal associative areas in response to their own names compared to meaningless noise (Laureys et al., 2004). Kotchoubey et al. (2005) also confirmed that MCS patients frequently yield auditory evoked potentials, indicating complex information processing.

1.5 Definition of Auditory Processing Deficits

Auditory processing deficits (APDs) have been defined in the literature in various ways. The American Speech-Language-Hearing Association (ASHA, 2005) defines central auditory processing deficit [(C)APD] as "difficulties in the perceptual processing of auditory information in the central nervous system and the neurobiological activity that underlies that processing and gives rise to the electrophysiological auditory potentials." This definition is supported by the American Academy of Audiology (AAA, 2010).

The APD special interest group of the British Society of Audiology (BSA, 2011) specifies that APD is not a result of failure to understand simple instructions that may occur secondary to conditions such as intellectual disabilities. BSA (2011) further defines APDs by specifying their characteristics, origins, impact on daily life, assessment procedures, and symptoms, as shown in ▶ Fig. 1.8.

The Canadian Interorganizational Steering Group for Speech-Language Pathology and Audiology (2012) has defined APD in terms of the International Classification of Functioning, Disability, and Health (ICF) as described by the World Health Organization (WHO, 2002). Their conceptualization of APD is illustrated in ▶ Fig. 1.9.

1.6 Prevalence of Auditory Processing Deficits

APD prevalence statistics depend on the specific criteria and procedures used for diagnosing deficits. The estimated prevalence is about 2 to 3%, with a male-to-female ratio of 2:1 (Chermark & Musiek, 1997).

Among brain-injured children, the prevalence may be 16% (Cockrell & Gregory, 1992). Among individuals with closed head injuries, APDs have

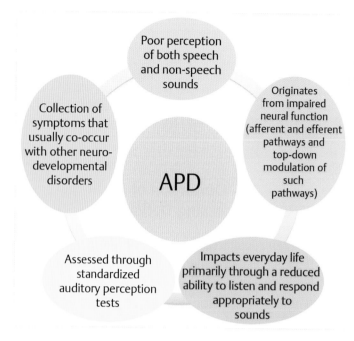

Poor perception of both speech and non-speech sounds

Collection of symptoms that usually co-occur with other neuro-developmental disorders

APD

Originates from impaired neural function (afferent and efferent pathways and top-down modulation of such pathways)

Assessed through standardized auditory perception tests

Impacts everyday life primarily through a reduced ability to listen and respond appropriately to sounds

Fig. 1.8 Illustration based on the definition of an auditory processing deficit (APD) provided by the APD special interest group of the British Society of Audiology (BSA, 2011). The BSA also states that an APD does not result from the failure to understand simple instructions in cases where auditory difficulties may be secondary to a primary deficit, such as an intellectual disability.

been reported in 58% of patients even after apparent recovery from an injury (Bergemalm & Lyxell, 2005). Two to 36% of adults older than 64 years may have APDs (Cooper & Gates, 1991), depending on the specific criteria used for determining a deficit, the age group, and the test procedures (▶ Fig. 1.10). More studies are necessary to determine the prevalence of APDs among children and adults using a well-specified test battery.

1.7 Multidisciplinary Evaluation

In some cases audiologists can provide sufficient assistance to minimize the impact of an APD on a patient's achievements in occupational, social, and educational environments. For example, an older adult may experience an APD in the presence or absence of a peripheral hearing loss. He or she may be struggling at work or at home when oral communication is necessary. Such a person can be fitted with hearing aids with integrated assistive listening technology. He or she can be provided with auditory training that drives the neural plasticity to improve speech comprehension in quiet and noisy surroundings. The training can be potentially completed using computerized techniques to drive both top-down and bottom-up plasticity, as explained in Chapter 9.

In other cases a multidisciplinary approach is likely to be more effective. For example, adults with traumatic brain injuries can benefit from an approach that is designed and coordinated by audiologists, speech-language pathologists, neurologists, physical therapists, and occupational therapists. Similarly, children who have APDs can benefit from collaboration among teachers, psychologists, speech-language pathologists, and audiologists.

1.8 Establishing Auditory Perceptual Deficits

Before proceeding with intervention, it is important to establish the existence of an APD and the specific subdomain or domains that are deficient. It is also important to establish the potential and actual impact of the deficit. A bright child may use higher cognitive strategies to cope with an APD. However, as the complexity of learning increases, the strategies may not be sufficient. Thus, even though initially the impact of the deficit may seem minimal, it is important to provide intervention designed to prevent future educational or social difficulties.

It is also important to rule out other potential causes, such as intellectual disabilities, that can lead to poor performance on auditory processing tasks. In this regard, the psychologist who may be involved in the evaluation of verbal or nonverbal intellectual abilities needs to be aware of the fact

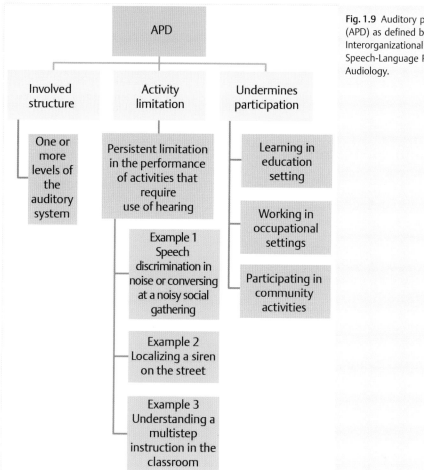

Fig. 1.9 Auditory processing deficit (APD) as defined by the Canadian Interorganizational Steering Group for Speech-Language Pathology and Audiology.

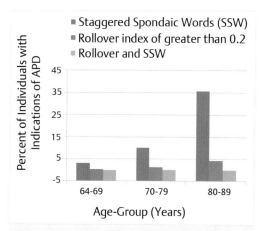

Fig. 1.10 Percent of older individuals with indications of auditory processing deficits (APDs) across different age groups depending on the tests used to determine APDs (based on Cooper & Gates, 1991).

that an APD may have a negative impact on the results of the tests, especially verbal tests. It is important to take all precautions to ensure that the child understands the task and the expected response. The testing needs to be conducted in a quiet environment. Very good performance on the nonverbal tasks in the presence of borderline or lower performance on verbal tasks suggests the possibility of an APD. Also during the testing the impact of an APD on working memory needs to be considered, as explained in Chapter 9.

A listener with a temporary or conductive peripheral hearing loss can have poor results on auditory processing tasks unless proper precautions are taken in selecting the test battery, administering the tests, and interpreting the results. The results of some auditory processing tasks are poor in the presence of hearing loss even after adjusting the presentation levels of stimuli to compensate for hearing loss. After the test is properly selected, the presentation levels need to be adjusted to ensure that the stimuli are audible but are not too loud, leading to discomfort and distortion. In interpreting the results, the data from individuals with hearing loss need to be considered in determining the presence of APDs. Refer to the case example in Chapter 16 for determination of APD in the presence of hearing loss.

1.9 Cross-linguistic Factors

Cultural, language, and dialect differences can affect the results of verbal auditory processing tasks. For example, in some languages, such as Spanish and Finnish, duration is a critical feature. Repetition of consonants tends to lengthen the phoneme duration of a sound and changes the meaning of the word (e.g., /ata/ vs. /atta/). Such differences do not exist in all languages. If possible, speech stimuli should be presented in the patient's native language. Some tests are available in several languages as discussed in Chapter 4.

If the use of speech-processing tasks is not possible, the use of nonverbal and objective measures of APDs is recommended, as discussed in Chapter 4. When these procedures are used, it is important to confirm that the listeners understand the instructions either through the use of interpreters or, if possible, by asking the patients to repeat what is expected from them.

1.10 Examples of Auditory Processing Deficits

Several types of APDs are possible, and many of these deficits can be evaluated using the procedures discussed in Chapters 4, 5, 6, and 7. Examples of some specific deficits that can lead to poor performance on a variety of auditory processing tasks are provided below.

1.10.1 Amusia or Tune Deafness or Dysmelodia

Individuals with amusia, or tune (or tone) deafness, have difficulty in appreciating, perceiving, or differentiating many aspects of musical melody. The Montreal Battery of Evaluation of amusia has been designed to diagnose individuals with this disorder (Peretz, Champod, & Hyde, 2003). The test evaluates pitch discrimination and other aspects of musical perception. Some individuals with congenital amusia show severe deficits in processing pitch variations, in recognizing music, in singing, and in tapping in time to music (Ayotte, Peretz, & Hyde, 2002).

Another available test is the Distorted Tunes Test (DTT) (Fry, 1948). The test expects listeners to decide if the presented short, familiar melodies are played correctly or not. Using this test, listeners can be identified as being tune deaf or as having dysmelodia. Family histories of tune deaf individuals suggest an autosomal dominant trait with variable penetrance (Kalmus & Fry, 1980). Tune-deaf individuals perform significantly poorly on temporal patterning tasks, including pitch and duration patterns, and show significantly poor gap detection ability compared to age-matched controls (Jones, Zalewski, Brewer, Lucker, & Drayna, 2009). In some individuals with pitch deafness, perception of nonpitched drum timbres or rhythm and beat processing can be normal (Phillips-Silver, Toiviainen, Gosselin, & Peretz, 2013).

Auditory training designed to improve the identification of pitch direction in syllables and piano tones can improve pitch perception in individuals with congenital amusia showing neural plasticity (Liu, Jiang, Francart, Chan, & Wong, 2013).

1.10.2 Diplacusis

Some individuals perceive the same tone as being different in pitch in the two ears. Such differing perception, referred to as *diplacusis,* can interfere with music perception. In one investigation consisting of 241 musicians, approximately 7% of musicians reported diplacusis, and it could be documented through measurements in 18% of musicians (Jansen, Helleman, Dreschler, & de Laat, 2009). The disorder can cause a musician to play out of tune.

As noted in Rawool (2012a), diplacusis can be evaluated and documented using an adaptive procedure by presenting tonal signals alternating to the right and left ears. First, the subject should be requested to match the loudness of a clearly audible tone (e.g., 40 dB SL [sensation level]) presented to one ear to that of the same frequency (e.g., 1000 Hz) tone presented to the other ear. The examiner can vary the loudness in the other ear around 40 dB SL in 1 dB steps to get loudness match. Using the same loudness levels in two ears, the pitch in one ear is kept constant by presenting the same frequency. The frequency in the other ear is then adjusted in 1 Hz steps around 1000 Hz to obtain a pitch match. In the presence of diplacusis, the pitch deviation between the ears can be expressed as a percentage of the reference frequency. For example, if a 1000 Hz tone presented to the right ear is matched to the pitch of a 1025 Hz tone, the pitch deviation is 2.5% (Jansen et al., 2009).

1.10.3 Phonagnosia

The term *phonagnosia* refers to the inability to recognize familiar or famous voices. Clinical and radiologic findings suggest that damage to the inferior and lateral parietal regions in the right hemisphere can lead to difficulty in recognizing familiar voices, whereas temporal lobe damage to either the right or left hemisphere can lead to difficulties in discriminating between unfamiliar voices (Van Lancker, Cummings, Kreiman, & Dobkin, 1988).

In some patients with congenital phonagnosia, impairment is apparent in recognizing famous voices and in learning the recognition of new voices. However, performance can be normal in recognizing vocal emotions and processing environmental sounds, speech, and music (Garrido et al., 2009). In cases with frontotemporal lobar degeneration, phonagnosia can be accompanied by severe deficit in recognizing faces with relatively good ability to recognize musical instruments and environmental sounds (Hailstone, Crutch, Vestergaard, Patterson, & Warren, 2010).

1.11 Potential Causes of Auditory Processing Deficits

The cause of APDs in children is not always known. Some factors that could lead to deficits are listed in case history forms presented in the appendixes of Chapter 3 and Chapter 4. Examples of some of these factors are provided in the following section.

1.11.1 Genetic Factors

Some auditory processing skills and deficits appear to be related to genetic factors (see Chapter 13 and Chapter 14). For example, children with *PAX6* mutations have difficulty localizing sounds and recognizing speech in noise. The anterior commissure of the corpus callosum is small in some of these children, which can lead to deficits in interhemispheric transfer of auditory stimuli (Bamiou et al., 2007).

1.11.2 Prenatal Factors

Prenatal exposure to various substances can have a negative impact on the neural development of a fetus, as discussed in Chapter 2. An example of this is fetal alcohol spectrum disorder (FASD) (http://www.cdc.gov/NCBDDD/fasd/facts.html), which is associated with deficits in the central nervous system function and hearing. Tone-evoked magnetoencephalography (MEG) has revealed significantly longer M100 and M200 latencies in FASD children ages 3 to 6 years with normal hearing compared to normal age-matched peers (Stephen et al., 2012). These findings show slower processing of auditory stimuli in children with FASD.

1.11.3 Perinatal Factors

Perinatal factors such as prematurity and low birth weight can lead to APDs. For example, preterm birth is associated with longer I–III and III–V interpeak intervals of the ABR in children between the ages of 4 and 6 years compared to age-matched control participants (Hasani & Jafari, 2013). These results show slower processing of auditory stimuli in children with a history of preterm birth. Adolescents (ages 9 to 16 years) with a history of preterm birth may show academic achievements, receptive vocabulary, and receptive language that are comparable to normal age-matched peers. However, they may continue to show a different neural activation pattern for auditory stimuli, such as sentences, suggesting the need for continuation of educational accommodations (Barde, Yeatman, Lee, Glover, & Feldman, 2012).

1.11.4 Exposure to Ototoxins

For information related to ototoxins, refer to Chapter 16. Various APDs can occur following ototoxin exposure. For example, cannabis users have reduced MMN amplitudes in response to frequency deviations (1000 vs. 1200 Hz) when compared to matched controls (▶ Fig. 1.11). In addition, the MMN amplitudes in response to duration deviations are smaller in long-term cannabis users compared to control groups and short-term cannabis users (Greenwood et al., 2014). The performance of long-term cannabis users is significantly poorer than controls on verbal learning tasks (Yücel et al., 2008).

Cannabis use in adolescence and early adulthood may lead to premature changes in cortical

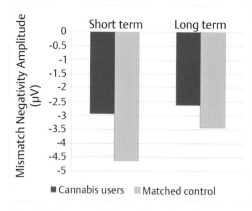

Fig. 1.11 Mean amplitudes of the mismatch negativity (MMN) peak response in cannabis (marijuana) users. The standard tones (82%) had a frequency of 1000 Hz; the deviant tones, 1200 Hz. The tones were presented at 80 dB SPL (based on Greenwood et al., 2014).

gyrification, including decreased concavity of the sulci and thinner sulci in the right frontal lobe that are normally apparent in older adults due to the aging process (Mata et al., 2010). Bilateral reduction of hippocampal and amygdala volumes (Yücel et al., 2008) and smaller cerebellar white matter volume (Solowij et al., 2011) are associated with long term heavy use of cannabis.

1.11.5 Structural Brain Defects

Several defects are possible within the auditory pathways, as discussed in several chapters. For example, individuals with agenesis of the corpus callosum can show deficits on several auditory processing tasks, including localization, dichotic listening, and phonological processing, leading to academic difficulties (Temple, Jeeves, & Vilarroya, 1990). The posterior midbody/isthmus region of the corpus callosum appears to be shorter in boys with dyslexia compared to a control group. This region includes the interhemispheric fibers from the primary and secondary auditory cortices (von Plessen et al., 2002).

1.11.6 Neurologic Conditions

Several neurologic conditions can lead to APDs. For example, individuals with multiple sclerosis show temporal processing deficits and difficulty in recognizing speech in noise (Valadbeigi et al., 2013). For additional information, refer to Chapter 5.

1.11.7 Metabolic Disorders

In some metabolic disorders, such as adrenoleukodystrophy, the I–V interpeak interval of the ABR can become progressively longer with worsening of the condition. In addition, demyelination of auditory nerves and extensive loss of neurons has been noted within the auditory pathways (Kaga, Tokoro, Tanaka, & Ushijima, 1980).

1.11.8 Brain Trauma

Brain injuries can occur due to various reasons, including strokes, occupational injuries such as those occurring in the military, sport-related injuries, including concussions, and injuries resulting from surgical procedures. For example, sport-related concussions can lead to APDs in some athletes (Turgeon, Champoux, Lepore, Leclerc, & Ellemberg, 2011).

In some cases of brain injury, partial or complete recovery is possible due to neuroplasticity. For example, a professional jazz guitarist suffered from temporal lobe epilepsy due to an arteriovenous cerebral malformation. To address the epileptic seizures, the left temporal lobe was removed in 1980, which resulted in loss of interest in music. However, a detailed study in 2007 revealed that the subject had completely recovered his musical ability, showing very high neuroplasticity (Galarza et al., 2014). In some of these cases, auditory training can drive some of the recovery or enhance the speed of recovery.

1.11.9 Auditory Processing Deficit Secondary to Other Conditions

APD can occur as a secondary result of other conditions, including peripheral hearing loss (see Chapter 3) and aging (see Chapter 17). The central auditory system shows tonotopic reorganization and neural hyperactivity due to reduced output from the cochlea. When a region in the cochlea is dead or silent following loss of outer and inner hair cells, the subset of neurons that correspond to the particular region or frequencies do not receive any stimulation. After a few weeks these neurons begin to respond to frequencies that are associated with cochlear regions surrounding the damaged area. Such tonotopic reorganization is apparent in the cochlear nucleus (Kaltenbach, Czaja, & Kaplan, 1992), inferior colliculus (Salvi, Wang, & Powers, 1996), and auditory cortex (Robertson & Irvine, 1989; Willott, Aitkin, & McFadden, 1993). One possible mechanism for this reorganization is functional activation of preexisting excitatory synapses with a potential for being tuned to several different frequencies (Wang, Caspary, & Salvi, 2000).

The central auditory system also appears to compensate for the reduced cochlear output due to noise-induced hearing loss by increasing the gain or by becoming hyperactive. One reason for the hyperactivity may be the loss of gamma-aminobutyric acid (GABA)–mediated inhibition (Salvi, Wang, & Ding, 2000; Szczepaniak & Møller, 1995). Other excitatory and inhibitory neurotransmitters may be involved in increasing the gain (Suneja, Potashner, & Benson, 1998). The increased gain can lead to hyperacusis (difficulty tolerating moderate sounds) and/or tinnitus.

1.12 Impact of Auditory Processing Deficit

1.12.1 Oral Language Acquisition

In most cases oral language is mainly acquired through mostly spontaneous input of speech stimuli to the auditory system. When the auditory system is deficient in processing speech sounds, language acquisition can be delayed or disordered, depending on the severity of the deficit (see Chapter 14). Specific aspects of inefficient auditory cortical processing can be ameliorated through training (Heim, Keil, Choudhury, Thomas Friedman, & Benasich, 2013). Not all children with language delays or disorders have APDs. Several other causes can result in language disorders.

1.12.2 Reading Difficulties

Normal ability to process auditory stimuli is important because reading requires the reader to make connections between the auditory and visual representations of letters and words. In some cases deficits in auditory processing can lead to reading difficulties (see Chapter 14). Some individuals with dyslexia show difficulties in discriminating frequency, rise time, and duration of auditory stimuli. They also show deficits in detecting amplitude and frequency modulation (reviewed in Hämäläinen, Salminen, & Leppänen, 2013).

1.12.3 Learning Disability

Isolated auditory-phonologic processing disorders have been reported in some children with learning disabilities (Jerger, Martin, & Jerger, 1987). Up to 40% of children with language-based learning problems have abnormal ABRs to speech stimuli (Banai, Abrams, & Kraus, 2007). APDs have been reported in 43.3% of children referred to a learning disability clinic, and in 25% of these cases APDs co-occur with dyslexia. These findings suggest that children with learning disabilities should be screened for APDs (Iliadou, Bamiou, Kaprinis, Kandylis, & Kaprinis, 2009). Such children can continue to struggle in academic settings unless their APDs are addressed through intervention.

1.12.4 Music Perception

Children with APDs have significantly lower musical meter percentile scores than age-matched normal-hearing peers (Olakunbi, Bamiou, Stewart, & Luxon, 2010). The occurrence of relatively long notes and the repetition of melodic phrases are considered important cues to meter (regular beats) perception in a piece of music (Steedman, 1977).

1.12.5 Psychosocial Status

Children with APDs report significantly more emotional and overall health issues compared to children without APDs. Parents of children with APDs are more likely to report that their children have greater psychosocial difficulties compared to parents of children in the control group. More specifically, parents of children with APDs express concerns about their children's reduced emotional health, poor or inappropriate behaviors, and difficulty in adapting to school environments (Kreisman, John, Kreisman, Hall, & Crandell, 2012).

1.12.6 Vocational Performance and Outcomes

APDs have the potential to minimize job efficiency and productivity, depending on the particular job and the listening and communication demands in the profession. APDs may also increase stress levels at work and may lead to slower recovery from fatigue. The extent to which workers are able to recover from fatigue and distress at work can predict psychosomatic complaints, emotional exhaustion, sleep problems, and duration of absences due to sick leave (de Croon, Sluiter, & Frings-Dresen, 2003; Sluiter, de Croon, Meijman, & Frings-Dresen, 2003).

As noted in Rawool (2012b), one dominant model used in examining the relationship between work and health is the job demand-control (JDC) model or the job strain model (Karasek, 1979), which may be applicable to workers with APD. Four types of occupations are identified in the JDC model. The first type is referred to as a "high stress" job that is highly demanding but offers low control to the worker over his or her work situation and tasks. The second type is the "active" job, which is also highly demanding but offers a high level of control to the worker. The third type is the "passive" job, which is low in both demand and control, and the fourth type is the "low stress" job, which is low in demand and offers a high degree of control. Lack of control regardless of whether the job has high or low demands is associated with increased risk of poor health.

Individuals with APDs may experience high stress along with low control due to their deficit given that many jobs involve the use of efficient communication. The stress can be higher for those who work in noisy and/or reverberant environments. For example, individuals with peripheral hearing impairment more often report their jobs as being the high-stress (high demand and low control) type compared to a control group. In addition, hearing-impaired individuals with high-stress jobs more frequently report poor physical health status and psychological well-being (Danermark & Gellerstedt, 2004).

Rawool (2012) has presented a comprehensive model for supporting individuals with hearing loss in the workplace. Similar models (Kramer, Allessie, Dondorp, Zekveld, & Kapteyen, 2005) can be applied to workers with APDs. In managing workers with APDs, specific attention should be given to the following elements: the noise level perceived by the worker, reverberation in the work environment, the need to detect and differentiate sounds, the need to communicate in noise, the effort required in processing auditory stimuli, and the degree of control the worker perceives in job situations.

1.13 Comorbid Disorders

Children with APDs can have other comorbid disorders. Examples include language-related disorders, such as reading, writing, and learning deficits. Children with attention deficit hyperactivity disorder (ADHD) can have comorbid APDs due to various reasons, including shared structures involved in attention and auditory processing or genetic factors. In some cases an underlying APD may appear as an attention deficit, as the child may struggle in focusing attention on auditory stimuli that are hard to process. For more information, refer to Chapter 13.

1.14 Demands from Caregivers and Patients

Parents and families who are more familiar with their children's listening difficulties may visit several professionals in seeking a diagnosis and a solution. In some cases parents may seek second or even third opinions before gaining needed assistance leading to improved function in the child. Similarly, older adults may express their listening difficulties and may not get properly diagnosed until the correct test is administered that is sensitive to their specific deficit. It is important to pay close attention to the specific complaints of the patient and to administer proper tests to ensure accurate diagnosis and treatment. In most cases it is fair to assume that if the parents and patient have concerns about listening difficulties, the listening difficulty exists in some form. In a very few cases, such as when compensation is being sought (see Chapter 16), the difficulties may be exaggerated.

1.15 Reimbursement for Services

Reimbursement for services is available from a variety of sources and vary depending on specific regions. In some countries, health care services are offered free of charge. For example, in the United States, services written into individualized education plans may be reimbursed at least partially by school districts. Often parents seek diagnostic services from a facility outside the school system and may be successful in receiving reimbursement from school districts.

The Current Procedural Terminology (CPT) codes for a behavioral central auditory processing evaluation in the United States are 92620 and 92621. The CPT code 92620 provides reimbursement for the first hour of administration, interpretation, and provision of results. Up to eight additional 15-minute increments can be billed under the 92621 code. Separate codes exist for electrophysiological test procedures and acoustic reflex tests.

1.16 Service Delivery for Auditory Processing Deficits

The key elements of services for individuals with APDs are shown in ▶ Fig. 1.12.

1.16.1 Usefulness of Tests for Diagnosing Auditory Processing Deficits

Several considerations, including those shown in ▶ Fig. 1.13, can be helpful in the determination of

usefulness of tests (Newman, Browner, & Cummings, 2001). In determining the accuracy of tests, clinical decision analysis matrices can be used, as described in Chapter 4. In determining reliability, inter- and intraobserver and test−retest reliability should be considered. The variability due to test readministration and learning effects should also be taken into account. The impact of test results on clinical decisions and outcomes should be considered. For example, does the test administration serve a purpose in terms of guiding treatment decisions or establishing need for special accommodation or determining the need for workers'

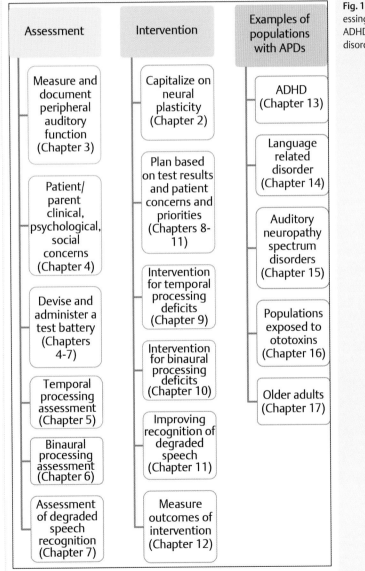

Fig. 1.12 Addressing auditory processing deficits in clinical practice. ADHD, attention deficit hyperactivity disorder.

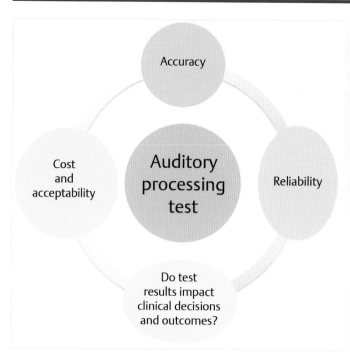

Fig. 1.13 Considerations for determining usefulness of tests used in diagnosing auditory processing deficits.

compensation? The test should be cost effective, should be acceptable to both clinicians and patients, and should have minimal risks associated with it.

1.16.2 Efficacy and Effectiveness of Intervention

Although randomized controlled trials (RCTs) are assumed to provide the best evidence for efficacy of treatment, estimates of treatment effects in well-designed observational studies may not necessarily be quantitatively smaller than or qualitatively different from those apparent from RCTs (Benson & Hartz, 2000; Britton et al., 1998; Concato, Shah, & Horwitz, 2000). Possible improvements in methodologies from more precise test instruments, sophisticated choices of datasets, and better statistical methods may reduce the differences between randomized controlled and observational studies. Although randomized controlled designs have many strengths, judging effectiveness of treatment entirely based on the study design may be unscientific. Assumptions that RCTs trials are the best may lead to inattention to the limitations of such studies and the strengths of observational studies (Concato, 2013). Due to the heterogeneous nature of APD populations, the efficacy demonstrated in RCTs may not necessarily generalize to patients seen in natural clinical settings. Thus, RCTs may demonstrate efficacy, but treatment may not be effective for a specific patient. On the other hand, RCTs may demonstrate lack of efficacy, but a theoretically sound treatment may lead to effective outcomes for a patient. In some cases single case trials may provide better evidence of effectiveness if the characteristics of a specific patient are similar to those published in a single case study. For more information, see Chapter 12.

1.17 Future Trends

Foldable stretchable electrode arrays have been developed that can noninvasively monitor neural activity. The electrodes incorporate silicon electronics that are capable of conforming to curved shapes and achieving mechanical properties similar to skin. The intimate contact of such stretchable electrode arrays allows efficient electrical coupling and high-fidelity measurements with very good signal-to-noise ratio. The stretchable, skinlike membranes are like temporary transfer tattoos and include not only electrode arrays but also electronics, a power supply, and communication components for interfacing with computers or other devices (Kim et al., 2011). These electronic tattoos are being commercialized by MC10 Inc., Cambridge, MA, USA (http://www.mc10inc.com/

digital-health/remote-monitoring/) as bio-stamps that are attached to the user's skin using something similar to a rubber stamp. Use of such epidermal electronic systems can allow recording of neural activity in natural environments and along with sophisticated signal-processing algorithms may enhance our knowledge about the specific neural networks or ensembles that are involved in specific auditory processing skills, such as gap detection and localization. Such knowledge in turn may provide better insights into APDs.

In the future, results of ongoing studies are likely to lead to a well-designed battery for diagnosing APDs. Better treatment approaches are expected to emerge due to advances in technology and advanced knowledge about normal and disordered processing within the auditory system.

1.18 Review Questions

1. Describe the various parts of the afferent and efferent auditory system. Discuss the amygdala and its relevance to the processing of auditory stimuli.

2. What are some approaches for measuring loudness perception in clinical environments? What is the potential impact of hearing loss on loudness perception? How can older age affect loudness perception? What is the impact of temporal lobe pathology on the results of the alternate loudness balance test?

3. Your patient has Alzheimer's disease and peripheral hearing loss. What can you do to predict his maximum comfortable loudness levels at 1000 and 2000 Hz before fitting hearing aids?

4. What does the term *auditory scene analysis* refer to? Describe two tasks related to auditory scene analysis.

5. Discuss how auditory processing can occur without active attention with examples. Can auditory processing occur in the presence of a damaged auditory cortex? What are the limitations of such processing?

6. Discuss supportive evidence for documentation of auditory processing in patients in persistent vegetative and minimally conscious states.

7. Discuss various definitions of auditory processing deficits (APDs). Which definition do you prefer?

8. Review specific APDs, including tune deafness, diplacusis, and phonagnosia.

9. Discuss potential causes and effects of APDs.

10. Discuss future trends that could improve our understanding of the auditory processing system and related deficits.

References

[1] American Academy of Audiology (AAA). (2010). Clinical practice guidelines: Diagnosis, treatment, and management of children and adults with central auditory processing disorder. Retrieved from http://www.audiology.org/resources/documentlibrary/Documents/CAPD%20Guidelines%208–2010.pdf.

[2] American Speech-Language-Hearing Association (ASHA). (2005). (Central) auditory processing disorders (technical report). Retrieved from http://www.asha.org/docs/html/TR2005–00043.html.

[3] Ayotte, J., Peretz, I., & Hyde, K. (2002). Congenital amusia: A group study of adults afflicted with a music-specific disorder. Brain, 125(Pt 2), 238–251.

[4] Bamiou, D. E., Free, S. L., Sisodiya, S. M., Chong, W. K., Musiek, F., Williamson, K. A., et al. (2007). Auditory interhemispheric transfer deficits, hearing difficulties, and brain magnetic resonance imaging abnormalities in children with congenital aniridia due to PAX6 mutations. Archives of Pediatrics & Adolescent Medicine, 161(5), 463–469.

[5] Banai, K., Abrams, D., & Kraus, N. (2007). Sensory-based learning disability: Insights from brainstem processing of speech sounds. International Journal of Audiology, 46(9), 524–532.

[6] Barde, L. H. F., Yeatman, J. D., Lee, E. S., Glover, G., & Feldman, H. M. (2012). Differences in neural activation between preterm and full term born adolescents on a sentence comprehension task: Implications for educational accommodations. Dev Cogn Neurosci, 2(Suppl 1), S114–S128.

[7] Benson, K., & Hartz, A. J. (2000). A comparison of observational studies and randomized, controlled trials. The New England Journal of Medicine, 342(25), 1878–1886.

[8] Bergemalm, P. O., & Lyxell, B. (2005). Appearances are deceptive? Long-term cognitive and central auditory sequelae from closed head injury. International Journal of Audiology, 44(1), 39–49.

[9] Boly, M., Faymonville, M.-E., Peigneux, P., Lambermont, B., Damas, P., Del Fiore, G., et al. (2004). Auditory processing in severely brain injured patients: Differences between the minimally conscious state and the persistent vegetative state. Archives of Neurology, 61(2), 233–238.

[10] Bregman, A. S. (1990). Auditory scene analysis. Cambridge, MA: MIT Press.

[11] British Society of Audiology (BSA). (2011). Position statement: Auditory Processing Disorder (APD). Retrieved from http://www.thebsa.org.uk/wp-content/uploads/2014/04/BSA_APD_PositionPaper_31March11_FINAL.pdf.

[12] Britton, A., McKee, M., Black, N., McPherson, K., Sanderson, C., & Bain, C. (1998). Choosing between randomised and non-randomised studies: A systematic review. Health Technology Assessment, 2(13), i–iv, 1–124.

[13] Brodmann, K. (2006). Vergleichende Lokalisationslehre der Großhirnrinde in ihren Prinzipien dargestellt auf Grund des Zellenbaues (Barth, Leipzig, 1909). In L. J. Garey (Ed. & Trans.), Brodmann's localization in the cerebral cortex. New York, NY: Springer. Retrieved from http://www.appliedneuroscience.com/Brodmann.pdf (original work published in 1909).

[14] Canadian Interorganizational Steering Group for Speech-Language Pathology and Audiology (CISG). (2012). Canadian guidelines on auditory processing disorder in children and adults: Assessment and intervention. Retrieved from http://www.canadianaudiology.ca/assets/docs/Canadian_Guidelines_on_Auditory_Processing_Disorder_in_Children_and_Adults_EN_2012_new-site.pdf.

[15] Chermark, G. D., & Musiek, F. E. (1997). Central auditory processing disorders: New perspectives. San Diego, CA: Singular Publishing Group.

[16] Cockrell, J. L., & Gregory, S. A. (1992). Audiological deficits in brain-injured children and adolescents. Brain Injury, 6(3), 261–266.

[17] Concato, J. (2013). Study design and "evidence" in patient-oriented research. American Journal of Respiratory and Critical Care Medicine, 187(11), 1167–1172.

[18] Concato, J., Shah, N., & Horwitz, R. I. (2000). Randomized, controlled trials, observational studies, and the hierarchy of research designs. The New England Journal of Medicine, 342 (25), 1887–1892.

[19] Cooper, J. C., Jr, & Gates, G. A. (1991). Hearing in the elderly—the Framingham cohort, 1983-1985: Part II. Prevalence of central auditory processing disorders. Ear and Hearing, 12 (5), 304–311.

[20] Da Costa, S., van der Zwaag, W., Miller, L. M., Clarke, S., & Saenz, M. (2013). Tuning in to sound: Frequency-selective attentional filter in human primary auditory cortex. The Journal of Neuroscience, 33(5), 1858–1863.

[21] Danermark, B., & Gellerstedt, L. C. (2004). Psychosocial work environment, hearing impairment and health. International Journal of Audiology, 43(7), 383–389.

[22] Davis, H., & Goodman, A. C. (1966). Subtractive hearing loss, loudness recruitment and decruitment. The Annals of Otology, Rhinology, and Laryngology, 75(1), 87–94.

[23] de Croon, E. M., Sluiter, J. K., & Frings-Dresen, M. H. W. (2003). Need for recovery after work predicts sickness absence: A 2-year prospective cohort study in truck drivers. Journal of Psychosomatic Research, 55(4), 331–339.

[24] Drayna, D., Manichaikul, A., de Lange, M., Snieder, H., & Spector, T. (2001). Genetic correlates of musical pitch recognition in humans. Science, 291, 1969-1672.

[25] Engelien, A., Huber, W., Silbersweig, D., Stern, E., Frith, C. D., Döring, W., et al. (2000). The neural correlates of 'deaf-hearing' in man: Conscious sensory awareness enabled by attentional modulation. Brain, 123(Pt 3), 532–545.

[26] Fowler, E. P. (1936). A method for the early detection of otosclerosis: A study of sounds well above threshold. Arch Otolaryngol, 24(6), 731–741.

[27] Fry, D. B. (1948). An experimental study of tone deafness. Speech, 2, 1-7.

[28] Galarza, M., Isaac, C., Pellicer, O., Mayes, A., Broks, P., Montaldi, D., et al. (2014). Jazz, guitar, and neurosurgery: The Pat Martino case report. World Neurosurgery, 81(3-4), e1–e7.

[29] Garrido, L., Eisner, F., McGettigan, C., Stewart, L., Sauter, D., Hanley, J. R., et al. (2009). Developmental phonagnosia: A selective deficit of vocal identity recognition. Neuropsychologia, 47(1), 123–131.

[30] Greenwood, L.-M., Broyd, S. J., Croft, R., Todd, J., Michie, P. T., Johnstone, S., et al. (2014). Chronic effects of cannabis use on the auditory mismatch negativity. Biological Psychiatry, 75(6), 449–458.

[31] Hailstone, J. C., Crutch, S. J., Vestergaard, M. D., Patterson, R. D., & Warren, J. D. (2010). Progressive associative phonagnosia: A neuropsychological analysis. Neuropsychologia, 48(4), 1104–1114.

[32] Hämäläinen, J. A., Salminen, H. K., & Leppänen, P. H. T. (2013). Basic auditory processing deficits in dyslexia: Systematic review of the behavioral and event-related potential/field evidence. Journal of Learning Disabilities, 46(5), 413–427.

[33] Hasani, S., & Jafari, Z. (2013). Effect of infant prematurity on auditory brainstem response at preschool age. Iran J Otorhinolaryngol, 25(71), 107–114.

[34] Heim, S., Keil, A., Choudhury, N., Thomas Friedman, J., & Benasich, A. A. (2013). Early gamma oscillations during rapid auditory processing in children with a language-learning impairment: Changes in neural mass activity after training. Neuropsychologia, 51(5), 990–1001.

[35] Hoon, A. H., Jr, & Reiss, A. L. (1992). The mesial-temporal lobe and autism: Case report and review. Developmental Medicine and Child Neurology, 34(3), 252–259.

[36] Iliadou, V., Bamiou, D.-E., Kaprinis, S., Kandylis, D., & Kaprinis, G. (2009). Auditory processing disorders in children suspected of learning disabilities—a need for screening? International Journal of Pediatric Otorhinolaryngology, 73(7), 1029–1034.

[37] Jansen, E. J. M., Helleman, H. W., Dreschler, W. A., & de Laat, J. A. P. M. (2009). Noise induced hearing loss and other hearing complaints among musicians of symphony orchestras. International Archives of Occupational and Environmental Health, 82(2), 153–164.

[38] Jerger, J. F. (1960). Observations on auditory behavior in lesions of the central auditory pathways. A.M.A. Archives of Otolaryngology, 71, 797–806.

[39] Jerger, S., Martin, R. C., & Jerger, J. (1987). Specific auditory perceptual dysfunction in a learning disabled child. Ear and Hearing, 8(2), 78–86.

[40] Jones, J. L., Zalewski, C., Brewer, C., Lucker, J., & Drayna, D. (2009). Widespread auditory deficits in tune deafness. Ear and Hearing, 30(1), 63–72.

[41] Kaga, K., Shindo, M., & Tanaka, Y. (1997). Central auditory information processing in patients with bilateral auditory cortex lesions. Acta Oto-Laryngologica (Supplementum), 532, 77–82.

[42] Kaga, K., Tokoro, Y., Tanaka, Y., & Ushijima, H. (1980). The progress of adrenoleukodystrophy as revealed by auditory brainstem evoked responses and brainstem histology. Archives of Oto-Rhino-Laryngology, 228(1), 17–27.

[43] Kalmus, H., & Fry, D. B. (1980). On tune deafness (dysmelodia): Frequency, development, genetics and musical background. Annals of Human Genetics, 43(4), 369–382.

[44] Kaltenbach, J. A., Czaja, J. M., & Kaplan, C. R. (1992). Changes in the tonotopic map of the dorsal cochlear nucleus following induction of cochlear lesions by exposure to intense sound. Hearing Research, 59(2), 213–223.

[45] Karasek, R. A. (1979). Job demands, job decision latitude and mental strain: Implications for job redesign. Adm Sci Q, 24, 285–308.

[46] Kim, D.-H., Lu, N., Ma, R., Kim, Y. S., Kim, R. H., Wang, S., et al. (2011). Epidermal electronics. Science, 333(6044), 838–843.

[47] Koelsch, S., Heinke, W., Sammler, D., & Olthoff, D. (2006). Auditory processing during deep propofol sedation and recovery from unconsciousness. Clinical Neurophysiology, 117 (8), 1746–1759.

[48] Kotchoubey, B., Lang, S., Mezger, G., Schmalohr, D., Schneck, M., Semmler, A., et al. (2005). Information processing in severe disorders of consciousness: Vegetative state and minimally conscious state. Clinical Neurophysiology, 116(10), 2441–2453.

[49] Kramer, S. E., Allessie, G. H. M., Dondorp, A. W., Zekveld, A. A., & Kapteyn, T. S. (2005). A home education program for older adults with hearing impairment and their significant others: A randomized trial evaluating short- and long-term effects. International Journal of Audiology, 44(5), 255–264.

[50] Kreisman, N. V., John, A. B., Kreisman, B. M., Hall, J. W., & Crandell, C. C. (2012). Psychosocial status of children with auditory processing disorder. Journal of the American Academy of Audiology, 23(3), 222–233, quiz 234.

[51] Kumar, S., von Kriegstein, K., Friston, K. J., & Griffiths, T. D. (2013). A dynamic system for the analysis of acoustic features and valence of aversive sounds in the human brain. Advances in Experimental Medicine and Biology, 787, 463–472.

[52] Laureys, S., Perrin, F., Faymonville, M. E., Schnakers, C., Boly, M., Bartsch, V., et al. (2004). Cerebral processing in the minimally conscious state. Neurology, 63(5), 916–918.

[53] LeDoux, J. (2007). The amygdala. Current Biology, 17(20), R868–R874.

[54] Liu F., Jiang C., Francart T., Chan A. H., Wong P. C. (2013). Training Mandarin-speaking amusics to recognize pitch direction: Pathway to treat musical disorders in congenital amusia? J Acoust Soc Am, 134(5), 4064.

[55] Mata, I., Perez-Iglesias, R., Roiz-Santiañez, R., Tordesillas-Gutierrez, D., Pazos, A., Gutierrez, A., et al. (2010). Gyrification brain abnormalities associated with adolescence and early-adulthood cannabis use. Brain Research, 1317, 297–304.

[56] Mencher, G. T., Clack, T. D., & Rupp, R. R. (1973). Decruitment and the growth of loudness in the ears of brain-damaged adults. Cortex, 9(4), 335–345.

[57] Newman, T. B., Browner, W. S., & Cummings, S. R. (2001). Designing studies of medical tests. In S. B. Hulley, S. R. Cummings, W. S. Browner, D. Grady, N. Hearst, & T. B. Newman (Eds.), Designing clinical research: An epidemiologic approach (pp. 175-191). Philadelphia, PA: Lippincott, Williams & Wilkins.

[58] Oh, J., Kwon, J. H., Yang, P. S., & Jeong, J. (2013). Auditory imagery modulates frequency-specific areas in the human auditory cortex. Journal of Cognitive Neuroscience, 25(2), 175–187.

[59] Olakunbi, D., Bamiou, D.-E., Stewart, L., & Luxon, L. M. (2010). Evaluation of musical skills in children with a diagnosis of an auditory processing disorder. International Journal of Pediatric Otorhinolaryngology, 74(6), 633–636.

[60] Peretz, I., Champod, A. S., & Hyde, K. (2003). Varieties of musical disorders. The Montreal battery of evaluation of amusia. Annals of the New York Academy of Sciences, 999, 58–75.

[61] Perrin, F., García-Larrea, L., Mauguière, F., & Bastuji, H. (1999). A differential brain response to the subject's own name persists during sleep. Clinical Neurophysiology, 110 (12), 2153–2164.

[62] Petkov, C. I., & Sutter, M. L. (2011). Evolutionary conservation and neuronal mechanisms of auditory perceptual restoration. Hearing Research, 271(1-2), 54–65.

[63] Phillips-Silver, J., Toiviainen, P., Gosselin, N., & Peretz, I. (2013). Amusic does not mean unmusical: Beat perception and synchronization ability despite pitch deafness. Cognitive Neuropsychology, 30(5), 311–331.

[64] Portas, C. M., Krakow, K., Allen, P., Josephs, O., Armony, J. L., & Frith, C. D. (2000). Auditory processing across the sleep-wake cycle: Simultaneous EEG and fMRI monitoring in humans. Neuron, 28(3), 991–999.

[65] Rawool V. W. (1998a). Categorical loudness perception in normal and hearing impaired subjects. Journal of the Acoustical Society of America, 103, 2977-2978.

[66] Rawool, V. W. (1998b). Loudness growth in older (70+years) hearing impaired individuals. Paper presented at the annual convention of the American Auditory Society, Los Angeles, CA.

[67] Rawool, V. W. (2001). Can maximum comfortable loudness levels in hearing impaired listeners be predicted from ipsilateral acoustic reflex thresholds recorded with high frequency probes? Scandinavian Audiology, 30(2), 96–105.

[68] Rawool, V. W. (2012a). Comprehensive audiological, tinnitus, and auditory processing evaluations. In V. W. Rawool (Ed.), Hearing conservation: In occupational, recreational, educational, and home settings (pp. 106-135). New York, NY: Thieme.

[69] Rawool, V. W. (2012b). Support for workers with noise induced hearing loss. In V. W. Rawool (Ed.), Hearing conservation: In occupational, recreational, educational, and home settings (pp. 266-282). New York, NY: Thieme.

[70] Ress, D., & Chandrasekaran, B. (2013). Tonotopic organization in the depth of human inferior colliculus. Front Hum Neurosci, 7, Article ID 586, 1-10.

[71] Robertson, D., & Irvine, D. R. (1989). Plasticity of frequency organization in auditory cortex of guinea pigs with partial unilateral deafness. The Journal of Comparative Neurology, 282(3), 456–471.

[72] Romanski, L. M., Clugnet, M. C., Bordi, F., & LeDoux, J. E. (1993). Somatosensory and auditory convergence in the lateral nucleus of the amygdala. Behavioral Neuroscience, 107 (3), 444–450.

[73] Ruby, P., Caclin, A., Boulet, S., Delpuech, C., & Morlet, D. (2008). Odd sound processing in the sleeping brain. Journal of Cognitive Neuroscience, 20(2), 296–311.

[74] Salvi, R. J., Wang, J., & Ding, D. (2000). Auditory plasticity and hyperactivity following cochlear damage. Hearing Research, 147(1-2), 261–274.

[75] Salvi, R. J., Wang, J., & Powers, N. L. (1996). Plasticity and reorganization in the auditory brainstem: implications for tinnitus. In G. Reich & J. Vernon (Eds.), Proceedings of the Fifth International Tinnitus Seminar (pp. 457-466). Portland, OR: American Tinnitus Association.

[76] Sluiter, J. K., de Croon, E. M., Meijman, T. F., & Frings-Dresen, M. H. W. (2003). Need for recovery from work related fatigue and its role in the development and prediction of subjective health complaints. Occupational and Environmental Medicine, 60(Suppl 1), i62–i70.

[77] Solowij, N., Yücel, M., Respondek, C., Whittle, S., Lindsay, E., Pantelis, C., et al. (2011). Cerebellar white-matter changes in cannabis users with and without schizophrenia. Psychological Medicine, 41(11), 2349–2359.

[78] Steedman, M. J. (1977). The perception of musical rhythm and metre. Perception, 6(5), 555–569.

[79] Stephen, J. M., Kodituwakku, P. W., Kodituwakku, E. L., Romero, L., Peters, A. M., Sharadamma, N. M., et al. (2012). Delays in auditory processing identified in preschool children with FASD. Alcoholism, Clinical and Experimental Research, 36(10), 1720–1727.

[80] Strainer, J. C., Ulmer, J. L., Yetkin, F. Z., Haughton, V. M., Daniels, D. L., & Millen, S. J. (1997). Functional MR of the primary auditory cortex: An analysis of pure tone activation and tone discrimination. American Journal of Neuroradiology, 18(4), 601–610.

[81] Suneja, S. K., Potashner, S. J., & Benson, C. G. (1998). Plastic changes in glycine and GABA release and uptake in adult brain stem auditory nuclei after unilateral middle ear ossicle removal and cochlear ablation. Experimental Neurology, 151(2), 273–288.

[82] Szczepaniak, W. S., & Møller, A. R. (1995). Evidence of decreased GABAergic influence on temporal integration in the inferior colliculus following acute noise exposure: A study of evoked potentials in the rat. Neuroscience Letters, 196(1-2), 77–80.

[83] Temple, C. M., Jeeves, M. A., & Vilarroya, O. O. (1990). Reading in callosal agenesis. Brain and Language, 39(2), 235–253.

[84] Turgeon, C., Champoux, F., Lepore, F., Leclerc, S., & Ellemberg, D. (2011). Auditory processing after sport-related concussions. Ear and Hearing, 32(5), 667–670.

[85] Valadbeigi, A., Weisi, F., Rohbakhsh, N., Rezaei, M., Heidari, A., & Rasa, A. R. (2013). Central auditory processing and word discrimination in patients with multiple sclerosis. European Archives of Oto-Rhino-Laryngology, 271, 2891-2896.

[86] Van Lancker, D. R., Cummings, J. L., Kreiman, J., & Dobkin, B. H. (1988). Phonagnosia: A dissociation between familiar and unfamiliar voices. Cortex, 24(2), 195–209.

[87] von Plessen, K., Lundervold, A., Duta, N., Heiervang, E., Klauschen, F., Smievoll, A. I., et al. (2002). Less developed corpus callosum in dyslexic subjects—a structural MRI study. Neuropsychologia, 40(7), 1035–1044.

[88] Wang, J., Caspary, D., & Salvi, R. J. (2000). GABA-A antagonist causes dramatic expansion of tuning in primary auditory cortex. Neuroreport, 11(5), 1137–1140.

[89] Warren, R. M., Obusek, C. J., & Ackroff, J. M. (1972). Auditory induction: Perceptual synthesis of absent sounds. Science, 176(4039), 1149–1151.

[90] Willott, J. F., Aitkin, L. M., & McFadden, S. L. (1993). Plasticity of auditory cortex associated with sensorineural hearing loss in adult C57BL/6J mice. The Journal of Comparative Neurology, 329(3), 402–411.

[91] Winer, J. A., & Schreiner, C.E. (Eds.). (2005). The inferior colliculus. New York: Springer.

[92] World Health Organization (WHO). (2002). Towards a common language for functioning, disability and health: ICF. Geneva, Switzerland.

[93] Yücel, M., Solowij, N., Respondek, C., Whittle, S., Fornito, A., Pantelis, C., et al. (2008). Regional brain abnormalities associated with long-term heavy cannabis use. Archives of General Psychiatry, 65(6), 694–701.

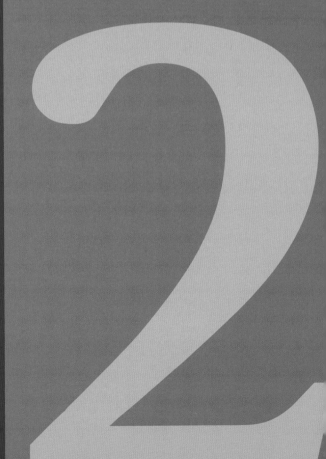

Chapter 2

Maturation and Plasticity of the Neural Auditory System

2 Maturation and Plasticity of the Neural Auditory System

The term *neural plasticity* refers to the ability of the nervous system to systematically change with physiological and behavioral consequences. Neural plastic changes can occur at the molecular, cellular, systems, and cognitive levels. As an example of plasticity at the molecular level, sympathetic neurons, which are conventionally considered as being noradrenergic or cholinergic, are also capable of expressing putative peptide transmitters including substance P. At the cellular level, neural connections, or synapses, can change. At the systems level, changes can occur in neurochemical systems due to changes in neurotransmitter expressions. Changes can occur at cognitive levels following intensive training. There appears to be a transition of neural plasticity with a sensory-driven plasticity in childhood to a cognitively driven plasticity in the adult years (Kral & Eggermont, 2007). The exact period of transition may vary, depending on a variety of factors. The changes driven by neural plasticity can be divided into various categories, as shown in ▶ Fig. 2.1.

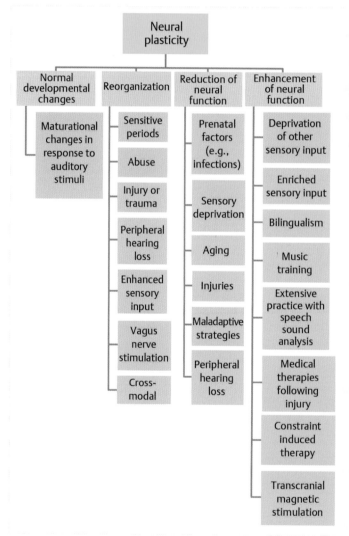

Fig. 2.1 Examples of categories of neural plasticity.

2.1 Normal Developmental (Maturational) Changes

The auditory system begins to develop in early embryonic life and follows a complex process involving several parallel occurrences. The embryo has three layers: endoderm, mesoderm, and ectoderm. The ectoderm gives rise to both neural tissue and skin. In the initial stages of development, the otic placode, a thickening of the ectoderm in the area of the developing hindbrain, is formed.

Fifteen days after fertilization, a primitive streak divides the embryonic disc, which leads the way for development of the ectodermal-lined primitive groove and primitive fold. The primitive groove deepens into a primitive pit, which forms the neural groove and neural fold. The ectodermal-lined neural folds come together to close off the neural groove, which forms the neural tube. The neurons that form the central auditory system are produced within the ventricular portion of the neural tube. From this area they migrate to their final site in the brain. During migration, neurons begin to send out axons that are guided toward the target site by chemical molecules produced by the target structures (Fekete & Campero, 2007). These molecules are detected by receptors on the exploring growth cones that form the tips of the growing neurons. Other types of molecules ensure that the axons make contact with the appropriate region of the target structure (e.g., at the base of the inner hair cells and not at the tip).

Animal studies suggest that the first auditory neurons give rise to the cochlear nucleus, the superior olivary complex, and the medial geniculate nucleus. The neurons that are produced slightly later give rise to the inferior colliculus and auditory cortex. In humans all the subcortical auditory structures and the precursor of the cerebral cortex or the cortical plate are recognizable at the 8th fetal week. Hair cells are innervated by the spiral ganglion cells by the 14th week. Axons from the thalamus begin to connect with the cortical plate during the 21st week of gestation. Myelination of the auditory nerve and the major brainstem pathways begins at the 26th week of gestation, around the time that fetal responses to sounds can be measured. Myelination is necessary for rapid conduction of action potentials through the nerve fibers. A week later, during the 27th week of gestation, the temporal lobe, which includes the auditory cortex, can be recognized as a distinct feature (Moore & Linthicum, 2007). With functional magnetic resonance imaging (fMRI), infants show a fully active language-related neural substrate in both hemispheres at the age of 2 days. However, intrahemispheric functional structural connections within this substrate are immature, with strong connections apparent only between the two hemispheres (Perani et al., 2011).

During normal development there is approximately 50% overproduction of neurons and synapses in mammals (Janowsky, 1993). This is followed by a 20 to 80% loss of neurons and retraction of related synapses in different cortical regions (Buss, Sun, & Oppenheim, 2006; Huttenlocher, 1990; Huttenlocher & Dabholkar, 1997; Huttenlocher, de Courten, Garey, & Van der Loos, 1982). Such loss is most likely related to competition for resources and is controlled by input and/or reorganization in response to environmental stimuli (Changeux & Danchin, 1976). Reorganization depends on auditory, visual, olfactory, somatosensory, kinesthetic, and autonomic inputs.

Some reorganization may occur to correct connectivity errors or to improve connectivity and thus enhance the response of the brain to specific and useful environmental input. For example, all infants can discriminate between sounds that occur in a variety of languages. However, depending on the specific language input, the ability to discriminate some sounds that do not occur in the child's mother tongue is lost. As a specific example, English-speaking adults show poorer performance on Mandarin alveolo-palatal affricate-fricative discrimination than Mandarin-speaking adults. If contrast discrimination is evaluated in infants exposed to English or Mandarin languages, results show that the performance on native language speech sound contrasts improves significantly between the ages of 6 and 12 months, whereas performance on nonnative contrasts decreases. Such functional diversity exists across different languages, including Japanese (Kuhl et al., 2006; Tsao, Liu, & Kuhl, 2006).

2.1.1 Maturational Changes in Response to Auditory Stimuli

During postnatal development, auditory function can be mapped using behavioral or electrophysiological approaches. Behavioral responses during

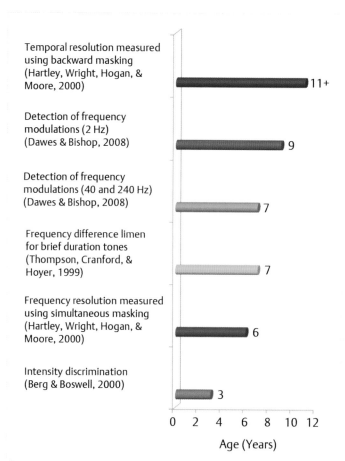

Fig. 2.2 Age (in years) at which adult-like performance is apparent on some of the auditory processing skills. Note that the age depends on the specific task used in assessing the processing skills.

various auditory tasks and some electrophysiological measures, such as late auditory evoked potentials, are influenced by maturation. Diffusion tensor imaging (DTI) data from children between 9 and 11 years of age show that the brain regions correlating with auditory processing vary according to the specific auditory processing skills (Schmithorst, Holland, & Plante, 2011).

Behavioral auditory perceptual skills develop over different time periods, but most skills appear to mature between the ages of 7 and 11 years. The specific age at which adultlike performance is apparent depends on the specific auditory processing skill and response task (▶ Fig. 2.2). However, on many auditory tasks some children in the age range of 6 to 7 years show adultlike performance (Moore, Cowan, Riley, Edmondson-Jones, & Ferguson, 2011). An example of the effect of age on speech recognition in noise is shown in ▶ Fig. 2.3. As apparent in the figure, younger children require a better signal-to-noise ratio to recognize 50% of the speech signal than do older children. The

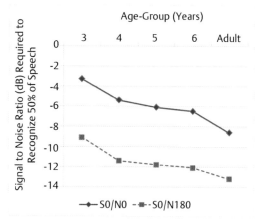

Fig. 2.3 The average signal-to-noise ratio (dB) required to recognize 50% of speech across different age groups. The noise is classroom noise presented at 60 A-weighted decibels (dBA). S0/N0: Both speech and classroom noise are presented in front of the listener. S0/N180: Speech is presented in front and noise from behind (based on Schafer et al., 2012).

difference between 6-year-old children and adults is not significant, suggesting maturation of speech recognition in noise at age 6 (Schafer et al., 2012).

2.2 Reorganization of Neural Function

2.2.1 Experience or Sensory Input

As noted previously, during development, the auditory system can organize itself depending on the sensory input to the auditory system.

Sensitive Periods

The neural system shows maximum plasticity during the *sensitive* periods, during which altered experience can change neuronal response properties and related behaviors. The plasticity during sensitive periods allows optimal function of brain circuits to match the infant's environment so that the child can understand and maximize the benefit from the immediate auditory environment, including the specific language or languages spoken at home. The sensitive period of development during which language can be learned with ease lasts for about 3.5 years. This matches the period around which synaptic density appears to peak in the auditory cortex (Huttenlocher, 2000).

The latency of the P1 peak of the cortical auditory evoked potentials decreases to within normal limits after receiving auditory stimulation through cochlear implants in children who receive the implants before the age of 3.5 years. Children who receive implants after this age but before the age of 7 years show mixed cortical development, with some children showing normal latencies of the P1, whereas others show longer latencies even after several years of cochlear implant use (Sharma & Dorman, 2006; Sharma, Dorman, & Spahr, 2002a,b; Sharma, Dorman, Spahr, & Todd, 2002).

Influence of Context

Input to the auditory system is also shaped by the context in which the sound stimulation occurs. Nine-month-old American infants can easily learn phonemes and words in Mandarin Chinese if they are given an opportunity to interact with a live Chinese speaker. This ease in learning is not apparent if the same sounds are delivered by television or audiotapes (Kuhl, Tsao, & Liu, 2003) with no opportunities for interactions.

Sensitive Periods of Music Perception

Sensitive periods are also apparent for music perception. Initially, infants respond in a similar way to the music of any culture. With experience, their perceptual abilities become increasingly focused on the style of music to which they have been exposed. Six-month-old infants show sensitivity to rhythmic variations in the music of different cultures, but at the age of 12 months, they show a culture-specific bias. However, the perception of rhythms in foreign music can be improved in 12-month-old infants by exposing them to that particular type of music (Hannon & Trehub, 2005).

2.2.2 Reorganization of Neural Function Due to Abuse

Young adults with histories of parental verbal aggression in childhood show a reduction in fractional anisotropy in the arcuate fasciculus connecting the Wernicke and frontal areas, suggesting an impact of emotionally abusive language on the development of the auditory association cortex. Exposure to parental verbal aggression may attenuate the degree of pruning necessary to refine neural structures and lead to an increase in the volume of gray matter in the left superior temporal gyrus (Tomoda et al., 2011).

2.2.3 Reorganization Due to Injury

In the presence of injuries, the cortex is usually reorganized; the type of reorganization depends on the type and extent of the injury. Because of the neural plasticity of the developing brain, injury during the early developmental period can disturb normal development. Loss of specific neural resources can impair some functions, including auditory, linguistic, visuospatial, and affective processing. The timing, extent, location, and specificity of the injury and the timing, specificity, and quality of any intervention measures determine the magnitude and duration of the impairment and the reorganization of the underlying neural substrates related to the specific functions.

2.2.4 Reorganization Due to Peripheral Hearing Loss

The normal auditory cortex shows some tonotopic organization. If the high-frequency cochlear areas toward the base of the cochlea are destroyed using ototoxic substances, the input to the most caudal regions is eliminated. This leads to a reorganization of the auditory cortex in about 2 to 3 months. The areas previously responding only to high-frequency tones begin to respond to midfrequency tones (Schwaber, Garraghty, & Kaas, 1993). In humans the areas near the frequencies with maximum high-frequency hearing loss show better frequency discrimination ability compared to those without hearing loss, suggesting cortical reorganization (Kluk & Moore, 2006; Moore & Vinay, 2009). In addition, high-frequency hearing loss is associated with improved amplitude modulation detection at lower frequencies (Moore & Vinay, 2009), which may be due to the added contribution of the high-frequency neural areas to the detection at lower frequencies.

Temporary reorganization can be demonstrated by inducing temporary hearing loss. Munro and Blount (2009) fitted adults with normal hearing with earplugs in one ear. After 7 days of regular use of the earplug, the level required to elicit the acoustic reflex in the fitted ear was decreased by 5 to 7 dB compared to baseline levels before the fitting. The lowering or improvement of acoustic reflex thresholds may have occurred due to reorganization of the neural system in the form of increased gain of incoming stimuli to maintain baseline neural activity. After discontinuing the use of the earplug, the acoustic reflex thresholds returned to the baseline levels. These findings suggest that the use of earplugs in individuals with hypersensitivity to sounds may worsen hyperacusis.

2.2.5 Reorganization Due to Enhanced Sensory Input

Reorganization of the neural pathways can occur following increased sensory input. For example, when individuals with normal hearing are provided with low-gain hearing aids in one ear for 5 days, acoustic reflex thresholds are elevated compared to baseline levels prior to the fitting of hearing aids, suggesting reorganization of the neural system in the form of decreased gain for incoming stimuli (Munro & Merrett, 2013). Such reorganization may be helpful for improving tolerance to loud sounds for patients with hyperacusis.

2.2.6 Reorganization Following Vagus Nerve Stimulation

Vagus nerve stimulation (VNS) triggers the release of neuromodulators, such as acetylcholine and norepinephrine. The synergistic action of multiple neuromodulators in the cerebral cortex and other brain regions following VNS appears to drive neural plasticity. Patients suffering from tinnitus who are not on medications that interfere with acetylcholine and norepinephrine release (e.g., norepinephrine agonists) show benefit from electrical stimulation of the vagus nerve. To derive the benefit, VNS is paired with tones excluding the tones matching the tinnitus frequency. The benefit appears in the form of less distress from tinnitus and reduction of perceived tinnitus (De Ridder, Vanneste, Engineer, & Kilgard, 2014).

2.2.7 Cross-Modal Reorganization

Cross-modal plasticity occurs when a cortical area is deprived of sensory stimulation and that area is then recruited by another sensory system. For example, auditory cortices of congenitally deaf individuals tend to show larger N1 visual evoked potentials over the frontal and anterior temporal areas in response to peripheral visual motion compared to normal-hearing individuals; this effect is not apparent in individuals who become deaf after the age of 4 years (Neville & Lawson, 1987; Neville, Schmidt, & Kutas, 1983). Age of onset of sensory deprivation due to deafness appears to be a critical variable determining whether or not cross-modal reorganization will occur (Buckley & Tobey, 2011).

Precursors to Cross-Modal Reorganization

Cross-modal reorganization is partially mediated by the transient connections between the various cortical areas, including the auditory, visual, and tactile cortices (Dehay, Bullier, & Kennedy, 1984; Frost, 1984; Innocenti & Clarke, 1984). A precursor to cross-modal reorganization may be a failure of the development of connections between primary and secondary auditory cortices leading to the decoupling of the higher auditory cortex from the secondary auditory cortex. These connections allow top-down modulatory input from the higher order auditory cortex to the secondary auditory cortex (Kral, 2007; Kral & Eggermont, 2007). The activity of the cortical loops between higher order and association auditory cortices is reflected in the N1 component of the cortical auditory evoked potentials. This component is absent in children who receive cochlear implants after the sensitive periods, suggesting some degree of decoupling due to long-term auditory deprivation (Eggermont & Ponton, 2003; Kral, 2007; Kral & Eggermont, 2007; Sharma et al., 2007). Such decoupling might allow higher auditory cortices to connect with areas that are devoted to other sensory modalities (Gilley, Sharma, & Dorman, 2008; Sharma, Gilley, Dorman, & Baldwin, 2007), leading to cross-modal reorganization.

Cross-Modal Reorganization Due to Auditory Deprivation

Functional MRI shows activation of the auditory cortex to visual stimuli in deaf individuals (Finney, Clementz, Hickok, & Dobkins, 2003; Finney, Fine, & Dobkins, 2001). Some regions normally devoted to auditory stimuli may be involved in the detection of rare (oddball) tactile-frequency changes embedded in a stream of frequent (standard) tactile frequency stimuli in deaf individuals (Levänen & Hamdorf, 2001). Similarly, some individuals with prelingual deafness report somatosensory sensations in response to acoustic input immediately following activation of cochlear implants (Eisenberg, 1982; McFeely, Antonelli, Rodriguez, & Holmes, 1998); such sensations are not reported by postlingually deafened patients (McFeely et al., 1998). The use of auditory cortices in deaf individuals for enhanced processing of visual or tactile stimuli is not related to the use of sign language but is related to the presence of severe or worse hearing loss (Finney et al., 2001; Neville & Lawson, 1987).

Impact of Cross-Modal Reorganization on Auditory Processing

If another sensory modality recruits auditory cortical processing areas, stimulation of auditory system through a cochlear implant may not allow normal amounts of cortical resources for speech processing, creating a specific auditory processing deficit. Auditory stimulation of children who receive cochlear implants before the age of 3.5 years activates the auditory areas in the temporal lobe, whereas children who are implanted after the age of 3.5 years show maximum activation in the parietal region, which is involved in multisensory or multimodal processing (Gilley et al., 2008).

The right temporal lobe is involved in the processing of suprasegmental speech features. Individuals with cochlear implants need to rely on such suprasegmental features because of the lack of fine structure detail in the speech signals processed by cochlear implants. Larger amplitudes of N1 evoked potential over the right temporal lobe in response to visual stimuli in prelingually deaf individuals suggest that these areas are recruited by visual modality. Furthermore, such large amplitudes are associated with poorer speech perception. Such a relationship is not apparent in individuals who acquire severe to profound hearing loss later in life (Buckley & Tobey, 2011) because cross-modal organization in these individuals is likely to be absent due to the presence of sufficient auditory sensory stimulation early in life. For similar reasons, individuals with a low resting metabolic rate of the temporal cortices compared to other cortical areas before cochlear implantation tend to have good speech-processing abilities after cochlear implantation. Individuals showing resting temporal cortical metabolic rates similar to other cortical areas before cochlear implants, suggesting cortical reorganization due to cross-modal plasticity, tend to fail to achieve high speech-processing abilities following implantation (D. S. Lee et al., 2001; J. S. Lee et al., 2003; Oh et al., 2003). The consequences of cross-modal reorganization are not restricted to auditory processing deficits; deficits in the integration of auditory and visual modes can also occur (Bergeson, Pisoni, & Davis, 2005; Gilley, Sharma, Mitchell, & Dorman, 2010; Schorr, Fox, van Wassenhove, & Knudsen, 2005).

Cross-Modal Reorganization Due to Blindness

Sensory deprivation due to blindness can lead to cross-modal plasticity. For example, fMRI shows activation of the visual cortex to tactile stimuli, such as braille letters, in blind individuals (Sadato, Okada, Honda, & Yonekura, 2002). Individuals who become blind early in life leading to sensory deprivation to visual cortices show somatosensory/visual cross-modal plasticity, but those who become blind later in life do not show such cross-modal organization (Cohen et al., 1999; Lewis & Maurer, 2005; Sadato et al., 2005; Voss et al., 2004).

2.3 Reduction of Neural Function

Under certain circumstances neural function can be reduced. Some of these circumstances are presented below.

2.3.1 Reduction of Neural Function Due to Prenatal Factors

Prenatal Exposure to Toxic Substances

Prenatal exposure to potentially toxic substances, such as antiepileptic drugs, including valproic acid, can increase the risk of neural tube defects (Wyszynski et al., 2005). Other antiepileptic drugs, such as phenytoin, are associated with an increased risk of other anomalies (reviewed in Ornoy, 2006). Heavy prenatal exposure to cocaine can lead to poor memory and deficits in information processing (Jacobson, Jacobson, Sokol, Martier, & Chiodo, 1996). Prenatal cocaine exposure of more than 3 days per week during the first trimester leads to an increase in the I–III, I–V, and III–V interpeak latencies of the auditory brainstem response compared to nonexposed control children. Similarly, infants with prenatal exposure to opiates show increased III–V interpeak latencies (Lester et al., 2003).

Prenatal alcohol exposure has a negative impact on the brain at all stages of development, from neurogenesis to myelination, resulting in cognitive and behavioral problems, including deficits in executive functioning and motor control (reviewed in Riley, Infante, & Warren, 2011). Exposure of the fetal and neonatal brain to nicotine through smoking or nicotine replacement therapy (NRT) has detrimental effects on cholinergic modulation of the developing brain, including the survival of neurons and synaptogenesis. Such alterations can lead to auditory-cognitive dysfunction (Dwyer, Broide, & Leslie, 2008). Similar affects are apparent in cases of fetal solvent syndrome due to excessive prenatal exposure to organic solvents, such as toluene from commercially available spray cans. Ear abnormalities, developmental delays, postnatal microcephaly (Pearson, Hoyme, Seaver, & Rimsza, 1994), language impairments, and cerebellar dysfunction are apparent in children with fetal solvent exposure (reviewed in Bowen & Hannigan, 2006).

Fetal Exposure to Infections

Exposure to various infections during the prenatal period can have a negative impact on neural development. Examples of such infections are cytomegalovirus, herpes simplex virus, toxoplasmosis, and acquired immunodeficiency disease (AIDS).

Other Prenatal Factors

Other factors that can have a negative impact on neural development and function are nutritional deficiency, vitamin (e.g., vitamin B_9) and mineral (e.g., iron) deficiencies, and hormonal abnormalities, including thyroid hormone deficiency, excessive use of corticosteroid hormones, and lack of folic acid supplements. Folate, or vitamin B_9, is found in dark green leafy vegetables, orange juice, beans, nuts, asparagus, and strawberries. Folic acid is the synthetic form of folate. During pregnancy, folate requirements increase partially because of fetal development. Pregnant women are also more likely to be deficient in cobalamin, or vitamin B_{12}, than nonpregnant women. A paired management strategy, including folic acid and vitamin B_{12} maternal and paternal supplementation, has been recommended to reduce the risk of neural tube defects (Reynolds, 2014; Safi, Joyeux, & Chalouhi, 2012).

2.3.2 Reduction of Neural Function Due to Sensory Deprivation

If the input to the auditory system is minimized during the sensitive period due to permanent hearing impairment of a congenital nature or acquired impairment due to conditions such as meningitis or temporary hearing impairment due to otitis media or reduced sensory input due to child abuse or neglect, organization of neurons can be profoundly affected in a negative manner with a resultant dysfunction in the ability to process acoustic stimuli.

Children who suffer from chronic otitis media over a period of several years are deprived of optimal auditory input in childhood. Such children can suffer from auditory processing deficits even after full recovery of hearing in the later years. School-age children with a history of conductive hearing loss due to otitis media with effusion in the first 3 years of life show elevated contralateral acoustic reflex thresholds and prolonged latencies of the wave V component of the auditory brainstem response, suggesting alterations in the auditory brainstem pathways (Gravel et al., 2006).

When the otitis media is severe enough to cause degraded signal delivery to the auditory system, children are at a risk for developing lasting auditory processing deficits. Because animal models suggest that asymmetric, degraded input to the auditory system can lead to serious alterations to the structure and function of binaural processing neural circuits, auditory sensitivity in both ears should be considered to estimate the risk of auditory processing deficits in children with chronic otitis media (Whitton & Polley, 2011). Children ranging in age from 8 to 12 years with a history of secretory otitis media in the first 5 years of life along with surgical placement of bilateral ventilation tubes perform poorly on dichotic digits and gap detection tasks. In addition, the performance of children in public schools is worse than those in private schools (Borges, Paschoal, & Colella-Santos, 2013) perhaps due to lower socioeconomic status and poorer access to health care for children in public schools. Some investigators have suggested that only those children who have a cumulative experience of otitis media with effusion of more than half the time during the first 5 years show binaural processing deficits (Hogan & Moore, 2003).

Implications of Sensory Deprivation Research

Overall, the research shows that sensory deprivation can be one of the causes of auditory processing deficits. Thus, one strategy is to minimize sensory deprivation. Every attempt should be made to minimize sensory deprivation during periods of both unilateral and bilateral episodes of otitis media to prevent auditory processing deficits. This includes prompt medical attention for children who suffer from conditions such as otitis media. Children who do not appear to respond to medical or surgical treatment and suffer from intermittent hearing loss should be fitted with minimal gain amplification. Parents and teachers should be trained on watching for the signs of minimal hearing loss due to otitis media so they can prompt the use of amplification when necessary to avoid sensory deprivation to the auditory system and to minimize speech, language, and educational delays.

For children who are socially isolated due to abusive types of situations, society and social workers need to be more vigilant in reporting such abuse, and law enforcement needs to be more vigilant in following up on reports. When necessary, such children should be placed in situations where they can receive maximum sensory input for adequate development of their neural systems.

For children with both unilateral and bilateral hearing loss, prompt amplification and intervention should be provided to ensure proper development of the central auditory system. In some cases, such as congenital auditory processing deficits and auditory neuropathy spectrum disorder (see Chapter 15), the input to the auditory system can be aberrant and thus can negatively affect the function of the central auditory pathways. Therefore, early intervention is important in maximizing normal maturation of the auditory system.

Critical Period

The reduction in function occurring during the sensitive period can be reversed during the *critical* period by introducing normal or enriched sensory experiences. The critical period is somewhat longer than the sensitive period.

The critical period for language development appears to last until the age of 7 years. Acquisition of a new language after this period is difficult without previous exposure to that language. Congenitally deaf children introduced to sound after the age of 7 years show abnormal processing of auditory stimuli, suggesting significant reduction of neuroplasticity after this period. More specifically, deaf children who receive cochlear implants after the age of 7 years show abnormal P1 response of the cortical auditory evoked potentials. The abnormal responses last even after several years of cochlear implant use (Sharma, Dorman, & Kral, 2005).

Critical periods may also exist for nonspeech stimuli, such as music. Individuals with early music training beginning before age 8 years are more likely to show absolute pitch (the ability to identify or recreate a given musical note without a reference tone) skills compared to those with later initiation of music training after the age of 8 years (▶ Fig. 2.4), suggesting a critical period for acquiring absolute pitch (Deutsch, Henthorn, Marvin, & Xu, 2006).

2.3.3 Reduction of Neural Function Due to Aging

With aging, the central auditory system can change even in the absence of peripheral hearing loss. Investigators have reported primary degeneration of the spiral ganglion (cell bodies of the auditory nerve fibers) or loss of fibers that can occur even in the absence of loss of sensory hair cells (Felder & Schrott-Fischer, 1995; Felix, Johnsson, Gleeson, & Pollak, 1990). Neuronal loss has been reported in the cochlear nucleus, inferior colliculus, medial geniculate body, and temporal lobe

(Brody, 1976; Hansen & Reske-Nielsen, 1965; Kirikae, Sato, & Shitara, 1964).

Konigsmark and Murphy (1972) found a relation between age and a decrease in the volume of the cochlear nucleus that appeared to be associated with changes in axon size and degree of myelination. Degenerative changes in the myelin sheaths and axis cylinders have also been reported (Hansen & Reske-Nielsen, 1965). Other degenerative

changes, such as cell size and cell shape irregularities, and the possible accumulation of lipofuscin pigments have been observed in the cochlear nucleus, superior olivary nucleus, inferior colliculus, medial geniculate body, and inferior olive (Brody, 1976; Kirikae et al., 1964; Konigsmark & Murphy, 1972). Progressive loss of dendritic mass without obvious clinical symptoms, especially in the frontal and temporal cortex, has been reported with aging (Scheibel & Scheibel, 1975). Such changes can lead to the reduction of neural function with aging.

2.3.4 Reduction of Neural Function Due to Injuries

A focal brain injury to the auditory cortex can reduce normal function due to lost or impaired input from the damaged areas.

Unilateral Brain Injuries

The right hemisphere appears to be involved in constructing an overall picture from spatially placed stimuli, whereas the left hemisphere is involved in paying attention to the details within an overall pattern (Fink et al., 1996; Martinez et al., 1997). An illustration of these deficits for visual stimuli is provided in ► Fig. 2.5. Thus, in general,

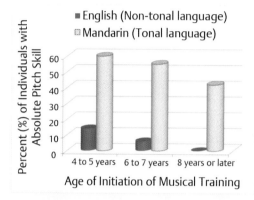

Fig. 2.4 Percentage of individuals who obtained a score of at least 85% correct (no semitone errors allowed) on the test of absolute pitch as a function of onset of music training (based on Deutsch et al., 2006).

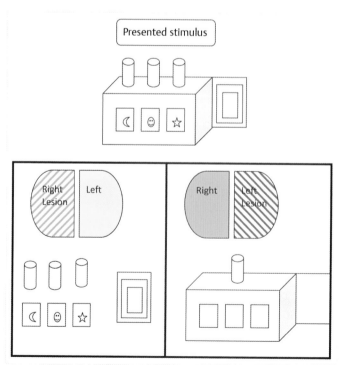

Fig. 2.5 Illustration of a highly simplified model of outcomes of right versus left hemisphere damage on perception. With right hemisphere damage, the details of the image are perceived but there is difficulty in integrating the entire image. With left hemisphere damage, the overall image is perceived, but the details are missing, suggesting that the left hemisphere allows perception of details.

for visual stimuli, adults with injury to the right hemisphere regions have difficulty with spatial integration. They can identify the parts of spatial forms but have difficulty integrating the parts into an overall pattern. Patients with left hemisphere injuries tend to generate the overall pattern but miss the details within a pattern. If the brain injury occurs at a very early stage in development, then the deficits tend to be less severe due to the neural plasticity within a developing brain. However, some deficits in performing complex tasks may continue to persist in later stages of development (Akshoomoff, Feroleto, Doyle, & Stiles, 2002).

The fine temporal structure of the speech signal is processed by the left temporal lobe (Friederici & Alter, 2004). Thus, damage to the left temporal lobe may make it difficult to perceive subtle speech cues necessary for speech perception and language development. Extraction of the overall meaning of the message relies on the suprasegmental features of speech, which are processed by the right temporal lobe (Meyer, Alter, Friederici, Lohmann, & von Cramon, 2002). Under degraded listening conditions, some fine structures in the speech signal are missing or altered; under such conditions, speech perception may depend heavily on the functional status of the right temporal lobe (Boatman et al., 2006; Liikkanen et al., 2007; Shtyrov et al., 1998). Thus, acquired focal injuries to the right temporal lobe may make it difficult to perceive degraded speech. However, as discussed in Chapter 8, speech perception is complex, and many different brain regions are involved in speech perception. Also, some patients may use cognitive strategies to perceive speech under degraded listening conditions.

Individuals with right hemisphere lesions of adult onset often show aprosodic or monotonous and uninflected speech. Similar difficulties are apparent in children diagnosed with nonverbal learning disability (Voeller, 1986; Weintraub & Mesulam, 1983). This suggests lower capacity for reorganization of the right hemisphere functions, including prosody and spatial integration.

2.3.5 Reduction of Neural Function Due to Maladaptive Compensatory Strategies

After unilateral brain damage, reliance on the less-affected body side may limit the propensity of individuals to engage in behaviors that can promote function of the impaired side. This is referred to as *learned nonuse.* Individuals employing learned nonuse show greater dysfunction than what can be expected based on the sustained damage (reviewed in Taub, 2012).

Another example of a maladaptive compensatory strategy is when a person with bilateral hearing loss wears a hearing aid in only one ear. In this case the sensory input to the aided ear is reestablished by the hearing aid, but the unaided ear is deprived of similar auditory input. Over time the speech recognition scores of some individuals become progressively poorer in the unaided ear when compared to those in the aided ear, as shown in ▶ Fig. 2.6 (Silman, Gelfand, & Silverman, 1984). In individuals who are fitted monaurally, up to 25% show significant worsening of speech recognition ability in the unfitted ear over a period of 5 years, whereas only 6% of individuals fitted with binaural hearing aids show significant worsening of speech recognition skills over the same period (Hurley, 1999). This functional decline can be reversed after fitting a hearing aid in the unaided ear (Silman, Silverman, Emmer, & Gelfand, 1992), but such improvement may not occur in all cases (Gelfand, 1995).

2.3.6 Reduction of Neural Function Due to Peripheral Hearing Loss

As noted previously, sensory deprivation can reduce neural function. High-frequency hearing loss is associated with a lower volume of auditory

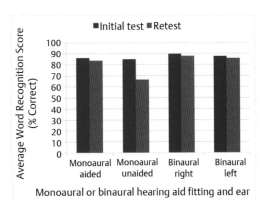

Fig. 2.6 Reduced neural function due to monoaural auditory deprivation in individuals with binaural hearing loss and fitted with a hearing aid in one ear. The word recognition scores in the unaided ear become worse over time (based on Silman et al., 1984).

cortex gray matter, along with increased cerebrospinal fluid in the same area, indicating atrophy of the auditory cortex with hearing loss. Such atrophy can lead to a reduction of neural function (Eckert, Cute, Vaden, Kuchinsky, & Dubno, 2012).

2.4 Enhancement of Neural Function

Neural function can be enhanced through various procedures, including enriched sensory input and medical therapies. The underlying mechanisms for enhancement of brain function after training or treatments include creation of new neurons (neurogenesis) and new neuronal connections. Formation of new neurons continues in adulthood (reviewed in Lazarov & Marr, 2013). Some factors can suppress neurogenesis, including high levels of stress, probably due to increased release of glucocorticoid. Factors that enhance neurogenesis include physical activity and learning experience.

2.4.1 Enhancement of Auditory Function Due to Deprivation of Other Sensory Input

Blind individuals who are deprived of visual sensory input show enhanced perception in other sensory modalities. These include finer tactile discrimination (Norman & Bartholomew, 2011), superior auditory pitch discrimination, better spatial sound localization, better spatial navigation, superior speech discrimination, and better performance on verbal recall tasks.

Totally blind listeners show better auditory distance discrimination in simulated anechoic and reverberant virtual rooms. They appear to use the decrease in sound level as a function of distance more effectively than do sighted listeners. In addition, they are also able to use the direct sound-to-reverberant sound ratio cue more effectively (Kolarik, Cirstea, & Pardhan, 2013). Blind listeners are also substantially better than sighted listeners in perceiving sound motion. The minimum audible movement angle of blind listeners is about half of what is necessary for sighted listeners (Lewald, 2013). Older blind listeners are better than age-matched sighted peers at recognizing time-compressed (fast) speech (Gordon-Salant & Friedman, 2011).

Pitch and melody discrimination is significantly better in blind listeners compared to matched controls and is related to cortical thickness of occipital areas showing adaptive plasticity (Voss & Zatorre, 2012). Magnetic source imaging shows that the auditory cortex is enlarged by a factor of 1.8 in blind adults compared to sighted controls. In addition, the latency of the N1 m component is significantly shorter in blind adults compared to the control group (Elbert et al., 2002).

2.4.2 Enriched Sensory Input

Neural plasticity allows enhancement of auditory function by enriching the input to the auditory system through systematic auditory training. The key characteristics of the training that drive enhanced function are repetition, consolidation period, and salience. The input needs to be repeated sufficiently and to be salient to induce plasticity. Short-term behavioral changes may be apparent in the absence of neural changes, such as an increase in synaptic number. To induce neural changes, sufficient repetition of the training stimuli is necessary. The stimuli should be presented at clearly audible but safe presentation levels to the listener. Overall, high-intensity stimuli appear to lead to long-term potentiation, although in some cases long-term potentiation may be enhanced at low test stimulus intensities (Jeffery, 1995). Other aspects of enriched input are discussed in Chapters 8 through 11. Enriched sensory input is most efficient at a younger age in enhancing neural function.

Although there are critical periods during childhood, some input-dependent plasticity continues during the adult period. The residual plasticity in adulthood does allow correction of perceptual dysfunction or processing deficits through training or acquisition of lost functions such as speech following injuries to the central systems, including stroke. In one study younger and older adults were trained for 100 sessions, with each session lasting for 1 hour, on a set of various memory and six perceptual speed tasks. Control groups in the study did not receive any training but were assessed before and after the training duration. Training affected several metrics of DTI and increased the anterior area of the corpus callosum, as seen on a structural MRI. The effect was similar in younger and older adults. These findings suggest training induced plasticity of the white matter macrostructure. Such findings show that reduced interhemispheric connectivity can be enhanced through training (Lövdén et al., 2010).

2.4.3 Bilingualism

Bilinguals show a widespread cognitive advantage in other areas, including executive processing and nonlinguistic inhibitory control (reviewed in Hilchey & Klein, 2011). Bilingualism enhances attention and cognitive control for children (Bialystok, 2001) and older adults (Bialystok, Craik, Klein, & Viswanathan, 2004; Bialystok, Craik, & Ryan, 2006). Because of continued practice in focusing attention on the relevant language and ignoring or inhibiting interference from a second language (Green, 1998), bilingual children develop attention control earlier than age-matched controls. Because of this experience in attention control, the auditory system of bilingual individuals becomes more efficient and flexible in processing sounds. Children with exposure to more than one language regardless of active use or nonuse of a second language are better at learning the phonological patterns of a new language (Kuo & Anderson, 2012).

Adolescent bilinguals show enhanced encoding in the auditory brainstem response of the fundamental frequency of the speech syllable /da/ presented in quiet and in the presence of multitalker babble (Krizman, Marian, Shook, Skoe, & Kraus, 2012). The perception of fundamental frequency is important for auditory scene analyses or segregation of auditory streams. At the cortical level, second language acquisition increases the density of gray matter in the inferior parietal cortex. The increase in gray matter density is positively related to the level of proficiency in the second language (Mechelli et al., 2004).

Exposure and mastery of more than one language can delay the onset of dementia in old age (Craik, Bialystok, & Freedman, 2010). In one study, case histories of individuals who were referred to a memory clinic with cognitive complaints were evaluated. Fifty-one percent of these individuals were bilingual. When all other measures were controlled, the bilingual individuals showed symptoms of dementia 4 years later than monolinguals (Bialystok, Craik, & Freedman, 2007).

2.4.4 Music Training

Music training can lead to neural and cognitive advantages for processing of auditory stimuli. Musicians show better encoding of acoustic stimuli, including music and speech stimuli. For more information on the enhancement of neural function due to music, see Chapter 8.

2.4.5 Extensive Practice with Speech Sound Analysis

The left pars opercularis is larger in professional phoneticians than matched controls, suggesting plastic changes in the Broca area due to extensive training with speech sound analyses. In addition, the amount of phonetic transcription training is positively correlated with the area of the left pars opercularis (Golestani, Price, & Scott, 2011). This region is important for phonologically based working memory, as shown by repetitive transmagnetic stimulation that disrupts phonologically based working memory for a visually presented word (Nixon, Lazarova, Hodinott-Hill, Gough, & Passingham, 2004).

2.4.6 Enhancement through Medical Therapies following Injury

Spontaneous functional recovery after injury is marked by following phases with partial overlap. Recovery from injury can be enhanced at each phase by external interventions, including medical therapies.

1. Initially, debris is cleared, cells are repaired, and metabolism and neuronal function is reestablished in existing neurons. Neurons that resume metabolic function may still exhibit deficient neurotransmission partially due to dysfunctional spines. Activators of the noradrenergic, dopaminergic, and cholinergic systems can promote and stabilize functional plasticity during this phase.
2. Axonal growth, spine remodeling, and spine activation begins following clearance of debris. Neural plasticity during this phase can be enhanced through growth factors and attenuators of axonal growth inhibition.
3. Finally, new neural networks are established and consolidated. Cortical stimulation and physical therapy can enhance recovery during this phase.

2.4.7 Constraint-Induced Therapy

Constraint-induced therapy is usually effective in cases with unilateral brain damage in promoting the function of the impaired side. For example, a patient is asked to wear a restraining mitt on the less-affected side and is provided with repetitive practice in performing tasks with the hemiplegic hand (Wolfe et al., 2006). Constraint-induced therapy is a good example of how changes in behavior can improve brain function due to neural plasticity.

2.4.8 Transcranial Magnetic Stimulation

Transcranial magnetic stimulation (TMS) allows noninvasive stimulation of the brain. The technique has the potential to modulate cortical excitability and enhance the effects of rehabilitation efforts following brain injury (Harris-Love, 2012). For more information on TMS, see Chapter 8.

2.5 Future Trends

In the future the occurrence of many of the preventable birth defects will be minimized through improved prevention, surveillance, prenatal screening, and counseling programs. Examples of preventable birth defects include congenital rubella syndrome, folic acid–preventable spinal bifida and anencephaly, fetal alcohol syndrome, Down syndrome, and defects associated with maternal diabetes (Kancherla, Oakley, & Brent, 2014).

Sensory cortical prostheses are being developed to not only restore normal neurologic function but also to augment or expand natural perceptual capabilities. For example, perception of infrared light is usually beyond the sensory capabilities of rats. However, rats can learn to perceive otherwise invisible infrared light and make use of this information. The perception is achieved through a neuroprosthesis that links the output of a head-mounted infrared sensor to the somatosensory cortex through intracortical microstimulation. The infrared perception does not compromise the original tactile representations in the somatosensory cortex (Thomson, Carra, & Nicolelis, 2013). In the future such prostheses may allow us to hear sounds that are considered outside the normal hearing range.

2.6 Review Questions

1. Define the term *neural plasticity*. Discuss reorganization within the central nervous system during neural development. Also, discuss and differentiate between sensitive periods and critical periods of sensory development.
2. Discuss the effect of sensory deprivation or abuse during sensitive periods. What are the implications of sensory deprivation research for auditory processing deficits?
3. Discuss prenatal factors that can lead to the reduction of neural function.
4. Discuss the reduction of neural function as a result of the aging process, focal injuries to the auditory cortex, maladaptive compensatory strategies, and peripheral hearing loss.
5. Discuss the reorganization of neural function due to injury, peripheral hearing loss, enhanced sensory input, and vagus nerve stimulation.
6. What is cross-modal reorganization, and what are its precursors? Review cross-modal organization following auditory deprivation. What is the potential impact of cross-modal reorganization on auditory processing? Discuss cross-modal organization due to blindness.
7. What are the underlying mechanisms for enhancement of neural function? Discuss the enhancement of auditory function due to deprivation of other sensory input.
8. Discuss the enhancement of auditory function through enriched sensory input. What are the effects of bilingualism, music training, and extensive practice with speech sound analyses on auditory function?
9. How can medical therapies enhance neural function following injury? Discuss constraint-induced therapy and transcranial magnetic stimulation with reference to enhancement of neural function following injury.
10. Discuss future trends in the prevention of reduction of neural function during development and augmentation of sensory capabilities following development.

References

[1] Akshoomoff, N. A., Feroleto, C. C., Doyle, R. E., & Stiles, J. (2002). The impact of early unilateral brain injury on perceptual organization and visual memory. Neuropsychologia, 40(5), 539–561.

[2] Berg, K. M., & Boswell, A. E. (2000). Noise increment detection in children 1 to 3 years of age. Perception & Psychophysics, 62(4), 868–873.

[3] Bergeson, T. R., Pisoni, D. B., & Davis, R. A. O. (2005). Development of audiovisual comprehension skills in prelingually deaf children with cochlear implants. Ear and Hearing, 26(2), 149–164.

[4] Bialystok, E. (2001). Bilingualism in development: Language, literacy, and cognition. New York, NY: Cambridge University Press.

[5] Bialystok, E., Craik, F. I. M., & Freedman, M. (2007). Bilingualism as a protection against the onset of symptoms of dementia. Neuropsychologia, 45(2), 459–464.

[6] Bialystok, E., Craik, F. I. M., Klein, R., & Viswanathan, M. (2004). Bilingualism, aging, and cognitive control: Evidence from the Simon task. Psychology and Aging, 19(2), 290–303.

[7] Bialystok, E., Craik, F. I. M., & Ryan, J. (2006). Executive control in a modified antisaccade task: Effects of aging and bilingualism. Journal of Experimental Psychology: Learning, Memory, and Cognition, 32(6), 1341–1354.

[8] Boatman, D. F., Lesser, R. P., Crone, N. E., Krauss, G., Lenz, F. A., & Miglioretti, D. L. (2006). Speech recognition impairments in patients with intractable right temporal lobe epilepsy. Epilepsia, 47(8), 1397–1401.

[9] Borges, L. R., Paschoal, J. R., & Colella-Santos, M. F. (2013). (Central) auditory processing: The impact of otitis media. Clinics (Sao Paulo), 68(7), 954–959.

[10] Bowen, S. E., & Hannigan, J. H. (2006). Developmental toxicity of prenatal exposure to toluene. The AAPS Journal, 8(2), E419–E424.

[11] Brody, H. (1976). An examination of cerebral cortex and brain stem aging. In R. D. Terry & S. Gershon (Eds.), Neurobiology of aging. New York, NY: Raven Press.

[12] Buckley, K. A., & Tobey, E. A. (2011). Cross-modal plasticity and speech perception in pre- and postlingually deaf cochlear implant users. Ear and Hearing, 32(1), 2–15.

[13] Buss, R. R., Sun, W., & Oppenheim, R. W. (2006). Adaptive roles of programmed cell death during nervous system development. Annual Review of Neuroscience, 29, 1–35.

[14] Changeux, J. P., & Danchin, A. (1976). Selective stabilisation of developing synapses as a mechanism for the specification of neuronal networks. Nature, 264(5588), 705–712.

[15] Cohen, L. G., Weeks, R. A., Sadato, N., Celnik, P., Ishii, K., & Hallett, M. (1999). Period of susceptibility for cross-modal plasticity in the blind. Annals of Neurology, 45(4), 451–460.

[16] Craik, F. I. M., Bialystok, E., & Freedman, M. (2010). Delaying the onset of Alzheimer disease: bilingualism as a form of cognitive reserve. Neurology, 75(19), 1726–1729.

[17] Dawes, P., & Bishop, D. V. M. (2008). Maturation of visual and auditory temporal processing in school-aged children. Journal of Speech, Language, and Hearing Research, 51(4), 1002–1015.

[18] Dehay, C., Bullier, J., & Kennedy, H. (1984). Transient projections from the fronto-parietal and temporal cortex to areas 17, 18 and 19 in the kitten. Experimental Brain Research, 57(1), 208–212.

[19] De Ridder, D., Vanneste, S., Engineer, N. D., & Kilgard, M. P. (2014). Safety and efficacy of vagus nerve stimulation paired with tones for the treatment of tinnitus: A case series. Neuromodulation, 17, 170-179.

[20] Deutsch, D., Henthorn, T., Marvin, E., & Xu, H. (2006). Absolute pitch among American and Chinese conservatory students: Prevalence differences, and evidence for a speech-related critical period. The Journal of the Acoustical Society of America, 119(2), 719–722.

[21] Dwyer, J. B., Broide, R. S., & Leslie, F. M. (2008). Nicotine and brain development. Birth Defects Research. Part C, Embryo Today, 84(1), 30–44.

[22] Eckert, M. A., Cute, S. L., Vaden, K. I., Jr, Kuchinsky, S. E., & Dubno, J. R. (2012). Auditory cortex signs of age-related hearing loss. Journal of the Association for Research in Otolaryngology, 13(5), 703–713.

[23] Eisenberg, L. S. (1982). Use of the cochlear implant by the prelingually deaf. The Annals of Otology, Rhinology & Laryngology. Supplement, 91(2 Pt 3), 62–66.

[24] Eggermont, J. J., & Ponton, C. W. (2003). Auditory-evoked potential studies of cortical maturation in normal hearing and implanted children: Correlations with changes in structure and speech perception. Acta Oto-Laryngologica, 123(2), 249–252.

[25] Elbert, T., Sterr, A., Rockstroh, B., Pantev, C., Müller, M. M., & Taub, E. (2002). Expansion of the tonotopic area in the auditory cortex of the blind. The Journal of Neuroscience, 22(22), 9941–9944.

[26] Fekete, D. M., & Campero, A. M. (2007). Axon guidance in the inner ear. The International Journal of Developmental Biology, 51(6-7), 549–556.

[27] Felder, E., & Schrott-Fischer, A. (1995). Quantitative evaluation of myelinated nerve fibres and hair cells in cochleae of humans with age-related high-tone hearing loss. Hearing Research, 91(1-2), 19–32.

[28] Felix, H., Johnsson, L. G., Gleeson, M., & Pollak, A. (1990). Quantitative analysis of cochlear sensory cells and neuronal elements in man. Acta Oto-Laryngologica. Supplementum, 470, 71–79.

[29] Fink, G. R., Halligan, P. W., Marshall, J. C., Frith, C. D., Frackowiak, R. S., & Dolan, R. J. (1996). Where in the brain does visual attention select the forest and the trees? Nature, 382(6592), 626–628.

[30] Finney, E. M., Clementz, B. A., Hickok, G., & Dobkins, K. R. (2003). Visual stimuli activate auditory cortex in deaf subjects: Evidence from MEG. NeuroReport, 11, 1425-1427.

[31] Finney, E. M., Fine, I., & Dobkins, K. R. (2001). Visual stimuli activate auditory cortex in the deaf. Nature Neuroscience, 4(12), 1171-1173.

[32] Friederici, A. D., & Alter, K. (2004). Lateralization of auditory language functions: A dynamic dual pathway model. Brain and Language, 89(2), 267-276.

[33] Frost, D. O. (1984). Axonal growth and target selection during development: Retinal projections to the ventrobasal complex and other "nonvisual" structures in neonatal Syrian hamsters. Journal of Comparative Neurology, 230(4), 576-592.

[34] Gelfand, S. A. (1995). Long-term recovery and no recovery from the auditory deprivation effect with binaural amplification: Six cases. Journal of the American Academy of Audiology, 6(2), 141-149.

[35] Gilley, P. M., Sharma, A., & Dorman, M. F. (2008). Cortical reorganization in children with cochlear implants. Brain Research, 1239, 56-65.

[36] Gilley, P. M., Sharma, A., Mitchell, T. V., & Dorman, M. F. (2010). The influence of a sensitive period for auditory-visual integration in children with cochlear implants. Restorative Neurology and Neuroscience, 28(2), 207-218.

[37] Golestani, N., Price, C. J., & Scott, S. K. (2011). Born with an ear for dialects? Structural plasticity in the expert phonetician brain. Journal of Neuroscience, 31(11), 4213-4220.

[38] Gordon-Salant, S., & Friedman, S. A. (2011). Recognition of rapid speech by blind and sighted older adults. Journal of Speech, Language, and Hearing Research, 54(2), 622-631.

[39] Gravel, J. S., Roberts, J. E., Roush, J. et al. (2006). Early otitis media with effusion, hearing loss, and auditory processes at school age. Ear and Hearing, 27(4), 353-368.

[40] Green, D. W. (1998). Mental control of the bilingual lexico-semantic system. Bilingualism: Language and Cognition, 1, 67-81.

[41] Hannon, E. E., & Trehub, S. E. (2005). Tuning in to musical rhythms: Infants learn more readily than adults. Proceedings of the National Academy of Sciences of the United States of America, 102(35), 12639-12643.

[42] Hansen, C. C., & Reske-Nielsen, E. (1965). Pathological studies in presbycusis: Cochlear and central findings in 12 aged patients. Archives of Otolaryngology, 82, 115-132.

[43] Harris-Love, M. (2012). Transcranial magnetic stimulation for the prediction and enhancement of rehabilitation treatment effects. Journal of Neurologic Physical Therapy, 36(2), 87-93.

[44] Hartley, D. E., Wright, B. A., Hogan, S. C., & Moore, D. R. (2000). Age-related improvements in auditory backward and simultaneous masking in 6- to 10-year-old children. Journal of Speech, Language, and Hearing Research, 43(6), 1402-1415.

[45] Hilchey, M. D., & Klein, R. M. (2011). Are there bilingual advantages on nonlinguistic interference tasks? Implications for the plasticity of executive control processes. Psychonomic Bulletin and Review, 18(4), 625-658.

[46] Hogan, S. C. M., & Moore, D. R. (2003). Impaired binaural hearing in children produced by a threshold level of middle ear disease. Journal of the Association for Research in Otolaryngology, 4(2), 123-129.

[47] Hurley, R. M. (1999). Onset of auditory deprivation. Journal of the American Academy of Audiology, 10(10), 529-534.

[48] Huttenlocher, P. R. (1990). Morphometric study of human cerebral cortex development. Neuropsychologia, 28(6), 517-527.

[49] Huttenlocher, P. R. (2000). Synaptogenesis in human cerebral cortex and the concept of critical periods. In N. A. Fox, L. A. Leavitt, & J. G. Warhol (Eds.), The role of early experience in infant development. St. Louis, MO: Johnson & Johnson Pediatric Institute.

[50] Huttenlocher, P. R., & Dabholkar, A. S. (1997). Regional differences in synaptogenesis in human cerebral cortex. Journal of Comparative Neurology, 387(2), 167-178.

[51] Huttenlocher, P. R., de Courten, C., Garey, L. J., & Van der Loos, H. (1982). Synaptogenesis in human visual cortex—evidence for synapse elimination during normal development. Neuroscience Letters, 33(3), 247-252.

[52] Innocenti, G. M., Clarke, S. (1984). Bilateral transitory projection to visual areas from auditory cortex in kittens. Brain Research, 316(1), 143-148.

[53] Jacobson, S. W., Jacobson, J. L., Sokol, R. J., Martier, S. S., Chiodo, L. M. (1996). New evidence for neurobehavioral effects of in utero cocaine exposure. Journal of Pediatrics, 129(4), 581-590.

[54] Janowsky, J. S. (1993). The development and neural basis of memory systems. In M. Johnson (Ed.), Brain development and cognition: A reader. Cambridge, MA: Blackwell.

[55] Jeffery, K. J. (1995). Paradoxical enhancement of long-term potentiation in poor-learning rats at low test stimulus intensities. Experimental Brain Research, 104(1), 55-69.

[56] Kancherla, V., Oakley, G. P., Jr., Brent, & R. L. (2014). Urgent global opportunities to prevent birth defects. Seminars in Fetal and Neonatal Medicine, 19, 153-160.

[57] Kirikae, I., Sato, T., & Shitara, T. (1964). A study of hearing in advanced age. Laryngoscope, 74, 205-220.

[58] Kluk, K., & Moore, B. C. J. (2006). Dead regions in the cochlea and enhancement of frequency discrimination: Effects of audiogram slope, unilateral versus bilateral loss, and hearing-aid use. Hearing Research, 222(1–2), 1-15.

[59] Kolarik, A. J., Cirstea, S., & Pardhan, S. (2013). Evidence for enhanced discrimination of virtual auditory distance among blind listeners using level and direct-to-reverberant cues. Experimental Brain Research, 224(4), 623-633.

[60] Konigsmark, B. W., & Murphy, E. A. (1972). Volume of the ventral cochlear nucleus in man: Its relationship to neuronal population and age. Journal of Neuropathology and Experimental Neurology, 32(2), 304-316.

[61] Kral, A. (2007). Unimodal and cross-modal plasticity in the "deaf" auditory cortex. International Journal of Audiology, 46(9), 479-493.

[62] Kral, A., & Eggermont, J. J. (2007). What's to lose and what's to learn: Development under auditory deprivation, cochlear implants and limits of cortical plasticity. Brain Research Reviews, 56(1), 259-269.

[63] Krizman, J., Marian, V., Shook, A., Skoe, E., & Kraus, N. (2012). Subcortical encoding of sound is enhanced in bilinguals and relates to executive function advantages. Proceedings of the National Academy of Sciences of the United States of America, 109(20), 7877-7881.

[64] Kuhl, P. K., Stevens, E., Hayashi, A., Deguchi, T., Kiritani, S., & Iverson, P. (2006). Infants show a facilitation effect for native language phonetic perception between 6 and 12 months. Developmental Science, 9(2), F13-F21.

[65] Kuhl, P. K., Tsao, F. M., & Liu, H. M. (2003). Foreign-language experience in infancy: Effects of short-term exposure and social interaction on phonetic learning. Proceedings of the National Academy of Sciences of the United States of America, 100(15), 9096-9101.

[66] Kuo, L. J., & Anderson, R. C. (2012). Effects of early bilingualism on learning phonological regularities in a new language. Journal of Experimental Child Psychology, 111(3), 455-467.

[67] Lazarov, O., & Marr, R. A. (2013). Of mice and men: Neurogenesis, cognition and Alzheimer's disease. Frontiers in Aging Neuroscience, 5, 43.

[68] Lee, D. S., Lee, J. S., Oh, S. H., et al. (2001). Cross-modal plasticity and cochlear implants. Nature, 409(6817), 149–150.

[69] Lee, J. S., Lee, D. S., Oh, S. H., et al. (2003). PET evidence of neuroplasticity in adult auditory cortex of postlingual deafness. Journal of Nuclear Medicine, 44(9), 1435–1439.

[70] Lester, B. M., Lagasse, L., Seifer, R., et al. (2003). The Maternal Lifestyle Study (MLS): Effects of prenatal cocaine and/or opiate exposure on auditory brain response at one month. Journal of Pediatrics, 142(3), 279–285.

[71] Levänen, S., & Hamdorf, D. (2001). Feeling vibrations: Enhanced tactile sensitivity in congenitally deaf humans. Neuroscience Letters, 301(1), 75–77.

[72] Lewald, J. (2013). Exceptional ability of blind humans to hear sound motion: Implications for the emergence of auditory space. Neuropsychologia, 51(1), 181–186.

[73] Lewis, T. L., & Maurer, D. (2005). Multiple sensitive periods in human visual development: Evidence from visually deprived children. Developmental Psychobiology, 46(3), 163–183.

[74] Liikkanen, L. A., Tiitinen, H., Alku, P., Leino, S., Yrttiaho, S., & May, P. J. C. (2007). The right-hemispheric auditory cortex in humans is sensitive to degraded speech sounds. NeuroReport, 18(6), 601–605.

[75] Lövdén, M., Bodammer, N. C., Kühn, S., et al. (2010). Experience-dependent plasticity of white-matter microstructure extends into old age. Neuropsychologia, 48(13), 3878–3883.

[76] Martinez, A., Moses, P., Frank, L., Buxton, R., Wong, E., & Stiles, J. (1997). Hemispheric asymmetries in global and local processing: Evidence from fMRI. NeuroReport, 8(7), 1685–1689.

[77] McFeely, W. J., Jr., Antonelli, P. J., Rodriguez, F. J., & Holmes, A. E. (1998). Somatosensory phenomena after multichannel cochlear implantation in prelingually deaf adults. American Journal of Otolaryngology, 19(4), 467–471.

[78] Mechelli, A., Crinion, J. T., Noppeney, U., et al. (2004). Neurolinguistics: Structural plasticity in the bilingual brain. Nature, 431(7010), 757.

[79] Meyer, M., Alter, K., Friederici, A. D., Lohmann, G., & von Cramon, D. Y. (2002). fFMRI reveals brain regions mediating

slow prosodic modulations in spoken sentences. Human Brain Mapping, 17(2), 73–88.

[80] Moore, D. R., Cowan, J. A., Riley, A., Edmondson-Jones, A. M., & Ferguson, M. A. (2011). Development of auditory processing in 6- to 11-yr-old children. Ear and Hearing, 32(3), 269–285.

[81] Moore, J. K., & Linthicum, F. H., Jr. (2007). The human auditory system: A timeline of development. International Journal of Audiology, 46(9), 460–478.

[82] Moore, B. C. J., & Vinay, S. N. (2009). Enhanced discrimination of low-frequency sounds for subjects with high-frequency dead regions. Brain, 132(Pt 2), 524–536.

[83] Munro, K. J., & Blount, J. (2009). Adaptive plasticity in brainstem of adult listeners following earplug-induced deprivation. Journal of the Acoustical Society of America, 126(2), 568–571.

[84] Munro, K. J., & Merrett, J. F. (2013). Brainstem plasticity and modified loudness following short-term use of hearing aids. Journal of the Acoustical Society of America, 133 (1), 343–349.

[85] Neville, H. J., & Lawson, D. (1987). Attention to central and peripheral visual space in a movement detection task. 3III. Separate effects of auditory deprivation and acquisition of a visual language. Brain Research, 405(2), 284–294.

[86] Neville, H. J., Schmidt, A., & Kutas, M. (1983). Altered visual-evoked potentials in congenitally deaf adults. Brain Research, 266(1), 127–132.

[87] Nixon, P., Lazarova, J., Hodinott-Hill, I., Gough, P., & Passingham, R. (2004). The inferior frontal gyrus and phonological processing: An investigation using rTMS. Journal of Cognitive Neuroscience, 16(2), 289–300.

[88] Norman, J. F., & Bartholomew, A. N. (2011). Blindness enhances tactile acuity and haptic 3-D shape discrimination. Attention, Perception, and Psychophysics, 73(7), 2323–2331.

[89] Oh, S. H., Kim, C. S., Kang, E. J., et al. (2003). Speech perception after cochlear implantation over a 4-year time period. Acta Otolaryngologica, 123(2), 148–153.

[90] Ornoy, A. (2006). Neuroteratogens in man: An overview with special emphasis on the teratogenicity of antiepileptic drugs in pregnancy. Reproductive Toxicology, 22(2), 214–226.

[91] Pearson, M. A., Hoyme, H. E., Seaver, L. H., & Rimsza, M. E. (1994). Toluene embryopathy: Delineation of the phenotype and comparison with fetal alcohol syndrome. Pediatrics, 93 (2), 211–215.

[92] Perani, D., Saccuman, M. C., Scifo, P., et al. (2011). Neural language networks at birth. Proceedings of the National Academy of Sciences of the United States of America, 108(38), 16056–16061.

[93] Reynolds, E. H. (2014). The neurology of folic acid deficiency. Handbook of Clinical Neurology, 120, 927–943.

[94] Riley, E. P., Infante, M. A., & Warren, K. R. (2011). Fetal alcohol spectrum disorders: An overview. Neuropsychology Review, 21(2), 73–80.

[95] Sadato, N., Okada, T., Honda, M., & Yonekura, Y. (2002). Critical period for cross-modal plasticity in blind humans: A functional MRI study. Neuroimage, 16(2), 389–400.

[96] Sadato, N., Okada, T., Honda, M., et al. (2005). Cross-modal integration and plastic changes revealed by lip movement, random-dot motion and sign languages in the hearing and deaf. Cerebral Cortex, 15(8), 1113–1122.

[97] Safi, J., Joyeux, L., & Chalouhi, G. E. (2012). Periconceptional folate deficiency and implications in neural tube defects. Journal of Pregnancy, Article ID 295083, 1-9.

[98] Schafer, E. C., Beeler, S., Ramos, H., Morais, M., Monzingo, J., & Algier, K. (2012). Developmental effects and spatial hearing in young children with normal-hearing sensitivity. Ear and Hearing, 33(6), e32–e43.

[99] Scheibel, M. E., & Scheibel, A. B. (1975). Structural changes in the aging brain. In H. Brody, D. Harman, & J. M. Ordy (Eds.), Aging, Vol. 1. New York: Raven Press.

[100] Schmithorst, V. J., Holland, S. K., & Plante, E. (2011). Diffusion tensor imaging reveals white matter microstructure correlations with auditory processing ability. Ear and Hearing, 32(2), 156–167.

[101] Schorr, E. A., Fox, N. A., van Wassenhove, V., & Knudsen, E. I. (2005). Auditory-visual fusion in speech perception in children with cochlear implants. Proceedings of the National Academy of Sciences of the United States of America, 102 (51), 18748–18750.

[102] Schwaber, M. K., Garraghty, P. E., & Kaas, J. H. (1993). Neuroplasticity of the adult primate auditory cortex following cochlear hearing loss. American Journal of Otolaryngology, 14(3), 252–258.

[103] Sharma, A., & Dorman, M. F. (2006). Central auditory development in children with cochlear implants: Clinical implications. Advances in Otorhinolaryngology, 64, 66–88.

[104] Sharma, A., Dorman, M. F., & Kral, A. (2005). The influence of a sensitive period on central auditory development in children with unilateral and bilateral cochlear implants. Hearing Research, 203(1-2), 134–143.

[105] Sharma, A., Dorman, M. F., & Spahr, A. J. (2002a). Rapid development of cortical auditory evoked potentials after early cochlear implantation. NeuroReport, 13(10), 1365–1368.

[106] Sharma, A., Dorman, M. F., & Spahr, A. J. (2002b). A sensitive period for the development of the central auditory system in children with cochlear implants: Implications for age of implantation. Ear and Hearing, 23(6), 532–539.

[107] Sharma, A., Dorman, M., Spahr, A., & Todd, N. W. (2002). Early cochlear implantation in children allows normal development of central auditory pathways. Annals of Otology, Rhinology, and Laryngology Supplment, 189, 38–41.

[108] Sharma, A., Gilley, P. M., Dorman, M. F., & Baldwin, R. (2007). Deprivation-induced cortical reorganization in children with cochlear implants. International Journal of Audiology, 46(9), 494–499.

[109] Shtyrov, Y., Kujala, T., Ahveninen, J., et al. (1998). Background acoustic noise and the hemispheric lateralization of speech processing in the human brain: Magnetic mismatch negativity study. Neuroscience Letters, 251(2), 141–144.

[110] Silman, S., Gelfand, S. A., & Silverman, C. A. (1984). Late-onset auditory deprivation: Effects of monaural versus binaural hearing aids. Journal of the Acoustical Society of America, 76(5), 1357–1367.

[111] Silman, S., Silverman, C. A., Emmer, M. B., & Gelfand, S. A. (1992). Adult-onset auditory deprivation. Journal of the American Academy of Audiology, 3(6), 390–396.

[112] Taub, E. (2012). The behavior-analytic origins of constraint-induced movement therapy: An example of behavioral neurorehabilitation. Behavior Analyst, 35(2), 155–178.

[113] Thompson, N. C., Cranford, J. L., & Hoyer, E. (1999). Brief-tone frequency discrimination by children. Journal of Speech, Language, and Hearing Research, 42(5), 1061–1068.

[114] Thomson, E. E., Carra, R., & Nicolelis, M. A. (2013). Perceiving invisible light through a somatosensory cortical prosthesis. Nature Communications, 4, 1482–1495.

[115] Tomoda, A., Sheu, Y. S., Rabi, K., et al. (2011). Exposure to parental verbal abuse is associated with increased gray matter volume in superior temporal gyrus. Neuroimage, 54(Suppl 1), S280–S286.

[116] Tsao, F. M., Liu, H. M., & Kuhl, P. K. (2006). Perception of native and non-native affricate-fricative contrasts:

Cross-language tests on adults and infants. Journal of the Acoustical Society of America, 120(4), 2285–2294.

[117] Voeller, K. K. (1986). Right-hemisphere deficit syndrome in children. American Journal of Psychiatry, 143(8), 1004–1009.

[118] Voss, P., Lassonde, M., Gougoux, F., Fortin, M., Guillemot, J.-P., & Lepore, F. (2004). Early- and late-onset blind individuals show supra-normal auditory abilities in far-space. Current Biology, 14(19), 1734–1738.

[119] Voss, P., & Zatorre, R. J. (2012). Occipital cortical thickness predicts performance on pitch and musical tasks in blind individuals. Cerebral Cortex, 22(11), 2455–2465.

[120] Weintraub, S., & Mesulam, M. M. (1983). Developmental learning disabilities of the right hemisphere: Emotional, interpersonal, and cognitive components. Archives of Neurology, 40(8), 463–468.

[121] Whitton, J. P., & Polley, D. B. (2011). Evaluating the perceptual and pathophysiological consequences of auditory deprivation in early postnatal life: A comparison of basic and clinical studies. Journal of the Association for Research in Otolaryngology, 12(5), 535–547.

[122] Wolf, S. L., Winstein, C. J., Miller, J. P., et al; EXCITE Investigators. (2006). Effect of constraint-induced movement therapy on upper extremity function 3 to 9 months after stroke: The EXCITE randomized clinical trial. Journal of the American Medical Association, 296(17), 2095–2104.

[123] Wyszynski, D. F., Nambisan, M., Surve, T., Alsdorf, R. M., Smith, C. R., & Holmes, L. B. Antiepileptic Drug Pregnancy Registry. (2005). Increased rate of major malformations in offspring exposed to valproate during pregnancy. Neurology, 64(6), 961–965.

Chapter 3

Assessing and Documenting Peripheral Auditory Status

3 Assessing and Documenting Peripheral Auditory Status

Before initiating auditory processing tests, it is important to assess and document the peripheral auditory status of each individual. This chapter provides an overview of key components of a peripheral audiological evaluation in the context of diagnosing auditory processing deficits. Several variables (e.g., test environment) that can influence test results are also discussed, as the same variables can influence the outcomes of auditory processing tests. Audiologists usually administer a complete peripheral auditory test battery consisting of the following tests:
- Air conduction thresholds
- Bone conduction thresholds
- Speech recognition thresholds
- Speech recognition scores in quiet
- Tympanometry to assess middle ear function
- Acoustic reflex thresholds
- Otoacoustic emissions (OAEs)

3.1 Auditory Thresholds

Most of the information related to determination of tonal thresholds in this chapter is adopted from Rawool (2012a). It is included here to provide a complete picture of audiological assessments. The key component of documenting auditory sensitivity is determination of auditory thresholds for a series of tones at various frequencies. The threshold is the softest hearing level (HL) that the examinee responds to on at least 50% of the test trials presented at decreasing HLs. The accuracy of air conduction thresholds is critical because these thresholds are used for a variety of purposes:
- To determine if the listener has normal sensitivity or hearing loss
- To determine the type and severity of any hearing loss and the possible cause of hearing loss. In some retrocochlear pathologies, such as acoustic tumors, the initial presenting symptom is hearing loss (Hart, Gardner, & Howieson, 1983).
- To determine the presentation level to be used in each ear for various auditory processing tests
- To consider hearing loss during the interpretation of test results. Peripheral hearing loss can affect the results of central auditory processing

tests (Miltenberger, Dawson, & Raica, 1978). Corrections may be necessary when interpreting the results of some tests in the presence of even a mild hearing loss (Neijenhuis, Tschur, & Snik, 2004).

3.1.1 Audiograms

Auditory thresholds can be either plotted in a graphic format or recorded in a table.

Graphic Representation

The thresholds obtained during audiological monitoring can be recorded on a graph called an audiogram (▶ Fig. 3.1). The horizontal axis represents the frequency (Hz) of sounds, and the vertical axis represents the stimulus level, referred to as the decibel hearing level (dB HL). As an example, in ▶ Fig. 3.1, the softest sounds that the patient responded to on at least 50% of the test trials at the frequency of 500 Hz was 45 dB HL; the softest sound he responded to at the frequency of 4000 Hz was 50 dB HL.

When the graphic form is employed, thresholds for the right ear are plotted on the audiogram using a circle, and those for the left ear are plotted using a cross, as shown in ▶ Fig. 3.1. If there is no response at the maximum output of the

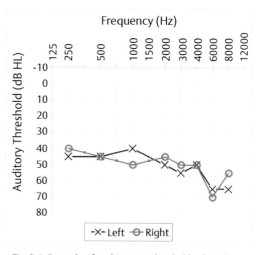

Fig. 3.1 Example of audiometric thresholds plotted on an audiogram (adapted from Rawool, 2012a).

audiometer, an arrow is attached to the lower outside corner of the symbol and drawn downward and at approximately 45 degrees outward from the vertical ruling—to the right for left-ear symbols and to the left for right-ear symbols. Other symbols used during audiometry (American Speech-Language-Hearing Association [ASHA], 1990) are shown in ► Fig. 3.2.

		Right	Left	Unspecified
Air conduction	Unmasked			
	Unmasked, no response at the intesity limit of the audiometer			
	Masked			
	Masked, no response at the intensity limit of the audiometer			
Bone conduction	Mastoid placement, unmasked			
	Mastoid placement, unmasked, no response at the intesity limit of the audiometer			
	Mastoid placement, masked			
	Mastoid placement, masked, no response at the intesity limit of the audiometer			
	Forehead placement, unmasked			
	Forehead placement, unmasked no response at the intesity limit of the audiometer			
	Forehead placement, masked			
	Forehead placement, masked, no response at the intensity limit of the audiometer			
Sound field				S

Fig. 3.2 Audiogram symbols recommended by the American Speech-Language-Hearing Association (1990).

Tabular Representation

The thresholds obtained from audiological testing can also be recorded in a tabular format. ▶ Table 3.1 shows the audiometric test results represented in ▶ Fig. 3.1. Representation of thresholds in a tabular format allows easier comparison of audiograms obtained from one patient over several years.

3.1.2 Hearing Level versus Sound Pressure Level

Plotting audiograms in hearing levels versus sound pressure levels (SPLs) allows easier interpretation of normal versus impaired hearing (▶ Fig. 3.3). In panel A of ▶ Fig. 3.3 (HL), it is easier to see how much of a hearing loss above the normal range is occurring at each frequency and that the hearing loss is worst at 4000 Hz compared to other frequencies, suggesting a notch that is typically apparent in individuals who are exposed to hazardous noise. In most cases audiograms are plotted using hearing levels. During hearing aid fittings, audiograms are sometimes plotted using sound pressure levels, as shown in panel B of ▶ Fig. 3.3. Note that when plotted in dB HL (▶ Fig. 3.3 a), the Y-axis values are reversed so that −10 appears on top of the axis.

Table 3.1 Audiometric Thresholds Represented in Fig. 3.1

Ear	Frequency (Hz)							
	250	500	1000	2000	3000	4000	6000	8000
Left	45	45	40	50	55	50	65	65
Right	40	45	50	45	50	50	70	55

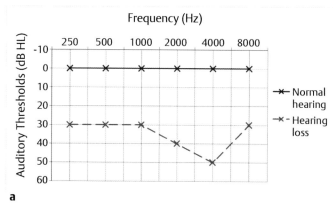

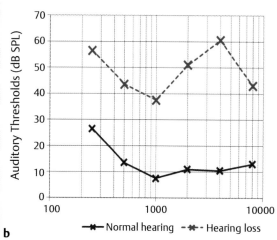

a

b

Fig. 3.3 Plotting of audiometric thresholds in hearing level (HL, part a) and sound pressure level (SPL, part b) (adapted from Rawool, 2012a).

3.1.3 Air Conduction versus Bone Conduction Thresholds

Air conduction testing is conducted by using supra-aural earphones (▶ Fig. 3.4) or insert earphones (▶ Fig. 3.5). During air conduction testing, sounds travel through the outer, middle, and inner ear (▶ Fig. 3.6). Thus, abnormalities in any of the three parts can yield elevated auditory thresholds.

Supra-aural earphones are often used during testing. However, these types of earphones can collapse the ear canals of some individuals, including infants, young children, and older adults, causing an artificial elevation of auditory thresholds. Use of insert earphones can prevent ear canal collapse, thereby revealing true auditory sensitivity through air conduction.

For regular use of insert earphones, it is important to identify ear canals that prevent achievement of an adequate fit with insert earphones. The insert earphones need to be fitted deeply in the canals. The occlusion effect at 250 and 500 Hz is significantly lower with deep insertion compared to shallow insertion (Dean & Martin, 2000). Besides preventing ear canal collapse, insert earphones provide greater interaural attenuation, better attenuation of background noise entering the ear canal, and better infection control. However, in the presence of excessive wax, the wax can block the tubing and cause artificial elevation of thresholds.

Bone conduction testing is conducted by placing a bone vibrator (▶ Fig. 3.7) on the front of the forehead (▶ Fig. 3.8) or on the mastoid (▶ Fig. 3.9) (behind the ears). During bone conduction testing, an attempt is made to bypass the outer and middle ear, allowing direct stimulation of the inner ear (▶ Fig. 3.10). Thus, bone conduction testing allows evaluation of the integrity of the inner ear in the presence of outer and middle ear pathologies. Because we hear most external sounds through air conduction, air conduction thresholds reflect the disability that can result from elevation of auditory thresholds. An individual who has abnormal air conduction thresholds will have difficulty hearing external sounds even if he or she has normal bone conduction thresholds.

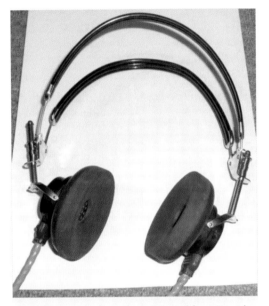

Fig. 3.4 Supra-aural earphones (adapted from Rawool, 2012a).

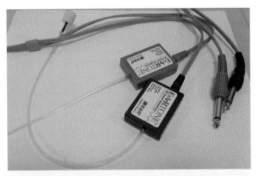

Fig. 3.5 Insert earphones (adapted from Rawool, 2012a).

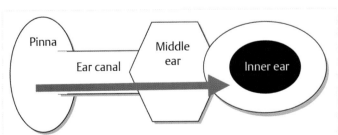

Fig. 3.6 Path of sound during air conduction testing (adapted from Rawool, 2012a).

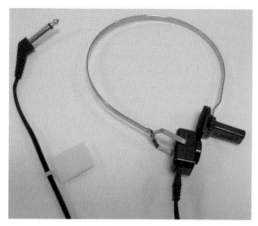

Fig. 3.7 Bone conduction vibrator (adapted from Rawool, 2012a).

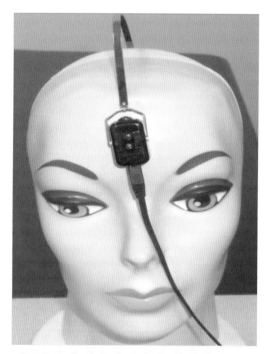

Fig. 3.8 Forehead placement for bone conduction testing (adapted from Rawool, 2012a).

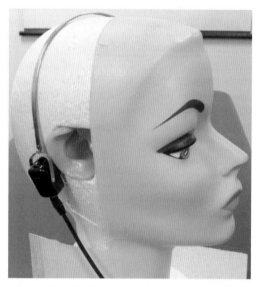

Fig. 3.9 Mastoid placement for bone conduction testing (adapted from Rawool, 2012a).

3.2 Audiogram Classifications

Audiograms can be classified using a variety of factors, including the severity of the hearing loss, the location of the underlying pathology responsible for the hearing loss (the type of hearing loss), the audiometric configuration, the modality of the hearing loss (unilateral vs. bilateral), and the symmetry of the hearing loss (▸ Fig. 3.11).

3.2.1 Severity of Hearing Loss

Different criteria have been used to describe the severity of hearing loss. Most frequently, average thresholds at 0.5, 1.0, and 2.0 kHz are used to determine the severity of hearing loss. The criteria that are generally used in describing the severity of hearing loss in adults are presented in ▸ Table 3.2. In some cases when a worker is seeking compensation for hearing loss, the severity is expressed in terms of percentage of hearing loss. For information on calculating the percentage of hearing loss, refer to Rawool (2012b).

3.2.2 Type of Hearing Loss

Based on the approximate location of dysfunction in the ear, hearing loss can be classified as conductive, sensorineural, or mixed.

Conductive Hearing Loss

In conductive hearing loss, when stimuli are delivered directly to the inner ear through the bone conduction vibrator, thresholds are within normal limits, suggesting normal inner ear function. However, when stimuli are delivered through headphones or the air-conduction path, the thresholds are elevated or are outside the normal limits, suggesting abnormality within the conductive pathway or the outer and middle ear. There are

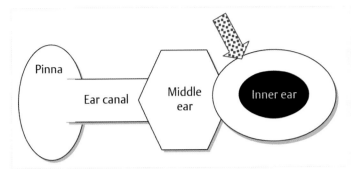

Fig. 3.10 Major path of sound during bone conduction testing (adapted from Rawool, 2012a).

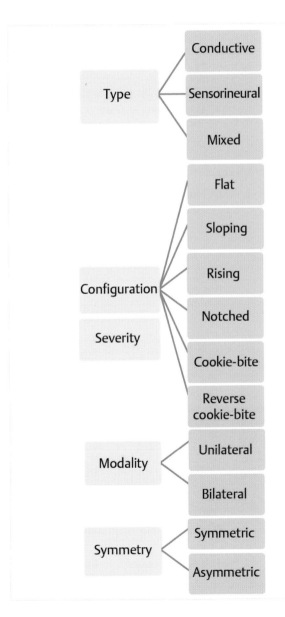

Fig. 3.11 Audiogram classification (adapted from Rawool, 2012a).

several causes of conductive hearing loss, including excessive cerumen in the outer ear canal, fluid in the middle ear, fixation of one of the bones in the middle ear (otosclerosis), disarticulation of the ossicular chain, and cholesteatoma. ► Fig. 3.12 shows the audiogram of a child with permanent conductive hearing loss in the left ear due to invasive cholesteatoma leading to destruction of the ossicular chain.

Table 3.2 Severity of Hearing Loss Based on Audiometric Thresholds

Description of Severity of Hearing Loss	Average of Thresholds at 0.5, 1.0, and 2 kHz (dB HL)
Mild	26 to 40
Moderate	41 to 55
Moderately severe	56 to 70
Severe	71 to 90
Profound	>90

Abbreviation: HL, hearing loss. Adapted from Rawool, 2012a.

Sensorineural Hearing Loss

In sensorineural hearing loss, both air and bone conduction thresholds are outside the normal limits and are similar, suggesting that the abnormality is in the inner ear or beyond. Sensorineural hearing loss can be further classified as sensory or neural. If the damage can be diagnosed as being located within the inner ear, the hearing loss is considered sensory. Hearing loss induced by noise or ototoxins usually tends to be at least initially sensory in nature. Other causes of sensory hearing loss are Ménière disease, viral infections, genetic hearing loss, and autoimmune conditions. If the hearing loss is due to abnormality beyond the inner ear, the hearing loss is considered neural. As an example, hearing loss caused by an auditory nerve tumor can be considered neural. Further classifications of sensorineural hearing loss are possible, as discussed in Chapter 15. ► Fig. 3.13 shows an audiogram of an 85-year-old man with sensorineural hearing loss.

Mixed Hearing Loss

In mixed hearing loss, both air and bone conduction thresholds are outside the normal limits, but bone conduction thresholds are better than air conduction thresholds. Stated differently, when an attempt is made to present stimuli directly to the inner ear by bypassing the outer and middle ear,

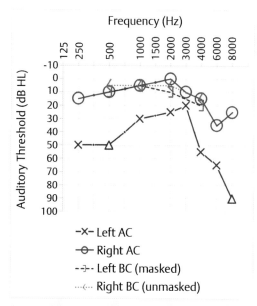

Fig. 3.12 Example of a permanent conductive hearing loss in the left ear. The blue triangles show left ear air conduction thresholds obtained by presenting masking noise to the right ear to minimize the participation of the right ear in left ear results.

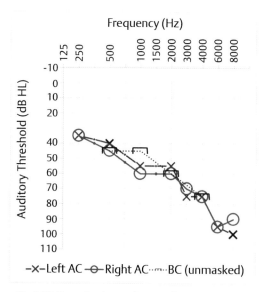

Fig. 3.13 Example of an audiogram showing sensorineural hearing loss in both ears.

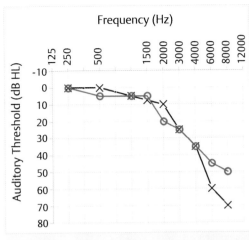

Fig. 3.14 Audiogram of a 52-year-old woman showing a sharply sloping configuration in the right ear from 1500 Hz and a precipitous sloping configuration in the left ear from 2000 Hz (adapted from Rawool, 2012a).

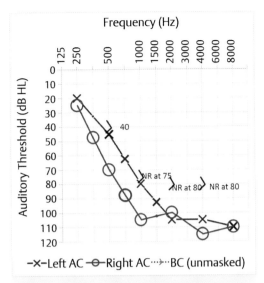

−✕−Left AC −⊖−Right AC ···⊁···BC (unmasked)

Fig. 3.15 Example of an audiogram of an 80-year-old man with precipitously sloping hearing loss between 250 and 1000 Hz. NR, no response at the limits of the audiometer.

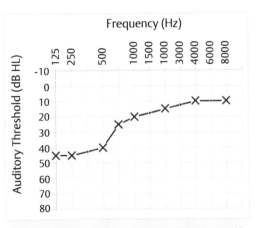

Fig. 3.16 Example of an audiogram from a 27-year-old individual showing a rising configuration based on Humes, Tharpe, and Bratt (1984). In this graph it is assumed that the thresholds are from the left ear.

the person is able to hear better than when stimuli are presented through the outer ear. Mixed hearing loss can result from the presence of pathologies in both the conductive (outer and middle ear) and sensorineural (inner ear) mechanisms.

3.2.3 Audiometric Configurations

Flat

When auditory thresholds are similar across the test frequency range, the audiometric configuration is described as being flat. In ▶ Fig. 3.1, the hearing loss in the right ear is relatively flat up to the frequency of 4000 Hz.

Sloping

When auditory thresholds are better in the lower frequencies and continue to get worse with higher frequencies, the audiogram is referred to as having a sloping configuration. When the thresholds become worse by about 6 to 10 dB with each octave, the hearing loss is described as gradually sloping. When the thresholds become worse by 11 to 15 dB with each octave, the hearing loss is described as sharply sloping. When the thresholds become worse by more than 16 dB with each octave, the hearing loss is described as being precipitously sloping. ▶ Fig. 3.14 shows an audiogram from a 52-year-old woman with sharply sloping hearing loss in the right ear and precipitously sloping hearing loss in the left ear. ▶ Fig. 3.15 shows the

audiogram of an 80-year-old man with a precipitous slope between 250 and 1000 Hz.

Rising

When thresholds are worse at lower frequencies but get better with increasing frequencies, the audiogram is considered to have a rising configuration (▶ Fig. 3.16). The audiogram in ▶ Fig. 3.16 is based on the audiometric thresholds of a 27-year-old participant (Humes, Tharpe, & Bratt, 1984). In ▶ Fig. 3.16, it is assumed that the thresholds are from the left ear. In cases where the slope of the rising portion of the audiogram is more than 25 dB per octave, the severity of the loss may be underestimated for test frequencies close to the rising portion of the audiogram (Humes et al., 1984). In such cases, the upward spread of excitation in the cochlea may allow the listeners to detect the presented lower frequency tones by capitalizing on the better sensitivity at the higher adjacent frequency.

Notched

In notched configuration, the thresholds are worse at 3 or 4 or 6 kHz but better at lower and higher

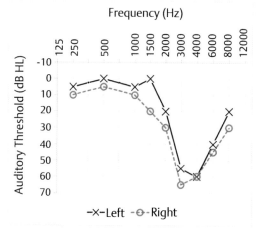

Fig. 3.17 Example of a notched audiogram of a 47-year-old man with a history of noise exposure during military service (adapted from Rawool, 2012a).

frequencies. ▶ Fig. 3.17 shows a notched audiogram of a 47-year-old man with a history of noise exposure during service in the army. The exact definition for identification of the presence of an audiometric notch varies among investigators (▶ Table 3.3). A high-frequency notch with a history of hazardous noise exposure is suggestive of a noise-induced hearing loss (McBride & Williams, 2001). However, in 11% of cases a notch can occur without any history of noise exposure (Nondahl et al., 2009).

Cookie-Bite or Saucer-shaped

When auditory thresholds are worse in the middle frequencies compared to those in the lower and higher frequencies, the pattern is referred to as a cookie-bite configuration. ▶ Fig. 3.18 is the audiogram of a woman with congenital hearing loss showing a cookie-bite configuration.

Reverse Cookie-Bite

In a reverse cookie-bite configuration, the auditory thresholds are normal or near normal in the middle frequencies and worse in the lower and higher frequencies, as represented in left ear air conduction thresholds in ▶ Fig. 3.12.

3.2.4 Modality

Unilateral Hearing Loss

When hearing is normal in one ear in the presence of hearing loss in the other, the loss can be considered unilateral. Medical referrals should be initiated for unilateral hearing loss to determine the cause and appropriate treatment unless the cause

Table 3.3 Criteria Used for Detecting a Notched Audiogram

Study	Criteria
Coles, Lutman, & Buffin (2000)	Thresholds worse by at least 10 dB at 3, 4, or 6 kHz than those at 1 or 2 kHz and 6 or 8 kHz
McBride & Williams (2001)	Narrow or V-shaped notch: Only one frequency in the depth of the notch and the depth is at least 15 dB. Wide or U-shaped notch: More than one frequency in the depth of the notch, depth of 20 dB, and thresholds better by at least 10 dB at the high frequency end
Dobie & Rabinowitz (2002)	Notch index (NI): NI is obtained by subtracting the average thresholds at 1 and 8 kHz from the average thresholds at 2, 3, and 4 kHz. NI > 0 dB may indicate the presences of a bulge or a notch.
Hoffman, Ko, Themann, Dillon, & Franks (2006)	Thresholds worse by at least 15 dB at 3, 4, or 6 kHz than the average thresholds at 0.5 and 1.0 kHz and the thresholds at 8 kHz better by at least 5 dB than the worst threshold at 3, 4, or 6 kHz.

Adapted from Rawool, 2012a.

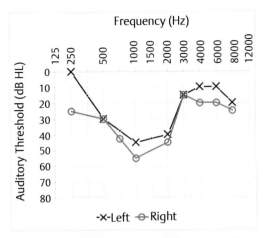

Fig. 3.18 Example of an audiogram of a woman with congenital hearing loss with a cookie-bite configuration (adapted from Rawool, 2012a).

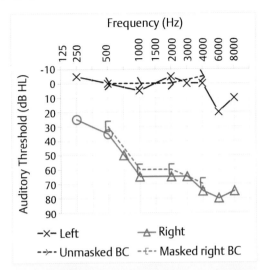

Fig. 3.19 Audiogram of a woman with sudden unilateral sensorineural hearing loss in the right ear and tinnitus in both ears (adapted from Rawool, 2012a). BC, bone conduction.

is already known. ▶ Fig. 3.19 shows the audiogram of a woman with a sudden sensorineural hearing loss in the right ear and continuous tinnitus in both ears.

Bilateral Hearing Loss

When hearing loss is apparent in both ears, the hearing loss is considered bilateral (▶ Fig. 3.13).

3.2.5 Symmetry

Symmetric Hearing Loss

When hearing loss in both ears is similar, the hearing loss is considered symmetric (▶ Fig. 3.13).

Asymmetric Hearing Loss

When hearing loss in the two ears is different, the hearing loss can be described as asymmetric. Medical referral should be initiated for asymmetrical hearing loss. In the United Kingdom, a difference of 20 dB at 0.5, 1, 2, or 4 kHz is used as a criterion for asymmetry; in the United States, a difference of 15 dB in the average thresholds of 0.5, 1, 2, and 3 kHz is used as a criterion for asymmetry to determine the need for medical referral. Using a criterion of 15 dB or more difference in the average thresholds at 0.5, 1, 2, and 4 kHz, approximately 1% of the general nonnoise-exposed U.K. population between the ages of 18 and 80 years have asymmetric audiometric configurations (Lutman & Coles, 2009). ▶ Fig. 3.20 shows an asymmetric

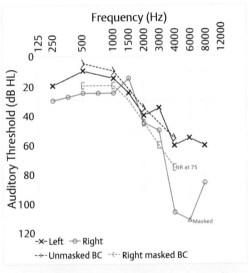

Fig. 3.20 Audiogram of a 54-year-old carpenter with asymmetric hearing loss at and above 4000 Hz. The man had a history of occupational noise exposure and a history of ear infections and mastoidectomy on the right side (adapted from Rawool, 2012a). BC, bone conduction.

audiogram of a 54-year-old carpenter with a history of occupational noise exposure and a history of ear infections and mastoidectomy on the right side. His postmedical referral magnetic resonance image on the right side revealed a tumor in the right mastoid space that was surgically removed and found to be benign.

3.2.6 Onset

Sudden Onset

If a significant hearing loss occurs suddenly, it is described as a sudden hearing loss. Such a hearing loss can occur following exposures to sudden loud noises, such as bomb blasts or firecrackers, or due to unknown causes. An example of a sudden sensorineural hearing loss in one ear is shown in ▶ Fig. 3.19.

Slowly Progressing

If the hearing continues to deteriorate over a longer period, the loss can be described as progressive. Hearing loss caused by occupational noise exposure or aging usually slowly progresses over time.

Congenital

If the hearing loss is noted at or during the neonatal period, it is referred to as congenital.

3.2.7 Classifications Based on More than One Audiogram

Hearing loss can be classified based on more than one audiogram.

Progressing or Worsening

If audiograms obtained sequentially at specific periods show worsening of auditory sensitivity, the hearing loss can be characterized as progressing or worsening. In some types of syndromes (e.g., Usher), hearing loss is progressive in nature. Some ototoxic medications can cause progressive hearing loss.

Fluctuating

In some cases the hearing can appear to become better, then become worse again over time. This type of hearing loss is described as fluctuating. Audiograms showing fluctuating but progressive hearing loss are presented in Chapter 16. Examples of diseases or conditions in which fluctuation in auditory sensitivity are apparent are auditory neuropathy/spectrum disorders (see Chapter 15), Ménière disease, and middle ear infections. ▶ Fig. 3.21 shows audiometric thresholds of a man obtained in 2007 at the age of 73 years and in 2012 at the age of 78 years. He had stapedectomy surgeries in 1978 and 1980 to address

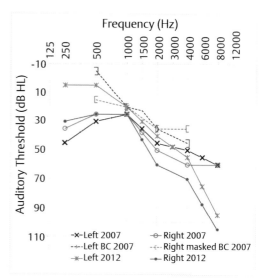

Fig. 3.21 Example of an audiogram of a man with fluctuating auditory sensitivity. Note the improvement in thresholds at 250 and 500 Hz in the left ear and the worsening of thresholds at 6000 and 8000 Hz in both ears from the age of 73 to 78 years. The man had stapedectomies in 1978 and 1980 to address his otosclerosis. BC, bone conduction.

bilateral otosclerosis. In the left ear an improvement in auditory thresholds is apparent at 250 and 500 Hz, but a deterioration of auditory sensitivity is apparent at 6000 and 8000 Hz. The right ear also shows significant deterioration at 6000 and 8000 Hz over the period of 5 years. Deterioration at higher frequencies may be partly due to aging and partly due to cochlear otosclerosis (Redfors & Möller, 2011).

3.3 Preparations Prior to Testing

3.3.1 Scheduling for Assessment of Peripheral Auditory Sensitivity

Determination of peripheral auditory sensitivity should be done just prior to the auditory processing test battery. This is especially important in cases where the hearing loss is unstable or fluctuates over time. As mentioned previously, the results of peripheral auditory sensitivity are important in determining the presentation levels of stimuli for the central assessments and for interpretation of the results.

3.3.2 Ensuring a Sufficiently Quiet Test Environment

The test environment needs to be sufficiently noise-free to allow accurate threshold measurements. High ambient noise levels can cause artificial elevation of auditory thresholds. In practice it is difficult to have an environment that is completely noise-free. Therefore, several agencies have specified maximum permissible noise levels for audiometric testing, as shown in ▶ Table 3.4.

Ideally, testing should be conducted in a quiet environment that does not exceed the maximum sound pressure levels specified in the American National Standards Institute/American Standards Association (ANSI/ASA) S3.1–1999 (2008), shown in ▶ Table 3.4. The maximum noise levels permitted by the U.S. Occupational Safety and Health Administration (OSHA, 1983) for supra-aural earphones are higher and can interfere in establishing very low thresholds, such as −10 dB HL in young adults. It is important to monitor the noise levels at 125 and 250 Hz even though these frequencies are not included in testing. High noise levels at these frequencies can elevate thresholds at higher frequencies due to upward spread of masking. Upward spread of masking occurs because the traveling wave in the cochlea always moves from the base to the apex, and the maximum excitation for low frequencies occurs at the apex. Thus, when the ear is stimulated with low-frequency noise, the related traveling wave, while moving toward the apex, can cause masking of high-frequency tones whose excitation patterns are located toward the base.

A sound-treated (treated with special sound attenuating and sound absorbing materials) double-wall booth is ideal for testing because it allows attenuation of even transient bursts of loud sounds, such as jet airplanes flying by. When speech audiometric testing is being conducted, the best practice is to have sound treatment for both the patient and examiner areas (▶ Fig. 3.22). Manufacturers often provide sound absorption and noise reduction data for their sound booths that can be used in determining if the noise levels in the booth will be within the maximum permissible noise levels specified by the ANSI/ASA (2008) standards. However, in evaluating the data provided by manufacturers, whether or not the data were obtained using standard testing procedures and with the air ventilation system on should be considered. Adequate ventilation and temperature control in the booth is necessary to minimize fatigue and discomfort that can affect thresholds during testing. The booths should be properly installed to achieve the attenuation characteristics provided by the manufacturers.

Table 3.4 Maximum Acceptable/Permissible Sound Pressure Levels for Audiometric Test Rooms

Octave band center frequency (Hz)	Supra-aural and Insert OSHA (1983)	Supra-aural Earphones ANSI S3.1–1999[1]		Insert Earphones ANSI S3.1–1999[2]	
		For 0 dB HL testing	For −10 dB HL testing	For 0 dB HL testing	For −10 dB HL testing
125		49	39	78	68
250		35	25	64	54
500	40	21	11	50	40
1000	40	26	16	47	37
2000	47	34	24	49	39
4000	57	37	27	50	40
8000	62	37	27	56	46

[1] Reaffirmed by ANSI October 2008. If 250 Hz is included in the test frequency range, noise levels at 125 and 250 Hz should be 10 dB lower.
[2] Reaffirmed by ANSI, October 2008). If 250 Hz is included in the test frequency range, noise levels at 125 and 250 Hz should be 11 dB lower.
Abbreviations: ANSI, American National Standards Institute; HL, hearing level; OSHA, Occupational Safety and Health Administration.

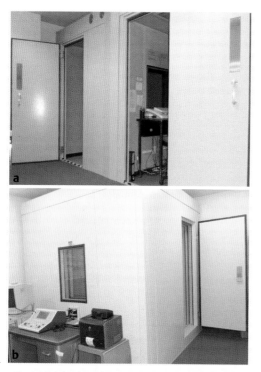

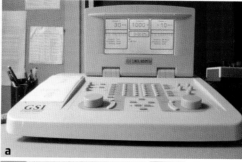

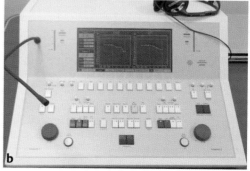

Fig. 3.23 (a,b) Examples of two audiometers.

Fig. 3.22 (a) A sound-treated booth setup for both patient and examiner rooms. (b) A double-wall booth.

3.4 Calibration of Equipment

All equipment used for audiometric testing should be calibrated on an annual basis, and the calibration should be checked on a daily basis. Some types of audiometric equipment allow calibration of sound pressure levels in each individual ear canal. Calibration serves several purposes, including ensuring that the signals are delivered accurately at the presentation levels specified by the equipment, that they are delivered at the frequencies specified by the equipment, and that the signals are relatively distortion free as specified by various standards. In measuring OAEs, the signals are calibrated in each ear canal to ensure accuracy of signal delivery and measurement of response amplitude and noise floors. In calibrating various pieces of audiometric equipment, including middle ear analyzers, the relevant standards should be used. As an example of equipment calibration, a brief review of audiometric calibration for tonal and speech signals for earphones is provided in the following section. Additional calibration procedures are employed for calibrating noise signals used for masking or other purposes and for stimuli delivered through bone conduction transducers and in the sound field.

3.5 Audiometric Functional Checks and Calibration

Audiometric testing should not begin until the audiometer (▶ Fig. 3.23) is properly calibrated and is determined to be in good working condition. Failure to ensure a calibrated audiometer can lead to inaccurate auditory thresholds. Three types of audiometric calibration procedures should be conducted: functional checks, acoustic calibrations, and exhaustive calibrations.

3.5.1 Daily Functional Checks

The functional operation of the audiometer should be checked at the beginning of each day of testing and at each facility where the testing is being conducted. The daily check should have the following components.

Visual Check

- Earphone cushions: Check the earphone cushions for any cracks or stiffness. The cushions should be cleaned periodically and replaced when cracks appear or when they are stiff.
- Cords: Check the cords for any discontinuities.

- Correct connections: Check to see if all earphone jacks are connected properly (e.g., the right jack is connected to the right earphone).

Listening Check

- Leave the equipment on for any recommended warm-up time before performing a listening check.
- Check for distortions: Listen to the output of the audiometer at both soft and moderately loud levels to ensure that there are no distortions or unwanted sounds mixed with the presented pure tone or speech signals.
- Check for acoustic crosstalk: Place one earphone on one ear and present tones through the other earphone. Check to see if the tones are audible in the earphone placed on the ear. If the tone is audible, recheck to see if the right and the left earphones are plugged into the corresponding jacks. Sometimes crosstalk can occur even after accurate plugging of headphones, although with new audiometers, this is less likely to occur.

Threshold or Biological Check

During the threshold check, the examiner makes sure that the output of the audiometer at each test frequency has not changed on the day of testing. This can be accomplished by using the following procedures.

- Test a person with known stable hearing and compare the individual's thresholds with his or her previously established reference or baseline thresholds. It is better to have the reference audiograms of at least two individuals available for comparison in case one person is absent or experiences elevated thresholds due to illness or other factors. In such cases, a second person with known stable hearing can be used to perform a calibration check on the audiometer.
- Use a bioacoustic simulator (also known as an electroacoustic ear), an instrument that simulates a human subject or ear. The earphones are placed on the simulator, and the thresholds are determined for the simulator as they will be established for an individual.

The best practice is to temporarily remove and/or recalibrate (exhaustive calibration) the audiometer if the daily biological test results differ from the baseline audiogram by more than 5 dB at 500 to 4000 Hz, or more than 10 dB at 6000 Hz, as required by the U.S. Navy (Navy and Marine Corps Public Health Center [NMCPHC], 2008). Such recalibrations will allow fairly accurate documentation of test results on an ongoing basis and are easier with modern digital audiometers and calibration equipment. Modern calibration equipment can automatically correct the reference equivalent threshold sound pressure levels (RETSPLs) and test supra-aural and insert earphones, extended frequency earphones, bone vibrators, and speakers based on limits in the ANSI standard specifications for audiometers. Examples of such equipment include the ACS 100 software from Audiological Service and Supply Company (AUSSCO) (Palantine, IL) and the AUDit with System 824 from Larson Davis Inc. (Depew, NY). Spare audiometers should be available in cases when an audiometer cannot be immediately recalibrated due to a lack of calibration equipment or expertise.

Record Results

A record of the daily functional checks should be maintained using a checklist. The best practice is to keep biologic calibrations available for review (upon request) for up to 5 years.

3.5.2 Annual Acoustic Calibration Checks

A sound level meter, an octave band filter set, and a National Bureau of Standards (NBS) 9A coupler are necessary to perform the acoustic calibration checks. The calibrating equipment itself needs to be adequately calibrated on an annual basis. The acoustic calibration has two components, a sound pressure output check and a linearity check.

Sound Pressure Output Check

During this check, the earphone is coupled to the microphone of the sound level meter through a coupler. The audiometer is then set to provide 70 dB HL at each of the test frequencies. The expected sound pressure levels indicated on the sound level meter are shown in the last rows in ▶ Table 3.5 for TDH-39 earphones from Telephonics ® A Griffon Company (Farmingdale, NY) and in ▶ Table 3.6 for TDH-49 earphones. The RETSPLs (dB re 20 μPa) for insert earphones are shown in ▶ Fig. 3.24 (ANSI/ASA S3.6–2010). Best practice is to perform exhaustive calibrations when the output levels are outside the range specified in standards.

Table 3.5 Levels for Checking Sound Pressure Output of the Audiometer for TDH-39 Earphones (ANSI/ASA S3.6–2010) Using the NBS-9A Coupler

Frequency	125 Hz	250 Hz	500 Hz	750 Hz	1000 Hz	1500 Hz	2000 Hz	3000 Hz	4000 Hz	6000 Hz	8000 Hz	Speech
Reference dB SPL for 0 dB HL (reference equivalent threshold SPLs)	45.0	25.5	11.5	8.0	7.0	6.5	9	10	9.5	15.5	13	19.5
Audiometric dial setting	70	70	70	70	70	70	70	70	70	70	70	70
Expected dB SPL output with the audiometric dial set at 70 dB HL	115.0	95.5	81.5	78.0	77.0	76.5	79	80	79.5	85.5	83	89.5

Abbreviations: ANSI/ASA, American National Standards Institute/American Standards Association; HL, hearing level; SPL, sound pressure level. From Telephonics ® A Griffon Company (Farmingdale, NY).

Table 3.6 Levels for Checking Sound Pressure Output of the Audiometer for TDH-49 and -50 earphones (ANSI/ASA S3.6–2010) Using the NBS-9A Coupler

Frequency	125 Hz	250 Hz	500 Hz	750 Hz	1000 Hz	1500 Hz	2000 Hz	3000 Hz	4000 Hz	6000 Hz	8000 Hz	Speech
Reference dB SPL for 0 dB HL (reference equivalent threshold SPLs)	47.5	26.5	13.5	8.5	7.5	7.5	11.0	9.5	10.5	13.5	13.0	20.0
Audiometric dial setting	70	70	70	70	70	70	70	70	70	70	70	70
Expected dB SPL output with the audiometric dial set at 70 dB HL	117.5	96.5	83.5	78.5	77.5	77.5	81.0	79.5	80.5	83.5	83.0	90.0

Abbreviations: ANSI, ASA, American National Standards Institute/American Standards Association; HL, hearing level; SPL, sound pressure level. From Telephonics ® A Griffon Company (Farmingdale, NY).

Linearity Check

The purpose of this check is to ensure that the attenuator of the audiometer is functioning properly. With the earphone still coupled to the microphone of the sound level meter through the coupler, a 1000 Hz tone is presented at 70 dB HL. The sound levels are then noted for each 10 dB decrement from 70 to 10 dB. For each 10 dB decrement in the hearing level dial, a 10 dB decrement in the sound level is expected. Linearity check can also be performed using a voltmeter connected to the earphone terminals and viewing a linear decrease in voltage with each 10 dB decrease in hearing level.

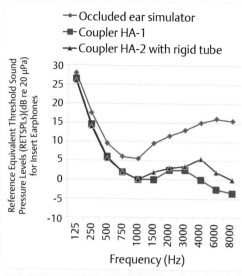

Fig. 3.24 Reference equivalent threshold sound pressure levels for insert earphones based on American National Standards Institute/American Standards Association (ANSI/ASA) S3.6–2010.

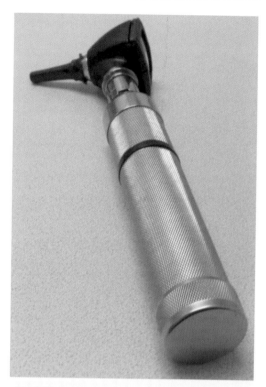

Fig. 3.25 An otoscope (adapted from Rawool, 2012a).

Record Results

A record of the results of acoustic calibration should be maintained in tabular formats.

3.5.3 Exhaustive Calibration

Exhaustive calibrations involve resetting the output of the audiometer to meet the ANSI standards. Exhaustive calibrations of the audiometer as specified in ANSI/ASA S3.6–2010 should be performed annually or when the audiometer appears to be out of calibration as indicated by a malfunction or aberrant results from patients. As noted previously, new equipment can allow exhaustive calibrations on site for digital audiometers within a short time period. The record of the date on which each exhaustive calibration was performed should be carefully noted.

Calibration Record Retention

The best practice is to maintain all calibration records for at least 5 years (National Institute for Occupational Safety and Health [NIOSH], 1998), including the results of the daily functional checks.

3.6 Case-History

A detailed case history form for adults is presented in the appendix at the end of this chapter. A case history form specifically designed for individuals (mainly children) referred for auditory processing evaluations is shown in the appendix of Chapter 4. A detailed history is important in determining the potential cause of hearing loss; it can also provide insights into the factors that increase the risk of auditory processing deficits.

3.7 Otoscopic Examination

An otoscopic examination should be performed before the test procedures (▶ Fig. 3.25). During the examination, both the eardrum and the ear canal should be observed for any signs of drainage and occluding cerumen. In the presence of drainage or occluding cerumen, the best practice is to postpone the evaluation until cerumen management is completed given that these conditions can elevate thresholds. In addition, the pinna should be pressed gently to mimic the positioning of supra-aural earphones to visualize any possibility of ear canal collapse, which can lead to poor test–retest reliability and artificial elevation of thresholds (Mahoney & Luxon, 1996). If ear canal collapse is apparent, the best practice is to use insert

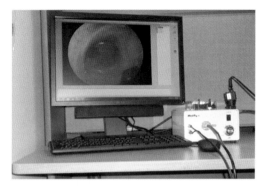

Fig. 3.26 A video-otoscope.

earphones for determining air conduction thresholds. When possible, a video-otoscope (▶ Fig. 3.26) should be used, which can allow individuals to visualize the conditions of their ear canals and eardrums. Such visualization can motivate them to follow any recommendations for medical management.

3.8 Test Procedures

The most current standard for manual procedures for determination of auditory thresholds is the ANSI S3.21–2004 standard, which was reaffirmed by ANSI in April 2009. This standard is a revision of ANSI S3.21–1978.

3.8.1 Instructions

The individual should be asked to remove any jewelry or eyeglasses because such items can make accurate placement of headphones difficult and cause discomfort. In addition, the individual should remove gum or tobacco given that chewing can make it difficult to hear sounds near thresholds. Cellphones and pagers should be turned off because they can interfere with and prolong the testing.

Instructions for the Test Procedure

Proper instructions (▶ Table 3.7) are extremely important for establishing accurate thresholds and completing the test in an efficient manner without the need for retest. If the person uses hearing aids, instructions should be provided prior to their removal. Hearing aids should then be removed prior to earphone placement.

Table 3.7 Instructions to the Patient before Determining Auditory Thresholds and Related Goals (adapted from Rawool, 2012a)

Goal	Instructions
Describe the purpose of the test.	We need to determine the softest sounds you can hear in each ear.
Inform the individual what to expect to reduce anxiety.	You will be hearing tones/beeps; some are going to be easy to hear, and some are going to be really soft. Some sounds will be high pitched, and some will be lower in pitch. We will test one ear at a time.
Tell the individual how to respond.	Please press this button (or raise your hand) as soon as you hear the tones/beeps, and let the button go (or lower your hand) as soon as the tones/beeps stop.
Emphasize the need for paying attention and responding to sounds near thresholds.	Please pay close attention and respond to any tones/beeps you hear, regardless of how soft they are.
Give an opportunity to ask questions.	Do you have any questions?
Make the individual feel comfortable in the booth (some individuals feel claustrophobic in the booth; others may feel fatigued during the test).	If you have any questions/concerns during testing or need a break, please feel free to speak. I can hear you from the other side.
For individuals with severe to profound hearing loss, confirm the comprehension of instructions.	Please tell me what you are supposed to do during the test procedures.

3.8.2 Earphone Placement

With supra-aural earphones, the earphone should be centered over the ear canal. Insert earphones should be placed relatively deeply in the canal.

3.8.3 Characteristics of Tones

The presented tones should be 1 to 2 seconds in duration, and the interval between successive presentations should be longer than the duration of tones and should be varied so that the timing of the tonal presentation cannot be predicted by the subject. During tonal presentations, the examiner should make sure that the examinee cannot visually see or receive any cues about when each tone is being presented.

3.8.4 Familiarization to the Listening and Response Task

The frequency of 1000 Hz is generally used during the familiarization phase. Two approaches have been suggested for familiarizing the subject with the task:

- Present the tone at a hearing level of 30 dB HL. If a clear or quick response occurs, threshold search can begin. If there is no response, then present the tone at 50 dB HL and at increments of 10 dB above 50 dB HL until a clear and quick response is apparent. The step size of 10 dB beyond 50 dB HL will minimize the possibility of presentation of the tones at uncomfortable loudness levels. A clear response indicates that the individual knows what to listen for and how to respond.
- Set the intensity dial at the softest level (−10 or 0 dB HL) and turn it continuously on. Slowly increase the sound pressure level until a clear response is apparent. Turn off the tone for a minimum period of 2 seconds, then present it again at the same level. If a clear response is apparent, familiarization is complete. If there is no response, repeat the procedure.

3.8.5 Frequencies to Be Tested

Air conduction thresholds are usually determined at 250, 500, 1000, 2000, 3000, 4000, 6000, and 8000 Hz. The thresholds at 750 and 1500 Hz are also determined if the difference in thresholds at 500 and 1000 or 1000 and 2000 Hz is greater than 15 dB HL. Bone conduction thresholds are usually determined at 500, 1000, 2000, and 4000 Hz, which is usually sufficient for determination of the type of hearing loss.

3.8.6 Order

If information is available, it is advantageous to test the better ear first given the task is easier when the tones are easily audible. To maintain consistency in the testing approach, testing should begin with the frequency of 1000 Hz and should proceed to higher frequencies. After thresholds at all higher frequencies are determined, the threshold should be reestablished at 1000 Hz to

determine the reliability of thresholds. If the reestablished thresholds at 1000 Hz differ by more than 5 dB, then the lower of the two thresholds may be accepted, but thresholds should be reestablished for at least one more frequency. If thresholds continue to differ by more than 5 dB, it may be better to reinstruct the individual before proceeding. Finally, thresholds are established at 500 and 250 Hz.

3.8.7 Level of Tonal Presentations

The level of the first presentation of tone should be 10 dB below the level at which the subject responded during the familiarization procedure. After each response, the level is decreased by 10 dB, and after each failure to respond, the tone is increased by 5 dB. This procedure is illustrated in ▶ Fig. 3.27.

3.8.8 Manual Determination of Threshold

The lowest hearing level at which a response is apparent on at least 50% of ascending trials with at least two responses out of three tonal presentations at the same level is considered the threshold. In ▶ Fig. 3.27, during the familiarization procedure, the subject provided a clear response at 30 dB HL. Thus, the level of the first presentation was 10 dB below 30 dB, or 20 dB. The subject did not respond at 20 dB. Therefore, the second presentation of the tone occurred at 5 dB higher, or 25 dB level. The subject responded to 25 dB HL. Thus, during the third trial, the level was lowered by 10 dB, and the tone was presented at 15 dB HL. There was no

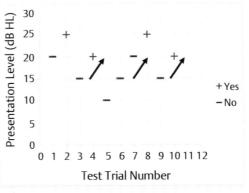

Fig. 3.27 Procedure for determining auditory thresholds (adapted from Rawool, 2012a).

response to the 15 dB tone. Thus, the level was raised to 20 dB on the fourth trial, and the subject responded. On the fifth trial, the level was lowered by 10 dB, and there was no response to 10 dB HL. On the sixth trial, the level was raised by 5 dB, and the subject did not respond to 15 dB HL. On the seventh trial, the level was raised by another 5 dB, and the subject still did not respond to 20 dB HL. Thus, on the eighth trial, the level was raised by another 5 dB, and the subject responded to 25 dB HL. On the ninth trial, the level was dropped by 10 dB to 15 dB HL, and there was no response. Thus, on the 10th trial, the level was increased by 5 dB, and the subject responded. Because the lowest level at which the subject responded on two out of three ascending trials (trials where the tone level was increased) was 20 dB, the threshold of the subject is 20 dB HL.

3.8.9 Automatic Determination of Thresholds Using Microprocessor-based or Computerized Audiometers

Computerized audiometers are programmed to follow the same procedures that are used during manual audiometry. Thus, after each response the level is decreased by 10 dB, and after each failure to respond, the tone is increased by 5 dB. All individuals cannot perform well with automatic audiometry. In such cases, it is necessary to use manual override to obtain valid thresholds. The advantage of computerized audiometry is that several individuals can be tested simultaneously. Some agencies require the use of microprocessor audiometers (e.g., the U.S. Navy for all active duty personnel) except in evaluating difficult-to-test patients (NMCPHC, 2008).

3.8.10 Use of Masking

When there is a wide difference in thresholds between the two ears, the hearing in the better ear can lead to underestimation of hearing loss in the worse ear. Thus, the better ear should be masked to eliminate its participation. An audiogram of a child suspected of having an auditory neuropathy spectrum disorder in one ear is shown in ▶ Fig. 3.28. In this case, masked thresholds have not been obtained. If hearing aids are fitted using unmasked thresholds, and the true thresholds are worse than the unmasked thresholds, the child may not benefit from hearing aids. Masked

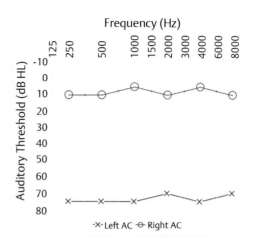

Fig. 3.28 Example of unmasked air conduction thresholds of a child with auditory neuropathy in the left ear. The child's distortion product otoacoustic emissions are shown in ▶ Fig. 3.42. AC, air conduction.

thresholds can be obtained in even young children by initially desensitizing them to the masking noise. The masking noise should be first introduced at lower levels and should be slowly raised to achieve adequate masking. The child should be discouraged from responding to masking noise and should be reinforced only when a response is provided for test tones. During visual or conditioned play audiometry, it may be necessary to recondition some children to the tonal or speech signals in the presence of the masking noise. For detailed masking procedures, refer to Yacullo (1996).

3.8.11 Potential Sources of Unreliable Thresholds

1. The examiner: Variations in content and delivery of instruction, placement of earphones, and variation in testing techniques, including masking procedures, can result in poor inter- and intratest reliability.
2. Calibration of test equipment: Failure to regularly and properly calibrate test equipment can increase test–retest threshold variability.
3. Test environment: Excessive noise in the test environment or uncomfortable test environment due to poor temperature control, causing excessive heat or cold, can lead to unreliable thresholds.
4. Characteristics of the examinee:
   • The dynamic nature of auditory sensitivity: Minor fluctuations in physiological activity

(e.g., moving around in the chair) can lead to minor fluctuations in thresholds. The presence of tinnitus can add to these fluctuations.

- Motivation: If the listener is motivated to make the hearing loss more severe, he or she may wait for the tones to become clearly loud before responding.
- Psychological and emotional state: Fatigue, anxiety, and physical sickness of the patient can interact with the examiner's experience and demeanor. If the audiologist is viewed as either an impersonal authority figure or an adversary, the listener may not fully cooperate.

3.8.12 Postponing Examination and Rescheduling

In some cases, in order to achieve valid results, it is necessary to postpone testing and reschedule a patient for another day to obtain a valid audiogram. Invalid test results are suggested by one or more of the following characteristics:

- Too much test–retest variability: Test–retest difference at 1000 Hz is 10 dB or more.
- Inconsistent response patterns: Thresholds vary greatly on ascending and descending trials of tonal presentation.
- False responses: These can consist of either the patient's responding in the absence of tonal presentation (false-positive) or not responding to a tone to which a clear and immediate response was apparent during previous trials (false-negative).

Other examples of when rescheduling is necessary are the presence of occluding cerumen in the ear canals, discharging ears, and signs of excessive fatigue.

3.8.13 Hygiene and Infection Control

It is important to maintain proper hygiene around the test area and to control for the spread of any infections. After testing, headphones, including earphone cushions, should be cleaned carefully with disinfection wipes. It is important to wipe surfaces that are touched by patients, such as chair armrests and response buttons.

Nondisposable otoscopic specula that are contaminated by ear drainage or blood can be first cleaned and then sterilized by soaking them in 2% glutaraldehyde or 7.5% hydrogen peroxide solution for 10 hours. Another option is to use an autoclave, which can sterilize the specula through high-pressure steam at 121°C (about 250°F) for 10 to 20 minutes. It may not be easy to determine ear drainage or blood in the presence of cerumen. Thus, sterilization of nondisposable specula is preferred (American Academy of Audiology Infection Control Task Force, 2003).

When there is an indication of a clear ear canal and a lack of blood or fluid drainage, specula should be cleaned of any visible organic matter such as cerumen with cotton swabs, washed with soap and water, and dried, then soaked in 70% alcohol for 10 to 20 minutes. If there is no time to soak the pieces between patients, after washing with soap and water the pieces can be wiped thoroughly with an alcohol-soaked cotton ball, rinsed with water, then dried. If this is done, at the end of each day the pieces should be soaked in 70% alcohol for 10 minutes (Texas Department of State Health Services, 2009).

3.8.14 Determination of Referrals

Some characteristics of patients or baseline audiograms that will need a medical referral are as follows:

1. Recent or chronic history of pain and drainage in one or both ears (American Academy of Otolaryngology–Head and Neck Surgery [AAO-HNS], 1997) because this suggests the possibility of current or chronic middle ear pathology that needs to be treated or managed, especially before fitting and use of hearing aids or hearing protection devices
2. History of dizziness; severe, persistent tinnitus; sudden, fluctuating, or rapidly progressive hearing loss; or a feeling of fullness or discomfort in one or both ears within the preceding 12 months. These symptoms are associated with ear pathologies and need to be treated or managed.
3. Asymmetric or unilateral hearing loss: In the presence of an asymmetric or unilateral hearing loss, a full evaluation is necessary to determine the type and degree of hearing loss and to treat or manage any underlying pathology, such as an acoustic nerve tumor.

3.8.15 Periodic Monitoring of Auditory Sensitivity

Annual audiometric evaluations are recommended for individuals with hearing loss to monitor auditory sensitivity and to make any needed alterations to hearing aids or other devices, such as cochlear implants (see Chapter 14). The risk of hearing loss increases with age. Thus, all individuals over the age of 60 years should receive annual audiological evaluations.

3.8.16 Review of Annual Audiograms

Annual audiograms should be compared to previous audiograms to determine significant changes in auditory sensitivity at any frequency and in one or both ears. Such changes should be noted in reports and explained to the patient.

Significant Threshold Shift

The NIOSH (1998) recommends a criterion of a change of 15 dB or more at any of the test frequencies for determining worsening of auditory thresholds.

3.9 Audiological Monitoring of Patients with Ototoxic Drug Exposure

Early detection of ototoxic hearing loss is important because such detection can allow a reduction in the drug dose or a change in the prescribed medication. When this is not possible, early detection can provide an opportunity for early aural rehabilitation and counseling related to the coping strategies for the progressive nature of the loss.

The auditory thresholds of patients who are scheduled to receive drugs with a high incidence of ototoxicity should be monitored. Such patients can be identified by medical personnel who are prescribing the drugs and/or monitoring the patients' pathology or by pharmacists dispensing the medications.

3.9.1 Baseline/Reference Audiometry

Ideally, a baseline audiogram should be obtained before initiation of any ototoxic drug. When this is not possible, the baseline audiogram can be obtained within 72 hours of initiation of aminoglycosides. However, chemotherapeutic drugs such as cisplatin can damage hearing after a single dose. Thus, baseline audiometry should be performed

before the administration of the first dose. A complete audiometric test battery can allow the documentation of thresholds, word recognition scores, OAEs, and the type of hearing loss if present before administration of the drugs. Test reliability should be assessed by repeating some parts of the tests (e.g., word recognition score in one ear, threshold determination at some frequencies). A history of tinnitus should also be noted. If tinnitus is present during baseline testing, it should be carefully investigated and documented. If patient illness or related fatigue is a major factor, the key information that should be recorded is the audiometric thresholds in the range of 0.25 to 8 kHz. When possible, thresholds should be documented for up to 20 kHz (ASHA, 1994).

3.9.2 Monitoring Audiometry

These evaluations mainly involve pure tone thresholds. For chemotherapeutic drugs, the periodic evaluations can occur before each dose; for aminoglycosides, these can occur once or twice weekly depending on the dose schedule. In the presence of significant changes, a retest should be performed to confirm the changes and to reduce false-positive rates (ASHA, 1994). Transient evoked OAEs (TEOAEs) may reveal cochlear damage before it is seen on an audiogram. A complete tinnitus evaluation is important for those patients who complain of an increase in the severity of preexisting tinnitus, as well as those who complain of onset of tinnitus during treatment, because tinnitus onset can be associated with chemotherapy and certain ototoxic antibiotic treatments (Dille et al., 2010).

3.9.3 Posttreatment Completion Audiometry

The monitoring test schedule should continue for as long as threshold changes are apparent on the audiogram. The recommended schedule is every week for chemotherapeutic drugs and every 2 days for aminoglycosides.

3.9.4 Long-term Follow-up Audiometry

Long-term follow-up testing at approximately 3 and 6 months is recommended to confirm that hearing is stable (ASHA, 1994) because the related deterioration in hearing can occur 6 months or even years following drug exposure (Al-Khatib, Cohen, Carret, & Daniel, 2010; Kolinsky, Hayashi, Karzon, Mao, & Hayashi, 2010). Patients who receive radiation to the posterior fossa and are fitted with hearing aids are at higher risk for late-onset deterioration of hearing (Kolinsky et al., 2010). If threshold deterioration is apparent during follow-up tests, weekly tests are recommended until the hearing becomes stable (ASHA, 1994).

3.9.5 Significant Threshold Shifts

There is a critical need for international consensus on ototoxicity assessment criteria (Neuwelt & Brock, 2010). In the interim, the following criteria can be used for determining significant changes in auditory sensitivity provided that the changes are confirmed by retest (ASHA, 1994):
- Worsening of thresholds by more than 20 dB at any single frequency
- Worsening of thresholds by more than 10 dB at any two consecutive test frequencies
- Previous response obtained close to the limits of the audiometer changing to "no response" status at three consecutive test frequencies, specifically at high frequencies

3.9.6 Extended High-Frequency Testing

Some investigators have recommended determination of a sensitive range of ototoxicity (SRO) for each individual. The SRO is defined as the highest frequency in the 0.25 to 20 kHz range at which threshold is 100 dB SPL or less and the six consecutive lower frequencies in one-sixth octave steps (Fausti et al., 1999) or three consecutive lower frequencies in one-third octave steps. The best overall test performance for detecting ototoxicity has been noted by using a criterion of a 10 dB or greater shift at two or more adjacent frequencies tested in one-sixth octave steps in the SRO (Konrad-Martin et al., 2010). Because these protocols have been mainly tested using drug-induced otoxicity, further research is necessary to see if they might be applicable to audiometric threshold shifts caused by other ototoxins.

For frequencies between 9 and 14 kHz, test–retest variability can be within 10 dB. In addition, false-positive rates indicating a change in ultra-high-frequency thresholds in patients who were not exposed to ototoxic drugs is reportedly low in young and older adults when testing is conducted in the hospital ward under controlled conditions. However, test–retest variability is generally greater in young children (Konrad-Martin et al., 2005).

3.10 Speech Audiometry

In selecting material for speech audiometry for bilingual listeners, the language proficiency should be considered. Self-rated English proficiency is a good predictor of English word recognition in quiet for bilingual listeners (Shi, 2013). An 11-point scale (0–10) called the Language Experience and Proficiency Questionnaire (LEAP-Q) has been validated for obtaining listeners' proficiency ratings in English or other languages. Although self-reported proficiency is generally predictive of language ability, for prediction on performance on specific tasks, language history should be taken into account (Marian, Blumenfeld, & Kaushanskaya, 2007). If the individual is not proficient in English, materials in the native language should be used for testing. Such materials are available in several different languages (see Chapter 4). It should also be noted that bilingual individuals may perform well in quiet, but in noise their performance may be poor if the spoken materials are presented in the nonnative language. In addition, differences in dialects can lead to poor performance. Ideally, phonetic features of the dialect should be considered when scoring a client's performance (Shi & Canizales, 2013).

Two speech audiometric tests are usually included in a regular audiological evaluation: the speech recognition threshold and speech recognition scores. For detailed information about these procedures, refer to Gelfand (2001a). A brief description is provided below.

3.10.1 Speech Recognition Thresholds

The speech recognition threshold (SRT) is the softest level at which the examinee can recognize half of spondee (bisyllabic words with equal emphasis on both syllables) words accurately through insert or supra-aural earphones or through bone conduction. For adults the response task involves repetition of the presented words. Children can be asked to point to pictures representing the spondee words. Children younger than 2 years can be asked to point to body parts or other familiar objects. Listeners are encouraged to guess the word when they are not sure of what is being said.

The SRT is usually within 8 to 10 dB of the average tonal thresholds at 0.5, 1, and 2 kHz (Chaiklin & Ventry, 1965) or at 0.5 and 1 kHz (Chaiklin & Ventry, 1965; Jahner, Schlauch, & Doyle, 1994). However, audiometric configuration should be taken into account in predicting the SRT based on pure tone thresholds (Carhart & Porter, 1971). If the audiogram has a steep slope, the SRT can be similar to the average thresholds at 500 and 1000 Hz. In the presence of a precipitous slope, the SRT may be similar to the best threshold, which can be either 500 or 250 Hz. Thus, the test is useful in confirming the accuracy of pure tone thresholds at these frequencies.

In patients with nonorganic hearing loss the pure tone average (PTA)–SRT difference often exceeds 10 dB (Chaiklin & Ventry, 1965). Thus, the PTA-SRT difference can be used to determine the possible presence of a nonorganic component. SRTs obtained with the ascending procedure provide the largest difference in SRT and PTA in the presence of pseudohypacusis (Conn, Ventry, & Woods, 1972). Thus, an ascending approach with an initial level of −10 dB HL is recommended in determining SRTs (Schlauch, Arnce, Olson, Sanchez, & Doyle, 1996).

Establishing SRTs using an ascending approach at the beginning of the audiological test battery minimizes opportunities for the patient to establish a loudness reference based on tonal stimuli that are used during air or bone conduction testing. In cases of unilateral hearing loss, no responses from one ear in the presence of normal SRTs in the other ear is suggestive of nonorganic pathology. In the presence of a true hearing asymmetry, the need for masking should be evaluated after establishing ear-specific bone conduction thresholds, and, if necessary, masked SRTs should be obtained.

3.10.2 Speech Recognition Scores

Speech recognition scores (SRSs) are determined by presenting speech materials (syllables, words, or sentences) to the listeners at the most comfortable listening levels or at the average conversational levels or several different levels. The listener is expected to repeat the stimuli or point to written or pictorial versions of the stimuli. The percent of correctly repeated sentences, words, or phonemes is computed to determine the SRS.

Materials Used for Determination of Speech Recognition Scores

Several different speech materials, including nonsense syllables, words, sentences, and paragraphs, are available for speech recognition tests. The most commonly used materials are the Central Institute for the Deaf W-22 (CID W-22) and the Northwestern University Auditory Test No. 6 (NU-6) word lists. These tests have listeners repeat what is heard by adding a carrier phrase before each word, such as "You will say…" or "Say the word…." Each test includes multiple lists, with 50 relatively familiar monosyllabic words in each list. The words in each list are phonetically or phonemically balanced.

Phonetic Balance

Phonetic balance means that the relative frequency of the phonemes in each list is assumed to be similar to the distribution of speech sounds in English. The words in the four 50-word lists in the CID W-22 words are phonetically balanced based on analyses of 100,000 words in newsprint in the early 1920s (Dewey, 1923) and analyses of spoken English embedded in business telephone conversations (French, Carter, & Koenig, 1930).

Phonemic Balance

It is hard to achieve true phonetic balance because the acoustic properties of speech sounds vary based on the sounds preceding and following them. Thus, a more achievable goal is to have phonemic balance in different word lists. To achieve phonemic balance, each initial consonant, each vowel, and each final consonant should appear with the same frequency of occurrence within each word list. Thorndike and Lorge (1944) compiled a list of 30,000 words and reported the frequency of occurrence of each word per million words. Lehiste and Peterson (1959) selected 1263 monosyllabic words occurring at least once per million words from the Thorndike and Lorge (1944) list. The words consisted of consonant-vowels-consonant sequence. They then determined the frequency with which each initial, medial, and final phoneme occurred in the set of the 1263 words. They created 10 lists of 50 monosyllabic words. Each single list of 50 words was constructed in such a way that each phoneme had the same frequency of occurrence as noted in the total pool of 1263 words. The original lists were revised several times, and the current version of the list is known as the NU-6 word lists (Tillman & Carhart, 1966). The recordings of these lists are available with female and male voices. The average word recognition scores obtained with four of the NU-6 word lists are shown in ▶ Fig. 3.29 for individuals with normal hearing and those with hearing loss as a function of presentation levels (Tillman & Carhart, 1966).

Test Materials for High-Frequency Hearing Loss

Individuals who have hearing loss limited to high frequencies may perform well on commonly used speech recognition materials partially due to re-cordings by male speakers of some of the materi-als. Although most speech sounds occur in the frequency range below or around 4000 Hz, sounds such as /s/ and /z/ have energy up to 10,000 Hz (Boothroyd, Erickson, & Medwetsky, 1994). The bandwidth for the /s/ phoneme is up to 4000 or 5000 for male speakers but above 9000 Hz for fe-male speakers (Stelmachowicz, Pittman, Hoover, & Lewis, 2001). New speech materials such as the Widex Office of Research in Clinical Amplification Nonsense Syllable Test (ORCA-NST) have been

developed to allow better assessment of speech recognition by individuals with hearing loss and to document the benefit of hearing aids that attempt to compensate for hearing loss at higher frequen-cies by extending the bandwidth of hearing aids or through frequency compression. The ORCA-NST items consist of C-V-C-V-C nonsense syllables, allowing presentation of each consonant in initial, medial, and final positions. The listener is asked to verbally repeat each stimulus item. Presentation of stimuli is randomized through computer control. The scoring is completed by the computer, which allows for quick analysis by phoneme class. The test reportedly has high test–retest reliability for both individuals with normal hearing and those with hearing loss (Kuk et al., 2010).

Materials for Children

Several materials are available for children. The most commonly used materials are the Word Intel-ligibility by Picture Identification (WIPI) test (Ross & Lerman, 1970), the 50-item Phonetically Bal-anced Kindergarten (PBK-50) word lists (Haskins, 1949), and the Northwestern University Children's Perception of Speech (NU-CHIPS) test (Elliott & Katz, 1980). Children are asked to point to the pic-ture representing the word in the WIPI (six foils) and NU-CHIPS (four foils) tests. Several other tests are available, including those shown in ▶ Table 3.8. A revised version of the Early Speech Perception (ESP) test (Geers & Moog, 1989) is available from the Central Institute for the Deaf. The CID ESP test (2012) (http://www.cid.edu/ProfOutreachIntro/EducationalMaterials.aspx) is designed for pro-foundly deaf children. The test kit includes a box of toys, full-color picture cards, scoring forms, revised manual, and a CD.

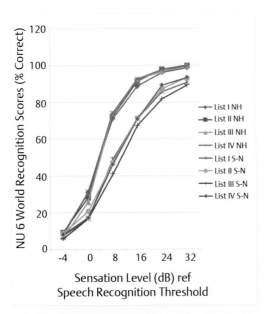

Fig. 3.29 Northwestern University Auditory Test No. 6 (NU-6) word recognition scores (percentage correct) as a function of presentation level in individuals with normal hearing (NH) and with sensorineural (S-N) hearing loss (based on Tillman & Carhart, 1966). The results are presented for four different word lists.

Table 3.8 Speech Recognition Tests for Children

Test Title	Study	Auditory Language Age
Early Speech Perception	Geers & Moog (1989)	Below 2 years
NU-CHIPS	Elliott & Katz (1980)	2 to 5 years
WIPI	Ross & Lerman (1970)	4 to 6 years
PBK-50	Haskins (1949)	5 to 8 years
NU-6	Tillman & Carhart (1966)	Above 8 years

Purposes of Speech Recognition Score Determination

SRS can serve several purposes, including the following:

1. To determine how well the person understands speech produced at average conversation levels in quiet surroundings. For such determination, the selected speech materials are presented at 45 to 50 dB HL. Such scores can be obtained with and without hearing aids to assess, document, and demonstrate the benefit from hearing aids, cochlear implants, or other assistive listening technologies. To determine if the improvement with hearing aids is significant, 95% critical differences should be taken into account (Thornton & Raffin, 1978). An example of such determination is shown in ▶ Fig. 3.30. Note that the critical difference range is narrower for very low or very high scores. It is also narrower if, instead of 25 words, 50 words are used to determine the SRS (Thornton & Raffin, 1978).

2. To determine how well an individual with hearing loss can understand speech if it is presented at levels that are clearly audible and still comfortably loud to him to or her. This test simu-

lates someone speaking loudly to an unaided person with hearing loss. The SRSs obtained at maximum comfortable levels are also referred to as maximum word recognition, with the assumption that the scores will not improve with further increase in presentation levels. For patients with moderately severe or severe hearing loss, the highest phoneme recognition appears at a level that is 5 dB below their uncomfortable listening levels (Guthrie & Mackersie, 2009). If the person scores below 80% at 5 dB below his or her uncomfortable listening level, materials should be presented at higher presentation levels in 2 dB steps if such levels are tolerable to the patient to ensure that the obtained score is in fact the maximum possible score for the patient. SRSs are partially dependent on the degree of hearing loss. To determine if the maximum speech recognition score (SRSmax) is much lower than expected from the hearing loss, published cutoff criterion can be used, as shown in ▶ Fig. 3.31 and ▶ Fig. 3.32. Note that SRSs are expected to become worse with the increase in the degree of hearing loss (Dubno, Lee, Klein, Matthews, & Lam, 1995). If the patient's speech recognition score is worse than what is expected based on the 95% confidence levels, the scores are assumed to be affected by retrocochlear or central factors. The cutoff values can differ based on the specific criterion, the selected speech materials, the specific

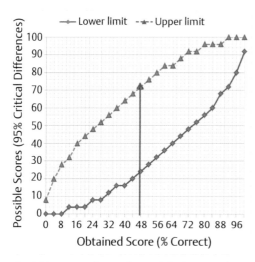

Fig. 3.30 Lower and upper limits of the 95% critical differences as a function of the obtained scores with the presentation of 25 words (half list) of the W-22 words (based on Thornton & Raffin, 1978). For a difference to be judged as true or significant, the score has to be outside the lower or upper limit. For example, if the unaided speech recognition score is 48%, the aided scores will have to be higher than 72% to yield a significant difference.

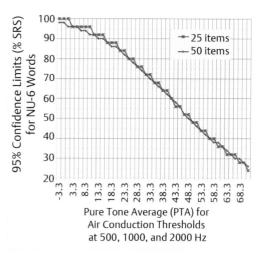

Fig. 3.31 NU-6 word recognition scores as a function of pure tone averages at 500, 1000, and 2000 Hz (based on Dubno, Lee, Klein, Matthews, & Lam, 1995).

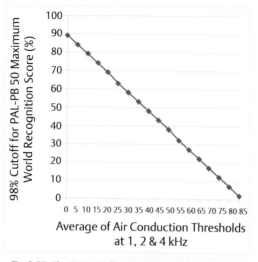

Fig. 3.32 The 98% cutoff values for maximum word recognition scores on the Harvard Psychoacoustics Lab (PAL-PB 50) word lists as a function of pure tone averages at 1, 2, and 4 kHz (based on Yellin, Jerger, & Fifer, 1989).

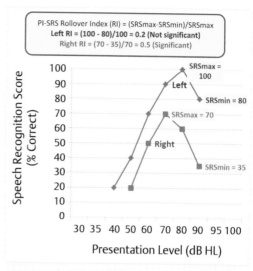

Fig. 3.33 Example of calculation of the performance intensity–speech recognition score (PI-SRS) rollover index for a hypothetical patient.

frequencies used in computing PTAs, and the age of participants in the study. In ▸ Fig. 3.31 the cutoff criterion is 95%, the speech material is NU-6 words, and the PTA is calculated using thresholds at 500, 1000, and 2000 Hz. In ▸ Fig. 3.32 the cutoff criterion is 98%, the speech material is Harvard Psychoacoustics Lab (PAL-PB) words, and the PTA is based on thresholds at 1000, 2000, and 4000 Hz (Yellin, Jerger, & Fifer, 1989). Word recognition scores can also vary somewhat based on whether the audiometric configuration is flat, gradually sloping, or sharply sloping (Gates, Cooper, Kannel, & Miller, 1990).

3. To rule out retrocochlear or central factors contributing to the SRS. Word recognition scores (WRSs) can be obtained at various presentation levels and plotted as a function of presentation level. This is commonly referred to as word recognition Performance Intensity (presentation level), or PI function. Based on these scores, a rollover index (RI) can be calculated using the following formula:

$$PI - SRS\ RolloverIndex = \frac{(SRS_{max} - SRS_{min})}{SRS_{max}}$$

where the minimum SRS (SRSmin) is the minimum score obtained at presentation levels higher than those used for yielding the maximum score (SRSmax). To obtain the SRSmin, the

words are usually presented up to a level of 90 dB HL or 110 dB SPL (Jerger & Hayes, 1977). Examples of calculations for the right and left ear of a hypothetical listener are shown in ▸ Fig. 3.33. For Harvard Psychoacoustics Lab (PAL-PB 50) words, a rollover index greater than 0.42 to 0.45 is suggestive of retrocochlear dysfunction (Dirks, Kamm, Bower, & Betsworth, 1977; Jerger & Hayes, 1977; Jerger & Jerger, 1971). For NU-6 words, a rollover index greater than 0.25 to 0.35 may be suggestive of retrocochlear dysfunction (Bess, Josey, & Humes, 1979; Meyer & Mishler, 1985). Although in younger adults higher rollover indices are more often observed in the presence of retrocochlear pathologies such as acoustic nerve tumors, an abnormal rollover index has also been reported in some older individuals suggestive of neural presbycusis (Gang, 1976).

WRSs obtained at several high presentation levels can be compared to those predicted by the articulation index (AI). The AI allows prediction of speech intelligibility based on a person's thresholds at each frequency. It is based on division of the entire frequency range into 20 different frequency bands in such a way that each frequency band makes equal contribution (5%) to understanding speech (French & Steinberg, 1947) in the presence of normal hearing. When a person has hearing loss, the ability to understand speech depends on the auditory thresholds in each of these frequency bands. Depending on the degree of hearing loss in each frequency band, the word recognition score predicted from the AI can vary from 0 to 100%. If the score is well below than that predicted from AI, retrocochlear or central pathology can be suspected. Older listeners whose WRSs fall below the predicted scores based on their auditory thresholds (▶ Fig. 3.30, Thornton & Raffin, 1978)should be considered for further testing for age-related auditory neuropathy (Gates, Feeney, & Higdon, 2003). Note that the data in the Thornton and Raffin (1978) study consisted of 4120 administrations of the CID W-22 word lists to hearing impaired listeners who were typically in the age range of 55 to 70 years.

4. To assist in hearing aid prescriptions. Following medical attention for ruling out retrocochlear pathology or addressing retrocochlear pathology, the PI-SRS function can provide useful information about the patient's optimum range of listening for providing hearing aid fittings (Boothroyd, 2008). For the hypothetical patient in ▶ Fig. 3.33, providing speech output greater than 70 dB HL or 90 dB SPL in the right ear may not result in improvement in SRSs. Auditory training in addition to hearing aid fitting may improve SRSs in the right ear. In the left ear the SRSs on the output of the hearing aid should be limited to 80 dB HL or 100 dB SPL where the scores are 100%. Additional gain can decrease the scores.

Variables Affecting Speech Recognition Scores

The outcomes of speech recognition testing are affected by several variables:

- Test environment (quiet, sound booth, etc.)
- Adequate calibration of test equipment used in delivering the materials
- Recorded versus monitored live-voice presentation. Recorded materials yield higher test–retest reliability compared to live-voice presentations. Commercial providers are expected to follow set standards in recording speech materials (Annex B of ANSI/ASA S3.6–2010). For example, the standard recommends a calibration signal at 1000 Hz and frequency response of +/−1 dB over the frequency range of 250 to 4000 Hz and +/−2 dB outside this range but within the range of 125 to 8000 Hz for recordings used with speech audiometers. The standard also specifies that

any inherent background noise on the recording should be at least 40 dB below the level of the calibration signal when measured with the sound level meter set at frequency weighting of C with a fast response time.

- Male versus female speakers
- The specific test or speech material used
- Use of a partial or full list. Full lists can improve test–retest reliability.
- Presentation level. With increasing presentation levels, speech recognition performance improves up to a certain level. A decrease in speech intelligibility can occur when levels are increased above 80 dB SPL even in individuals with normal hearing (French & Steinberg, 1947; Studebaker, Sherbecoe, McDaniel, & Gwaltney, 1999).
- Closed versus open response task. In the closed response task, the listener selects the response from a set of given alternatives. Depending on the materials, scores can be better with a closed response task compared to an open response task.
- Nonsense versus meaningful materials. Responses to meaningful materials can be influenced by use of top-down or cognitive strategies to yield a correct response.
- Use of sentence, word, or phoneme scoring

3.10.3 Speech Audiometry in the Presence of Background Noise

In real acoustic environments, there is often noise or reverberation in the background. In addition, some speakers may speak very rapidly. Such factors degrade the speech signal by the time it reaches the listener's ears. Thus, speech audiometric procedures are often performed in the presence of various types of background noise to estimate the ability of a listener to perceive speech in more realistic environments. These procedures are described in Chapter 7.

3.11 Tympanometry

Tympanometry is performed using a tympanometer, or middle ear analyzer (▶ Fig. 3.34), to evaluate the function of the middle ear and to confirm or rule out any conductive component to any hearing loss. A normal tympanogram is shown in the upper panel of ▶ Fig. 3.35. In the presence of some abnormal findings suggesting reduced mobility of the middle ear system or eardrum rupture, acoustic reflex tests cannot be conducted. Also, results of OAE testing should be interpreted with caution in the presence of middle ear dysfunction.

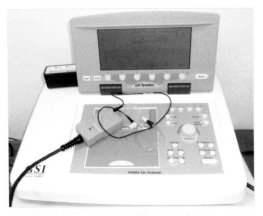

Fig. 3.34 Tympanometer/middle ear analyzer.

3.12 Acoustic Reflex Testing

Acoustic reflex tests are performed using a middle ear analyzer. The acoustic reflex occurs when relatively loud stimuli are presented to the ear. The acoustic reflex pathway is shown in Chapter 1.

3.12.1 Acoustic Reflex Thresholds

The softest stimulus level that causes a minimal recordable (specified) change in middle ear immittance is referred to as the acoustic reflex threshold (ART). The lower panel of ▶ Fig. 3.35 shows establishment of ARTs using a criterion of a minimum change of 0.02 ml in admittance for a probe frequency of 226 Hz. For the activator frequencies of 500 and 1000 Hz, the change in admittance at 80 dB HL was less than 0.02 ml. Using a 5 dB step size, the lowest level at which a change of at least 0.02 was apparent was 85 dB HL. Thus, in this case the ART is 85 dB HL for 500 and 1000 Hz. Note that for the probe frequency tone of 226 Hz, the middle ear system is mostly dominated by stiffness or compliance. Thus, the total middle ear admittance is mostly composed of compliance. Because the compliance of the middle ear can be calibrated with reference to the compliance of an equivalent volume of air in ml or CC, the middle ear admittance for a probe frequency of 226 Hz is sometimes reported in ml as shown in Fig. 3.35. For detailed discussions about these concepts, refer to the manufacture manuals or other extensive textbooks devoted to the topic of middle ear admittance. ARTs should be established at 500, 1000, and 2000 Hz using a 226 Hz probe tone in adults, although reflex thresholds can also be established using high-frequency probe tones (Rawool, 1998) and

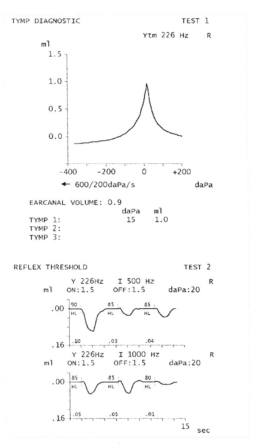

Fig. 3.35 Right ear tympanometric and acoustic reflex threshold test results of a 20-year-old woman.

broadband stimuli, such as clicks (Rawool, 1995). In normal-hearing individuals, ARTs can be recorded at levels between 85 and 100 dB SPL for pure tones and at approximately 20 dB lower levels for broadband stimuli (Gelfand, 1984).

3.12.2 Acoustic Reflex Decay

During the reflex decay test, a tone is presented continuously for 10 seconds at a level 10 dB above the reflex thresholds. The magnitude of the reflex response either stays the same or decreases over the 10-second period. Reflex decay or positive reflex decay is noted when the magnitude of the response decreases by 50% or more during the 10-second period, as shown in ▶ Fig. 3.36. In the presence of elevated ARTs, it is not always possible to conduct threshold decay testing due to the upper limit of presentation levels or loudness tolerance difficulties. For further applications of acoustic reflex tests, see Chapter 5.

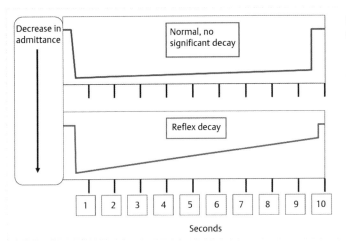

Fig. 3.36 Illustration of acoustic reflex decay.

3.12.3 Applications of Acoustic Reflex Test Results

Retrocochlear Pathologies

Acoustic reflex abnormalities, including reflex thresholds at elevated levels, absent reflexes, and positive reflex decay, are associated with retrocochlear pathologies in the ear receiving the stimulus tone. In the presence of hearing loss, ARTs that fall above the 90% range established for individuals without known retrocochlear pathologies should be considered as elevated (▶ Fig. 3.37). The expected range of ARTs for various air conduction thresholds is provided by Gelfand, Schwander, and Silman (1990). Consideration of positive findings on either or both reflex threshold or reflex decay tests has a hit rate of about 85% for retrocochlear pathologies and a relatively low false-positive rate of 11% (Silman & Silverman, 1991). The absence of acoustic reflexes in combination with a significant PI-SRS rollover is highly suggestive of auditory nerve dysfunction, including acoustic nerve tumor (Hannley & Jerger, 1981).

Auditory Neuropathy Spectrum Disorder

In cases with auditory neuropathy, acoustic reflexes are often absent in the presence of normal OAEs (see Chapter 15).

Nonorganic Hearing Loss

Because of the wide variability of ARTs in individuals with air conduction thresholds below 60 dB HL, it is difficult to differentiate between organic and

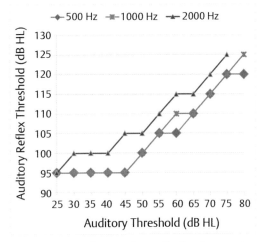

Fig. 3.37 Ninetieth percentile cutoff values for acoustic reflex thresholds (dB HL) at 500, 1000, and 2000 Hz as a function of auditory thresholds (dB HL). When the thresholds are below 25 dB HL, the 90th percentile cutoff values are 95 dB HL. For thresholds above 80 dB HL, absent reflexes are expected (based on Gelfand, Schwander, & Silman, 1990). Thresholds obtained above the specified values are considered to be elevated.

nonorganic hearing loss. For 60 dB HL or higher air conduction thresholds, nonorganic hearing loss is suspected when the patient's ARTs are below the admitted pure tone air conduction thresholds or below the ARTs specified in ▶ Fig. 3.38 (Gelfand, 2001b). For example, if the patient's audiogram shows an air conduction threshold of 75 dB HL, but his ARTs are established at 85 dB HL at 500, 1000, or 2000 Hz, the presence of nonorganic hearing loss should be considered. For complete evaluation

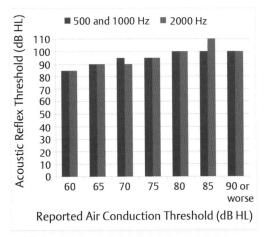

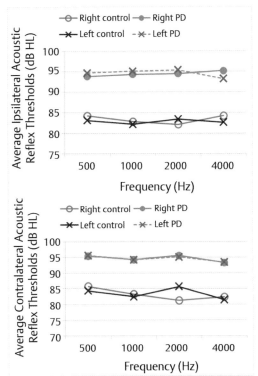

Fig. 3.38 Tenth percentile cutoff values for acoustic reflex thresholds (dB HL) for 60 dB HL and higher auditory air conduction thresholds (dB HL). If acoustic reflex thresholds are apparent below these values, nonorganic hearing loss is suspected (adapted from Rawool, 2012a, based on Gelfand, 2001b).

Fig. 3.39 Average ipsilateral and contralateral acoustic reflex thresholds from the right and left ears of children with phonological disorders (PD) and those with normal speech and language development (control) (based on Attoni, Quintas, & Mota, 2010).

procedures in the presence of suspected nonorganic hearing loss, refer to Rawool (2012c). Some individuals with a heightened sensitivity to sounds can yield ARTs at much lower levels than expected from their auditory thresholds. Auditory cortical damage can also yield ARTs at very low levels (e.g., 55 dB HL) (Downs & Crum, 1980).

Auditory Processing Deficits

Some individuals with auditory processing deficits show absent or elevated ARTs. In some children the abnormalities are apparent in both ipsilateral and contralateral reflex measurements (Lenhardt, 1981), whereas in other children the abnormalities are apparent only during the recording of contralateral reflex thresholds. In some cases the dysfunction within the auditory brainstem can be documented only with these tests, along with the auditory brainstem response measures. This is possible because some children with auditory processing deficits may use top-down processing to compensate for processing deficits on behavioral test measures. Such findings show the importance of conducting acoustic reflex testing in children referred for auditory processing evaluations (Allen & Allan, 2007, 2013). Children in the age range of 5 to 7 years with phonological disorders yield significantly higher ARTs compared to age-matched peers with normal speech and

language development. Average ipsilateral and contralateral ARTs from children with phonological disorders and age-matched peers are shown in ▶ Fig. 3.39 (Attoni, Quintas, & Mota, 2010). For the potential connection between auditory processing deficits and phonological or speech sound disorders, refer to Chapter 14.

As previously mentioned, in some cases with damage to the auditory cortex, ARTs may be apparent at very low stimulus presentation levels (e.g., 55 dB HL) perhaps due to the lack of inhibitory efferent influences (Downs & Crum, 1980).

3.13 Otoacoustic Emission Testing

OAEs are sounds generated in the cochlea and are recorded by presenting clicks or tonal stimuli to the ear. The equipment for measuring OAEs includes a probe tip assembly that is placed in the ear canal. The probe tip assembly has receivers for presenting stimuli to the ear and a microphone to pick up sounds elicited by the cochlea. The sounds picked up by the microphone are amplified and filtered to detect the emissions of interest. Background noise is minimized by applying signal averaging.

From a clinical standpoint, OAE testing is very useful because it allows quick evaluation at more discrete frequencies in an objective manner that is unaffected by fatigue factors. In addition, the only requirement from subjects is to sit still and not speak during the testing.

TEOAEs are elicited in response to stimuli of very brief duration (transients), such as clicks. Distortion product otoacoustic emissions (DPOAEs) are elicited by simultaneous presentation of two tones with different but relatively close frequencies that are referred to as primaries. The tone with lower frequency is referred to as f1, and the tone with higher frequency is referred to as f2. The ear generates different distortion products in response to the two tones, including 2f1-f2, 2f2-f1,and f2-f1. The distortion product (DP) 2f1-f2 has the largest amplitude (Gaskill & Brown, 1990), which allows for easier detection and is thus the most commonly measured DPOAE for clinical applications.

For clinical applications, DPOAEs are usually elicited for several different primary frequencies by holding the primary levels and frequency ratio constant. The amplitudes of the recorded DPOAEs are then plotted as a function of f2 (Gorga et al., 1997) or the geometric mean of the primaries (Lonsbury-Martin & Martin, 1990). The assumption underlying the plotting of DPOAEs as a function of f2 is that the level of the DPOAE reflects cochlear function near the f2 place (generator component) on the basilar membrane, where there is maximum overlap of excitation patterns generated by f1 and f2. However, when the distortion product (DP) frequency is lower than the f2 frequency, a proportion of the DP energy appears to travel to the characteristic place for that DP frequency and is reflected from there (Shaffer et al., 2003). This is referred to as the reflection component, and it can be larger than the generator component of DPOAE because energy traveling from the base to the DP characteristic place is amplified (Talmadge, Long, Tubis, & Dhar, 1999). The DPOAE fine structure (relatively large changes in DPOAE amplitudes with small changes in frequency) may be a result of the interaction of the generator and reflection components. When the frequencies of the primaries are changed, the phase of both the generator and reflection components is expected to change. However, the phase change is slower for the generator component compared to that for the reflection component. When the generator and the reflection components are in phase, DPOAE amplitudes can be expected to be larger; when they are out of phase, the magnitude is expected to be smaller, leading to the DPOAE fine structure. The DPOAE fine structure is indicative of a healthy cochlea and has been used for differential diagnosis of outer hair cell damage (Mauermannn, Uppenkamp, van Hengel, & Kollmeier, 1999). Use of rapidly sweeping tones has been proposed to obtain quicker estimates of DPOAE fine structure or to obtain estimates of DOPAE from the generator component uncontaminated by the reflection component (Long, Talmadge, & Lee, 2008).

3.13.1 Otoacoustic Emissions for Early Indication of Noise-induced Deterioration of the Cochlea

OAEs are useful in monitoring noise-induced deterioration of the cochlea if they can be measured initially or if there is enough room for recordable deterioration of OAEs (no floor effect). Significant reduction in DPOAEs obtained in half-octave bands centered at 1.4 to 6.0 kHz has been demonstrated following a 30-minute 85 dBC exposure to music in young adults in the absence of audiometric threshold shifts (Bhagat & Davis, 2008). In measuring noise levels, different types of weighting can be used including dBA or dBC. For description and use of such measures, refer to Rawool (2012). OAEs show reduction at more frequencies than audiometric thresholds, suggesting better sensitivity for detecting noise-induced damage (Helleman, Jansen, & Dresschler, 2010). Following impulse noise exposure, significant reduction in DPOAE amplitudes can occur in some ears with no changes in audiometric thresholds (Balatsouras et al., 2005). OAEs may also be useful in screening for susceptibility to noise-induced hearing loss, as individuals with low-level OAEs appear to be at a greater risk for noise-induced hearing loss (Job et al., 2009; Lapsley Miller, Marshall, Heller, & Hughes, 2006; Marshall et al., 2009).

3.13.2 Otoacoustic Emissions in Nonorganic Hearing Loss

If an individual suspected of nonorganic hearing loss has true thresholds that are within normal

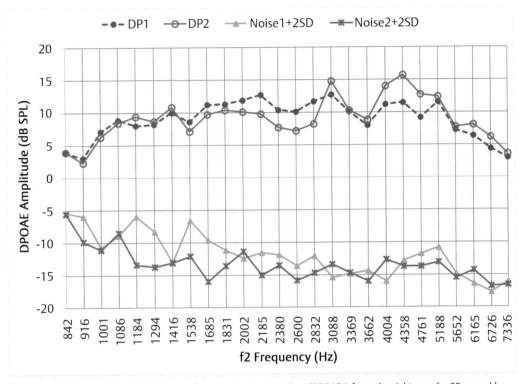

Fig. 3.40 Two recordings of distortion product otoacoustic emissions (DPOAEs) from the right ear of a 55-year-old woman with normal auditory sensitivity.

limits, OAE testing can quickly rule out hearing loss. ▶ Fig. 3.40 shows two test runs of DPOAEs from a 55-year-old woman using tones presented with an f1/f2 ratio of 1.22 at 65 and 55 dB SPL. The same data are shown in ▶ Fig. 3.41 for midoctave frequencies. At 2000 and 4000 Hz, a 9 dB DPOAE/ noise ratio is suggested as a criterion for assuming normal auditory sensitivity in older adults (Torre, Cruickshanks, Nondahl, & Wiley, 2003). Using this criterion, DPOAEs in ▶ Fig. 3.41 indicate normal sensitivity at 2000 and 4000 Hz. Application of the same strict criterion of +9 dB DPOAE/noise ratio (Dorn, Piskorski, Gorga, Neely, & Keefe, 1999; Gorga, Neely, & Dorn, 1999) to other frequencies also indicates normal sensitivity, ruling out the presence of a hearing loss.

DPOAEs are present in almost all normal ears and are absent in the presence of a sensory hearing loss of about 50 to 60 dB HL. Recording of OAEs in the presence of air conduction thresholds above 50 to 60 dB HL strongly suggests the presence of a nonorganic hearing loss, although in cases of auditory neuropathy spectrum disorder (see Chapter 15), OAEs can be normal.

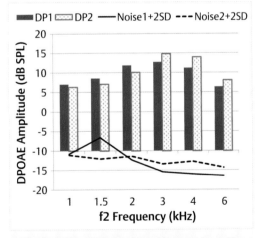

Fig. 3.41 DPOAE data from Fig. 3.40 plotted in half-octave bands.

In some noise-exposed workers, TEOAEs can be absent in the presence of normal audiometric thresholds due to subclinical cochlear damage (Attias et al., 1995; Prasher & Sulkowski, 1999). Even

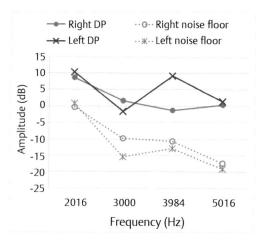

Fig. 3.42 DPOAEs plotted as a function of f2 in a child with unilateral neuropathy in the left ear. The child's unmasked auditory thresholds are shown in Fig. 3.28.

if OAEs may be present in a relatively small percentage of cases with noise exposure due to subclinical pathology, the objectivity of the test can encourage some patients with pseudohypacusis to yield more accurate air conduction thresholds following acoustic immittance and OAE tests (Balatsouras et al.; 2003; Kvaerner, Engdahl, Aursnes, Arnesen, & Mair, 1996).

3.13.3 Otoacoustic Emissions in Auditory Neuropathy Spectrum Disorders

As mentioned previously, normal OAEs are often recorded in the presence of audiometric hearing loss with auditory neuropathy spectrum disorder (ANSD), suggesting normal outer hair cell function in such cases. ► Fig. 3.42 shows the OAEs from a child with unilateral ANSD whose air conduction test results are shown in ► Fig. 3.28. Note the OAEs in the left ear in the presence of hearing loss. In such cases, acoustic reflexes are absent, or ARTs are elevated. For more information on ANSD, see Chapter 15.

3.13.4 Suppression of Otoacoustic Emissions with Contralateral Noise

In the presence of normal olivocochlear efferent function, OAEs are suppressed with the application of contralateral noise. When the efferent function is abnormal, OAE suppression is not observed. For a further description of the OAE suppression effect, see Chapter 6.

3.14 Future Trends

Many of the tests included in the peripheral audiological test battery are computerized. This includes automatic self-recorded audiometry, computerized presentation of speech materials, and automated response tracking. These procedures may further improve the delivery of stimuli and the accuracy of recording or responses. For ART testing, calibration of sound pressure levels in individual ear canals can improve test–retest reliability. More sophisticated signal-processing algorithms may improve the ability to detect auditory thresholds using OAEs and to more reliably record suppression of emissions with application of contralateral noise.

3.15 Review Questions

1. Why is it necessary to perform a peripheral audiological evaluation before conducting an auditory processing evaluation?
2. Discuss the various schemes used in classifying audiograms.
3. How do audiologists ensure a quiet test environment?
4. How do audiologists ensure that the audiometer is adequately calibrated? What is the purpose of the calibration?
5. List the potential sources of unreliable auditory thresholds.
6. What are the potential effects of linguistic and dialect differences on the results obtained with speech audiometry? How can you assess the English language proficiency of your patient?
7. Review the different purposes of documenting speech recognition scores in quiet.
8. Discuss the variables that can negatively affect speech recognition scores.
9. What are the potential effects of auditory nerve tumors, auditory neuropathy spectrum disorders, and auditory processing deficits on acoustic reflex thresholds?
10. What types of otoacoustic emission findings are expected in children with hearing loss due to auditory neuropathy spectrum disorder and individuals with nonorganic hearing loss?

APPENDIX A (adapted from Rawool, 2012a)

Identification

Name:_____

    Age: _____ Date of birth: _____ Gender: _____

    Employee number: _____ Job code: _____ Dept.: _____

    Occupation title: _____ Duration of current occupation: _____

    Second current job: _____

    Does the second job expose you to noise or other ototoxic substance exposure: _____

    Test date: _____ Test time: _____ Hours since last noise exposure: ___

    Test type: Baseline/periodic/exit

    Education: Highest level attained: _____

    Ethnicity: _____

    Native language: _____ Handedness: Left _____ Right _____

    If your native language is other than English, are you fluent in English? Yes _____ No ____

    If you are exposed to noise during work, provide the following information:

Noise exposure information

Noise monitoring results: _____ dB(A) TWA _____ % dose peak exposure levels: ____

Do you feel that you have temporary hearing loss at the end of the workday? (frequently, sometimes, no)

During the last week, were you exposed to
- a noise level over 85 dB(A) (not sure/yes/no/duration)
- noise with shocks or impulses (yes/no/duration)
- other disturbing noise (yes/no/duration)
- ultrasounds (yes/no/duration)
- Does noise interfere with your ability to work?

Do you have any hobbies that expose you to loud noises (loud music/band/concerts, hunting/shooting, motorcycles, car racing, other loud vehicles, using power tools, other) ?

_____

Have you ever been previously exposed to hazardous noise or other ototoxins in an occupational setting?

Yes _____ No _____

    If yes, where? Military service: _____

State any other occupation: _____

Hearing protection device use

Do you wear hearing protection devices during your current job?

Yes_____ No_____ Sometimes _____% of the time

Type of hearing protection worn: _____

Have you worn hearing protection devices during previous jobs with hazardous noise exposure? Yes _____

No _____ Sometimes ____%

Type of hearing protection worn: _____

Do you wear hearing protection devices during any recreational noise exposure?

Not applicable _____Yes _____ No_____ Sometimes _____% of the time

Type of hearing protection worn: _____

Occupational ototoxin exposure

Are you exposed to or have been exposed to the substances noted on the next page during work?

Have you been exposed to excessive heat during work? Yes _____ No _____

If yes, approximate % of time: _____

Have you been exposed to vibrations during work? Yes _____ No _____ Frequency _____

If yes, approximate % of time: _____

Medical history

Have you ever consulted an ear, nose, and throat specialist before? Yes _____ No _____

    Have you ever had ear surgery? Yes _____ No_____

Potential Ototoxin	Yes	No	Current Job	Current Second Job	Previous Job
Asphyxiant (carbon monoxide)					
Metals					
Arsenic					
Organic tin					
Mercury and derivatives					
Manganese					
Solvents					
Carbon disulfide					
Ethylbenzene					
n-propylbenzene					
n-hexane					
p-xylene					
Styrene or methylstyrenes					
Toluene					
Trichloroethylene					
Other chemicals					
Hydrogen cyanide					
Diesel fuel					
Kerosene fuel					
Jet fuel					
JP-8 fuel					
Organophosphate pesticides					
Chemical warfare nerve agents					
Radiation					

If yes, please list the date, the ear, and procedures, if known:

_____

Did you ever experience any of the following? If so, please state the duration and severity:

1. Earaches: Yes_____ No _____ Which ear(s) _____ Frequency _____ Severity _____
2. Draining in ears: _____
3. Noises, ringing, or buzzing in your ear(s): _____
   - Do you hear ringing or tinnitus at the end of the work-day? (frequently, sometimes, no)
   - How bothersome is your tinnitus? (highly, somewhat, minimally, not at all)
4. Dizziness (vertigo): _____
5. Nausea: _____
6. Chronic headaches: _____
   - Do you get headaches at the end of each workday? Yes _____ No _____
7. Concussion or severe blows on the head: _____
8. Mastoiditis: _____
9. Meningitis: _____

10. Pneumonia: _____

11. Frequent colds or respiratory infections: _____

12. Allergies: _____

13. Diabetes: _____

14. Heart disease: _____

15. High cholesterol: _____

16. Cerebrovascular disease: _____

17. Kidney problems: _____

18. Liver problems: _____

19. Hypothyroidism: _____

20. Hyperlipidemia: _____

21. Hypertension: _____

22. Stroke: _____

23. Arthritis: _____

24. Chronic lung disease: _____

25. Viral/bacterial infections: _____

26. Cancer: _____

27. Seizures: _____

28. White fingers (poor circulation of blood to fingers further aggregated by exposure to cold): _____

Did you ever use any of the following or any other medications over a prolonged period of time?

Aspirin: Yes _____ No _____

Diuretics: Yes _____ No _____

Chemotherapeutic agents: Yes _____ No _____

Aminoglycosides: Yes _____ No_____

Coumadin or other blood thinners: Yes _____ No _____

Did you ever use any other medications over a prolonged period of time?

If yes, please list the medications and their purposes: _____

Are you currently taking any medications regularly? Yes _____ No _____

If yes, please list the medications and their purposes: _____

Do you smoke? Yes _____ No _____ If yes, how frequently? _____

Do you use any other recreational drugs? Yes_____ No _____ If yes, how frequently? ___

How is your general health now? Good _____ Fair _____ Poor _____

Family history of hearing loss

Is there any history of hearing problems in your family? Yes _____ No _____

If yes, please describe who and the age of onset of hearing difficulties.

_____

How do you hear in the following situations?

Quiet: Good ___ Fair ____ Poor

Noisy: Good ___ Fair ____ Poor

How well do you understand conversation when someone is speaking at a fast or slow rate?

Fast rate: Good ___ Fair ____ Poor

Slow rate: Good ___ Fair ____ Poor

Hearing history

(Fill in this section, only if you think you have a hearing impairment.)

When did you first notice your problem? _____

In which ear? Right _____ Left _____ Both _____

Did the problem appear: Suddenly _____ Gradually with progression _____

How do you think your hearing problem started? _____

Hearing aid/assistive device use history

Fill in this section only if you have worn or currently wear hearing aids and/or assistive listening devices.)

Do you wear an aid or hearing aids now? Yes _____ No _____

Is your hearing aid satisfactory? Yes _____ No _____

How frequently do you wear your current aid(s)? _____

Have you worn another hearing aid in the past? Yes _____ No _____

How long have you been wearing the hearing aid(s)? _____

Do you use any other assistive listening device(s)? Yes ____ No _____

If yes, specify each and the satisfaction with each. _____

Rehabilitation history

Have you ever had speechreading training? Yes _____ No _____

Have you ever had auditory training? Yes _____ No _____

If you have had any other type of training to improve your communication, please describe:

Describe your current auditory difficulties and impact on personal and social life. If applicable, also describe how your hearing difficulties impact work or education.

References

[1] Allen, P., & Allan, C. (2007). Auditory processing disorders: Putting the neural back into sensorineural hearing loss. In R. C. Seewald & J. M. Bamford (Eds.), A sound foundation through early amplification. Stafa, Switzerland: Phonak.

[2] Allen, P., & Allan, C. (2014). Auditory processing disorders: Relationship to cognitive processes and underlying auditory neural integrity. International Journal of Pediatric Otorhinolaryngology, 78, 198-208.

[3] Al-Khatib, T., Cohen, N., Carret, A.-S., & Daniel, S. (2010). Cisplatinum ototoxicity in children, long-term follow up. International Journal of Pediatric Otorhinolaryngology, 74(8), 913–919.

[4] American Academy of Audiology Infection Control Task Force. (2003). Infection control in audiological practice. Audiology Today, 15, 12–19.

[5] American Academy of Otolaryngology–Head Neck Surgery (AAO-HNS). (1997). Otologic referral criteria for occupational hearing conservation programs. Alexandria, VA: AAO-HNS Foundation Inc.

[6] American National Standards Institute/Acoustical Society of America (ANSI/ASA). (2009). Methods for manual pure tone threshold audiometry, S3.21–2004 (R2009). New York: Author.

[7] American National Standards Institute (ANSI). (2010). ANSI S3.6-2010 (revision of ANSI S3.6–2004): American standard specifications for audiometers. New York: Author.

[8] American National Standards Institute/Acoustical Society of America (ANSI/ASA). (2008). ANSI/ASA S3.1–1999. (R 2008): Maximum permissible ambient noise levels for audiometric test rooms. New York: Author.

[9] American Speech-Language-Hearing Association (ASHA), Committee on Audiologic Evaluation. (1990). Guidelines for audiometric symbols. ASHA Supplnt, 32(2, Suppl), 25–30.

[10] American Speech-Language-Hearing Association. (1994). Audiologic management of individuals receiving cochleotoxic drug therapy [Guidelines]. Retrieved from http://www.asha.org/policy/GL1994-00003/.

[11] Attias, J., Furst, M., Furman, V., Reshef, I., Horowitz, G., & Bresloff, I. (1995). Noise-induced otoacoustic emission loss with or without hearing loss. Ear and Hearing, 16(6), 612–618.

[12] Attoni, T. M., Quintas, V. G., & Mota, H. B. (2010). Auditory processing, acoustic reflex and phonological expression. Brazilian Journal of Otorhinolaryngology, 76(6), 753–761.

[13] Balatsouras, D. G., Kaberos, A., Korres, S., Kandiloros, D., Ferekidis, E., & Economou, C. (2003). Detection of pseudohypacusis: A prospective, randomized study of the use of otoacoustic emissions. Ear and Hearing, 24(6), 518–827.

[14] Balatsouras, D. G., Tsimpiris, N., Korres, S., Karapantzos, I., Papadimitriou, N., & Danielidis, V. (2005). The effect of impulse noise on distortion product otoacoustic emissions. International Journal of Audiology, 44(9), 540–549.

[15] Bess, F. H., Josey, A. F., & Humes, L. E. (1979). Performance intensity functions in cochlear and eighth nerve disorders. American Journal of Otology, 1(1), 27–31.

[16] Bhagat, S. P., & Davis, A. M. (2008). Modification of otoacoustic emissions following ear-level exposure to MP3 player music. International Journal of Audiology, 47(12), 751–760.

[17] Boothroyd, A. (2008). The performance/intensity function: An underused resource. Ear and Hearing, 229(4), 479–491.

[18] Boothroyd, A., Erickson, F. N., & Medwetsky, L. (1994). The hearing aid input: A phonemic approach to assessing the spectral distribution of speech. Ear and Hearing, 15(6), 432–442.

[19] Carhart, R., & Porter, L. S. (1971). Audiometric configuration and prediction of threshold for spondees. Journal of Speech and Hearing Research, 14(3), 486–495.

[20] Chaiklin, J. B., & Ventry, I. M. (1965). Patient errors during spondee and pure tone threshold measurement. Journal of Auditory Research, 5, 219-320.

[21] Coles, R. R., Lutman, M. E., & Buffin, J. T. (2000). Guidelines on the diagnosis of noise-induced hearing loss for medicolegal purposes. Clinical Otolaryngology and Allied Sciences, 25(4), 264–273.

[22] Conn, M., Ventry, I. M., & Woods, R. W. (1972). Pure-tone average and spondee threshold relationship in simulated hearing loss. Journal of Auditory Research, 12, 234–239.

[23] Dean, M. S., & Martin, F. N. (2000). Insert earphone depth and the occlusion effect. American Journal of Audiology, 9 (2), 131–134.

[24] Dewey, G. (1923). Relative frequency of English speech sounds. Cambridge, MA: Harvard University Press.

[25] Dille, M. F., Konrad-Martin, D., Gallun, F., et al. (2010). Tinnitus onset rates from chemotherapeutic agents and ototoxic antibiotics: Results of a large prospective study. Journal of the American Academy of Audiology, 21(6), 409–417.

[26] Dirks, D. D., Kamm, C., Bower, D., & Betsworth, A. (1977). Use of performance-intensity functions for diagnosis. Journal Speech and Hearing Disorders, 42(3), 408–415.

[27] Dobie, R. A., & Rabinowitz, P. M. (2002). Change in audiometric configuration helps to determine whether a standard threshold shift is work-related. Spectrum, 19(Suppl 1), 17.

[28] Dorn, P. A., Piskorski, P., Gorga, M. P., Neely, S. T., & Keefe, D. H. (1999). Predicting audiometric status from distortion product otoacoustic emissions using multivariate analyses. Ear and Hearing, 20(2), 149–163.

[29] Downs, D. W., & Crum, M. A. (1980). The hyperactive acoustic reflex: Four case studies. Archives of Otolaryngology, 106 (7), 401–404.

[30] Dubno, J. R., Lee, F. S., Klein, A. J., Matthews, L. J., & Lam, C. F. (1995). Confidence limits for maximum word-recognition scores. Journal of Speech and Hearing Research, 38 (2), 490–502.

[31] Elliott, L. L., & Katz, D. (1980). Development of a new children's test of speech descrimination [technical manual]. St. Louis, MO: Auditec.

[32] Fausti, S. A., Henry, J. A., Helt, W. J., et al. (1999). An individualized, sensitive frequency range for early detection of ototoxicity. Ear and Hearing, 20(6), 497–505.

[33] French, N. R., Carter, C. W., Jr., & Koenig, W., Jr. (1930). The words and sounds of telephone conversations. Bell System Technical Journal, 9, 290–324.

[34] French, N. R., & Steinberg, J. C. (1947). Factors governing the intelligibility of speech sounds. Journal of the Acoustical Society of America, 19, 90–119.

[35] Gang, R. P. (1976). The effects of age on the diagnostic utility of the rollover phenomenon. Journal of Speech and Hearing Disorders, 41(1), 63–69.

[36] Gaskill, S. A., & Brown, A. M. (1990). The behavior of the acoustic distortion product, 2f1-f2, from the human ear and its relation to auditory sensitivity. Journal of the Acoustical Society of America, 88(2), 821–839.

[37] Gates, G. A., Cooper, J. C., Jr., Kannel, W. B., & Miller, N. J. (1990). Hearing in the elderly: The Framingham cohort, 1983–1985. Part I. Basic audiometric test results. Ear and Hearing, 11(4), 247–256.

[38] Gates, G. A., Feeney, M. P., & Higdon, R. J. (2003). Word recognition and the articulation index in older listeners with probable age-related auditory neuropathy. Journal of the American Academy of Audiology, 14(10), 574–581.

[39] Geers, A. E., & Moog, J. S. (1989). Evaluating speech perception skills: Tools for measuring benefits of cochlear implants, tactile aids, and hearing aids. In E. Owens & D. K. Kessler (Eds.), Cochlear implants in young deaf children (pp. 227–256). Boston: College-Hill Press.

[40] Gelfand, S. A. (1984). The contralateral acoustic reflex threshold. In S. Silman (Ed), The acoustic reflex: Basic principles and clinical applications (pp. 137–186). Orlando, FL: Academic Press.

[41] Gelfand, S. A. (2001a). Speech audiometry. In S. A. Gelfand (Ed.), Essentials of audiology (2nd ed.). New York: Thieme.

[42] Gelfand, S. A. (2001b). Nonorganic hearing loss. In S. A. Gelfand (Ed), Essentials of audiology (2nd ed., pp. 219–255). New York: Thieme.

[43] Gelfand, S. A., Schwander, T., & Silman, S. (1990). Acoustic reflex thresholds in normal and cochlear-impaired ears: Effects of no-response rates on 90th percentiles in a large sample. Journal of Speech and Hearing Disorders, 55(2), 198–205.

[44] Gorga, M. P., Neely, S. T., & Dorn, P. A. (1999). Distortion product otoacoustic emission test performance for a priori criteria and for multifrequency audiometric standards. Ear and Hearing, 20(4), 345–362.

[45] Gorga, M. P., Neely, S. T., Ohlrich, B., Hoover, B., Redner, J., & Peters, J. (1997). From laboratory to clinic: A large-scale study of distortion product otoacoustic emissions in ears with normal hearing and ears with hearing loss. Ear and Hearing, 18(6), 440–455.

[46] Guthrie, L. A., & Mackersie, C. L. (2009). A comparison of presentation levels to maximize word recognition scores. Journal of the American Academy of Audiology, 20(6), 381–390.

[47] Hannley, M., & Jerger, J. (1981). PB rollover and the acoustic reflex. Audiology, 20(3), 251–258.

[48] Hart, R. G., Gardner, D. P., & Howieson, J. (1983). Acoustic tumors: Atypical features and recent diagnostic tests. Neurology, 33(2), 211–221.

[49] Haskins, H. (1949). A phonetically balanced test of speech discrimination for children. Unpublished master's thesis, Northwestern University, Evanston, IL.

[50] Helleman, H. W., Jansen, E. J. M., & Dreschler, W. A. (2010). Otoacoustic emissions in a hearing conservation program: General applicability in longitudinal monitoring and the relation to changes in pure-tone thresholds. International Journal of Audiology, 49(6), 410–419.

[51] Hoffman, H. J., Ko, C. W., Themann, C. L., Dillon, C. F., & Franks, J. R. (2006). Reducing noise-induced hearing loss (NIHL) to achieve U.S. healthy people 2010 goals. American Journal of Epidemiology, 163(Suppl), S122-S122. Abstract retrieved from http://aje.oxfordjournals.org/content/163/suppl_11/S1.full.pdf + html.

[52] Humes, L. E., Tharpe, A.M., & Bratt, G. W. (1984). Validity of hearing thresholds obtained from the rising portion of the audiogram in sensorineural hearing loss. Journal of Speech and Hearing Research, 27(2), 206–211.

[53] Jahner, J. A., Schlauch, R. A., & Doyle, T. (1994). A comparison of American Speech-Language Hearing Association guidelines for obtaining speech-recognition thresholds. Ear and Hearing, 15(4), 324–329.

[54] Jerger, J., & Hayes, D. (1977). Diagnostic speech audiometry. Archives of Otolaryngology, 103(4), 216–222.

[55] Jerger, J., & Jerger, S. (1971). Diagnostic significance of PB word functions. Archives of Otolaryngology, 93(6), 573–580.

[56] Job, A., Raynal, M., Kossowski, M., et al. (2009). Otoacoustic detection of risk of early hearing loss in ears with normal audiograms: A 3-year follow-up study. Hearing Research, 251(1-2), 10–16.

[57] Kolinsky, D. C., Hayashi, S. S., Karzon, R., Mao, J., & Hayashi, R. J. (2010). Late onset hearing loss: A significant complication of cancer survivors treated with cisplatin containing chemotherapy regimens. Journal of Pediatric Hematology and Oncology, 32(2), 119–123.

[58] Konrad-Martin, D., Helt, W. J., Reavis, K. M., et al. (2005). Ototoxicity: Early detection and monitoring. ASHA Leader. Retrieved from http://www.asha.org/Publications/leader/2005/050524/050524b.htm.

[59] Konrad-Martin, D., James, K. E., Gordon, J. S., et al. (2010). Evaluation of audiometric threshold shift criteria for ototoxicity monitoring. Journal of the American Academy of Audiology, 21(5), 301–314, quiz 357.

[60] Kuk, F., Lau, C. C., Korhonen, P., Crose, B., Peeters, H., & Keenan, D. Development of the ORCA nonsense syllable test. Ear and Hearing, 31(6), 779–795.

[61] Kvaerner, K. J., Engdahl, B., Aursnes, J., Arnesen, A. R., & Mair, I. W. (1996). Transient-evoked otoacoustic emissions: Helpful tool in the detection of pseudohypacusis. Scandinavian Audiology, 25(3), 173–177.

[62] Lapsley Miller, J. A., Marshall, L., Heller, L. M., & Hughes, L. M. (2006). Low-level otoacoustic emissions may predict susceptibility to noise-induced hearing loss. Journal of the Acoustical Society of America, 120(1), 280–296.

[63] Lehiste, I., & Peterson, G. E. (1959). Linguistic considerations in the study of speech intelligibility. Journal of the Acoustical Society of America, 31, 280–286.

[64] Lenhardt, M. L. (1981). Childhood central auditory processing disorder with brainstem evoked response verification. Archives of Otolaryngology, 107(10), 623–625.

[65] Long, G. R., Talmadge, C. L., & Lee, J. (2008). Measuring distortion product otoacoustic emissions using continuously sweeping primaries. Journal of the Acoustical Society of America, 124(3), 1613–1626.

[66] Lonsbury-Martin, B. L., & Martin, G. K. (1990). The clinical utility of distortion-product otoacoustic emissions. Ear and Hearing, 11(2), 144–154.

[67] Lutman, M. E., & Coles, R. R. A. (2009). Asymmetric sensorineural hearing thresholds in the non-noise-exposed UK population: A retrospective analysis. Clinical Otolaryngology, 34(4), 316–321.

[68] Mahoney, C. F., & Luxon, L. M. (1996). Misdiagnosis of hearing loss due to ear canal collapse: A report of two cases. Journal of Laryngology and Otology, 110(6), 561–566.

[69] Marian, V., Blumenfeld, H. K., & Kaushanskaya, M. (2007). The Language Experience and Proficiency Questionnaire (LEAP-Q): Assessing language profiles in bilinguals and multilinguals. Journal of Speech, Language, and Hearing Research, 50(4), 940–967.

[70] Marshall, L., Lapsley Miller, J. A., Heller, L. M., et al. (2009). Detecting incipient inner-ear damage from impulse noise with otoacoustic emissions. Journal of the Acoustical Society of America, 125(2), 995–1013.

[71] Mauermann, M., Uppenkamp, S., van Hengel, P. W., & Kollmeier, B. (1999). Evidence for the distortion product frequency place as a source of distortion product otoacoustic emission (DPOAE) fine structure in humans: 2. Fine structure for different shapes of cochlear hearing loss. Journal of the Acoustical Society of America, 106(6), 3484–3491.

[72] McBride, D., & Williams, S. (2001). Characteristics of the audiometric notch as a clinical sign of noise exposure. Scandinavian Audiology, 30(2), 106–111.

[73] Meyer, D. H., & Mishler, E. T. (1985). Rollover measurements with Auditec NU-6 word lists. Journal of Speech and Hearing Disorders, 50(4), 356–360.

[74] Miltenberger, G. E., Dawson, G. J., & Raica, A. N. (1978). Central auditory testing with peripheral hearing loss. Archives of Otolaryngology, 104(1), 11–15.

[75] National Institute for Occupational Safety and Health (NIOSH). (1998). Criteria for a recommended standard: Occupational Noise Exposure–Revised Criteria 1998 (Pub. No. 98–126). Cincinnati, OH: Author.

[76] Navy and Marine Corps Public Health Center (NMCPHC). (2008). Navy and Marine Corps Public Health Center technical manual NMCPHC–TM 6260.51.99–2. Navy Medical Department Hearing Conservation Program procedures. Portsmouth, VA: Author.

[77] Neijenhuis, K., Tschur, H., & Snik, A. (2004). The effect of mild hearing impairment on auditory processing tests. Journal of the American Academy of Audiology, 15(1), 6–16.

[78] Neuwelt, E. A., & Brock, P. (2010). Critical need for international consensus on ototoxicity assessment criteria. Journal of Clinical Oncology, 28(10), 1630–1632.

[79] Nondahl, D. M., Shi, X., Cruickshanks, K. J., et al. (2009). Notched audiograms and noise exposure history in older adults. Ear and Hearing, 30(6), 696–703.

[80] Occupational Safety and Health Administration (OSHA). (1983). 29 CFR 1910.95 OSHA. Occupational noise exposure; hearing conservation amendment; final rule, effective 8 March 1983 (Fed. Reg. 48:9738–9785). Washington, DC: U.S. Department of Labor.

[81] Prasher, D., & Sułkowski, W. (1999). The role of otoacoustic emissions in screening and evaluation of noise damage. International Journal of Occupational Medicine and Environmental Health, 12(2), 183–192.

[82] Rawool, V. W. (1995). Ipsilateral acoustic reflex thresholds at varying click rates in humans. Scandinavian Audiology, 24(3), 199–205.

[83] Rawool, V. W. (1998). Effect of probe frequency and gender on click-evoked ipsilateral acoustic reflex thresholds. Acta Otolaryngologica, 118(3), 307–312.

[84] Rawool, V. W. (2012a). Hearing conservation: In occupational, recreational, educational, and home settings. New York: Thieme.

[85] Rawool, V. W. (2012b). Worker's compensation for noise-induced hearing loss and forensic audiology. In V. W. Rawool (Ed.), Hearing conservation: In occupational, recreational, educational, and home settings (pp. 242–265). New York: Thieme.

[86] Rawool, V. W. (2012c). Comprehensive audiological, tinnitus, and auditory processing evaluations. In V. W. Rawool (Ed.), Hearing conservation: In occupational, recreational, educational, and home settings (pp. 106–135). New York: Thieme.

[87] Redfors, Y. D., & Möller, C. (2011). Otosclerosis: Thirty-year follow-up after surgery. Annals of Otology, Rhinology, and Laryngology, 120(9), 608–614.

[88] Ross, M., & Lerman, J. (1970). A picture identification test for hearing-impaired children. Journal of Speech and Hearing Research, 13(1), 44–53.

[89] Schlauch, R. S., Arnce, K. D., Olson, L. M., Sanchez, S., & Doyle, T. N. (1996). Identification of pseudohypacusis using speech recognition thresholds. Ear and Hearing, 17(3), 229–236.

[90] Shaffer, L. A., Withnell, R. H., Dhar, S., Lilly, D. J., Goodman, S. S., & Harmon, K. M. (2003). Sources and mechanisms of DPOAE generation: Implications for the prediction of auditory sensitivity. Ear and Hearing, 24(5), 367–379.

[91] Shi, L. F. (2013). How "proficient" is proficient? Comparison of English and relative proficiency rating as a predictor of bilingual listeners' word recognition. American Journal of Audiology, 22(1), 40–52.

[92] Shi, L. F., & Canizales, L. A. (2013). Dialectal effects on a clinical Spanish word recognition test. American Journal of Audiology, 22(1), 74–83.

[93] Silman, S., & Silverman, C. A. (1991). Auditory diagnoses: Principles and applications. San Diego, CA: Academic Press.

[94] Stelmachowicz, P. G., Pittman, A. L., Hoover, B. M., & Lewis, D. E. (2001). Effect of stimulus bandwidth on the perception of /s/ in normal- and hearing-impaired children and adults. Journal of the Acoustical Society of America, 110(4), 2183–219.

[95] Studebaker, G. A., Sherbecoe, R. L., McDaniel, D. M., & Gwaltney, C. A. (1999). Monosyllabic word recognition at higher-than-normal speech and noise levels. Journal of the Acoustical Society of America, 105(4), 2431–2444.

[96] Talmadge, C. L., Long, G. R., Tubis, A., & Dhar, S. (1999). Experimental confirmation of the two-source interference model for the fine structure of distortion product otoacoustic emissions. Journal of the Acoustical Society of America, 105(1), 275–292.

[97] Texas Department of State Health Services. (2009). Infection control manual for ambulatory care clinics. Austin, TX: Author.

[98] Thorndike, E. L., & Lorge, L. (1944). The teacher's word book of 30,000 words. New York: Columbia University Press.

[99] Thornton, A. R., & Raffin, M. J. (1978). Speech-discrimination scores modeled as a binomial variable. Journal of Speech and Hearing Research, 21(3), 507–518.

[100] Tillman, T. W., & Carhart, R. (1966). An expanded test for speech discrimination utilizing CNC monosyllabic words: Northwestern University Auditory Test No. 6. (Tech. Rep. SAM-TR-66–55). Brooks AFB, TX: USAF School of Aerospace Medicine.

[101] Torre, P. III, Cruickshanks, K. J., Nondahl, D. M., & Wiley, T. L. (2003). Distortion product otoacoustic emission response characteristics in older adults. Ear and Hearing, 24 (1), 20–29.

[102] Yacullo, W. S. (1996). Clinical masking procedures. Needham Heights, MA: Allyn & Bacon.

[103] Yellin, M. W., Jerger, J., & Fifer, R. C. (1989). Norms for disproportionate loss in speech intelligibility. Ear and Hearing, 10 (4), 231–234.

Chapter 4

Screening and Diagnostic Procedures and Considerations

4 Screening and Diagnostic Procedures and Considerations

This chapter provides an overview of screening and diagnostic procedures. In addition, it reviews methods of selecting a test battery and variables that should be controlled or considered in administering and interpreting the test battery.

4.1 Case History

A careful case history can allow documentation of patient or parent concerns and provide guidance to the clinician for selecting an individualized test battery. The case history can also allow some insight into the possible causes of any processing deficits and offer documentation of the potential for other comorbid sensory deficits or disorders, such as attention deficit hyperactivity disorder (ADHD; see Chapter 13) or language-related disorders (see Chapter 14). An example of a case history form for adults is given in the appendix of Chapter 3. An example of a case history form designed primarily for children is shown in the appendix at the end of this chapter. The case history can be supplemented by a checklist to get an idea about specific auditory deficits, as seen in ▶ Table 4.1 and ▶ Table 4.2, and to document the impact of auditory processing deficits (APDs), as shown in ▶ Table 4.3. Note that a child can exhibit difficulties on the checklist in ▶ Table 4.3, but these difficulties can be caused by reasons other than APDs.

Clinicians may administer other questionnaires or complete additional checklists to document comorbid deficits or risks for other disorders due to APDs. For example, a child may have difficulty sustaining attention due to APDs. However, if the clinician suspects ADHD, checklists in Chapter 13 can be used. If the child is expected to be at risk for developing language delays or reading deficits or has comorbid language-related deficits (see Chapter 14), additional checklists can be used. An example of a checklist for children who are at risk for developing language-based reading disabilities is provided by Catts (1997). For older adults, several brief checklists or tools are available to document cognitive deficits (Lin, O'Connor, Rossom, Perdue, & Eckstrom, 2013).

4.2 Screening

Based on the case history, professionals, including speech-language pathologists, school nurses, social workers, educational psychologists, and pediatricians, may suspect the possibility of APDs and administer one of the screening procedures before referring a child for diagnostic testing. More research is needed on the sensitivity, specificity, and validity of some of these procedures. More specifically, the number of individuals who pass the screenings yet are found to have APD after diagnostic testing and those who are referred but are found to have no APD after diagnostic testing is still unknown.

4.2.1 Screening Questionnaires

Some of the screening instruments are questionnaires that are completed by the patient, parents, or teachers. These questionnaires are briefly described below. Detailed information can be found on the web by searching the name of each questionnaire.

Auditory Processing Domain Questionnaire

This scale attempts to assess listening skills, attention control, and language competencies of children in the age range of 7 to 17 years. The 52 items are divided into 4 categories: auditory processing, targeted auditory processing, attention control, and language (O'Hara, 2009).

Buffalo Model Questionnaire Revised (BMQ-R)

This questionnaire can be used for children ages 6 years and older, as well as adults. The 48 items included in the questionnaire are listed under 8 categories: decoding, noise, memory, various (includes attention, using language, ADHD, and anxiety), integration, organization, APD, and general. The general category includes items such as hypersensitivy to touch, eye contact with speaker, coordination, allergies, and math (Katz & Zalewski, 2011).

Children's Auditory Processing Performance Scale (CHAPPS)

CHAPPS, which comprises 36 questions, can be used for children 7 years and older. Teachers, parents, or older children can respond to the

Table 4.1 Checklist for Identifying the Possibility of an Auditory Processing Deficit

Auditory processing deficit characterized by scores < 3 in two or more of the following areas	Circle the number that corresponds to the best description of the individual person's (adult's or child's) behavior considering his or her developmental level.					

The person hears a sound but cannot see the source of the sound. One example is a cat meowing (or dog barking) outside the home. Another example is someone calling the person from out of sight. Can the person accurately tell where the sound is coming from?

Setting/ Observer	Never	Rarely	Some-times	Often	Always	Score
Home/parent or guardian	0	1	2	3	4	
School/teacher	0	1	2	3	4	
Any/self	0	1	2	3	4	

Average score for this question (binaural listening, localizing a sound source)

The person is in a crowded room with a lot of noise. Can the person ignore the noises and focus on someone talking to him or her?

Home/parent or guardian	0	1	2	3	4	
School/teacher	0	1	2	3	4	
Any/self	0	1	2	3	4	

Average score for this question (binaural interaction)

The person is watching TV. Someone enters the room and begins to talk to him or her. Can the person understand what is being said on the TV and understand what the person is saying without asking for repetition?

Home/parent or guardian	0	1	2	3	4	
School/teacher	0	1	2	3	4	
Any/self	0	1	2	3	4	

Average score for this question (stream segregation)

The person is in a room where there is a lot of noise. The noise could be due to several other people talking or music being played loudly. Someone begins to talk to the person. Can he or she understand what is being said without asking for repetition?

Home/parent or guardian	0	1	2	3	4	
School/teacher	0	1	2	3	4	
Any/self	0	1	2	3	4	

Average score for this question (spectrally degraded speech)

Someone is speaking very rapidly. Can the person understand the speaker without asking for repetition?

Home/parent or guardian	0	1	2	3	4	
School/teacher	0	1	2	3	4	
Any/self	0	1	2	3	4	

Average score for this question (temporally degraded speech)

Can the person clap hands in rhythm with songs or rhymes?

Home/parent or guardian	0	1	2	3	4	
School/teacher	0	1	2	3	4	

Table 4.1 continued

Auditory processing deficit character-ized by scores <3 in two or more of the following areas	Circle the number that corresponds to the best description of the individual person's (adult's or child's) behavior considering his or her developmental level.				
Any/self	0	1	2	3	4
Average score for this question (temporal pattern perception)					
Total auditory processing deficit score out of 24					

Table 4.2 Judging the Validity and Reliability of Ratings in Table 4.1

Do the assigned scores appear reliable? (Lack of too much discrepancy in the ratings assigned by different observers)	Y	N
Is there an overreporting bias as indicated by more than 3 "never" responses? Even individuals with auditory processing deficits are expected to sometimes respond well in difficult listening situations with the exception of those with auditory neuropathy spectrum disorders and hearing loss.	Y	N

Table 4.3 Auditory Processing Deficits Impact Questionnaire

Area of Assessment	Often	Sometimes	Rarely
Place a checkmark in the appropriate column to indicate the individual person's (adult's or child's) behavior considering his or her developmental level. Note that, although auditory processing deficits can lead to these behaviors, the behaviors can also occur in the absence of deficits.			
Makes errors in producing speech sounds			
Shows language delays			
Has reading difficulties			
Has writing difficulties			
Academic performance is lagging.			
Socialization is difficult.			
Has difficulty sustaining attention to verbal messages (e.g., stories)			
Responds slowly or with delay to verbal questions			
Makes errors in following oral instructions			
Has poor short-term memory			

questions using a seven-point Likert-type scale by comparing the child's listening skills to age-matched peers. The listening skills are rated in the presence of auditory and visual input, in quiet, in noise, and in ideal listening conditions. In addition, auditory memory sequencing skills and auditory attention span are evaluated. A total score is calculated, as well as scores for each condition. A study conducted by the authors of the scale demonstrated that children diagnosed with APD perform more poorly on this scale compared to age-matched peers (Smoski, Brunt, & Tannahill, 1992a,b).

Children's Home Inventory for Listening Difficulties: Parent and Student Versions (CHILD)

The parent version of this scale can be completed by caregivers or parents for children ages 3 to 12 years, and the child version can be completed by children ages 8 to 12 years. The scale includes questions focused on listening skills in various situations (Anderson & Smaldino, 2000).

Fisher's Auditory Problems Checklist

This checklist is for children ages 5 to 12 years. It includes 25 items on listening skills and related issues, such as attention. It is simpler to complete because it requires only the placement of a checkmark next to each item (Fisher, 1976).

Listening Inventories for Education (LIFE)

LIFE consists of three inventories: Student Appraisal of Listening Difficulty, Teacher Appraisal of Listening Difficulty, and Teacher Opinion and Observation List. The inventories can be used to document classroom listening situations that are challenging for the student and teacher's observations of the child's listening and learning behaviors. The student appraisal of listening difficulties is intended primarily for elementary school-aged children. To allow responses from children who are deficient in reading and writing skills, the stimulus items are picture based. Children can respond either verbally or by pointing to pictures. The revised LIFE-R inventories are appropriate for children ages 8 years and older. A French version of the LIFE-R is also available (Anderson & Smaldino, 1999).

Scale of Auditory Behaviors (SAB)

The SAB, which contains 12 questions, is intended to be used along with the Multiple Auditory Processing Assessment (MAPA) test battery. Parents or teachers can complete the questions, which address children's listening behaviors, academic difficulties, attention span, and organization skills. The scale can be used for children ages 8 to 11 years (Schow, Seikel, Brockett, & Whitaker, 2007).

Screening Checklist for Auditory Processing (SCAP)

This checklist covers 12 symptoms that are associated with APDs in children. The respondent places a checkmark next to each item that is applicable to the child (e.g., Has difficulty relating what is heard with what is seen). A score is then computed

by adding the checkmarks. A score of 6 or more on the SCAP suggests a risk for APD (Yathiraj & Maggu, 2013a).

Screening Instrument for Targeting Educational Risk (SIFTER)

SIFTER includes 15 questions that compare a child's performance to age-matched peers using a five-point scale. Areas covered are academics, attention, communication, class participation, and social behavior. A total score is calculated, in addition to the scores for each area. This questionnaire can be used for children in grades 1 through 5 or 6 (Anderson, 2004). The preschool version of SIFTER (Preschool SIFTER) is appropriate for children ages 3 to kindergarten. The Secondary SIFTER is appropriate for children in middle and high schools (Anderson & Matkin, 1996).

The Listening Inventory (TLI)

The Listening Inventory is designed for children between the ages of 4 and 17 years. Teachers or parents can complete the inventory by assigning a score on a scale of 0 to 5 for each statement. The statements are related to six areas: linguistic organization, decoding/language mechanics, attention/organization, sensory/motor, social/behavioral, and auditory processes. Index scores are derived for each area for comparison to criterion-based cutoff scores. According to the authors, the testing/scoring time is 15 minutes (Geffner & Ross-Swain, 2006).

4.2.2 Behavioral Screening Measures

Several screening measures and screening batteries are available. Some of these measures are discussed below.

Auditory Skills Assessment (ASA)

The ASA test (Geffner & Goldman, 2010) is designed to screen children ages 3 years, 6 months to 6 years and 11 years and can be administered in 5 to 15 minutes. A CD-ROM is used to present the stimuli. The following six listening tasks are included in the battery:
- Speech discrimination in babble: The test requires discrimination of speech sounds in words in the presence of background babble.

- Mimicry. This test requires repetition of spoken nonwords. Nonwords are constructed by grouping a string of English phonemes to sound like a word but have no meaning in English (e.g., dama).
- Rhyming: This test requires the listener to indicate if two words rhyme.
- Phoneme blending: This task requires the listener to say a word after presentation of phonemes.
- Tonal discrimination: This task requires the listener to indicate if two tones are from the same musical instrument.
- Tonal patterning: This task requires the listener to indicate which of the two tones was presented last.

Test of Auditory Perceptual Skills-3 (TAPS-3)

This test is administered with live voice and takes approximately 1 hour to administer. It has the following subsections: word discrimination, phonological segmentation, phonological blending, numbers forward, numbers reversed, word memory, sentence memory, auditory comprehension, and auditory reasoning. The test can be administered to children ages 4 to 19 years. The normative data for the test are based on more than 2000 listeners. An optional Auditory Figure-Ground task is included as a supplemental subtest presented via CD (Gardner, 2005).

Differential Screening Test for Processing (DSTP)

This screening instrument is designed to help professionals determine if diagnostic testing is necessary and the specific areas that should be addressed during diagnostic testing for children ages 6 to 12 years. The three levels of screened areas are acoustic, acoustic-linguistic, and linguistic. The subtests included in each of these three areas are shown in ▶ Fig. 4.1. The DSTP is administered via directions presented on a CD. The test examiner and the patient are required to wear headphones for the acoustic subtests. For the last subtest, eight picture cards are provided (Richard & Ferre, 2006).

SCAN-3

Different versions of this test are available for children and adults (Keith, 2009ab). Three tests are included in the screening portion of SCAN-3: gap detection, auditory figure-ground, and competing words–free recall (▶ Fig. 4.2).

- Gap detection: The gap detection task requires the listener to detect brief silent gaps of variable durations between tonal pairs. The listener is expected to indicate whether he or she heard one or two sounds. There are a total of 15 items, including 5 practice items. In the practice items, the gaps vary from 5 to 60 ms. In the test items, the duration of the gaps are 0, 2, 5, 10, 15, 20, 25, 30, and 40 ms. If the listener is able to hear two sounds for gaps less than 25 to 30 ms, he or she passes the task.
- Auditory figure-ground: The auditory figure-ground task is designed to screen the child's ability to understand words in the presence of multitalker babble, which is 8 dB softer than the target words. Two practice items and 20 test items are presented to each ear. The listener is expected to repeat the words. Cutoff criteria are provided for determining if the child passed the subtest in each ear.
- Competing words: The competing words subtest is a dichotic task in which two different words are simultaneously presented to each ear (e.g., right ear: dig; left ear: barn). The listener is expected to repeat both words in any order (free recall). Left and right ear and total scores are calculated. Cutoff criteria are provided for determining if the child passed the subtest.

Screening Test for Auditory Processing (STAP)

According to the developers (Yathiraj & Maggu, 2013b), this test battery takes approximately 12 minutes to administer and score. It includes four subtests for screening speech-in-noise perception, dichotic consonant-vowel (CV) perception, gap detection, and auditory memory (▶ Fig. 4.2). All subtests involving verbal stimuli are recorded in an Indian-English accent, thus making the test more applicable to listeners from India. However, there are several regional accents in India that could influence test outcomes. Further validation of this screening test is necessary.

- Speech-in-noise: The speech-in-noise subsection consists of 10 monosyllabic words presented monaurally in the presence of 8-talker English babble. To pass this subsection, the child needs to correctly repeat 6 of the 10 words.

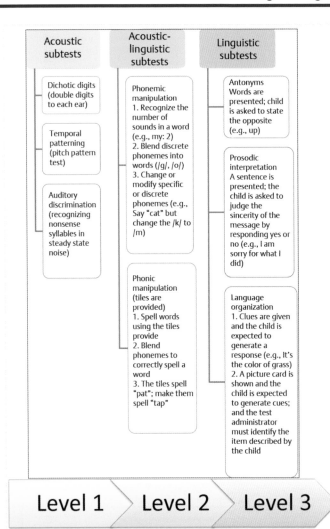

Fig. 4.1 Differential Screening Test for Processing (DSTP) (based on Richard & Ferre, 2006).

- Dichotic CV: The dichotic (different stimuli to each ear) CV pairs subsection consists of six CVs: /pa/, /ta/, /ka/, /ba/, /da/, and /ga/. Different pairs are presented simultaneously to each ear. To pass this subsection, the child needs to repeat four of the CVs presented to each ear correctly.
- Gap detection: The gap detection subtest consists of 12 test items, with 6 items presented to each ear. Each test item has a triad of 300 ms white noise, and one of the triads has a gap of 6 ms. To pass this subsection, the child needs to correctly identify the gaps in four of the six items presented to each ear.
- Auditory memory: The auditory memory section consists of four monosyllabic word sequences for a total of 16 words. To pass this subsection, the child needs to correctly repeat 12 of the 16 words.

4.2.3 Comparison of Screening Questionnaires and Behavioral Screening Measures

Yathiraj and Maggu (2013a) compared the results of the SCAP and STAP. A total of 400 children were screened using both measures. The SCAP was administered by teachers and the STAP, by audiologists. Out of the 400 children, 49 (12.3%) were considered to be at risk for APD based on SCAP results, and 64 (16%) were considered to be at risk using the STAP battery. A total of 31 children (7.75%) were considered to be at risk on both measures. In these children a significant correlation was noted between the SCAP and the auditory memory section of the STAP battery (Yathiraj & Maggu, 2013a). Such correlations can be expected

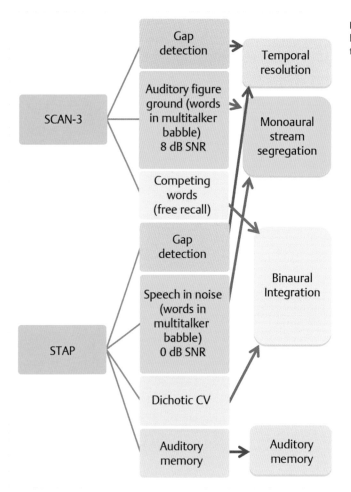

Fig. 4.2 Examples of screening test batteries and processes assessed by the subtests.

to depend on the specific questions included in the checklist and the specific tests in the screening test battery.

4.2.4 Validity of Screening Instruments

Many of the questionnaires outlined above have not been properly validated. Also, several of them require respondents to have an eighth-grade or higher reading level (Atcherson, Richburg, Zraick, & George, 2013). Complicating this is the level of knowledge and sophistication required of the respondents, who are usually the subjects' parents. A study by Yin et al. (2009) found that approximately 30% of parents in the United States have below-basic health literacy, and 68.4% are unable to correctly enter names and birth dates on a typical health insurance form. Thus, if parents are asked to complete APD questionnaires, they may not always understand the questions and may not wish to reveal that lack of understanding to clinicians. Asking the questions rather than having respondents complete a form may help, but the answers may be prone to interviewer bias.

Iliadoua and Bamioub (2012) investigated the clinical utility of CHAPPS in children around the age of 12 years. The scale was administered to 97 children. Diagnostic tests shown in ▶ Fig. 4.3 were administered to clinically referred children. The diagnosis of APD was based on poor performance on at least one of the verbal tests and two nonverbal tests shown in ▶ Fig. 4.3. Based on the diagnostic test batteries, referred children were assigned to APD and non-APD groups. The performance of the APD group was poorer than the non-APD group on the quiet, ideal, attention, and memory subscales of CHAPPS. The performance of the non-APD group was poorer than the performance of the normal-hearing group on the noise, multiple

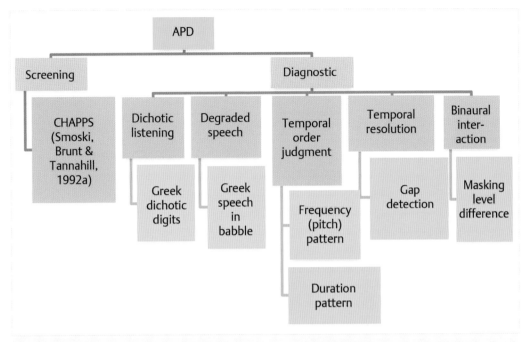

Fig. 4.3 Screening and diagnostic tests employed in the study conducted by Iliadou and Bamiou (2012). APD, auditory processing disorder.

inputs, and attention subscales. In addition, significant moderate to strong correlations were apparent between dichotic digits and duration pattern test results and the CHAPPS memory, attention, and total scores. The investigators concluded that CHAPPS may have clinical utility for detecting processing deficits in 12-year-olds.

Wilson et al. (2011) investigated the relationship between three tests used for screening for APD and four tests used in diagnosing the deficit (▶ Fig. 4.4) in children ranging in age from 6 to 14 years. They concluded that the CHAPPS, SIFTER, and TAPS-R can be useful in highlighting the concerns about a child but should not be used to determine the need for diagnostic evaluation. They found only weak to moderate correlations mainly between the short-term and working memory components of the TAPS-R test results and the dichotic digits and pitch pattern sequence test scores.

Lam and Sanchez (2007) investigated the sensitivity and specificity of four screening tests (▶ Fig. 4.5) by administering diagnostic tests to 23 children ranging in age from 7 to 10 years referred for auditory processing evaluations. They concluded that the competing sentence test from the SCAN-A (Keith, 1994) battery is practical with relatively low cost and ease of use. In addition, a cutoff

score for the left ear of 4 out of 10 correct responses yields a sensitivity of 89% and a specificity of 61%. Note that their diagnostic test battery included only dichotic listening tests, as shown in ▶ Fig. 4.5.

Based on factor analyses of SCAN (Keith, 1986), Domitz and Schow (2000) concluded that test batteries have better sensitivity and specificity than single screening tests.

4.3 Diagnoses

A test battery is usually used for diagnosing APDs. The tests included in the battery can be divided into three major domains: temporal processing (see Chapter 5), binaural processing (see Chapter 6), and degraded speech (see Chapter 7). Each of these domains can in turn be divided into several different subcategories, as described in the relevant chapters. In selecting tests, clinicians should consider the age, gender, specific functional deficits, memory and attentional capabilities, and cultural and linguistic background of each individual. Clinicians use various approaches for selecting the tests in the test batteries, as shown in ▶ Fig. 4.6. Readers are encouraged to carefully review Chapters 5, 6, and 7 before selecting tests.

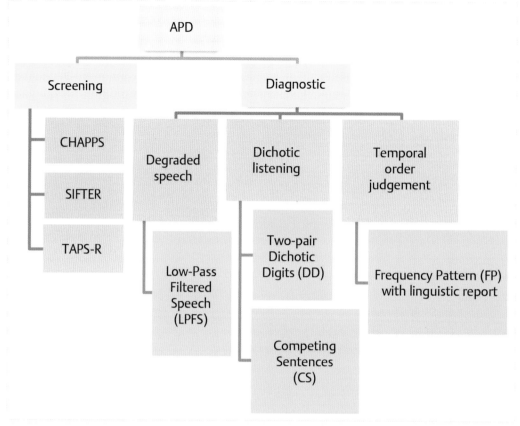

Fig. 4.4 Screening and diagnostic tests used by Wilson et al. (2011). APD, auditory processing disorder; CHAPS, Children's Auditory Processing Performance Scale; SIFTER, Screening Instrument for Targeting Educational Risk; TAPS-R, Test of Auditory Perceptual Skills-Revised.

4.3.1 Using Standard Test Batteries

Some investigators have compiled test batteries for ease of administration and scoring. In using the batteries, readers should note that some may place high demands on memory and may not necessarily tap into the specific APD experienced by each individual. A brief description of some of the test batteries is provided below. Detailed descriptions of the subtests and the auditory processing domains assessed by the subtests are provided in Chapters 5, 6, and 7.

Dutch Auditory Test Battery

This battery (Neijenhuis, Snik, Priester, van Kordenoordt, & van den Broek, 2002; Neijenhuis, Stollman, Snik, & Van der Broek, 2001) includes the tests shown in ▶ Fig. 4.7. The underlying processes assessed by the tests are also given in ▶ Fig. 4.7.

- Digit span: This task involves forward and backward recall of a series of digits.
- Dichotic digits: Digit triplets are presented simultaneously to both ears. The listener is expected to repeat the digits in any sequence (free recall).
- Categorical perception: This task requires the listener to identify and/or discriminate seven different stimuli derived from a continuum within a speech category (e.g., voice onset time).
- Words-in-noise: Monosyllabic words are presented in speech spectrum noise at signal-to-noise ratios of −2 and −5 dB. The noise is fixed at 65 dB sound pressure level (SPL) but is interrupted between words to minimize adaptation to the noise. The percentage of correctly repeated phonemes is calculated for each ear.
- Filtered speech: Filtered monosyllabic words with two frequency bands (a high pass band with a cutoff of 3000 Hz and a low pass band with a frequency cutoff of 500 Hz) are presented monaurally to each ear. The filter slope is 60 dB

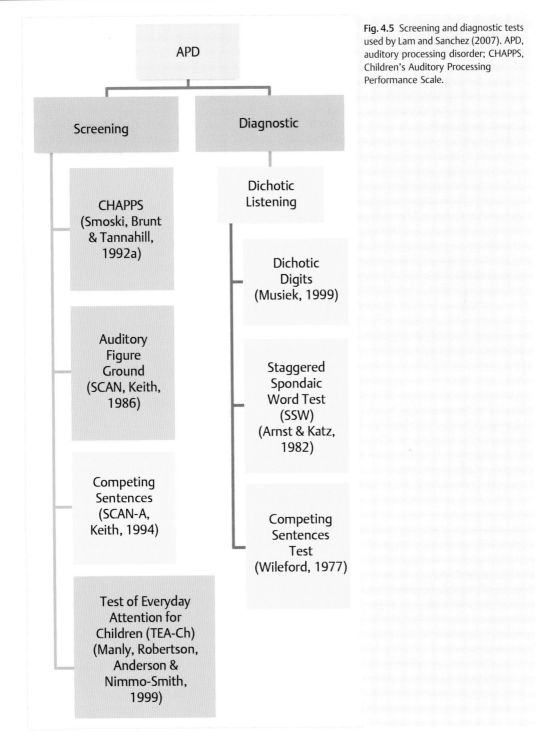

Fig. 4.5 Screening and diagnostic tests used by Lam and Sanchez (2007). APD, auditory processing disorder; CHAPPS, Children's Auditory Processing Performance Scale.

per octave. The percentage of correctly repeated phonemes is calculated for each ear.

- Binaural fusion: The same stimuli that are used in the filtered speech task are used in this task

except that the low pass band is presented to one ear and the high pass band to the other.

- Backward masking: Thresholds of a 20 ms 1000 Hz tone are determined adaptively in the

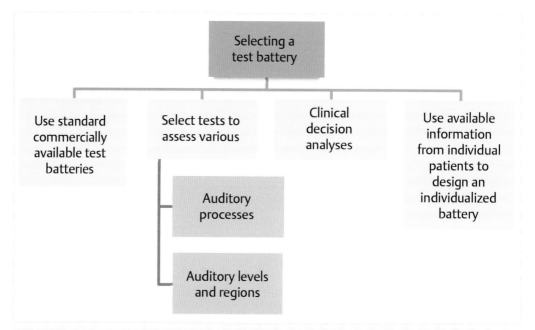

Fig. 4.6 Approaches used for determining tests to be included in a battery for assessment of auditory processing deficits.

presence of a 300 ms (600–1400 Hz centered on 1000 Hz) noise that immediately follows the tone. Although the backward masking task assesses a separate processing domain, the task lacks reliability because very few items are included in the test.

- Frequency pattern test: A series or sequences of three tones are presented with either low (880 Hz) or high (1122 Hz) frequencies. The duration of each tone is 150 ms, and the intertone interval is 200 ms. The percentage of correctly repeated sequences is then determined.
- Duration pattern test: A series of three tones are presented with either short (250 ms) or long (500 ms) duration tones. The interval between the tones is 300 ms. The percentage of correctly repeated sequences is then determined.
- Difference scores:
  ○ Binaural fusion versus monaural fusion of filtered speech: In both of these tasks, the common element is spectral closure to fill in the missing spectral information from approximately 500 to 3000 Hz. The difference score allows estimation of the efficiency of the binaural system to combine the information from the two ears. If the binaural fusion scores are

poorer than the monaural fusion scores, a binaural fusion deficit is suspected.
  ○ Right and left ear score difference on the dichotic digits task: This difference score allows the determination of any ear advantage or ear-specific deficit.

Multiple Auditory Processing Assessment (MAPA)

The MAPA test battery (Schow et al., 2007) includes five subtests and three supplemental subtests, as shown in ▶ Fig. 4.8. In addition to the following subtests, there are three supplemental tests on the MAPA CD: the duration patterns test, speech-in-noise test, and auditory fusion test (revised) for determining gap detection thresholds for clicks.

- MAPA Tap Test: In the Tap subtest, a series of taps are presented to the listener, and the listener is expected to report the number of taps heard after each series. The interstimulus interval between taps is 120 ms. Individuals with slower temporal processing may miss some of the taps and report fewer taps.
- MAPA Pitch Pattern Test: The test is similar to the pitch pattern test described in Chapter 5.

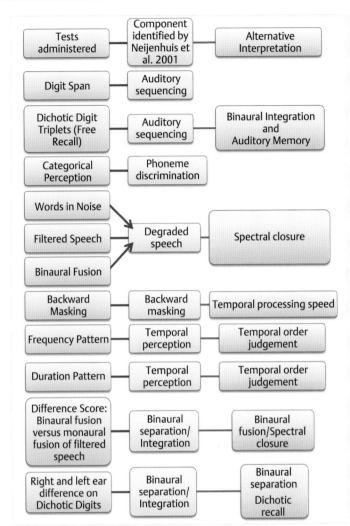

Fig. 4.7 Example 1 of auditory processing deficit components emerging from factor analyses (Neijenhuis et al., 2001).

However, each series has four stimuli (high-high-low-high) instead of the commonly used three stimuli. Only two frequencies referred to as high and low tones are used for each series. Four stimuli are used in each series instead of three to minimize ceiling effects. Reversals (e.g., stimulus: high-high-low-high; response: low-low-high-low) are considered accurate to minimize floor effects. The four-tone sequence may be more demanding on memory than the three-tone sequence.

- MAPA Dichotic Digits: This test is similar to the dichotic digits test described in Chapter 6. Three pairs of digits are presented to each ear, and the listener is asked to repeat the digits presented to the right ear first, then those in the left ear.

Double digits to each ear require the recall of four digits after the presentation of each series, whereas the presentation of triple digits requires the recall of six digits. Thus, due to the presentation of triplets to each ear, demands on auditory memory are expected to be greater.

- MAPA Competing Sentence Test: In this subtest, two sentences are presented simultaneously to each ear, and the listener is expected to repeat both sentences in a directed recall task. The listener is asked to repeat what is heard in the right ear first, then the left ear, or vice-versa.

MAPA administration and scoring time: According to Schow et al. (2007), the test takes approximately 21 minutes to administer and 5 minutes to score.

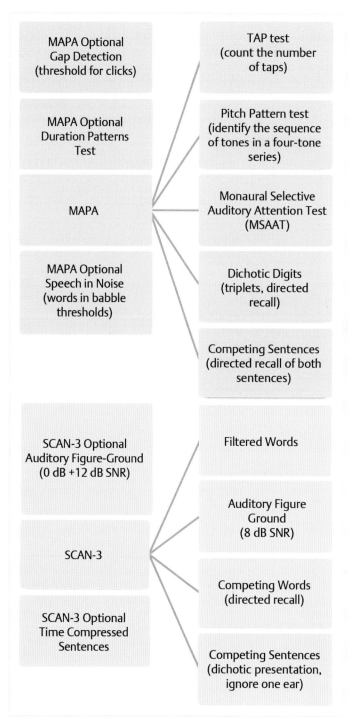

Fig. 4.8 Examples of diagnostic test batteries.

Obscure Auditory Dysfunction (OAD) Test Battery

Individuals with OAD have more difficulty understanding speech in noise than what is expected based on their pure tone thresholds. The patients also have difficulty learning to read or write during childhood. Similar findings can be seen in some individuals with APDs and those with auditory neuropathy spectrum disorder (ANSD, see Chapter 15). The test battery (Higson, Haggard, & Field, 1994; Saunders, Field, & Haggard, 1992) is described here as an example of how test selection and derived measures can be influenced by assumptions underlying the auditory deficit. The OAD test battery includes the following:

- OAD interview questionnaire: This questionnaire has three subsections. The first section includes general biographical questions, the second is designed to elicit general health information, and the third is related to specific symptoms and circumstances of auditory difficulties.
- Disability impact questions: Three questions related to the impact of auditory difficulties are taken from another hearing questionnaire (Lutman, Brown, & Coles, 1987): "(1) How often does any hearing problem you may have restrict your enjoyment of social and personal life, compared to others around you? (2) Do you get a feeling of being cut off from things because of difficulty in hearing? and (3) Do any difficulties you may have lead to embarrassment?" The response choices are never, rarely, quite often, and very often. The highest possible score is 12. A score of 6 or more indicates severe impact of the auditory deficit.
- Pseudo-free-field speech-in-noise test: This test includes the Bamford-Kowal-Bench (BKB, Bench, Kowal & Bamford, 1979) sentences (BKB sentences are based on natural language samples elicited from partially hearing impaired children), which are recorded in a sound-damped environment on an acoustic mannequin (dummy head), which makes them sound as though they are heard in a free field when presented through headphones (Gatehouse, 1989). The sentences are presented with a fixed level of white noise (65 dB SPL) and the level of the sentences is varied to determine the level necessary to recognize approximately 50% of the speech signal in two conditions: 1. Performance speech recognition threshold in noise (PSRTN): The listener is expected to repeat as much as each sentence as he or she hears. The audiologist determines the minimum sentence presentation level necessary

to achieve 50% recognition (e.g., PSRTN = 44 dBHL). (2) Self-assessed speech recognition threshold in noise (SSRTN): The listener guides the tester to adjust the presentation level of the sentences to allow the patient to "just understand all that is said." (e.g., SSRTN = 52 dBHL) The discrepancy in the results of the PSRTN and the SSRTN (e.g., PS-DIS = 52-44 = 8 dB) can suggest a deficit. Note that this task involves recognition of degraded speech.
- Dichotic listening test: In this test, two words are presented simultaneously to each ear. The listener is asked to focus attention on one ear and repeat any words in one of the following two categories: the semantic category of "food and drink items" and the phonetic category of words beginning with a given letter. Only words with unique phoneme-grapheme correspondence are used. Complex spellings, such as the word *psychological,* are excluded. This is a binaural separation task with a relatively high linguistic load.
- Masked thresholds for pure tones: In this test, the threshold for a 2 kHz tone is determined in the presence of a spectrally notched wide-band (0–8 kHz) noise centered at 2 kHz. The width of the notch is 1.2 kHz. This measure is expected to reflect the combined role of general sensory processing efficiency and frequency resolution.

SCAN-3

The SCAN-3 diagnostic test battery (Keith, 2009a, b) has four subtests, as shown in ▶ Fig. 4.8. In addition, the SCAN-3 CD has three optional tests: auditory figure-ground with 0 and 12 dB signal-to-noise ratio and time-compressed sentences.

- Auditory Figure-Ground + 8 dB: The test includes monosyllabic words that are presented in the background of multitalker babble at a signal-to-noise ratio of 8 dB.
- Filtered Words: This subtest includes monosyllabic words that are low-pass filtered using a frequency cutoff of 750 Hz. Spectral closure is required for successful performance on this task.
- Competing Words–Directed Ear: In this test, words are presented simultaneously to both ears, and the listener is asked to repeat the words in the specified order (e.g., right ear first, then left).
- Competing Sentences: In this test, two sentences are presented simultaneously to each ear, and the listener is expected to repeat the sentences in one ear and ignore those presented to the other.

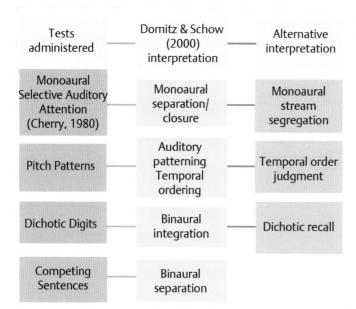

Tests administered	Domitz & Schow (2000) interpretation	Alternative interpretation
Monoaural Selective Auditory Attention (Cherry, 1980)	Monoaural separation/ closure	Monoaural stream segregation
Pitch Patterns	Auditory patterning Temporal ordering	Temporal order judgment
Dichotic Digits	Binaural integration	Dichotic recall
Competing Sentences	Binaural separation	

Fig. 4.9 Example 2 of auditory processing deficit components emerging after factor analyses (Domitz & Schow, 2000).

4.3.2 Considering Processes, Levels, and Regions Assessed by the Tests to Compile the Battery

The American Speech-Language-Hearing Association (ASHA, 2005) has recommended inclusion of tests in the battery that allow assessment of different auditory processes and different levels and regions of the central auditory system.

Examples of different processes are temporal resolution, temporal order judgment, binaural interaction, and binaural fusion. Some investigators have used a factor analytic approach to determine the major auditory processing components. The identified components vary depending on the specific tests used in the investigation. Examples of different components identified in various investigations are shown in ▶ Fig. 4.7 and ▶ Fig. 4.9.

The levels of the auditory system are the auditory nerve, brainstem, midbrain, and cortex. The regions are the left versus right auditory cortices and the corpus callosum.

As described in Chapters 5, 6, and 7, a wide variety of tests are possible. If too many tests are administered to a patient, however, the statistical probability of the patient yielding abnormal test results in the absence of a deficit increases. In addition, the administration of many tests does not guarantee that the patient's specific deficit will be identified. Similarly, if only one or two tests are administered, the patient's specific deficit may be

missed. A better approach is to use available information about the patient from various sources and carefully select a few tests. If the results show discrepancy in various measures, additional tests can be administered to guide in the selection of deficit-specific training.

4.3.3 Using Clinical Decision Analysis to Select the Test Battery

The term *clinical decision analysis* (CDA) refers to a systematic analytical approach to allow the best possible clinical decisions. At least in theory, CDA can lead to the selection of the most effective test batteries. CDA evaluates data to determine the relative presence and absences of disorders and whether or not the test results are positive or negative. The key terms related to CDA are described below:

Clinical Decision Matrix

A matrix similar to that shown in ▶ Table 4.4 is generally used during CDA.

If a person with an auditory processing deficit is identified as having a disorder, this is considered a true positive (TP), or a "hit." If the same person is determined by a test as not having the disorder, this is considered a false negative (FN), or a "miss." In other words, the test missed the correct identification of the disorder. Minimizing false-negative

Table 4.4 Matrix for Clinical Decision Analyses

Test Results	Does the person actually have the disorder?		Total Number
	Yes	No	
Positive, indicating presence of disorder	True positive (TP)/hit	False positive (FP)/false alarm	Total test positive
Negative, indicating absence of the disorder	False negative (FN)/miss	True negative (TN)/ correct rejection	Total test negative
	Total patients with the disorder	Total individuals without the disorder	Total sample

results is important when the disorder can have serious effects, such as social isolation in older adults and language delays, reading deficits, and poor academic performance in children.

If a person does not have a disorder, but the test results indicate the presence of one, this is referred to as a false positive (FP). Minimizing false-positive results is considered important when the costs of intervention are relatively high, and the impact on life of the disorders is relatively low. If the test results indicate the absence of a disorder when the person does not have the disorder, this is referred to as a true negative (TN), or correct rejection.

In addition to the above terms, the terms *sensitivity* and *specificity* are usually used to describe the accuracy of tests.

Sensitivity

Sensitivity refers to the probability that a test will correctly identify those with a particular disorder. It is calculated using the following equation:

$$\text{Sensitivity} = \frac{TP}{P} \times 100 = \left[\frac{TP}{(TP + FN)} \right] \times 100$$

where *TP* is the number of indviduals with the disorder yielding true positive results, *P* is the total number of individuals with the disorder evaluated using the test, and *FN* is the number of individuals with false negative results. For example, let us assume that a test is administered to a total of 50 individuals who are known to have auditory processing disorders, the test results are positive (true Positive or TP) for 40 of the patients and negative (false negative or FN) for 10 of the individuals. In this case, the sensitivity is [(40/50) × 100] = 80%.

Specificity

Specificity refers to the probability that a test will correctly reject those who do not have a particular disorder. It is calculated using the following equation:

$$\text{Specificity} = \frac{TN}{N} \times 100 = \left(\frac{TN}{(TN + FP)} \right) \times 100$$

where *TN* is the number of normal individuals yielding true negative results, *N* is the total number of normal individuals evaluated, and *FP* is the number of individuals with false positive results. For example, if we assume that an APD test is administered to 50 normal individuals who do not have any auditory processing disorders, the test results are negative (true negative or TN) in 45 of these individuals and positive (false positive or FP) in 5 of the patients, then the specificity is [(45/50) × 100] = 90%.

The sensitivity and specificity of a test can vary with disease prevalence. Overall, lower specificity is expected in populations with higher prevalence of the disorder. A change in prevalence from the lowest to highest value can lead to a change in sensitivity or specificity from 0 to 40% (Leeflang, Rutjes, Reitsma, Hooft, & Bossuyt, 2013). The variation is probably partially related to the fact that the severity of a disorder can vary from mild to severe to profound in patients.

Positive Predictive Value

The positive predictive value (PPV) attempts to determine the probability that a person with positive test results actually has the disorder. In other words, if the person is in the TP cell in the matrix in ▶ Table 4.4, then what is the probability that the person actually belongs to the TP cell? This is calculated using the following equation:

$$\text{PPV} = \left[\frac{TP}{(TP + FP)} \right] \times 100$$

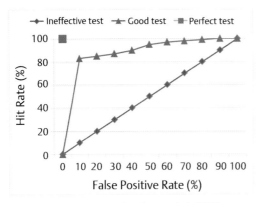

Fig. 4.10 Receiver operating characteristic (ROC) curves for three hypothetical tests.

where PPV is positive predictive value, TP is the number of individuals with true positive results, and FP is the number of individuals with false positive results.

In this case, the number of true positives are divided by the total number of positive results.

Negative Predictive Value

The negative predictive value (NPV) attempts to determine the probability that a person with negative test results actually does not have a particular disorder. The NPV is calculated using the following equation:

$$NPV = \left[\frac{TN}{(FN + TN)} \right] \times 100$$

where *NPV* is negative predictive value, *TN* is the number of individuals with true negative results, and *FN* is the number of individuals with false negative results.

In this case, the number of true negatives are divided by the total number of negative results.

PPV and NPV are also partially dependent on the prevalence of the disorder in the population that is being tested. If the selected population has a high prevalence of the disorder, the probability that the people who test positive actually have the disease is higher than if the test were performed on populations with low prevalence. Performing the same test on populations with a higher prevalence can increase PPVs and decrease NPVs.

Sensitivity, specificity, PPV, and NPV are often reported in test manuals. These values can be expected to differ depending on the populations used during the standardized procedures, the test conditions, and the test administrators.

Receiver Operating Characteristic Curves

When the test result scores yield ordinal or continuous values, several sensitivity and specificity values are possible, depending on the specific criteria used to determine a pass or refer outcome. For example, on the dichotic digits test, scores of 0 to 100% are possible for each ear. If 70% correct is used as a passing criterion for adults, the sensitivity and specificity can be different than when an 88% criterion is used for passing. If a criterion is selected to yield very high sensitivity, it can lead to low specificity.

The trade-off between sensitivity and specificity can be plotted on a graph called the receiver operating characteristic (ROC) curve. To plot the curve, the investigator selects several cutoff criteria and calculates the true- and false-positive rates for each selected criterion. The ROC curve is created by showing false-positive rates on the X-axis as a function of True positive or Hit rates on the Y-axis. An example of an ROC curve is shown in ▶ Fig. 4.10 for three hypothetical tests that yield test scores from 0 to 100% (e.g., speech recognition scores). The area under the ROC curve (A') ranges from 0.5 for tests with no diagnostic value to 1.0 for perfect tests. Thus, the area under the ROC curve summarizes the overall accuracy and can be used to compare various tests.

Applying Clinical Decision Analysis to Auditory Processing Test Selection

Some clinicians have applied CDA to determine the tests or test batteries that have the most efficacy and cost effectiveness. In one investigation (Singer, Hurley, & Preece, 1998), seven tests were administered to 90 children with normal learning and 147 children with a classroom learning disability (CLD). The children with CLD had normal speech and language skills but a history of reading difficulties and classroom learning problems identified through grade reports, teacher observations, and observations by speech-language pathologists and a psychologist. The following seven tests were administered in a sound-treated booth: binaural fusion, masking-level difference (MLD), filtered speech, time-compressed speech, dichotic digits, Staggered Spondaic Word (SSW), and the pitch pattern test. The hit rates from three of the tests are shown in ▶ Fig. 4.11. When hit rates, false-positive rates, and cost factors were considered,

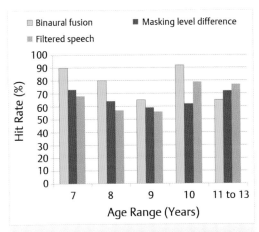

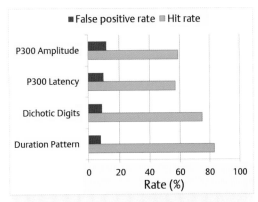

Fig. 4.11 Hit rates for the binaural fusion, masking level difference, and filtered speech tests in children with normal speech and language skills, a history of reading difficulties, and classroom listening difficulties. False-positive rates based on the performance of normal-hearing age-matched peers varied from 10 to 12% (based on Singer et al., 1998).

Fig. 4.12 Hit and false-positive rates for three tests using a population with lesions of the central auditory system and a normal-hearing control group (based on Hurley & Musiek, 1997).

the best test combination appeared to be either the binaural fusion and filtered speech tests or the binaural fusion and MLD tests. A CDA revealed that a combination of the binaural fusion and MLD tests would be the battery of choice for determining that a child with CLD has an auditory deficit when the test results are positive (Singer et al., 1998). This finding would apply for detecting APDs in children with CLD who have no speech and language delays, assuming that the seven tests administered were sufficient to track the major types of APDs. For example, the seven tests used in this investigation did not include any tests of temporal resolution (e.g., gap detection; see description under screening version of SCAN-3).

In another investigation (Hurley & Musiek, 1997), auditory processing tests were administered to three groups of participants: individuals with normal hearing (NH), those with sensorineural hearing loss (SNHL), and those with neurologically, radiologically, and/or surgically confirmed lesions of the central auditory nervous system (CANSLs). The tests under study were the dichotic digits, auditory duration pattern, and auditory evoked P300 potential. The hit rates for these tests are shown in ▶ Fig. 4.12. The duration pattern was the best overall test, with an A' of 0.93. The dichotic digits test revealed an A' of 0.90, and the P300 latencies revealed an A' of 0.84. The authors of the study cautioned against the generalization

of these results because all three tests were not administered to all of the participants, and the degree of lesions in listeners in the CANSLs was not controlled (Hurley & Musiek, 1997).

4.3.4 Synthesizing Patient-specific Information to Design a Test Battery

Information from the case history and checklists (▶ Table 4.1, ▶ Table 4.2, and ▶ Table 4.3) can suggest a probable cause and/or specific domain of APD. This information can be used to select a test battery. For example, for a child diagnosed with ANSD, temporal processing tests, including those that require the use of interaural timing cues (e.g., localization), are most likely to reveal APDs (see Chapter 15).

In compiling a test battery for a specific patient, the most important factor to consider is the specific complaint of the patient, parents, teachers, and significant others, as shown in the examples below. Often data are also available from questionnaires, evaluations, or screening instruments administered by other professionals, such as speech-language pathologists, psychologists, and pediatricians. These data can assist the audiologist in designing a test battery suitable for an individual child or adult. Some examples of such syntheses are presented below.

Case Example 1

The relevant information for this case is presented in ▶ Fig. 4.13. These findings suggest a phonology

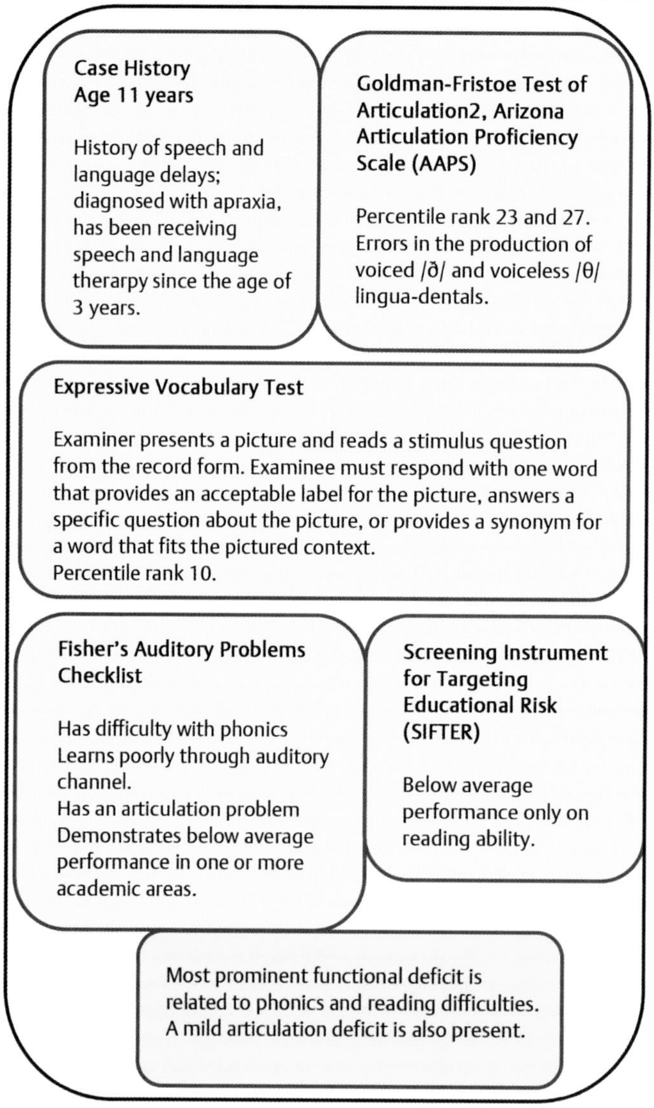

Fig. 4.13 Example of synthesis of information from various sources for a child with apraxia.

Case History Age 11 years

History of speech and language delays; diagnosed with apraxia, has been receiving speech and language therarpy since the age of 3 years.

Goldman-Fristoe Test of Articulation2, Arizona Articulation Proficiency Scale (AAPS)

Percentile rank 23 and 27. Errors in the production of voiced /ð/ and voiceless /θ/ lingua-dentals.

Expressive Vocabulary Test

Examiner presents a picture and reads a stimulus question from the record form. Examinee must respond with one word that provides an acceptable label for the picture, answers a specific question about the picture, or provides a synonym for a word that fits the pictured context. Percentile rank 10.

Fisher's Auditory Problems Checklist

Has difficulty with phonics Learns poorly through auditory channel. Has an articulation problem Demonstrates below average performance in one or more academic areas.

Screening Instrument for Targeting Educational Risk (SIFTER)

Below average performance only on reading ability.

Most prominent functional deficit is related to phonics and reading difficulties. A mild articulation deficit is also present.

problem. The available key information related to auditory processing is presented in ▶ Fig. 4.14. There is some discrepancy in the SCAN and DSTP test results probably because the SCAN was administered in a sound-treated booth, and the DSTP was administered in a therapy room. Overall, these results show no deficits in monaural sound segregation or dichotic listening measures, suggesting normal auditory processing capabilities. The most possible explanation for phonics and associated reading deficits is faulty mapping of oral sensory motor patterns (▶ Fig. 4.15), which can lead to reading difficulties noted on both the SIFTER and Fisher's auditory problem checklists (▶ Fig. 4.13). However, because the

child is referred for an auditory processing evaluation, the following tests could be useful in ruling out APDs.

Subjective Measures

- Gap detection thresholds for high-frequency stimuli, including 2000 and 4000 Hz: In children with language-related disorders, poor gap detection thresholds can occur at only higher frequencies.
- Temporal pattern sequence or duration pattern sequence: The child failed the DSTP pitch pattern task. Thus, it may be prudent to rule out a temporal sequencing deficit.

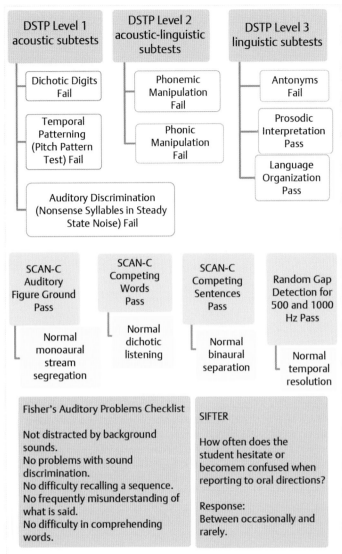

Fig. 4.14 Available information about auditory processing for the child with apraxia discussed in ▶ Fig. 4.13. DSTP, Differential Screening Test for Processing; SCAN-C, Test for Auditory Processing Disorders in Children.

- Binaural interaction: It will be useful to administer the MLD test to evaluate the ability of the two ears to work together.
- Spatial processing assessment: Although the child has performed well on the monaural segregation task, it may be useful to rule out a spatial processing deficit (see Chapter 6), which requires the use of two ears to separate target and background sounds.

Objective Measures

If this child is using top-down processing strategies to compensate for APDs, following objective measures may be useful.

- Temporal processing speed measure (see Chapter 5) to rule out slower processing
- Binaural summation (see Chapter 6) using acoustic reflex tests

Case Example 2

An 11-year-old boy was referred by his parents for listening difficulties in the classroom and poor academic performance in some subjects. The child was previously assessed using the SCAN battery and the random gap detection test with normal results. Upon inquiry, the child reported that he did not have listening difficulty with all of his teachers but only with some. When asked why he was

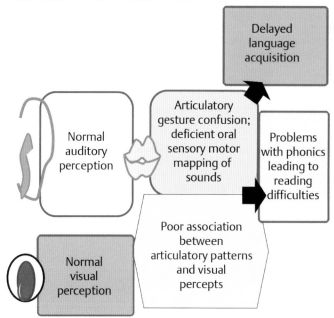

Fig. 4.15 Possible deficit area for the child with apraxia discussed in ▶ Fig. 4.13. Note that language acquisition is possible due to normal auditory perception, although it is delayed due to deficient oral sensory motor mapping of sounds.

having difficulty, he reported that some teachers appeared to speak at a very fast rate. This complaint suggests difficulty in processing rapid stimuli in the temporal domain. Thus, rate-induced facilitation (see Chapter 5) of the acoustic reflex was determined for the child. Most children show a minimum of 6 dB improvement in acoustic reflex thresholds (ARTs) with an increase in click rates from 50 to 100/s (see Chapter 5). In this case, a 10 dB improvement in thresholds was apparent in the right ear, but no improvement was apparent in the left ear. Although the right ear was showing normal temporal processing, the results of the left ear suggested either slower processing or a temporal integration deficit. Thus, for this child the auditory images from the right and the left ear may not be fused properly, leading to a blurred image of fast speech in a noisy and reverberant classroom. Such children can benefit from auditory training for the left ear, a frequency modulation (FM) device for the left ear in the classroom, and academic support for the specific subject where deficiencies are apparent.

Case Example 3

A 13-year-old girl was referred by her parents seeking a second opinion about her auditory difficulties. Previous tests at another clinic included the SCAN battery, the random gap detection test, ARTs, and the auditory brainstem response (ABR).

The child performed well on all behavioral tests. In addition, ARTs were within normal limits and all ABR peak and interpeak latencies were within normal limits. Additional advanced tests had ruled out any retrocochlear pathology. The previous test battery suggested that the girl does not have any deficit. However, the parents were concerned because the child continually increased the volume of TV at home to such an extent that even neighbors were complaining about the loudness. As a solution to this problem, the girl's parents purchased a new TV for the basement and instructed the child to watch the TV alone there. This arrangement allowed other family members to watch the TV at a normal volume in the living room. However, sometimes the TV was very loud in the basement and could be heard upstairs. The girl also reported difficulty in paying attention to teachers, and her educational performance was suffering.

In this case, although a test battery was administered, the child's auditory deficit was not captured. We suspected a temporal maintenance difficulty (see Chapter 5). Thus, tone decay, reflex decay, and suprathreshold adaptation tests (STAT; Jerger & Jerger, 1975) were performed. For a description of these tests, refer to Chapter 5. The testing revealed a marked decay during reflex decay testing only at 2000 Hz. The Carhart tone decay test results were within normal limits. However, the STAT results showed an inability to sustain the loud tones for a full minute at 500, 1000, and 2000 Hz. Note that, during reflex testing, the maintenance of reflex is expected over a period of 10 seconds, while during the STAT procedure, continuous response is expected over a period of 60 seconds.

The results were explained to the parents, and the child was asked to mute the TV temporarily when she felt that it was difficult to hear instead of turning up the volume. She was informed that louder sounds are more likely to appear to fade than softer sounds. The child reported that she perceived the classroom as being very noisy. Thus, an FM device was recommended in classroom settings for both ears, and the girl was informed to turn the device off momentarily when the sounds seemed to fade. These recommendations were successful in improving the child's academic performance and reducing the TV volume at home.

4.4 Objective Measures

Various objective measures, including acoustic reflex measures, otoacoustic emission suppression, and evoked potentials, can be used in assessing the central auditory system. Studies involving many of these measures are discussed in Chapters 5, 6, and 7.

4.4.1 Reasons for Including Objective Measures

There are several reasons for inclusion of objective measures in the auditory processing test battery, including the following:

- Objective measures are especially useful in ruling out the impact of cognitive variables on auditory test performance.
- For patients who are seeking special accommodations or monetary compensation, objective measures can strengthen the positive or negative results found during the testing (see Chapter 16).
- A combination of subjective and objective measures can guide in the selection of intervention approaches and better documentation of the effects of intervention.
- In some cases, only objective measures may be possible due to the young age of the patient or linguistic barriers.
- In some cases, objective measures are necessary to rule out serious pathologies, such as tumors, that need medical referrals.

4.4.2 Auditory Evoked Potentials and Fields

In response to sounds presented to ear(s), the auditory nervous system produces electrical signals or auditory evoked potentials and magnetic fields that can be picked up by surface electrodes placed on the head or magnetometers placed around the head. A brief description of some of the auditory evoked potentials and fields is presented here. Comparison of evoked potentials generated at various sites can allow for determination of the area of dysfunction. For example, a child may reveal a normal ABR but an abnormal middle latency response and slow cortical evoked potentials (Plyler & Harkrider, 2013). Several other types of evoked potentials can be recorded, including the steady-state evoked responses.

4.4.3 Auditory Brainstem Response

The response occurring within 7 to 8 miliseconds (msecs) following the stimulus onset is referred to as the auditory brainstem response if conventional averaging is used and the averaged waveform is displayed in the time domain. ABR relies on peak detection in a time-versus-amplitude plot. ABR amplitudes are measured in microvolts and ABRs can be elicited using clicks, tone bursts, or more complex stimuli such as speech.

The major peaks in the click- or tone-evoked ABR are labeled I to VII. Wave I is generated by portions of auditory nerve fibers closer to the inner hair cells, whereas wave II is generated by those closer to the brainstem. The other components have multiple contributions from the major auditory brainstem nuclei, including the cochlear nucleus, superior olivary complex, and inferior colliculus. These components probably reflect postsynaptic activity in major auditory brainstem nuclei. Click-evoked responses are assumed to reflect synchronous activation of onset-type neurons within the auditory system (reviewed in Hall, 1992).

Peripheral auditory sensitivity or threshold can be estimated by using the softest stimulus level at which wave V of the ABR is detected. The tonal ABR threshold in normal-hearing individuals is usually at 10 to 20 dB nHL (normal hearing level). In adults with sensorineural hearing loss, tone-evoked ABR thresholds are detected at 5 to 15 dB above behavioral thresholds (Stapells, 2002). The

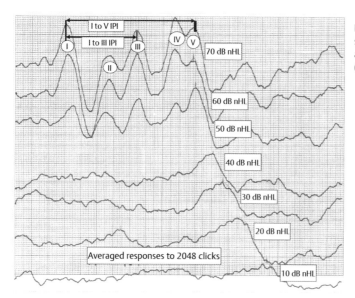

Fig. 4.16 Examples of auditory brainstem response (ABR) waveforms from a man with a normal auditory system (adapted from Rawool, 2012).

click-evoked ABR waveforms in ▶ Fig. 4.16 from a 29-year-old man suggest that he has hearing within normal limits, as wave V of the ABR is detectable at 10 dB nHL. In this case, ANSD and other retrocochlear pathologies can also be ruled out due to the presence of clear ABR waveforms from I to V and normal peak and interpeak latencies (I–III, III–V) at 70 dB nHL.

ABRs can be absent in the presence of auditory processing disorders (Lenhardt, 1981). Speech-evoked ABRs can be useful in assessing the processing of speech within the auditory brainstem and documenting effects of any intervention efforts (Anderson & Kraus, 2010).

4.4.4 Auditory Frequency Following Response

The frequency following response (FFR) is a sustained electrical potential that reveals precisely phase-locked responses of neural populations to low to midfrequency auditory stimuli. Human surface-recorded FFRs reflect phase-locked activity in neural elements in the rostral brainstem (Krishnan, 2007; Stillman, Crow, & Meshegian, 1978), including the cochlear nucleus, the lateral lemniscus, and the inferior colliculus. These responses encode critical speech features with marked selectivity to various sound sources. The responses are also amenable to top-down influences of attention to target stimuli. Age-related plasticity is also apparent in FFRs. The FFR may be useful

for investigating the "cocktail party" effect (Du, Kong, Wang, Wu, & Li, 2011), in which normal-hearing listeners can understand speech from a target speaker in the presence of several background noises, including speech from other talkers.

4.4.5 Auditory Middle Latency Response

As summarized in Rawool and Brouse (2010), auditory middle latency response (AMLR) is a far-field response that occurs between 10 and 90 ms following the onset of a transient auditory stimulus and can be recorded by placing electrodes on the scalp. The typical AMLRs in humans can be characterized by three negative (No, Na, Nb) and three positive (Po, Pa, Pb) components (Geisler, Frishkopf, & Rosenblith, 1958). Of these components, Pa is considered the most constant and reliable (Tucker & Ruth, 1996). It is also considered the most sensitive component for audiological assessments (Musiek & Geurkink, 1981). In adults, the Pa component occurs approximately 20 to 40 ms following stimulus onset (Jacobson & Grayson, 1988; Picton, Hillyard, Krausz, & Galambos, 1974). With moderately high-intensity stimuli of 70 to 75 dB nHL, Pa appears as a symmetric positivity over the central (Cz) and frontal (Fz) regions of the adult human scalp (Jacobson, 1994; Jacobson & Grayson, 1988; Jacobson & Newman, 1990). If the nasion is used as a reference electrode, Pa positivity appears to remain midline and symmetric regardless of the ear of stimulation (Jacobson & Grayson, 1988).

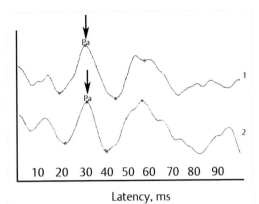

10 20 30 40 50 60 70 80 90

Latency, ms

Fig. 4.17 Examples of auditory middle latency responses from a young adult. The peak of Pa is marked. Waveform 1 was obtained without any contralateral noise. Waveform 2 was obtained with 30 dB normal hearing level (nHL) contralateral noise (adapted from Rawool & Brouse, 2010).

► Fig. 4.17 shows sample AMLR waveforms elicited with rarefaction clicks presented at 80 dB nHL, from one participant. The peak Pa is marked in the figure. Waveform 1 was obtained without any contralateral noise. Waveform 2 was obtained with contralateral noise of 30 dB nHL (Rawool & Brouse, 2010). The amplitude of the AMLR tends to be lower in children with APDs compared to their age-matched peers. Following an 8-week auditory training program, the amplitudes increase, suggesting that the AMLR can be useful in assessing auditory processing and documenting the benefits of intervention (Schochat, Musiek, Alonso, & Ogata, 2010).

Generator sources for the Pa waveform

There is some controversy about the generator sources of Pa (Cacace & McFarland, 2002). Portions of the primary auditory pathway, including the temporal lobe and thalamus, may contribute to the generation of the Pa waveform (Kaseda, Tobimatsu, Morioka, & Kato, 1991). Topographic studies (Cohen, 1982), magnetoencephalography source analyses (Borgmann, Ross, Draganova, & Pantev, 2001), and cortical recordings (Celesia & Puletti, 1969) also suggest that Pa is generated in the auditory cortex. However, Pa may be influenced by some deep midline brainstem generators (Cacace, Satya-Murti, & Wolpaw, 1990; Jacobson & Newman, 1990).

4.4.6 Late Evoked Potentials

These potentials are elicited later than the brainstem and middle latency responses with latencies greater than 80 ms. The responses can be elicited using various auditory stimuli. Several types of late responses can be elicited, including the P1-N1-P2 complex with latencies between 80 and 200 ms, the mismatch negativity (MMN) with latencies around 150-200 ms, and the P300 with latencies between 150 and 1000 ms (Stapells, 2002).

P1-N1-P2 is an obligatory response and can be recorded while allowing listeners to perform a quiet activity, such as watching a silent video during testing. This response is usually present in a healthy auditory system when subjects are awake, although developmental changes in morphology are apparent.

The MMN and the P300 are obtained with oddball paradigm presentations when a standard stimulus is presented frequently (80–90% of the time), and a deviant stimulus is presented rarely (10–20% of the time). The MMN response is automatic and does not require attention to the stimuli and thus is recorded in passive listening modes (Näätänen, Paavilainen, Rinne, & Alho, 2007).

During the recording of the P300, listeners are usually required to pay attention to the stimuli. For example, they can be asked to count the number of rare stimuli presented during the recording. This task requires them to discriminate between the rare (e.g., 1000 Hz tone bursts) and the frequently occurring (e. g., 500 Hz tone bursts) stimuli and to not respond to the frequent stimuli. The accuracy of the count of the rare stimuli can be used as an index of the amount of attention paid during the listening task.

The latencies of tone- and speech-evoked P300 responses are significantly delayed in children with specific language impairment compared to age-matched peers (Ors et al., 2002). Several other investigators have used late evoked potentials to assess auditory processing and relate such measures to speech perception. These studies are discussed in the chapters that follow.

4.4.7 Auditory-Evoked Magnetoencephalography

Magnetoencephalography (MEG) is a technique for mapping neural activity in the brain by recording magnetic fields produced by electrical currents. It allows direct assessment of neural events by recording the tiny magnetic signals generated from electrical currents traveling along activated

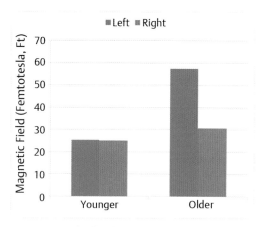

Fig. 4.18 Amplitudes (fT) of the M50 (P50m) response in younger (21–38 years) and older (56–84 years) adults elicited by presenting tone bursts to the right ear (based on Yamada et al., 2003).

neurons. The technique involves the use of highly sensitive magnetometers or gradiometers that are placed around the patient's head. A limitation of this technique is that any metal in the patient can distort the recorded signal.

The magnetic fields can be evoked by presenting auditory stimuli; such fields are referred to as auditory evoked fields (AEFs). Thus, AEFs are the magnetic counterpart of auditory evoked potentials. During the measurement of auditory evoked potentials, the electrical activity generated by neurons is recorded, while during the measurement of AEFs, the magnetic fields produced by the electrical activity are recorded.

The main generator sources of AEFs are the auditory and association cortices. The earliest cortical component of AEF is equivalent to the AMLR occurring between 30 and 50 ms after the stimulus onset. The early peaks are referred to as M30 and M50 and correspond to the Pa and Pb peaks of the AMLR. The amplitude of the contralateral M50 appears to enlarge with age, leading to an asymmetry between the right and left responses when the M50 is elicited by presenting tone bursts to the right ear (▶ Fig. 4.18). No such asymmetry is apparent in younger adults (Yamada et al., 2003). A possible reason for the enlargement of the contralateral M50 with aging is reduction of inhibitory feedback from the auditory cortex to the inferior colliculus and the medial geniculate body in the thalamus (Amenedo & Diaz, 1998). Other AEF responses are the M100, corresponding to the N1 peak of the auditory late response, which is frequently used in clinical applications. Later AEFs

are M150, M200, M300 (equivalent to P300), and M400. Some investigations incorporating AEFs are discussed in the chapters that follow.

4.4.8 Cortical Auditory Spectral Responses

The rhythmic electrical oscillations generated by the brain recorded using the electroencephalogram (EEG) can be divided into five frequency bands labeled using Greek letters. These bands are delta (δ), which includes frequencies less than 4 Hz; theta (θ), which includes frequencies from 4 to 7 Hz; alpha (α), with frequencies from 8 to 13 Hz; beta (β), with frequencies from 14 to 28 Hz; and gamma (γ), with frequencies above 29 Hz. These frequency bands are modulated by level of alertness (awake, drowsy, or asleep), sensory input, including auditory input, and cognitive tasks.

Speech Coding Due to Phase Locking in the Theta Range

Time–frequency analysis of single trials in response to standard speech stimuli (/ba/) with /da/ or /bi/ as deviant stimuli shows that the MMN results from phase synchronization of oscillations in the theta (θ)(4–7 Hz) band with less synchronization apparent in children than adults. The MMN appears to result from phase resetting in the theta frequency band rather than an increase in the power in the same band (Bishop & Hardiman, 2010; Bishop, Hardiman, & Barry, 2011). The M100 response elicited using MEG also reveals that in the presence of speech-shaped noise, low-frequency auditory cortical oscillations are consistently synchronized to the slow temporal modulations of speech even when the speech-to-noise ratio is relatively poor (Ding & Simon, 2013).

Gamma Band Responses and Auditory Processing

The gamma (γ) band can be further categorized as low gamma (30–60 Hz) and high gamma (60–150 Hz) due to functional and neurophysiological differences.

Low gamma contains phase-locked activity, such as the auditory steady-state response occurring at 40 Hz in response to auditory stimuli that are amplitude or frequency modulated at 40 Hz, including the FFR. Such phase-locked responses are obtained by averaging the responses in the time domain.

High gamma responses contain non-phase-locked components. If these responses are averaged in the time domain, they are invisible because the jitter in their latencies leads to cancellation of responses after averaging. Therefore, such spectral responses are recorded by averaging in the frequency domain (Gilley & Sharma, 2010). The temporal response is first transformed into the frequency domain through Fourier analysis, which decomposes the signal into sinusoidal component frequencies. The information about stimulus onset is preserved to allow comparison of the baseline pre- and post-stimulus EEG. Another type of analysis called wavelet transform allows transformation of the temporal waveforms into both the time and frequency domain.

Intracranial recordings of high gamma responses appear to be useful for assessing auditory processing (Cervenka, Nagle, & Boatman-Reicha, 2011). Robust gamma band responses in the range of 65 to 150 Hz are recordable within 50 to 120 ms following tonal onset. Maximum activity is apparent in the 75 to 110 Hz frequency range (Cervenka et al., 2013). Such gamma band responses appear to be useful in differentiating cortical areas associated with receptive and expressive speech processes in individual listeners. Tonal presentations lead to an increase in gamma band power in the primary auditory cortex, while presentation of words increases the gamma band power in the posterior temporal and parietal cortex. If the listener is asked to repeat the words, an increase in the gamma power is apparent in the lateral frontal and anterior parietal cortex (Towle et al., 2008).

4.5 Screening or Test Environment

When behavioral test batteries are administered in school environments, more children can show depressed scores compared to when the tests are administered in a sound-treated booth. The SCAN composite scores for six children obtained during school and audiometric booth administration are shown in ▶ Fig. 4.19 (Emerson, Crandall, Seikel, & Chermark, 1997). For tests that require listening to verbal or nonverbal stimuli in quiet or in the presence of noise, a sound-treated booth is preferred. The maximum permissible noise levels for audiometric testing are discussed in Chapter 3. The controlled background noise in such an environment along with presentation of stimuli via the audiometer allows more precise control over various parameters, including the signal-to-noise ratio and stimulus presentation levels. Precise

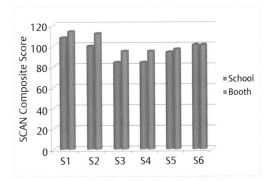

Fig. 4.19 SCAN composite scores for six participants during school and audiometric booth administration (based on Emerson et al., 1997).

documentation of deficits can improve diagnostic accuracy and allow better estimation of benefit following any intervention.

4.6 Equipment Calibration

Checking the calibration of audiometers on a daily basis is important for all tests (see Chapter 3). In addition, any CDs that are used for delivering stimuli should have calibration tones on them to allow precise control over presentation levels. Results of all auditory processing tests can vary greatly with variation in presentation levels. In addition, during dichotic tests, the administrator should ensure that the right and left channels are properly coupled to the right and left headphones and the right and left headphones are properly placed on the right and left ears. If errors are made, a right ear advantage may seem like a left ear advantage.

4.7 Test Reproducibility

As mentioned previously, test results can vary due to poor test environments or inadequate equipment calibrations. Test reproducibility can also vary depending on who is administering the test. An audiologist who is experienced in watching for patient fatigue or declining attention or false responses can get accurate results by controlling for these factors. An inexperienced audiologist may get different results due to the lack of sufficient controls. This can be referred to as interobserver variability. Some interobserver variability can exist even if two audiologists are equally experienced. Intraobserver variability refers to the difference in test results when the same administrator is administering the test at two different times. Tests that have low test–retest variability are preferred. Test–retest variability should also be considered when determining outcomes of intervention. A small improvement following intervention may not be a true improvement if it falls within the test –retest variability.

4.8 Patient Variables

Behavioral test results can be affected negatively by the lack of adequate attention, difficulty in sustaining attention through the test period, and fatigue. Patients should be carefully observed during test administration for signs of inattention or fatigue. A break period can be helpful for young children to control for both attention and fatigue. In addition, testing of young children should not be scheduled at the end of the school day given that they are more likely to be fatigued after school. Another strategy for controlling fatigue effects is to complete objective measures between different behavioral tests.

Motivation is another important factor to consider in administering tests. Poor motivation to complete the test can have a negative impact on outcomes. Children need to be verbally reinforced during tests by praising them for continuing to respond. In some adults, motivation to obtain an APD diagnosis may lead to exaggerated incorrect responses on some tasks. For example, one adult responded on the dichotic digits task by always replacing one of the four digits with 7. After he was informed that the digit 7 would never be presented and that when he is guessing, he should guess any other single digit, his performance was well within the normal range. The reasons to acquire a diagnosis of APDs can include special accommodation in educational or work settings or monetary compensation (see Chapter 16). Motivation can have a negative impact on the results of some objective tests given that the patient may not remain still during some procedures, such as acoustic reflex measures, which increases test –retest variability.

Overall health or medications can cause drowsiness in some patients. This is especially true for older adults. The evaluation should not be scheduled during nap periods for older adults. Participants should be told of the need for being fully awake during evaluations so that use of medications can be controlled when possible. Children with chronic otitis media (COM) may suffer from a general feeling of sickness during COM episodes, which can negatively affect test outcomes. If

possible, an evaluation should be performed when the child is feeling fairly well. It is also wise to postpone an evaluation if the child is suffering from sinusitis or another related condition until it is resolved.

Language competency can affect the results of tests that include speech stimuli requiring higher language competency. Some speech tasks, such as dichotic digits, do not require much language competency. For children who are suffering from language delays, nonverbal or objective tests should be administered to minimize the impact of a lack of language competency.

4.9 Consideration of Cultural/ Linguistic Background

In administering verbal subtests within a test battery, it is important to consider the linguistic background of the individual. Nonnative speakers can be expected to perform poorly on tests that are administered using stimuli in a nonnative language in the absence of any APDs. In addition, dialectal or accent differences can lead to poor performance. For example, published normative values for the SCAN and SCAN-C tests that are developed in the United States are not valid for direct application in the U.K. due to accent and word familiarity effects (Dawes & Bishop, 2007; Marriage, King, Briggs, & Lutman, 2001). Children in the United Kingdom show significantly worse performance on the filtered words and the auditory figure-ground subtests, and their composite scores are significantly worse. This can lead to higher false-positive rates unless correction values are applied to the normative values. Using speakers with local (e.g., British) accents may not always be an ideal solution due to regional variations in accents in each country (Dawes & Bishop, 2007).

4.9.1 Digit Triplet Test

For assessing speech perception in noise, the Digit Triplet Test (Smits, Kapteyn, & Houtgast, 2004) is available in several different languages, including British English (Hall, 2006), Dutch (Smits et al., 2004), French (Jansen, Luts, Wagener, Frachet, & Wouters, 2010), German (Zokoll, Wagener, Brand, Buschermöhle, & Kollmeier, 2012), Polish (Ozimek, Kutzner, Sek, & Wicher, 2009), Greek (HearCom deliverable D-1-6b, 2009), Swedish (Hällgren & Larsby, 2009), Russian, Turkish, and Spanish (Zokoll et al., 2013). The digit triplet test consists of the announcement "the digits" followed by digit triplets (e.g., 1–3-5) presented in a pseudo-random order in a background of speech spectrum noise. The listener is expected to select the correct digits heard using a number pad for automatic scoring. Thus, the test administrator does not need to be proficient in the selected language. All three digits have to be correct for a correct score on each item. The signal-to-noise ratio where half of the items (50%) are correct is determined using a one-up/one-down adaptive procedure. A total of 21 to 30 digit triplets are included in each list. One measurement lasts for about 3 to 6 minutes. The critical signal-to-noise ratios where 50% of the items are recognized correctly appear to vary somewhat depending on the language (Zokoll et al., 2013).

4.9.2 Matrix Test

The Matrix test (Hagerman, 1982) measures the patient's speech recognition threshold in quiet or noise using word scoring and an adaptive procedure. It is available in several languages, including British English (Hall, 2006), Danish (Wagener, Josvassen, & Ardenkjaer, 2003), French (Jansen et al., 2012), Polish (Ozimek, Warzybok, & Kutzner, 2010), Swedish (Hagerman, 1982), Spanish (Hochmuth et al., 2012), and Turkish (Zokoll et al., 2012). The test includes sentences that are difficult to predict (e.g., Karin gave two old buttons). The phoneme distribution corresponds to the specific language. The listener can repeat the stimuli for open format testing. However, if the audiologist is not familiar with the listener's native language, the test can be administered in a closed format. In this case, the 50 words included in the test are displayed on a computer screen, and the listener can select the words heard for automatic scoring.

4.9.3 Nonverbal and Objective Measures

A good solution for nonnative speakers is to rely heavily on nonverbal stimuli or to use highly familiar and very simple linguistic stimuli such as digits when necessary. In addition, if the instructions for response tasks are provided in English, the patient should be asked to restate what he or she is expected to do to ensure an understanding of the task. Objective measures using nonspeech stimuli can be useful in this context.

4.10 Interpretation of Test Results

All test results should be interpreted by compiling all available information and carefully following instructions in the test manuals. The results should be interpreted during the testing session to evaluate if other test measures are necessary. In addition, immediate interpretation allows an explanation of test results to the participants (or parents, in the case of children) following the session. Although a written report can be mailed to the parents following the session, parents may not always fully understand the results or implications. A face-to-face interpretation allows parents to ask questions for clarifications.

Test manuals should be carefully reviewed for interpretation, and the appropriate age norms should be applied. The cutoff criterion of worse than 2 standard deviations (SD) below the mean should be applied to both direct scores and difference scores. As previously mentioned, an example of a difference score is the difference between the scores from the right and left ears or the right ear advantage. For tests that do not yield normal distributions from normal-hearing populations, performance below the 10th percentile rank can be considered abnormal.

A score of worse than 2 SD below the mean in at least one ear on at least two different behavioral auditory processing tests has been suggested as a criterion for diagnosing APDs. Another recommendation is that if the performance on only one test is abnormal, it should be 3 SD below the normal limits (ASHA 2005). For tests that do not yield normal distributions from normal-hearing populations, performance below the 10th percentile rank in one of the tests or performance below the 25th percentile rank on two of the tests in the battery may be considered abnormal (Higson et al., 1994). Such interpretive criteria have limitations (Dillon, Cameron, Glyde, Wilson, & Tomlin, 2012). as shown in ▸ Table 4.5.

Besides using the results to reach a diagnosis, test results should be evaluated for patterns indicating areas showing strengths and weaknesses. Such patterns can help in selecting the areas and strategies for intervention. Certain patterns can also be useful in suggesting possible sites of lesion in central auditory pathways. It has been suggested that a pattern of poor performance across several tests in a test battery may be related to cognitive deficits (ASHA, 2005). The limitation of this interpretation is shown in ▸ Table 4.5.

Table 4.5 Limitations of criteria for Diagnosing an Auditory Processing Deficit or Interpreting Test Results

Criterion	Limitation	Example
Failure on more than one test in a test battery is necessary to diagnose APD.	The test battery may not include any test or may include only one test that is sensitive to the person's specific processing deficit.	A child may have a temporal maintenance deficit showing marked decay of temporal stimuli, but the test battery does not include a test of temporal maintenance.
If failure on only one test is used as a criterion, the performance of the individual should be 3 SD below the normal limits to diagnose APD	The battery may have only one test that is sensitive to the individual's specific processing deficit. Using a 3 SD criterion will require the person to have a profound deficit in the area.	A child may have only a dichotic listening deficit, and only one test in the battery may be designed to assess the deficit.
If a child shows deficit across several tests in a test battery, the deficit is more likely to be related to other issues, such as attention or memory deficits.	Tests in a test battery may be assessing the same underlying deficit that the child has.	All the tests in the test battery in ▶ Fig. 4.5 are designed to assess dichotic listening and binaural separation.
	Some basic processing deficits can have a negative impact on other test results unless proper controls are used.	A deficit on a gap detection (temporal processing domain) task can lead to difficulty in recognizing speech-in-noise and poor performance on auditory figure-ground task (degraded speech). The temporal resolution deficit apparent on the gap detection task may lead to poor performance on the masking level difference task (binaural interaction).

Abbreviations: APD, auditory processing deficit; SD, standard deviation.

4.11 Future Trends

Future studies are needed to explore several other auditory processing domains described in the following chapters on clinical populations. The outcomes of such studies are expected to refine available test batteries to allow the determination of specific processing deficits and their functional impact. The batteries will include both subjective and objective measures, including evoked potentials employing relatively cost-effective technologies that are becoming widely available. It may be possible in the future to extract auditory evoked high gamma activity from surface electrodes instead of intracranial electrodes due to application of improved signal-processing algorithms (Darvas, Rao, & Murias, 2013).

4.12 Review Questions

1. Discuss the importance of a case history in screening or diagnosing individuals who are suspected of having auditory processing deficits (APDs).

2. Review some screening questionnaires or checklists that have been used to screen individuals with APDs. How effective are such instruments in detecting individuals with APDs?

3. Review the checklist provided in ▶ Table 4.1 and ▶ Table 4.2. What types of underlying auditory processes are addressed by the questions on this checklist? Complete the checklist for a 6- or 7-year-old child with normal hearing. What are the results? How can you use the checklist in ▶ Table 4.3?

4. Review some behavioral screening test batteries used by clinicians. What aspects of auditory processes are included in these test batteries?

5. Discuss the various approaches used in selecting a diagnostic test battery for each patient. Which approach do you prefer? Why?

6. Review and compare some of the diagnostic test batteries. Assessments of which auditory processes are included in all test batteries?

7. Discuss the concepts of test sensitivity, specificity, positive predictive value, negative predictive value, and receiver operating

characteristic curves as they apply to clinical decision analyses for test selection.

8. Discuss the importance of including objective measures in a test battery. Briefly describe auditory evoked potentials and fields that can be used in assessing auditory processing skills.

9. Discuss several variables that can negatively impact test results. How can you control or accommodate for these variables?

10. Specify the procedures used in interpreting test results.

Appendix

Identifying information
Name: _____ Date of birth:_____ Age: ___
  Patient/parent/caregiver contact information: _____
  Handedness:
  Primary language spoken at home:
  Any other languages spoken by the patient:
  Competency of the patient/client in each language if more than one language is spoken at home:
  Age appropriate: Below age level:

Major concerns
  Specific auditory difficulties
  Specific communication difficulties
  When was the problem first noted?
  Family history (Place a checkmark where applicable. In case of family history, specify which member(s) is/are affected.)
  ___ Parents relatives before marriage
  ___ Family history of diabetes
  ___ Family history of kidney disease
  ___ Family history of thyroid problems
  ___ Family history of previous stillbirths or miscarriages
  ___ Family history of speech-language delays/disorders
  ___ Family history of reading difficulties
  ___ Family history of attention deficit hyperactivity disorder (ADHD)

Prenatal (during pregnancy) history
(Place a checkmark and specify the month of pregnancy where applicable.)
  ___ Rh immunoglobulin given
  ___ Rh or ABO incompatible
  ___ Amniocentesis
  ___ Bleeding
  ___ Anemia
  ___ Chickenpox exposure
  ___ Cytomegalovirus (CMV)
  ___ Diabetes
  ___ German measles or rubella exposure
  ___ Herpes virus
  ___ High blood pressure
  ___ Influenza
  ___ Measles exposure
  ___ Mumps exposure
  ___ Syphilis
  ___ Toxemia
  ___ Urinary infections
  ___ Other maternal illness (specify)

___ Medication (specify)
___ Smoking
___ Alcohol
___ Other recreational drugs (specify)
___ Exposure to radiation (provide details)
___ Chemical exposure (specify)
___ Trauma (specify)

Natal history
___ Not a full-term pregnancy (specify gestation age)
___ Induced pregnancy
___ Cesarean section
___ Asphyxia
___ Other (specify)

Newborn/postnatal period
___ Low birth weight (less than 5 lb or 2 kg) (specify)
___ Low APGAR score (specify)
___ Neonatal intensive care for more than 5 days
___ Breathing difficulties
___ Assisted ventilation
___ ECMO
___ High bilirubin levels (more than 15 mg/100 mL) requiring exchange transfusion
___ Congenital heart conditions
___ Congenital rubella
___ Congenital ear, nose, or throat defects (specify)
___ Other congenital defects (specify)
___ Paralysis
___ Seizures
___ Septicemia
___ Other medical conditions (specify)

Syndrome:
___ Neurofibromatosis
___ Osteopetrosis
___ Usher
___ Waardenburg
___ Alport
___ Pendred
___ Jervell and Lange-Nielson
___ Other (specify)

Neurodegenerative disorders:
___ Hunter syndrome
___ Other (specify)

Sensory motor neuropathy
___ Friedreich ataxia
___ Charcot-Marie-Tooth syndrome
___ Medications (e.g., gentamycin, tobramycin, furosemide, Lasix) (specify)
___ Chemotherapy

Infancy/childhood history
 ___ Vision problems (specify)
 ___ Balance/gait/dizziness problems (specify)
 ___ Cerebral palsy
 ___ Seizures
 ___ Auditory nerve or brain tumors
 ___ Head trauma/sports injuries to the head
 ___ Basal skull/temporal bone fractures requiring hospitalization
 ___ Swallowing/feeding difficulties (specify)
 ___ Meningitis
 ___ Encephalitis
 ___ Measles
 ___ Influenza
 ___ Rubella
 ___ Cytomegalovirus (CMV)
 ___ Chickenpox
 ___ Septicemia
 ___ Diabetes
 ___ Sickle cell disease
Current health (poor/fair/good/excellent):
Current medications:
Developmental milestones: Specify the age at which your child achieved the following milestones:
Sat alone:
Walked alone:
Showed stranger or separation anxiety:
Spoke first word:
Began to use two-word sentences:
Did the child seem to develop normally, but the development was interrupted? Yes/No
Specify possible reason: _____

Social development
How well does the child interact with family members and peers?

Known comorbid conditions
 ___ Attention deficit hyperactivity disorder (ADHD); specify type
 ___ Phonological disorders
 ___ Language delays/disorder
 ___ Reading deficits
 ___ Other

Educational performance
 How does the patient's educational performance compare to his or her peers?
 Does the patient perform poorly in any specific academic areas? Specify.
 Does the patient excel in any academic areas? Specify.
 Does the patient receive any special support services? Specify.
 Does the patient use any assistive listening technology? Specify.

Additional questions for adults:
Occupational performance: How is the patient's performance at work compared to coworkers? How do hearing difficulties affect performance? Are any assistive listening technologies being used?

Describe any previous intervention therapy efforts.

References

[1] Amenedo, E., & Díaz, F. (1998). Aging-related changes in processing of non-target and target stimuli during an auditory oddball task. Biological Psychology, 48(3), 235–267.

[2] American Speech-Language Hearing Association (ASHA). (2005). (Central) auditory processing disorders (No. TR2005–00043). Rockville, MD: Author. Retrieved from http://www.asha.org/docs/html/TR2005–00043.html.

[3] Anderson, K. (2004). Secondary Screening Instrument For Targeting Educational Risk (SIFTER). www.sifteranderson.com.

[4] Anderson, S., & Kraus, N. (2010). Sensory-cognitive interaction in the neural encoding of speech in noise: A review. Journal of the American Academy of Audiology, 21(9), 575–585.

[5] Anderson, K. L., & Matkin, N. (1996). Screening instrument for targeting educational risk in pre-school children (age 3 –kindergarten). Tampa, FL: Educational Audiology Association.

[6] Anderson, K., & Smaldino, J. (1999). Listening inventories for education: A classroom measurement tool. The Hearing Journal, 52(10), 74–76.

[7] Anderson, K. L., & Smaldino, J. J. (2000). Children's Home Inventory for Listening Difficulties (CHILD). Retrieved from http://www.phonakpro.com/content/dam/phonak/b2b/Pediatrics/Junior_Reports/Fitters/com_child_questionnaire_gb.pdf.

[8] Atcherson, S. R., Richburg, C. M., Zraick, R. I., & George, C. M. (2013). Readability of questionnaires assessing listening difficulties associated with (central) auditory processing disorders. Language, Speech, and Hearing Servives in Schools, 44 (1), 48–60.

[9] Bench, J., Kowal, A., & Bamford, J. (1979). The BKB (Bamford-Kowal-Bench) sentence lists for partially-hearing children. British Journal of Audiology, 13, 108-112.

[10] Bishop, D. V. M., & Hardiman, M. J. (2010). Measurement of mismatch negativity in individuals: A study using single-trial analysis. Psychophysiology, 47(4), 697–705.

[11] Bishop, D. V. M., Hardiman, M. J., & Barry, J. G. (2011). Is auditory discrimination mature by middle childhood? A study using time-frequency analysis of mismatch responses from 7 years to adulthood. Developmental Science, 14(2), 402–416.

[12] Borgmann, C., Ross, B., Draganova, R., & Pantev, C. (2001). Human auditory middle latency responses: Influence of stimulus type and intensity. Hearing and Research, 158(1-2), 57–64.

[13] Cacace, A. T., & McFarland, D. J. (2002). Middle-latency auditory evoked potentials: Basic issues and potential applications. In J. Katz (Ed.), Handbook of clinical audiology (5th ed. pp. 349-377). Philadelphia, PA: Lippincott, Williams & Wilkins.

[14] Cacace, A. T., Satya-Murti, S., & Wolpaw, J. R. (1990). Human middle-latency auditory evoked potentials: Vertex and temporal components. Electroencephalography and Clinical Neurophysiology, 77(1), 6–18.

[15] Catts, H. W. (1997). The early identification of language-based reading disabilities. Language, Speech, and Hearing Services in Schools, 28, 86–89.

[16] Celesia, G. G., & Puletti, F. (1969). Auditory cortical areas of man. Neurology, 19(3), 211–220.

[17] Cervenka, M. C., Franaszczuk, P. J., Crone, N. E., et al. (2013). Reliability of early cortical auditory gamma-band responses. Clinical Neurophysiology, 124(1), 70–82.

[18] Cervenka, M. C., Nagle, S., & Boatman-Reich, D. (2011). Cortical high-gamma responses in auditory processing. American Journal of Audiology, 20(2), 171–180.

[19] Cohen, M. M. (1982). Coronal topography of the middle latency auditory evoked potentials (MLAEPs) in man. Electroencephalography and Clinical Neurophysiology, 53(2), 231–23.

[20] Darvas, F., Rao, R. P. N., & Murias, M. (2013). Localized high gamma motor oscillations respond to perceived biologic motion. Journal of Clinical Neurophysiology, 30(3), 299–307.

[21] Dawes, P., & Bishop, D. V. M. (2007). The SCAN-C in testing for auditory processing disorder in a sample of British children. International Journal of Audiology, 46(12), 780–786.

[22] Dillon, H., Cameron, S., Glyde, H., Wilson, W., & Tomlin, D. (2012). An opinion on the assessment of people who may have an auditory processing disorder. Journal of the American Academy of Audiology, 23(2), 97–105.

[23] Ding, N., & Simon, J. Z. (2013). Adaptive temporal encoding leads to a background-insensitive cortical representation of speech. Journal of Neuroscience, 33(13), 5728–5735.

[24] Domitz, D. M., & Schow, R. L. (2000). A new CAPD battery—multiple auditory processing assessment: Factor analysis and comparisons with SCAN. American Journal of Audiology, 9(2), 101–111.

[25] Du, Y., Kong, L., Wang, Q., Wu, X., & Li, L. (2011). Auditory frequency-following response: A neurophysiological measure for studying the "cocktail-party problem." Neuroscience and Biobehavioral Reviews, 35(10), 2046–2057.

[26] Emerson, M. F., Crandall, K. K., Seikel, J. A., & Chermak, G. D. (1997). Observations on the use of SCAN to identify children at risk for central auditory processing disorder. Language, Speech, and Hearing Services in Schools, 28, 43–49.

[27] Fisher, L. I. (1976). Fisher auditory problem checklist. Cedar Rapids, IA: Grant Wood Area Educational Agency.

[28] Gardner, M. Y. (2005). Test of auditory processing skills–3. Austin, TX: Pro-Ed.

[29] Gatehouse, S. (1989). A pseudo free-field measure of auditory disability. British Journal of Audiology, 23(4), 317–322.

[30] Geffner, D., & Goldman, R. (2010). Auditory skills assessment. Mineapolis, MN: PsychCorp, Pearson.

[31] Geffner, D., & Ross-Swain, D. (2006). The listening inventory. Novato, CA: Academic Therapy Publications.

[32] Geisler, C. D., Frishkopf, L. S., & Rosenblith, W. A. (1958). Extracranial responses to acoustic clicks in man. Science, 128 (3333), 1210–1211.

[33] Gilley, P. M., & Sharma, A. (2010). Functional brain dynamics of evoked and event-related potentials from the central auditory system. SIG6. Perspectives on Hearing and Hearing Disorders: Research and Diagnostics, 14, 12–20.

[34] Hagerman, B. (1982). Sentences for testing speech intelligibility in noise. Scandinavian Audiology, 11(2), 79–87.

[35] Hall, J. W. III. (1992). Handbook of auditory evoked responses. Boston, MA: Allyn and Bacon.

[36] Hall, S. (2006). The development of a new English sentence in noise test and an English number recognition test (unpublished master's thesis). University of Southampton, U.K.

[37] Hällgren, M., & Larsby, B. (2009). The Swedish digit triplet test: Optimization and validation of broadband and telephone versions. Unpublished manuscript.

[38] HearCom deliverable D-1-6b. (2009). Development of a digit-triplet test in modern Greek. Retrieved from http://hearcom.eu/about/DisseminationandExploitation/deliverables/HearCom_D-1-6b_V2p.pdf.

[39] Higson, J. M., Haggard, M. P., & Field, D. L. (1994). Validation of parameters for assessing obscure auditory dysfunction—robustness of determinants of OAD status across samples and test methods. British Journal of Audiology, 28(1), 27–39.

[40] Hochmuth, S., Brand, T., Zokoll, M. A., Castro, F. Z., Wardenga, N., & Kollmeier, B. (2012). A Spanish matrix sentence test for assessing speech reception thresholds in noise. International Journal of Audiology, 51(7), 536–544.

[41] Hurley, R. M., & Musiek, F. E. (1997). Effectiveness of three central auditory processing (CAP) tests in identifying cerebral lesions. Journal of the American Academy of Audiology, 8(4), 257–262.

[42] Iliadou, V., & Bamiou, D. E. (2012). Psychometric evaluation of children with auditory processing disorder (APD): Comparison with normal-hearing and clinical non-APD groups. Journal of Speech, Language, and Hearing Research, 55(3), 791–799.

[43] Jacobson, G. P. (1994). Brain mapping of auditory evoked potentials. In J. Jacobson (Ed.), Principles and applications in auditory evoked potentials. Boston, MA: Allyn & Bacon.

[44] Jacobson, G. P., & Grayson, A. S. (1988). The normal scalp topography of the middle latency auditory evoked potential Pa component following monaural click stimulation. Brain Topography, 1(1), 29–36.

[45] Jacobson, G. P., & Newman, C. W. (1990). The decomposition of the middle latency auditory evoked potential (MLAEP) Pa component into superficial and deep source contributions. Brain Topography, 2(3), 229–236.

[46] Jansen, S., Luts, H., Wagener, K. C., Frachet, B., & Wouters, J. (2010). The French digit triplet test: A hearing screening tool for speech intelligibility in noise. International Journal of Audiology, 49(5), 378–387.

[47] Jansen, S., Luts, H., Wagener, K. C., et al. (2012). Comparison of three types of French speech-in-noise tests: A multi-center study. International Journal of Audiology, 51(3), 164–173.

[48] Jerger, J., & Jerger, S. (1975). A simplified tone decay test. Archives of Otolaryngology, 101, 403–407.

[49] Kaseda, Y., Tobimatsu, S., Morioka, T., & Kato, M. (1991). Auditory middle-latency responses in patients with localized and non-localized lesions of the central nervous system. Journal of Neurology, 238(8), 427–432.

[50] Katz, J., & Zalewski, T. (2011). Buffelo Model Questionnaire-Revised. Retrieved from http://www.audiologyisland.com/assets/CAPD-Questionnaire.pdf.

[51] Keith, R. W. (1986). SCAN: A screening test for auditory processing disorders. San Diego, CA: Psychological Corp.

[52] Keith, R. W. (1994). SCAN-A: A test for auditory processing disorders in adolescents and adults (2nd ed.). San Diego, CA: Psychological Corp.

[53] Keith, R. (2009a). SCAN-3: A tests for auditory processing disorders in adolescents and adults. San Antonio, TX: Pearson.

[54] Keith, R. (2009b). SCAN-3: C tests for auditory processing disorders for children. San Antonio, TX: Pearson.

[55] Krishnan, A. (2007). Frequency-following response. In R. F. Burkard, J. J. Eggermont, & M. Don (Eds.), Auditory evoked potentials: Basic principles and clinical application. Baltimore, MD: Lippincott, Williams & Wilkins.

[56] Lam, E., & Sanchez, L. (2007). Evaluation of screening instruments for auditory processing disorder (APD) in a sample of referred children. The Australian and New Zealand Journal of Audiology, 29, 26–39.

[57] Leeflang, M. M. G., Rutjes, A. W. S., Reitsma, J. B., Hooft, L., & Bossuyt, P. M. M. (2013). Variation of a test's sensitivity and specificity with disease prevalence. Canadian Medical Association Journal, 185(11), E537–E544.

[58] Lenhardt, M. L. (1981). Childhood central auditory processing disorder with brainstem. Arch Otolaryngol, 107(10), 623–625.

[59] Lin, J. S., O'Connor, E., Rossom, R. C., Perdue, L. A., & Eckstrom, E. (2013). Screening for cognitive impairment in older adults: A systematic review for the U.S. Preventive Services Task Force. Annals of Internal Medicine, 159(9), 601–612.

[60] Lutman, M. E., Brown, E. J., & Coles, R. R. (1987). Self-reported disability and handicap in the population in relation to pure-tone threshold, age, sex and type of hearing loss. British Journal of Audiology, 21(1), 45–58.

[61] Marriage, J., King, J., Briggs, J., & Lutman, M. E. (2001). The reliability of the SCAN test: Results from a primary school population in the UK. British Journal of Audiology, 35(3), 199–208.

[62] Musiek, F. E., & Geurkink, N. A. (1981). Auditory brainstem and middle latency evoked response sensitivity near threshold. Annals of Otology, Rhinology, and Laryngology, 90(3, Pt. 1), 236–240.

[63] Näätänen, R., Paavilainen, P., Rinne, T., & Alho, K. (2007). The mismatch negativity (MMN) in basic research of central auditory processing: A review. Clinical Neurophysiology, 118(12), 2544–2590.

[64] Neijenhuis, K., Snik, A., Priester, G., van Kordenoordt, S., & van den Broek, P. (2002). Age effects and normative data on a Dutch test battery for auditory processing disorders. International Journal of Audiology, 41(6), 334–346.

[65] Neijenhuis, K. A., Stollman, M. H., Snik, A. F., & Van der Broek, P. (2001). Development of a central auditory test battery for adults. Audiology, 40(2), 69–77.

[66] O'Hara, B. (2009). The Listening Questionnaire: A differential screening for auditory processing disorders. Retrieved from http://www.neuroaudiology.com/APDQ.pdf.

[67] Ors, M., Lindgren, M., Blennow, G., Nettelbladt, U., Sahlen, B., & Rosén, I. (2002). Auditory event-related brain potentials in children with specific language impairment. European Journal of Paediatric Neurology, 6(1), 47–62.

[68] Ozimek, E., Kutzner, D., Sek, A., & Wicher, A. (2009). Development and evaluation of Polish digit triplet test for auditory screening. Speech Communication, 51(4), 307–316.

[69] Ozimek, E., Warzybok, A., & Kutzner, D. (2010). Polish sentence matrix test for speech intelligibility measurement in noise. International Journal of Audiology, 49(6), 444–454.

[70] Picton, T. W., Hillyard, S. A., Krausz, H. I., & Galambos, R. (1974). Human auditory evoked potentials: 1. Evaluation of components. Electroencephalography and Clinical Neurophysiology, 36(2), 179–190.

[71] Plyler, E., & Harkrider, A. W. (2013). Serial auditory-evoked potentials in the diagnosis and monitoring of a child with Landau-Kleffner syndrome. Journal of the American Academy of Audiology, 24(7), 564–571.

[72] Rawool, V. W. (2012). Hearing conservation: In occupational, recreational, educational, and home settings. New York: Thieme.

[73] Rawool, V. W., & Brouse, M. V. (2010). Effect of contralateral noise on the click-evoked human auditory middle latency response. Hearing Review, 17(6), 24–27, 50–53.

[74] Richard, G., & Ferre, J. (2006). Differential screening test for processing. East Moline, IL: LinguiSystems.

[75] Saunders, G. H., Field, D. L., & Haggard, M. P. (1992). A clinical test battery for obscure auditory dysfunction (OAD): Development, selection and use of tests. British Journal of Audiology, 26(1), 33–42.

[76] Schochat, E., Musiek, F. E., Alonso, R., & Ogata, J. (2010). Effect of auditory training on the middle latency response in children with (central) auditory processing disorder. Brazilian Journal of Medical and Biological Research, 43(8), 777–785.

[77] Schow, R. L., Seikel, J. A., Brockett, J. E., & Whitaker, M. M. (2007). Multiple auditory processing assessment (test manual 1.0 version). St. Louis, MO: Auditec.

[78] Singer, J., Hurley, R. M., & Preece, J. P. (1998). Effectiveness of central auditory processing tests with children. American Journal of Audiology, 7, 73–84.

[79] Smits, C., Kapteyn, T. S., & Houtgast, T. (2004). Development and validation of an automatic speech-in-noise screening test by telephone. International Journal of Audiology, 43(1), 15–28.

[80] Smoski, W., Brunt, M., & Tannahill, J. (1992a). Children's auditory performance scale. Tampa, FL: Authors.

[81] Smoski, W. J., Brunt, M. A., & Tannahill, J. C. (1992b). Listening characteristics of children with central auditory processing disorders. Language, Speech, and Hearing Services in Schools, 23, 145–152.

[82] Stapells, D. (2002). Cortical event-related potentials to auditory stimuli. In J. Katz (Ed.), Handbook of clinical audiology (5th ed.). Philadelphia, PA: Lippincott, Williams & Wilkins.

[83] Stillman, R. D., Crow, G., & Moushegian, G. (1978). Components of the frequency-following potential in man. Electroencephalography and Clinical Neurophysiology, 44(4), 438–446.

[84] Towle, V. L., Yoon, H. A., Castelle, M., et al. (2008). ECoG gamma activity during a language task: Differentiating expressive and receptive speech areas. Brain, 131(Pt. 8), 2013–2027.

[85] Tucker, D. A., & Ruth, R. A. (1996). Effects of age, signal level, and signal rate on the auditory middle latency response. Journal of the American Academy of Audiology, 7(2), 83–91.

[86] Wagener, K., Josvassen, J. L., & Ardenkjaer, R. (2003). Design, optimization and evaluation of a Danish sentence test in noise. International Journal of Audiology, 42(1), 10–17.

[87] Wilson, W. J., Jackson, A., Pender, A., et al. (2011). The CHAPS, SIFTER, and TAPS-R as predictors of (C)AP skills and (C)APD. Journal of Speech, Language, and Hearing Research, 54(1), 278–29.

[88] Yamada, T., Nakamura, A., Horibe, K., et al. (2003). Asymmetrical enhancement of middle-latency auditory evoked fields with aging. Neuroscience Letters, 337(1), 21–24.

[89] Yathiraj, A., & Maggu, A. R. (2013a). Comparison of a screening test and screening checklist for auditory processing disorders. International Journal of Pediatric Otorhinolaryngology, 77(6), 990–995.

[90] Yathiraj, A., & Maggu, A. R. (2013b). Screening test for auditory processing (STAP): A preliminary report. Journal of the American Academy of Audiology, 24(9), 867–878.

[91] Yin, H. S., Johnson, M., Mendelsohn, A. L., Abrams, M. A., Sanders, L. M., & Dreyer, B. P. (2009). The health literacy of parents in the United States: A nationally representative study. Pediatrics, 124(Suppl. 3), S289–S298.

[92] Zokoll, M. A., Hochmuth, S., Fidan, D., Wagener, K. C., Ergenc, I., & Kollmeier, B. (2012). Speech intelligibility tests for the Turkish language. In Proceedings of the 15th Annual Conference of the German Audiology Society, Erlangen, Germany. Retrieved from http://akademikpersonel.kocaeli.edu.tr/dilek.fidan/bildiri/dilek.fidan12.09.2012_23.14.22bildiri.pdf.

[93] Zokoll, M. A., Hochmuth, S., Warzybok, A., Wagener, K. C., Buschermöhle, M., & Kollmeier, B. (2013). Speech-in-noise tests for multilingual hearing screening and diagnostics1. American Journal of Audiology, 22(1), 175–178.

[94] Zokoll, M. A., Wagener, K. C., Brand, T., Buschermöhle, M., & Kollmeier, B. (2012). Internationally comparable screening tests for listening in noise in several European languages: The German digit triplet test as an optimization prototype. International Journal of Audiology, 51(9), 697–707.

Chapter 5

Auditory Temporal Processing Assessment

5 Auditory Temporal Processing Assessment

Temporal processing refers to the processing of acoustic stimuli over time. It is very important for individuals to be able to understand speech in quiet and in background noise given that speech stimuli and other background sounds vary over time. Temporal processing can be measured across various categories with some overlap and differences in the underlying abilities across these categories. This chapter covers all issues related to temporal processing in the auditory system including those that have been reviewed previously (Rawool, 2006a; Rawool, 2006b).

5.1 Temporal Resolution

In measuring temporal resolution, the lower limit of the ability of the human auditory system to resolve time is assessed. Temporal resolution can be measured in several different ways.

5.1.1 Gap Detection Threshold

Gap detection threshold is the measurement of the minimum time gap necessary to perceive the presence of a gap, or time interval (▶ Fig. 5.1). When two stimuli are presented with a sufficient gap between them, the stimuli are perceived as two stimuli occurring one after other. Without the presence of a minimum time gap, the two stimuli occurring before and after the gap are perceived as one stimulus. Differences in stimulus spectral characteristics can cause some

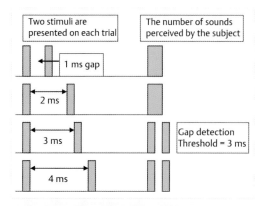

Fig. 5.1 Illustration of a gap detection threshold (adapted from Rawool, 2012).

variation in gap detection thresholds (Shailer & Moore, 1983).

Within-Channel Gap Detection Threshold

A within-channel gap detection threshold is the minimum gap necessary to detect gaps between sounds that are similar in spectrum (Hirsh, 1959; Purcell, John, Schneider, & Picton, 2004).

Across- or Between-Channel Gap Detection Threshold

An across- or between-channel gap detection threshold is the minimum gap necessary to detect gaps between sounds that are spectrally dissimilar (e.g., tone and noise; Heinrich, Alain, & Schneider, 2004; Hirsh, 1959).

Comparison of Gap Detection Thresholds Across and Within Channels

A schematic representation of the within- and between-channel gap detection paradigms is shown in ▶ Fig. 5.2. Within-channel gap detection requires detection of a discontinuity within a stimulus that is stimulating the same cochlear region before and after the gap. Across-channel gap detection requires comparison across different perceptual channels as the stimuli before and after the gap stimulate different cochlear regions (Phillips, Taylor, Hall, Carr, & Mossop, 1997). Across-channel gap detection thresholds are usually larger than within-channel gap detection thresholds (Hess, Blumsack, Ross, & Brock, 2012; Leigh-Paffenroth & Elangovan, 2011), and larger spectral disparity between the stimulus prior to the gap and the stimulus after the gap leads to larger gap detection thresholds (Phillips et al., 1997). ▶ Fig. 5.3 shows within-channel gap detection thresholds for broadband noise using the Gaps-in-Noise (GIN) test (Weihing, Musiek, & Shinn, 2007) and across- and within-channel gap detection thresholds across various sensation levels for a narrowband noise (Hess et al., 2012) using an adaptive procedure referred to as the Adaptive Test for Temporal Resolution (ATTR; Lister, Roberts, Krause, Debiase, & Carlson, 2011).

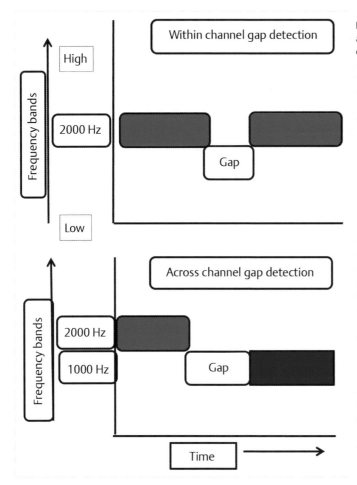

Fig. 5.2 Schematic of within- and across-channel gap detection paradigms.

Interaural Gap Detection

Interaural gap detection is the ability to detect gaps between sounds that are being presented to two ears. As an example, the Binaural Fusion Test developed by Musiek (Chermak & Lee, 2005) requires listeners to attend to pairs of noise bursts that are presented sequentially to each ear and are separated by gaps, or interpulse intervals (IPIs), that vary randomly from 0 to 100 ms, with a smallest step size of 5 ms. The ear that receives the first noise burst is also randomized to minimize guessing. The listener is required to respond by indicating whether one or two noise bursts were heard.

Comparison of Monaural and Interaural Gap Detection

When spectrally similar stimuli are used for both tasks, interaural gap detection thresholds are expected to be larger than monaural gap detection thresholds (Pollack, 1977). During monaural gap detection tasks, the same regions of the same cochlea are stimulated, which requires the detection of a discontinuity between the stimuli. During interaural gap detection, regions of the left and right cochlear are stimulated, which requires a comparison of the two stimuli at some central level. When a 4 kHz noise is presented, gaps as small as 4 to 5 ms can be detected during monaural gap detection protocols, whereas the gap detection thresholds can be as large as 17 ms during interaural gap detection protocols. In addition, during interaural gap detection procedures, gap detection thresholds can become larger with a decrease in duration of the leading stimulus (Phillips et al., 1997).

Effect of Stimulus Level on Gap Detection

When stimuli are presented near auditory thresholds, larger gaps are necessary for detecting gaps

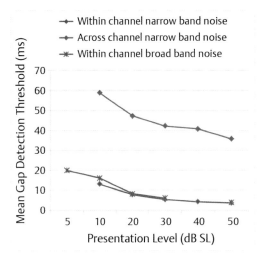

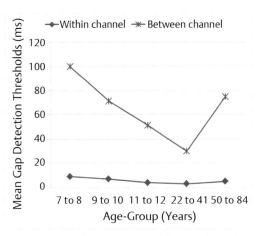

Fig. 5.3 Mean gap detection thresholds for narrowband noises across within- and between-channel conditions as a function of the stimulus presentation level (based on Hess, Blumsack, Ross, & Brock, 2012) and for within-channel broadband noise conditions (based on Weihing, Musiek & Shinn, 2007).

Fig. 5.4 Effect of age on within and between (across) channel gap detection using narrowband noise (based on Lister, Roberts, & Lister, 2011).

compared to when stimuli are presented at comfortable listening levels (▶ Fig. 5.3). With increasing stimulus levels, shorter gaps can be detected up to a certain level (Leigh-Paffenroth & Elangovan, 2011). In individuals with normal hearing, gap detection thresholds may not improve significantly beyond 30 dB sensation level (SL; Hess et al., 2012; Shailer & Moore, 1983).

Effect of Age on Gap Detection

Thresholds obtained with the ATTR show changes in gap detection thresholds across the lifespan that are more obvious for between-channel gap detection, as shown in ▶ Fig. 5.4. Thresholds for children recorded in ▶ Fig. 5.4 are averaged across left and right ears, and those for adults were obtained with diotic (same stimuli with gaps delivered to both ears) stimuli. Within-channel gap detection thresholds were for 2000 Hz narrowband noise. Across-channel gap detection thresholds involved detection of gaps between 2000 and 1000 Hz narrowbands of noise (Lister, Roberts, & Lister, 2011). Within-channel gap detection thresholds for 500 Hz tone pips are expected to be around 11.0 ms for infants, 5.6 ms for children, and 5.2 ms for adults (Trehub, Schneider, & Henderson, 1995).

Effect of Hearing Loss on Gap Detection

The ability to detect gaps in the presence of hearing loss is partially determined by the degree to which the stimuli used for the gap detection task vary randomly in amplitude and the sound level of the stimuli. Individuals with hearing loss generally show poorer gap detection when the sound pressure levels are similar to those used for measuring gap detection in normal individuals. At higher presentation levels or at sensation levels similar to those used in normal-hearing individuals, gap detection can be normal when the signal is clearly audible in some individuals with hearing loss (Fitzgibbons & Wightman, 1982; Glasberg, Moore, & Bacon, 1987; Hall, Grose, Buss, & Hatch, 1998; Moore, Glasberg, Donaldson, McPherson, & Plack, 1989). Even with optimal presentation levels, gap detection may be poor in some individuals with hearing loss (Fitzgibbons & Gordon-Salant, 1987), and it may be poor even if hearing is normal in the low-frequency regions and the hearing loss is limited to high-frequency areas (Feng, Yin, Kiefte, & Wang, 2010; Leigh-Paffenroth & Elangovan, 2011). Furthermore, when stimuli have random amplitude fluctuations (e.g., bands of noise), individuals with hearing loss have more difficulty in detecting gaps than do normal-hearing individuals (Fitzgibbons & Wightman, 1982). Because most individuals with significant hearing loss will hear environmental sounds at softer levels without amplification, they can be expected to have difficulty in detecting gaps in common noisy backgrounds without hearing aids (reviewed in Rawool, 2006).

Clinical Assessment of Within-Channel Gap Detection

Some of the tests for estimating within-channel gap detection thresholds are the Auditory Fusion Test–Revised (AFT-R), Random Gap Detection Threshold (RGDT), and GIN. All of these measures incorporate a practice test, which allows familiarization of the test material. They all are administered at comfortable listening levels because temporal resolution tends to be poorer at softer levels. When obtaining ear-specific data, care should be taken to keep the presentation level below the levels at which crossover of the stimuli to the other ear is possible. Children often have very good bone conduction sensitivity (−10 dB hearing level [HL] or better thresholds), which may allow crossover of signals at levels as low as 25 to 30 dB HL (Snyder, 1973), and the possibility of crossover is greater for broadband stimuli such as noise. With TDH-39 (Brännström & Lantz, 2010; Smith & Markides, 1981), TDH-49 (Sklare & Denenberg, 1987), or TDH-50 (Blackwell, Oyler, & Seyfried, 1991) earphones (from Telephonics ® A Griffon Company, Farmingdale, NY), low-frequency acoustic crossover is possible in some individuals at 50 dB HL. Acoustic crossover can be minimized using insert earphones (Munro & Contractor, 2010; Sklare & Denenberg, 1987) or presenting stimuli at or below 35 dB SL in individuals with normal hearing. Stimulus presentation levels of at least 25 to 35 dB SL are necessary for assessment of optimal gap resolution in individuals with sensory hearing loss (Fitzgibbons & Gordon-Salant, 1987).

Auditory Fusion Test–Revised (AFT-R)

The AFT-R, developed by McCrosky and Keith (1996), consists of pairs of tonal bursts that are varied in frequency from 250 to 4000 Hz. The bursts are presented with the gaps between the pairs of bursts or IPIs increasing in duration from 0, 2, 5, 10, 15, 20, 25, 30, and 40 ms (ascending), then decreasing in duration from 40 to 0 ms (descending). The listener's task is to judge whether one or two sounds are audible. When the listener hears the gap between the pulses, the pulses are identified as two ("2"). The perception of the tonal pair as a single sound ("1") suggests that the gap between the pair is not recognized. On

the ascending trial, the auditory fusion point is identified as that IPI that yields the last "1" response before the "2" responses. On the descending trial, it is that IPI that yields the first of two consecutive "1" responses. The average of the ascending and descending auditory fusion points is the auditory fusion threshold for that frequency or mode (right ear, left ear, or binaural). If the listener judged all pairs as single sounds up to the IPI of 40 ms, subtest 3 or the expanded test can be administered in which the IPIs are varied from 40 to 100 ms in 10 ms steps, and two additional pairs are presented with IPIs of 200 and 300 ms.

Normative data for the auditory fusion points are provided on the back of the test form for age groups ranging from 3 to 70 years. The mean auditory fusion thresholds and 1 standard deviation (SD) above mean data are shown in ▶ Fig. 5.5. Although the test does not directly measure gap detection thresholds, approximate gap detection thresholds can be estimated as the average of the minimal IPIs where the response "2" occurred on the ascending and descending trials. Significantly poor performance on the AFT-R has been reported in children with reading disorders, learning disabilities (McCroskey & Kidder, 1980), and articulation disorders (Scudder, 1978).

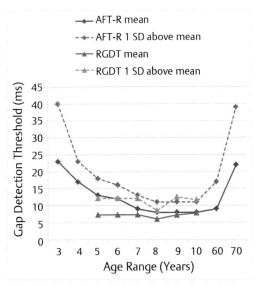

Fig. 5.5 Age effects on the Auditory Fusion Test –Revised (AFT-R) (based on McCroskey & Keith, 1996) and the random gap detection threshold test (RGDT) (based on Keith, 2000).

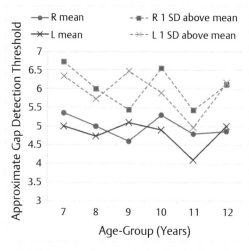

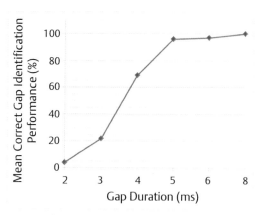

Fig. 5.6 Approximate gap detection thresholds on the Gaps-in-Noise (GIN) test across various age groups in children (based on Shinn, Chermark, & Musiek, 2009).

Fig. 5.7 Mean correct gap identification performance (percentage) of young normal-hearing adults at 50 dB sensation level (SL) (reference pure tone average) on the Gaps-in-Noise (GIN) test as a function of gap duration (based on Samelli & Schochat, 2008).

Random Gap Detection Test

The RGDT (Keith, 2000) is a less time-consuming (10 minutes) version of the AFT-R, described above. It includes pairs of clicks (1 ms white noise) and tonal bursts (duration 15 ms, 1.5 ms rise-fall time) with frequencies ranging from 500 to 4000 Hz. The interpulse intervals or gaps are varied from 0, 2, 5, 10, 15, 20, 25, 30, 35, and 40 ms in a random order. The listener's task is to verbally or manually (by holding up fingers) indicate if one or two sounds are perceived. The approximate gap detection threshold can be estimated from this test by determining the smallest interpulse interval, or gap, at which the listener perceives two stimuli. The expanded version, RGDT-EXP, includes gaps with additional interpulse intervals up to 300 ms.

The effect of age maturation on the RGDT is shown in ▶ Fig. 5.5. Workers exposed to solvents show poorer performance on the RGDT compared to nonexposed individuals (Fuente & McPherson, 2007). Children with previous language delays show poorer performance on the RGDT when compared to age-matched peers (Muluk, Yalçinkaya, & Keith, 2011).

Gaps-in-Noise

The GIN test, developed by Musiek et al. (2005), consists of a series of 6-second segments of broadband noise with zero to three gaps embedded within each segment. The white noise is generated via a computer and is uniformly distributed. The noise is turned on and off instantaneously to create gaps. The gaps vary in duration, from 2, 3, 4, 5, 6, 8, 10, 12, 15, and 20 ms. The shortest duration between two consecutive gaps is always greater than 500 ms. The interstimulus interval between noise segments is 5 seconds. The gap duration and the location of gaps within the noise are pseudorandomized. A total of 60 gaps are presented. Listeners are expected to press a button every time they hear a gap. Each response following an occurrence of a gap is considered a correct response. If a response occurs when there is no gap, a false-positive response is noted. The approximate gap detection threshold is defined as the shortest gap duration that is correctly identified at least four out of six times. The percentage of correct responses out of the total 60 gaps can also be calculated. Most investigators have administered the test at 50 dB SL with reference to the pure tone average (500, 1000, and 2000 Hz) in each ear.

Children who are 7 years or older can perform the GIN task without much difficulty with a performance similar to that of adults. The approximate gap detection thresholds of children in various age groups are shown in ▶ Fig. 5.6 (Shinn, Chermak, & Musiek, 2009). The mean correct responses of young adults as a function of gap duration on the GIN test are shown in ▶ Fig. 5.7 (Samelli & Schochat, 2008). Three indices can be derived from the GIN test: the approximate threshold, which is the lowest gap (ms) where at least four out of six gaps are correctly detected; the total percent correct response, which indicates the total number of gaps identified correctly out of the 60 presented gaps; and the psychometric function-derived from percent correct responses, which assesses performance for gaps of 4, 5, and 6 ms duration. Individuals with confirmed neurologic involvement show significantly poorer performance on all of these measures compared to normal-hearing listeners (Musiek et al., 2005). Using 1 SD above mean criteria, the approximate gap detection threshold cutoff appears to be 7 ms, and the total percent correct response cutoff criterion appears to be 72% for adults (Prem, Shankar, & Girish, 2012). Children with dyslexia and significant phonological awareness deficits show significantly poorer performance on the GIN compared to children with normal reading skills (Zaidan & Baran, 2013).

Comparison of Clinical Gap Detection Tests

Chermak and Lee (2005) compared the above three tests in a group of 10 normal-hearing children ranging in age from 7 to 11 years. The GIN test required 20 minutes for administration, which is longer than the 10 to 16 minutes required for other tests. However, the GIN test also yielded the smallest range and standard deviations and was thought to provide better specificity.

Impact of Poor Gap Detection Ability

Individuals with compromised central auditory nervous systems need larger gaps or intervals of time to detect gaps (Bamiou et al., 2006; Musiek et al., 2005). They may have difficulty in processing rapidly occurring elements in speech. Fast speech has smaller gaps, and poor temporal resolution can make it difficult to detect the small gaps, thus making it hard to separate sounds from each other. Gap detection thresholds also appear to be related to speech perception in noise (Feng et al., 2010; Glasberg & Moore, 1989). Real-life background sounds often fluctuate in intensity, allowing for better extraction of useful information from the signal of interest during the softer levels of background noise. The poor gap detection in some individuals may not allow them to take advantage of such gaps in background noise. Across-channel gap detection thresholds may be more sensitive to auditory processing deficits (APDs) in children compared to within-channel gap detection (Phillips, Comeau, & Andrus, 2010).

5.1.2 Detection of Temporal Modulation

Temporal modulation refers to a change in the stimulus over time. For example, a stimulus can change in amplitude over time (amplitude modulation). Listeners can be presented with two intervals with modulated and unmodulated signals, and their task is to select the interval that has the modulated signal (▶ Fig. 5.8 a). The characteristics of a modulating signal can be described with reference to modulation depth and rate. Modulation rate refers to the speed with which the change occurs. For example, if the amplitude of the signal changes very frequently over time, the modulation rate is considered to be high (▶ Fig. 5.8 b). Modulation depth refers to the degree of change. If the amplitude of the signal changes over time from very high to very low, then the signal is considered to have greater modulation depth (▶ Fig. 5.8 c). We need to have a minimum modulation depth to detect that a stimulus is modulated in some way. The listener's sensitivity can be measured in terms of the minimum modulation depth necessary to detect modulation. The modulation depth is usually expressed in decibels. For example, 0, −6, −12, and

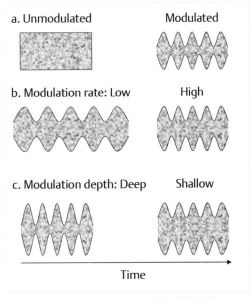

Fig. 5.8 (a–c) Schematic illustration of temporal modulation, modulation rate, and modulation depth.

−20 dB can correspond to 100, 50, 25, and 10% modulation. For signals with a high modulation rate, the modulation depth needs to be greater to detect that the signal is modulated compared to a signal with a low modulation rate (Lorenzi et al., 2001; Viemeister, 1979). High-functioning children with autism spectrum disorders need greater modulation depths to detect modulation at slow modulation rates compared to age-matched normal peers (Alcántara, Cope, Cope, & Weisblatt, 2012).

Impact of Poor Temporal Modulation Detection

Individuals with poor ability to detect temporal modulations may have difficulty in processing speech because many consonants have rapid intensity changes or amplitude modulations that must be perceived correctly for accurate recognition of the consonants. In addition, as stated above, normal-hearing individuals are able to take advantage of the fluctuations that occur in background noise that make it easier to listen to speech occurrences during the dips or softer levels in the noise. Individuals with poor abilities to detect temporal modulations in background noise may not be able to take advantage of the dips in noise to improve speech recognition in background noise and thus perform poorly on figure-ground (speech in noise) listening tasks. Individuals with auditory neuropathy perform significantly poorer than normal-hearing listeners on amplitude and frequency modulation detection tasks; these measures are correlated with speech recognition performance in noise (Narne, 2013).

Effect of Hearing Loss on Temporal Modulation Detection

Individuals with high-frequency hearing loss appear to have reduced sensitivity to high rates of modulation when compared to normal-hearing individuals, probably because of inaudible high frequencies (Bacon & Viemeister, 1985). Listeners with flat hearing loss appear to show modulation detection performance that is similar to that of individuals with normal hearing when stimuli are presented at equal sound pressure levels. When stimuli are presented at equal sensation levels to normal-hearing and hearing-impaired listeners, individuals with hearing loss appear to be good at detecting modulations (Bacon & Gleitman, 1992). Thus, temporal modulation detection appears to depend on the bandwidth audible to the listener. If the entire bandwidth is audible to the listener, temporal modulation detection is expected to be normal. If the high-frequency bands are inaudible, temporal modulation detection can be expected to be poorer. However, some listeners with hearing loss may show poor modulation detection, especially at high modulation rates, even for signals that are audible to them (Grant, Summers, & Leek, 1998).

5.2 Duration Discrimination

Duration discrimination threshold is the minimum difference in duration necessary to perceive that two otherwise identical stimuli are different in duration (Hellström & Rammsayer, 2004). Note that such duration discrimination is affected by temporal integration, which can make the sound with longer duration appear louder for stimuli that are shorter than about 200 to 300 ms. For tonal stimuli, duration discrimination can also be affected by changes in the frequency composition of the signal with changes in duration. In children, duration discrimination performance improves with age, and between the ages of 8 to 10 years, adultlike performance is apparent using three interval forced choice procedures (Elfenbein, Small, & Davis, 1993; Jensen & Neff, 1993). Duration discrimination is very important for accurate speech recognition. For example, the differentiation between unvoiced and voiced consonants partially depends on the duration of the vowel preceding the consonant. The duration is longer for voiced consonants than that for unvoiced consonants. Also, fricatives can be differentiated from affricates based on the difference in the duration of the fricative noises associated with these sounds (Dorman, Raphael, & Isenberg, 1980). Musicians show better duration discrimination than do nonmusicians (Güçlü, Sevinc, & Canbeyli, 2011).

5.2.1 Effect of Hearing Loss on Duration Discrimination

Some investigators have reported no effect of hearing loss (Grose, Hall, & Buss, 2004), whereas others have reported that duration discrimination is poorer in the presence of hearing loss (Irwin & Purdy, 1982). Effect of hearing loss on duration discrimination appears to depend on the duration of the standard stimulus. Just detectable durational increments in tonal complexes as a function of

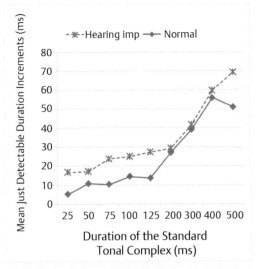

Fig. 5.9 Just detectable durational increments in tonal complexes as a function of the duration of the standard tonal complex (based on Bochner, Snell, & MacKenzie, 1988).

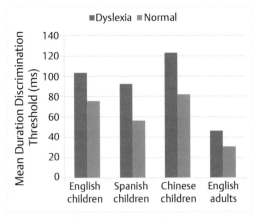

Fig. 5.10 Duration discrimination thresholds (ms) of children ages 7 to 13 years (based on Goswami et al., 2011) and adults ages 18 to 31 years (based on Thomson, Fryer, Maltby, & Goswami, 2006) with dyslexia and age- and language-matched normal-hearing peers for a standard duration of 400 ms. For children, the tonal frequency was 500 Hz; for adults, it was 1000 Hz.

the duration of a standard tonal complex for listeners with normal hearing and those with hearing impairments are shown in ► Fig. 5.9 (Bochner, Snell, & MacKenzie, 1988).

5.2.2 Effect of Pathology on Duration Discrimination

Individuals with left and right temporal lobe pathologies need larger differences in duration for detecting differences in duration between two stimuli compared to individuals in control groups. The differences are more obvious with a shorter standard duration stimulus (50 ms) compared to a larger standard duration stimulus (300 ms). The deviation from normal performance is more obvious in individuals with left temporal pathologies compared to those with right temporal lobe pathologies. In listeners with left temporal lobe pathologies, duration discrimination performance for the 50 ms standard stimulus is correlated with consonant discrimination (Thompson & Abel, 1992).

Children in ages 7 to 13 years with dyslexia show significantly poor duration discrimination (► Fig. 5.10) compared to their age- and language-matched peers (Goswami et al., 2011), and duration discrimination skills are significantly correlated with reading, spelling, and phonological skills (Thomson & Goswami, 2008). Adults

between the ages of 18 and 31 years with dyslexia also show poor duration discrimination skills compared to age-matched peers (► Fig. 5.10), with a significant correlation between duration discrimination and reading skills (Thomson, Fryer, Maltby, & Goswami, 2006).

5.3 Gap Duration Discrimination

Gap duration discrimination threshold is the minimum difference in the duration of two gaps that is necessary to perceive that the two gaps are different in duration. The two gaps can be created by using acoustic markers (e.g., brief tones) at the beginning and at the end of the gap. One of the gaps serves as the standard gap. The duration of the second gap is varied to determine the minimum difference in gap duration necessary to detect that the two gaps differ in duration (► Fig. 5.11).

5.3.1 Significance of Gap Duration Discrimination

Gap duration discrimination is important for discriminating fricatives and affricates, for identifying the presence or absence of a stop consonant in a consonant cluster, for detecting voicing of a stop

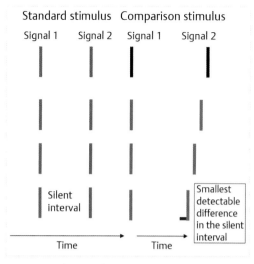

Fig. 5.11 Schematic showing gap duration discrimination.

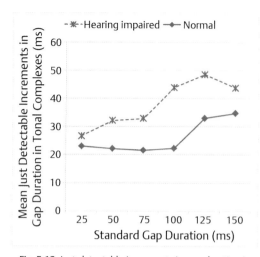

Fig. 5.12 Just detectable increments in gap duration in tonal complexes as a function of the standard gap duration (based on Bochner, Snell, & MacKenzie, 1988).

consonant in word-medial position, and for discriminating between single- and double-stop consonants (Dorman, Raphael, & Liberman, 1979). Children with attention deficit hyperactivity disorder (ADHD) need significantly larger differences in gap durations to detect differences in gap duration compared to age-matched normal peers (Himpel et al., 2009).

5.3.2 Effect of Hearing Loss on Gap Duration Discrimination

Hearing loss may (Irwin & Purdy, 1982) or may not (Grose et al., 2001) have any effect on gap duration discrimination. The effect of hearing loss on gap duration discrimination may depend on the gap duration of the standard stimulus, with the effect more apparent when the standard gap is very brief (Fitzgibbons & Gordon-Salant, 1994). Just detectable durational increments in gaps in tonal complexes as a function of the standard gap duration for listeners with normal hearing and those with hearing impairments are shown in ▶ Fig. 5.12 (Bochner, Snell, & MacKenzie, 1988).

5.4 Temporal Asynchrony

In a temporal asynchrony task, the temporal alignment of one or more of the frequency bands of two complex stimuli differs, and the listener is expected to differentiate between the two stimuli.

5.4.1 Temporal Asynchrony Detection Threshold

Thresholds can be measured for detecting asynchrony among complex signals composed of many sinusoidal components (Zera & Green, 1993a, 1995). The components either form a harmonic series or are uniformly spaced on a logarithmic frequency scale. In the standard synchronous stimulus, all components start and stop synchronously. In the comparison stimulus, asynchrony is created by starting (onset asynchrony) or stopping (offset asynchrony) only one or certain components slightly before or after the other components in the complex (▶ Fig. 5.13). The listener's task is to discriminate between the standard and the comparison stimulus. The asynchrony in turning the components "on" or "off" is varied. Temporal asynchrony detection thresholds can range from 0.2 to 2 ms, suggesting good acuity in detecting onset or offset differences in listeners with normal hearing (Zera & Green, 1993a). When all components of the complex signal are in phase, asynchrony detection is easier when compared to conditions where some components are out of phase (Zera & Green, 1995).

Temporal asynchrony detection thresholds determined using a pair of tones tend to vary as a function of the leading frequency. It is easier to detect onset asynchrony when the lower frequency tone begins earlier than the higher frequency tone compared to when the higher frequency tone

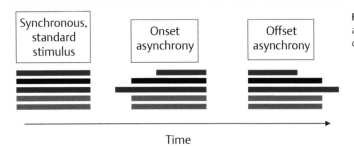

| Synchronous, standard stimulus | Onset asynchrony | Offset asynchrony |

Fig. 5.13 Schematic of temporal asynchrony. The color bands represent different frequencies or harmonics.

Time

begins earlier than the lower frequency tone (Wojtczak, Beim, Micheyl, & Oxenham, 2013a).

5.4.2 Temporal Asynchrony Discrimination

In this case, a standard asynchronous stimulus is created by linearly delaying successive components of a complex stimulus. Another asynchronous comparison stimulus is created by altering the temporal position of a single component in the complex relative to its temporal position in the standard stimulus (Zera & Green, 1993b). The listener's task is to discriminate between the standard and the comparison stimulus.

5.4.3 Significance of Temporal Asynchrony Measures

Detection and discrimination of temporal asynchrony are important for understanding speech in background noise or where more than one person is speaking at the same time. The rapid sequence of sounds in such environments is not always perceived as a coherent whole. The sounds may actually be divided into different groups according to their general attributes, such as loudness, perceived location, pitch, closeness to each other, and temporal synchrony of different frequency bands. The different frequency components from a particular sound source tend to start and finish together. Thus, if the different frequency bands start together, or have onset synchrony, they are detected as part of the same sound source; otherwise, they are perceived as separate auditory streams. The ability to detect and discriminate temporal synchrony allows us to concentrate on the signal of interest (e.g., a single speaker) while ignoring the signals that are not of interest (e.g., background music or other speakers in the background).

5.4.4 Effect of Hearing Loss on Temporal Asynchrony Detection

Effects of hearing loss on temporal asynchrony detection may depend on the particular asynchrony task. Some investigators have suggested that hearing loss does not appear to affect the ability to make use of relatively gross temporal asynchrony cues, suggesting good ability to group auditory objects into separate streams based on temporal asynchronies (Grose & Hall, 1996). However, some individuals with age-related hearing loss may show relatively poor temporal asynchrony detection ability (Wojtczak, Beim, Micheyl, & Oxenham, 2013b), which may lead to difficulties in grouping auditory objects.

5.5 Temporal Separation (Sequential Stream Segregation) or Stream Fusion

The term *stream fusion* or *coherence* refers to the perception of a single sound source in the presence of two alternating sounds. The term *sequential stream segregation, temporal separation,* or *fission* is used when the two sounds are perceived as two separate sounds that are occurring at the same time. Each of the perceived sounds in this case can be considered a stream (Moore & Gockel, 2012). Thus, during stream segregation, if the sounds differ in frequency, the individual does not recognize the sounds as a sound from a single source that is alternating in pitch. Instead, the listener hears two coexisting sounds.

In a temporal separation or stream fusion task, two sounds, tones A and B, that are different in some dimension (level, temporal modulation pattern, frequency, etc.) are presented in an alternating fashion to the ear. Both sounds are turned on and off in such a way that when the first sound is off, the second is on, and when the first sound is on, the second is off. The listener's task is to judge whether two separate sound sources are occurring simultaneously or if there is just one sound that is fluctuating in some way. For example, tone A can be fixed in frequency at 250 Hz. Tone B can be started with a frequency well above or below that of tone A, then its frequency can be swept toward that of tone A so that the frequency separation between the two tones decreases (▶ Fig. 5.14) in an exponential manner. Listeners are expected to indicate when they can no longer perceive tones A and B as two separate streams but perceive a single stream with a "gallop" rhythm. This is called the *fission boundary* (Rose & Moore, 1997). The minimal frequency separation at which listeners no longer perceptually perceive two streams or two sound sources is referred to as the *fusion threshold.*

Stream segregation is most likely when the differences in successive sounds are very large and stream fusion is most likely when the differences are very small. Between stream fusion and stream segregation, the perception can vary from one to two streams. The perception of fusion or segregation in alternating tone sequences appears to depend partly on the extent of overlap of the excitation patterns evoked by the successive sounds in the cochlea (Rose & Moore, 2000). However, several other differences in successive sounds can induce stream segregation, including temporal envelope, fundamental frequency, phase spectrum, and alternating presentation of successive sounds to left and right ears (Moore & Gockel, 2012).

Most acoustic environments have sounds that come from several coexisting sound sources. Our ability to segregate the sound streams from each source can help us focus on the signal of interest and recognize the signal (e.g., music in the background of noise). Lower fusion thresholds are associated with better speech recognition ability in the presence of competing speech stimuli (Mackersie, Prida, & Stiles, 2001).

5.5.1 Effect of Hearing Loss on Temporal Separation

Fusion thresholds for listeners with age-related hearing loss tend to be higher than those obtained from normal-hearing young adults (Mackersie et al., 2001). Mackersie (2003) recorded speech recognition scores of individuals with hearing loss by presenting sentences spoken by male and female speakers simultaneously and measured tonal fusion thresholds by varying frequency either below (ascending pattern) or above (descending pattern) the frequency of the fixed tone (1000 Hz). Speech recognition scores for male talkers were correlated with the ascending fusion thresholds, and those for female talkers were correlated with the descending fusion thresholds. These results show the importance of temporal streaming in the perceptual separation of male and female talkers.

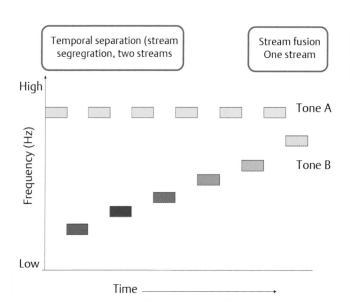

Fig. 5.14 Schematic showing temporal separation (stream segregation) and stream fusion (adapted from Rawool, 2013).

5.6 Temporal Ordering

Temporal ordering refers to our ability to accurately perceive the sequence of sounds. Most acoustic stimuli in nature follow one another. In speech, sounds appear in sequence with minimum gaps across sounds, and in music, notes are played in sequence. Thus, accurate temporal order judgment in the presence of minimal gaps across different sounds is necessary for accurate perception of speech. Otherwise, a child may say *aks* instead of *ask* or *nam* instead of *man*. Temporal ordering can be viewed and measured in several ways. Some children with dyslexia may have temporal processing deficits (see Chapter 14).

5.6.1 Temporal Order Threshold

This is the minimum time -gap between sound sequences necessary to perceive the order of incoming stimuli (e.g., clicks or tones) correctly on at least 75% of the test trials. This time gap is generally larger (15–20 ms) than the gap necessary to just perceive that there is a gap (2 ms) between two sounds (Hirsh, 1959). Furthermore, the minimum gaps necessary for accurate temporal order judgments increase with the number of stimuli in the sequence of items. Thus, the necessary gap is smaller when the order of only two stimuli is to be judged compared to when there are three stimuli in the sequence.

Spatial Temporal Order Threshold

In this procedure, stimuli (e.g., clicks) are presented one after another to each ear. The listeners' task is to indicate the order of the clicks by either pointing to the left or right ear or saying "first left ear, then right ear" or by indicating the order using a computer. The listeners can point to both ears when they perceive that the clicks are occurring at the same time in both ears. The interstimulus interval is varied to determine the minimum interstimulus interval at which correct order can be judged on at least 75% of trials. The mean spatial temporal order thresholds for clicks in children (Berwanger, Wittmann, von Steinbüchel, & von Suchodoletz, 2004) and adults (Fink, Ulbrich, Churan, & Wittman, 2006) are shown in ▸ Fig. 5.15. With increasing age, the performance of children improves and may reach adult values at around the age of 10 years (Berwanger et al., 2004).

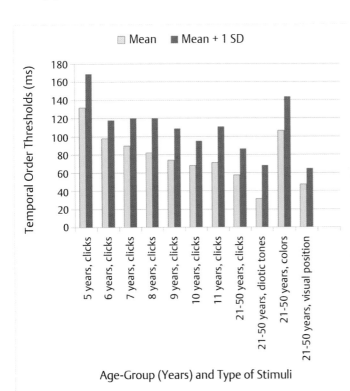

Fig. 5.15 Spatial temporal order thresholds (ms) in children for interaural clicks (based on Berwanger, Wittmann, von Steinbüchel, & von Suchodoletz, 2004) and for adults for interaural clicks. The last three columns show temporal order thresholds for adults for diotic tones (spectral order), visual colors, and visual position; based on Fink, Ulbrich, Churan, & Wittman, 2006) for comparison. Note that for adults, the lowest thresholds are apparent for diotic tones or spectral order.

Spectral Temporal Order Threshold

In this task, tones of different frequencies are presented to both ears one after the other (e.g., 500 Hz, 1500 Hz). The listeners indicate the order of the tones by saying "high" or "low" or using a computerized protocol. The interstimulus interval is varied to determine the minimum interstimulus interval at which the correct order can be reported on at least 75% of trials. As shown in ▶ Fig. 5.15, the temporal order detection thresholds are smaller for diotic tones than for interaural clicks. In addition, spectral temporal order thresholds show better test–retest reliability, and there is a significant correlation between spectral temporal order detection thresholds and phoneme discrimination. Therefore, in clinical settings, temporal order thresholds using tones are preferred over spatial (interaural) temporal order thresholds using clicks (Fink, Churan, & Wittman, 2005). Ear-specific spectral temporal order thresholds using tones can be determined by presenting the tones to only one ear at a time. In addition, spatial/spectral temporal order thresholds can be determined using stimuli differing in frequency to the two ears (Karnath, Zimmer, & Lewald, 2002).

Effect of Pathologies on Temporal Order Thresholds

Individuals who need larger time gaps to judge sound sequences accurately may have difficulty understanding rapid speech. Patients with injuries to the left cerebral hemisphere need larger gaps for accurate perception of temporal order (Efron, 1963; Swisher & Hirsh, 1972). Patients with circumscribed unilateral brain lesions due to strokes or hemorrhage documented by magnetic resonance imaging (MRI) or computed tomography (CT) often show poor performance on dichotic tasks for stimuli presented to the contralateral ear. Such patients perceive two narrowband noises differing in frequency presented to the two ears as occurring simultaneously when the sound in the ear contralateral to the lesion is leading by as much as 270 ms, whereas normal-hearing listeners perceive simultaneous presentation when the interstimulus interval is around 0 ms (Karnath et al., 2002). There is a moderate association of lesion size and temporal order thresholds in patients with brain-injuries (Wittmann, Burtscher, Fries, & von Steinbüchel, 2004).

5.6.2 Temporal Order Judgment

We can measure the ability of individuals to order sound sequences correctly after providing sufficient gaps between the sound sequences (Musiek, 1994; Warren, Obusek, Farmer, & Warren, 1969). Some individuals have difficulty in ordering sound sequences even after sufficient time gaps are provided between sounds. For example, if the sound sequence consists of variations in pitch (low-low-high), the individuals may report an incorrect sequence, such as high-low-high. Sound sequences that vary in duration or intensity can be used in such tasks (Pinheiro & Ptacek, 1971). Temporal order judgment can also be evaluated as a function of the interstimulus interval. ▶ Fig. 5.16 shows the performance of children with aphasia and age-matched normal peers as a function of the interstimulus interval between tonal bursts of 100 and 305 Hz (Tallal & Piercy, 1973). Children with aphasia show poor temporal judgment compared to normal children only when the interstimulus intervals are 305 ms or lower. Temporal order judgment tasks are partially dependent on good short-term memory, especially for longer tonal sequences.

Examples of two temporal order judgment tests that are available for clinical use are the Frequency Pattern Test and the Duration Pattern Test (Musiek, 1994; Noffsinger, Wilson, & Musiek, 1994). Before administering the tests, clinicians should ensure that the individual has understood the

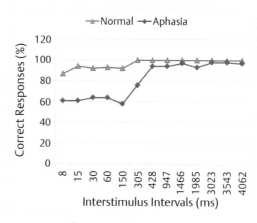

Fig. 5.16 Performance of children with aphasia and normal peers on a temporal order judgment task with tonal bursts of 100 and 305 Hz as a function of the interstimulus interval between the two tones (based on Tallal and Piercy, 1973).

instructions by using visual cues or gestures, if necessary. Practice test items are always used before administering the test items. The test scores are expressed in terms of the percentage of correctly identified patterns. In the presence of borderline normal performance, the test can be repeated to assess any practice-related improvements.

Frequency Pattern Test

The Frequency Pattern Test consists of 60 segments with three 200 ms tones in each segment, with a rise-fall time of 10 ms. The tones are separated from each other by a silent interval of 150 ms. The low tone has a frequency of 880 Hz, and the high tone has a frequency of 1122 Hz. These two frequencies are perceived as being equally loud; thus, listeners are forced to listen to the differences in pitch. The listeners' task is to identify each pattern verbally (e.g., high-low-low) and/or through humming. Ninety percent of normal-hearing young adults achieve 78% or better scores on this test (Musiek, 1994). Other suggested norms include a cutoff criterion of 40% for 8-year-old children, 65% for 9-year-old children, 72% for 10-year-old children, and 75% for older children and adults (Musiek, 2002). Working memory capacity is positively correlated with the Frequency (pitch) Pattern Test (Mukari, Umat, & Othman, 2010).

Duration Pattern Test

The Duration Pattern Test is similar to the Frequency Pattern Test except that listeners identify the pattern by specifying the duration of the tones (e.g., short-long-long). Each tone has the same frequency of 1000 Hz, but the duration is either long (500 ms) or short (250 ms). The tones are separated from each other by a 300 ms silent interval. Ninety percent of normal young adults achieve 73% or better scores on this test (Musiek, 1994).

Effect of Pathologies on Temporal Order Judgment

Some individuals with hemispheric or interhemispheric dysfunction show poor performance on temporal patterning tasks (Bamiou et al., 2006; Musiek, Baran, & Pinheiro, 1990; Musiek & Pinheiro, 1987). Workers exposed to solvents show poor performance on the frequency pattern test

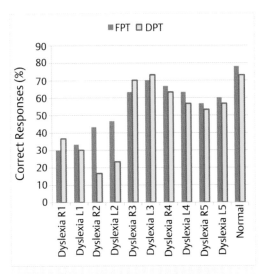

Fig. 5.17 Performance of 5 of 11 individuals with dyslexia (based on King, Lombardino, Crandell, & Leonard, 2003) on the frequency pattern test (FPT) and duration pattern test (DPT) for the right (R) and left (L) ears. Normal cutoff criteria are shown in the last columns based on Musiek (1994).

(Fuente & McPherson, 2007; Fuente, McPherson, & Cardemil, 2013). Some individuals with dyslexia (▶ Fig. 5.17) (King, Lombardion, Crandell, & Leonard, 2003), sport-related concussions (Turgeon, Champoux, Lepore, Leclerc, & Ellemberg, 2011), and temporal lobe epilepsy (Han et al., 2011) show poor performance on frequency and duration pattern tests.

Effect of Hearing Loss on Temporal Order Judgment

Individuals with hearing loss tend to show good performance on the duration pattern recognition task as long as the signal is audible to them (Musiek et al., 1990).

5.7 Temporal Pattern Discrimination

5.7.1 Pitch Pattern Discrimination

In this task, the ability of the individual to detect differences between two patterns is assessed. For example, the standard sequence may consist of two, four, six, or eight tones of different frequencies; in the deviant sequence, the frequency of one of the tones is varied (▶ Fig. 5.18). The listener's

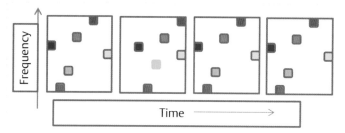

Fig. 5.18 Example of the temporal pattern discrimination task. In this example, the frequency of one of the tones is changed in the deviant tonal sequence (second block).

task is to indicate every time the deviant sequence is heard. The responses are tracked to determine the hit and false alarm rates. Musicians perform significantly better than nonmusicians on such a task (Boh, Herholz, Lappe, & Pantev, 2011).

5.7.2 Duration Pattern Discrimination

In this task, the ability of the individual to detect differences between two patterns is assessed. For example, the standard sound sequence may consist of 10 tones with durations of 40 ms. In the comparison stimulus, the duration of one of the tones can be varied to determine the smallest change in duration that leads to the perception of a temporal pattern that is different from the pattern of the standard stimulus (Espinoza-Varas & Watson, 1986). The task can be varied by asking listeners to detect changes in the duration of brief (40–50 ms) components or word-length (400–500 ms) tonal sequences.

5.8 Temporal Masking

Temporal masking refers to the ability of one sound (masker) to mask another sound (probe) that precedes and/or follows it (Elliott, 1962; Hartley & Moore, 2002). The shift in the threshold of the probe signal or the amount of masking produced by the masker is determined while adjusting the time interval between the probe and the masker. Temporal masking can be considered in three ways, as specified below.

5.8.1 Forward Masking

The masker is presented, and following a brief time delay the signal is presented. Thus, the masker can be considered as moving forward in time to mask the signal.

5.8.2 Backward Masking

In this case, the masker follows the signal after a brief time interval. Thus, the masker can be viewed as moving backward in time to mask the signal.

5.8.3 Combined Backward and Forward Masking

The signal is separated briefly in time by a masker that precedes it and another masker that follows it.

5.8.4 Variables Affecting the Amount of Temporal Masking

For listeners with normal hearing, most of the forward or backward masking effects occur when the masker is separated by the signal by less than 100 ms. Elliott (1971) identified the following variables that have an impact on the amount of temporal masking:

- The amount of masking is greater with closer temporal proximity of the signal and masker and is reduced with an increase in the time interval between the probe and the masker. Stated differently, the threshold shift of the probe signal is less when the probe and the masker are further apart in time.
- When the time interval between the signal and the masker is small, backward masking is greater than forward masking.
- Temporal masking is greater when the signal and masker are presented to the same ear (monotic) compared to when the signal and masker are presented to different ears (dichotic).
- When the signal and masker are closer in time, the duration of the masker has an effect on forward masking.
- More temporal masking occurs when the frequency of the probe is similar to the frequency of the masker.

5.8.5 Effect of Hearing Loss on Temporal Masking

Some investigators have reported that individuals with hearing loss yield more forward masking than predicted from results with normal-hearing individuals. In addition, the growth of forward masking with masker level tends to be steeper in individuals with hearing loss. The difference is more obvious for brief masker durations (Kidd, Mason, & Feith, 1984). The temporal masking function slopes for a given stimulus frequency tend to decrease with an increase in thresholds obtained with a 500 ms duration tone (Desloge, Reed, Braida, Perez, & Delhorne, 2011). Many listeners with moderate to severe sensorineural hearing loss show significant backward and forward masking, sometimes extending as far as 200 ms. Also, there are large individual differences in the degree and temporal extent of masking (Danaher, Wilson, & Pickett, 1978).

5.8.6 Impact of Abnormally Large Temporal Masking

Abnormally large temporal masking from adjacent sounds can affect the perception of speech. More specifically, forward masking effects appear to play a role in the perception of speech in quiet (Dreschler & Plomp, 1985). In average conversational speech, the intensity of sounds can vary by about 30 dB. If an individual demonstrates abnormally large temporal masking, this may result in frequent masking of a weaker sound when it is followed by a relatively intense sound (backward masking). There is also a correlation between forward masked thresholds and speech recognition in temporally interrupted noise. Higher forward masked thresholds are related to poor recognition of nonsense syllables in temporally interrupted noise in normal-hearing listeners. This correlation is most likely caused by poor recovery from forward masking effects, which minimizes the ability to take advantage of gaps in temporally interrupted noise (Dubno, Horwitz, & Ahlstrom, 2003).

Children with specific language impairment show more backward masking than do children with no such impairments (Wright et al., 1997). It should be noted that abnormally large temporal masking can also affect temporal separation or the ability to perceive two alternating sound sources as two sound streams because the sound from one source may mask the sound from another source occurring earlier or later in time.

5.9 Temporal Maintenance or Decay

Temporal maintenance refers to the ability of the auditory system to maintain the audibility of a continuous signal. If the signal is a tone, in addition to the audibility, maintenance of perception of tonality can be measured. Depending on the site of pathology, some patients cannot maintain the perception of tonality and audibility of the stimulus as well as is possible with a normal auditory system. The reduction in the ability to maintain the audibility of the tone is referred to as *tone decay*.

5.9.1 Threshold Tone Decay Test

Tone decay at or near threshold can be measured using various procedures. In most cases, the patient is asked to press a button immediately following the presentation of a tone at threshold (0 dB HL) and to let the button go as soon as he or she stops hearing the tone. As soon as the patient ceases to hear the tone, the presentation level of the tone is increased in 5 dB steps until the patient hears the tone. This procedure is repeated until the patient can continue to hear the tone for a full minute (Carhart, 1957). ▶ Fig. 5.19 shows the results of a tone decay test in a 21-year-old listener at 1000 Hz. The threshold in the left ear is 0 dB HL, and in the right ear it is 20 dB HL. As shown in ▶ Fig. 5.19, the tone was audible for a full minute at a sensation level of 10 dB in the left ear and 30 dB in the right ear (50 − 20), suggesting the possibility of subtle cochlear pathology in the right ear.

In the Rosenberg (1958, 1969) tone decay procedure, the presentation level of the tone is increased in 5 dB steps as described above, until 60 seconds are passed from the beginning of the test. The threshold shift that is apparent at the end of the 60 seconds is recorded as the amount of tone decay. Using this procedure, the listener in ▶ Fig. 5.19 shows a 10 dB decay in both the left and right ears. ▶ Fig. 5.20 shows the percent of patients showing 30 dB or more decay across cochlear, eighth nerve, brainstem, and temporal lobe pathologies using the Rosenberg (1958) test. As apparent in ▶ Fig. 5.20, patients with eighth nerve tumors often show tone decay (Antonelli, Bellotto, & Grandori, 1987). Some patients showing slow decay in the initial minute

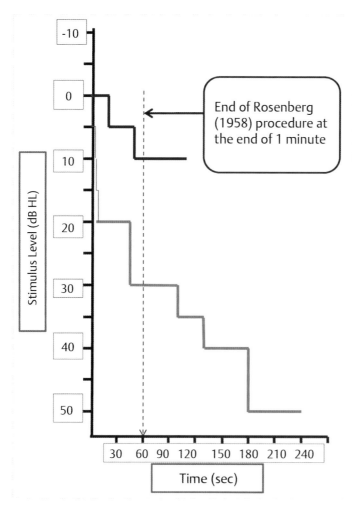

Fig. 5.19 Results of the tone decay test in the right and left ears at 1000 Hz in a young adult. The threshold is 0 dB hearing level (HL) in the left ear and 20 dB HL in the right ear. The decay for the left ear is 10 dB, and that for the right ear is 30 dB. Using the Rosenberg (1958, 1969) procedure, the decay is 10 dB in both ears, as indicated by the 10 dB threshold shift in both ears at the end of 1 minute.

End of Rosenberg (1958) procedure at the end of 1 minute

Stimulus Level (dB HL)

Time (sec)

can be missed using the Rosenberg (1958) technique (Parker & Decker, 1971). Tone decay tests can improve the accuracy in identifying vestibular schwannomas in the presence of hearing loss (Callan, Lasky, & Fowler, 1999).

5.9.2 Suprathreshold Tone Decay Test

In the Suprathreshold Adaptation Test (STAT), the tone is presented at 110 dB sound pressure level (SPL) for 1 minute, and the maintenance of audibility of the tone is determined. A lack of maintenance of audibility for 1 minute is suggestive of retrocochlear pathology (Jerger & Jerger, 1975). ▶ Fig. 5.20 shows the percent of patients showing decay on the STAT across cochlear, eighth nerve, brainstem, and temporal lobe pathologies (Antonelli, Bellotto, & Grandori, 1987).

5.9.3 Factors Determining Tone Decay

The critical factor determining tone decay may be the number, distribution, or timing of nerve spikes evoked by the tone. Tone decay appears to be associated with poor function of the inner hair cells and/or auditory neurons. Thus, in the presence of hearing loss, the degree of tone decay may provide an index of the functional status of the inner hair cells and/or neurons responsible for detecting the test tone (Huss & Moore, 2003).

5.9.4 Impact of Abnormal Tone Decay

Costello and McGee (1967) described two patients with abnormal tone decay and poor speech recognition skills in the presence of normal audiograms.

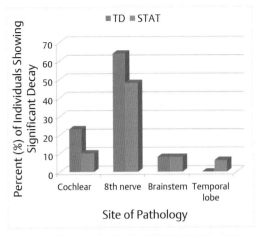

Fig. 5.20 The percentage of individuals showing 30 dB or more decay on the Rosenberg (1958) tone decay (TD) test and significant decay on the Jerger (1975) Suprathreshold Adaptation Test (STAT) across various sites of pathology (based on Antonelli, Bellotto, & Grandori, 1987).

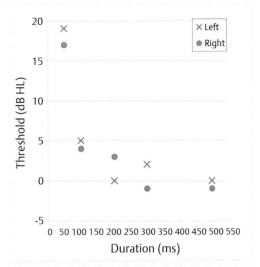

Fig. 5.21 Thresholds (dB HL) at 1000 Hz of a 21-year-old woman as a function of tonal duration obtained using the AC40 clinical audiometer shown in Chapter 3.

Some patients with hearing loss can perceive less audibility and clarity after using their hearing aids for a while, but after not using hearing aids for a period, the clarity and audibility may return (Goldberg, as cited in Green [1978]). Abnormal temporal maintenance, along with a reduced dynamic range, can lead to a frequent need for volume change on hearing aids and television in such patients (see Chapter 4 for an example).

5.10 Temporal Integration or Temporal Summation

Temporal integration or summation refers to the assumed ability of the auditory system to add up information over time or over duration up to a critical duration point. Temporal summation can be measured by presenting auditory stimuli near or above thresholds.

5.10.1 Temporal Summation at Thresholds

Temporal Summation at Threshold Due to an Increase in Stimulus Duration

In this case, the thresholds improve due to an increase in the duration of the stimulus (Pedersen & Salomon, 1977). The participant is expected to raise his or her hand or press a button whenever he or she hears a signal. Threshold is usually recorded as the softest signal to which the participant responds on at least two out of three ascending trials. As an example of this phenomenon, if an individual has a threshold of 15 dB for a stimulus lasting 20 ms, the threshold may be −5 dB for a stimulus that is 200 ms long. In this example, the threshold improved by 20 dB because of an increase in the duration of the stimulus. Thus, the auditory system appears to operate as an energy detector. A certain amount of energy is needed to detect the sound. This energy may be achieved by using higher intensity over a shorter duration or lower intensity over a longer duration. The ear appears to integrate energy over an integration time frame of about 200 ms. Thus, auditory thresholds do not improve much with an increase in stimulus duration beyond 200 ms. In fact, if the stimulus duration is too long (e.g., 2 minutes), the thresholds can become worse. This phenomenon is referred to as *adaptation.*

Some commercially available audiometers allow changes in the duration of tones. Thus, the thresholds can be measured by varying the duration of the tones to obtain a temporal integration function. ▶ Fig. 5.21 shows a temporal integration function at 1000 Hz for both the left and right ears for a 21-year-old woman obtained using the AC40 clinical audiometer (Interacoustics AS, Drejervaenget 8, DK-5610, Assens, Denmark). The thresholds in the right ear improved from 19 dB HL for a 50 ms tone to 0 dB for a 500 ms tone, showing an improvement of 19 dB. The threshold in the left ear improved from 17 dB for a 50 ms tone to −1 dB for a 500 ms tone, showing an improvement of 18 dB. Note that most of the improvement occurs when the duration of the tone is up to 200 to 300 ms. Increasing the duration beyond 300 ms does not lead to much more improvement. A more time-saving approach may be to measure the thresholds for brief duration tones (20 ms) and for long duration tones (500 ms), then to compare the difference between the two thresholds with age-appropriate norms. Children age 5 to 7 years show temporal integration similar to that of adults for higher frequencies (6500 Hz), but for lower frequencies, such as 1625 Hz, they show relatively more temporal integration due to higher thresholds for brief stimuli (e.g., 8 ms) (He, Buss, & Hall, 2010).

Temporal Summation at Threshold Due to an Increase in Stimulus Rate

In this case, the auditory thresholds improve due to an increase in stimulus rates (Beattie & Rochverger, 2001; Garner, 1947). This is partially because, at higher rates, more stimuli are presented within a shorter period. Thus, the energy is added over time. However, at very low rates (1 −4/s), thresholds may also improve due to more opportunities to detect the stimulus at higher rates (Garner, 1947). For example, when stimuli are presented at a rate of 4/s, there are four opportunities within 1 second to detect the stimulus, whereas there is only one opportunity within 1 second to detect the stimulus when stimuli are presented at a rate of 1/s.

5.10.2 Temporal Summation of Loudness at Suprathreshold Levels

Increase in Perceived Loudness Due to an Increase in the Duration of Suprathreshold Stimuli

When two equally intense stimuli of different durations are compared, the stimulus with longer duration is perceived as being louder because there is more energy in the long-duration stimulus (Buus, Florentine, & Poulsen, 1999; Miller, 1948). In this case, the participant is presented with signal pairs that are equally intense

but differ in duration and is expected to judge if the two stimuli appear equal or different in loudness.

Increase in the Perceived Loudness of Suprathreshold Stimuli Due to an Increase in the Stimulus Rate

When two equally intense stimuli of different stimulus rates are compared, the stimulus with the higher rate sounds louder (Darling & Price, 1989).

5.10.3 Effect of Hearing Loss on Temporal Summation

The improvement in auditory thresholds with increase in duration tends to be less in individuals with hearing loss than that apparent in normal-hearing listeners (Chung, 1982). Reduced temporal integration is more apparent at frequencies with the greatest hearing loss (Kidd, Mason, & Faith, 1984). Thus, the ability of the auditory system to integrate acoustic energy in brief sounds is reduced in the presence of hearing loss (Florentine, Fastl, & Buus, 1988; Hall & Fernandes, 1983; Watson & Gengel, 1969). Similarly, stimulus rate−induced improvement in auditory thresholds is reduced in individuals with hearing loss (Carlyon et al., 1990).

5.10.4 Impact of Abnormal Temporal Summation

Normal temporal summation can provide important cues for duration discrimination for very short sounds. As stated previously, duration discrimination is important for normal speech perception. Some individuals with temporal lobe pathologies have difficulty in detecting sounds of very short duration (1 ms), so their thresholds are elevated for such brief sounds (Baru & Karaseva, 1972). In addition, approximately one third of patients with abnormalities of the eighth nerve show increased temporal integration compared to normal-hearing participants (Pederson, 1976).

5.11 Precedence Effect or the Principle of the First Wavefront

A signal that precedes any other signals (e.g., echoes or reverberations) in time dominates our perception of the sound (Gardner, 1968; Yost & Soderquist, 1984). In other words, the auditory system suppresses signals that occur within about 40 ms after the earlier arriving sound, provided that the later occurring signals are quieter than the original signal. The precedent effect helps us in locating sounds in reverberant fields. If an individual has poor ability to fuse direct sounds with the early reflections of that sound, the listener may have difficulty in recognizing speech in reverberant environments (Roberts, Koehnke, & Besing, 2003). The performance on precedence effect localization tasks is correlated with speech recognition in the presence of a competing message (Cranford & Romereim, 1992). Precedence effect plays a role in sound localization as discussed in Chapter 6.

5.12 Interaural Temporal Processing

In addition to spatial gap detection discussed previously, several other interaural tasks involve temporal processing: sound localization, interaural time difference discrimination, masking level difference, binaural speech perception in quiet and noise, and rapidly alternating speech. These tasks are discussed in Chapter 6.

5.13 Time-Altered Speech Measures

In addition to nonspeech stimuli, speech stimuli can be used to assess temporal processing. For example, recognition of time-compressed speech is related to processing speed efficiency. Time-altered speech measures are discussed in Chapter 7.

5.14 Objective Temporal Measures

Various objective temporal measures can be used for assessing temporal processing in the auditory system, including stapedial reflex measures, auditory evoked potentials (AEPs), and magnetoencephalography (MEG). Picton (2013) provided a classification of AEPs based on how the responses occur as a function of changes in stimuli over time (▸ Fig. 5.22).

5.14.1 Temporal Summation in Acoustic Reflex Thresholds

An objective way to measure temporal summation or integration at suprathreshold levels is to measure acoustic reflex thresholds (ARTs) with stimuli of increasing duration or rates. The softest stimulus at which a recordable change in middle ear admittance is apparent on at least two out of three trials is considered the ART. Thresholds are established using commercially available clinical middle ear analyzers. During ART measures, the participant is expected to sit quietly and not move, talk, or swallow.

Stimulus Duration–Induced Improvement of Acoustic Reflex Thresholds

This is the improvement in ARTs apparent with an increase in the duration of stimuli (Cacace, Margolis, & Relkin, 1991; Moller, 1962). In this case, ARTs are determined for stimuli of varying duration.

Rate-induced Facilitation of Acoustic Reflex Thresholds

This is the improvement in ARTs apparent with an increase in the stimulus rates (Johnsen & Terkildsen, 1980; Rawool, 1995). ▸ Fig. 5.23 shows ARTs at various click rates obtained using 300 clicks (varying click-train duration) (Rawool, 1996a) or a fixed click-train duration (Rawool, 1995) in young adults. The differences in thresholds obtained between the faster and slower click rates can be referred to as rate-induced facilitation (RIF) of ARTs. Young children in the age range of 6 to 10 years show an RIF that is similar to young adults when click rates are changed from 50 to 100/s (Fielding & Rawool, 2002). The click RIF of ARTs can be measured using 1000 Hz probe tones in addition to the commonly used 226 Hz probe tones (Rawool, 1998a). Thus, it can also be measured in infants.

5.14.2 Objective Measures of Temporal Processing Speed

The speed with which stimuli are processed over time can be referred to as the *temporal processing speed*. ▸ Fig. 5.23 shows that the RIF of clicks in older adults is similar to that seen in young adults for click rates up to 150/s; at higher rates the RIF is lower in older adults (Rawool, 1996b). It appears that in the presence of a reduced temporal processing speed,

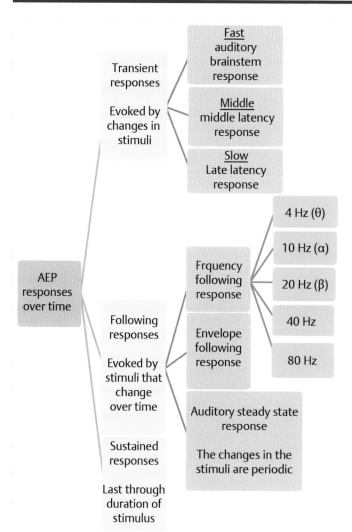

Fig. 5.22 Classification (Picton, 2013) of auditory evoked responses based on how the responses occur as a function of changes in stimuli over time.

some of the clicks presented at higher rates are missed, leading to a smaller RIF (▶ Fig. 5.24; Rawool, 2012). Thus, in the presence of slower processing speed, the click RIF of ARTs is reduced (Rawool, 1996b). The click RIF has not been evaluated in individuals with auditory processing difficulties but can serve as an indirect but objective measure of the temporal processing speed that is not influenced by linguistic or cognitive factors.

Direct Measures of Temporal Processing Speed

Direct measures of temporal processing speed are latencies of acoustic reflex measures and various AEPs, including the auditory brainstem response (ABR), middle latency response, and late evoked potentials. Longer latencies compared to age-matched peers suggest a slower processing speed. Longer latencies of different evoked potentials have been reported in various clinical populations. For example, children with specific language impairments show prolonged latencies of the P300 evoked with tones and speech stimuli compared to their age-matched peers (Ors et al., 2002).

Acoustic Reflex Latency

Acoustic reflex onset latencies can be specified as follows:

1. Initial or "10% on" latency: This is the period from signal onset to 10% of the maximum amplitude of the acoustic reflex.

2. Terminal or "90% on" latency: This is the period from signal onset to 90% of the maximum acoustic reflex amplitude.

Mean initial acoustic reflex latencies (10% on) for young adults, along with lower and higher limits for 95% of the population, are shown in ▶ Fig. 5.25 (Qiu & Stucker, 1998). Examples of latencies established at 500 and 1000 Hz from a young adult are shown in ▶ Fig. 5.26. The "10%

on" latency at 1000 Hz in this case is 106 ms on the first trial and 104 ms on the second trial. The "10% on" latency for 500 Hz is 110 ms on the first trial and 108 ms on the second trial. These latencies are within normal limits. An example of a very short latency is shown in ▶ Fig. 5.27. In this case, the 10% on latency is 8 ms, which is much shorter than the normal limits and is suggestive of heightened sensitivity to loud sounds, although there is no hyperacusis or abnormal sensitivity to loud sounds in this particular case. If clicks are used as stimuli, the reflex latencies cannot be established in some of the population if the click rate is 50/s (Qiu & Stucker, 1998). Thus, if clicks are used as stimuli, the click rate should be 100/s or higher. Acoustic reflex latencies are significantly longer in children with autism compared to age-matched peers (Lukose, Brown, Barber, & Kulesza, 2013).

5.14.3 Objective Measures of Temporal Response Maintenance (Decay)

Temporal response maintenance can be thought of as the ability of the auditory system to continue to evaluate high-level stimuli without fatigue. This ability can be evaluated using the stapedial reflex decay test. The most common procedure for measuring stapedial reflex decay involves presentation of stimuli 10 dB above the reflex threshold for 10 seconds and recording the response (▶ Fig. 5.28). The testing is usually conducted at 500 and

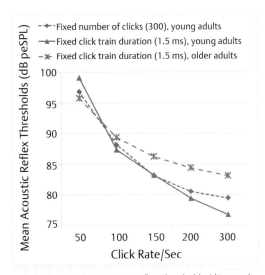

Fig. 5.23 Average acoustic reflex thresholds (dB sound pressure level [SPL]) in young adults obtained using 300 clicks (based on Rawool, 1996a) and 1.5-second click-train duration (based on Rawool, 1995) and in older adults using 1.5 ms click-train duration (based on Rawool, 1996b) at various click rates.

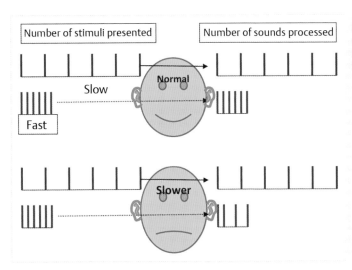

Fig. 5.24 Illustration of processing of stimuli by individuals with normal and slower processing speeds (adapted from Rawool, 2012).

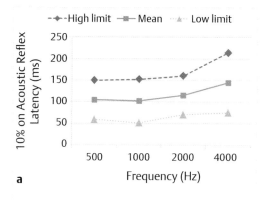

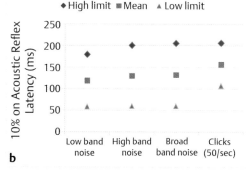

Fig. 5.25 Mean acoustic reflex "10% on" latencies (ms) across tones of various frequencies (a) and across different broadband stimuli (b) and 95% limit values from young normal-hearing adults (based on Qiu and Stucker, 1998).

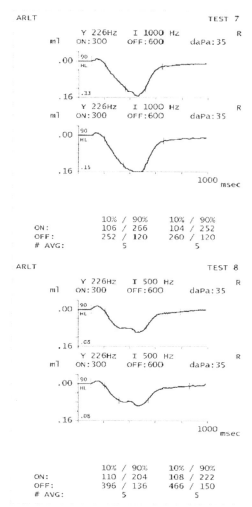

Fig. 5.26 Example of objective measurement of the temporal processing speed for loud stimuli using the acoustic reflex latency test. Latencies were established for a 21-year-old woman for 1000 and 500 Hz tones presented ipsilaterally at 10 dB above the acoustic reflex thresholds. Each waveform is obtained by averaging data over five trials. Two waveforms are shown for each of the test frequencies. The on and off reflex latencies are displayed below the waveforms.

1000 Hz given that reflex decay is frequently apparent at higher frequencies in normal-hearing individuals. More than 50% reduction in the acoustic reflex amplitude over a period of 10 seconds at 500 and 1000 Hz is indicative of abnormal decay. An example of a reflex decay pattern is shown in ▶ Fig. 5.29.

Although traditionally reflex decay has been measured over a fixed time period (10 s), it can also be measured using a fixed number of stimuli, such as 1000 clicks (Rawool, 1996c). When the reflex is recorded by presenting 1000 clicks at the rates of 50 or 100/s at 95 or 105 dB HL, the reflex decays in about 5 to 10% of individuals tested. The reflex amplitude increases over time in about 5 to 10% of individuals, suggesting tough ears (ears that are at a lower risk for noise-induced hearing loss). In the remaining subjects, the amplitude either remains steady or fluctuates over time (▶ Fig. 5.30). Examples of fluctuating and increasing reflex amplitudes are shown in ▶ Fig. 5.31.

Effect of Lesions on Acoustic Reflex Decay

The percentage of individuals showing abnormal stapedial reflex decay across lesions at various sites in the auditory pathway is shown in ▶ Fig. 5.32 (Antonelli, Bellotto, & Grandori, 1987). Stapedial reflex decay is abnormal in patients with subclinical and clinical hypothyroidism and

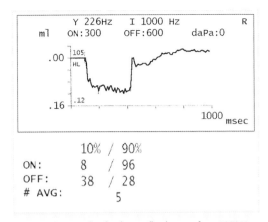

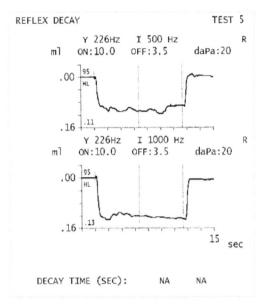

10% / 90%

ON: 8   / 96
OFF: 38 / 28
AVG: 5

Fig. 5.27 Example of a short reflex latency for a 1000 Hz tone obtained from a 60-year-old listener. The very short latency may be indicative of heightened sensitivity to loud sounds. The reflex attained 10% of maximum amplitude within 8 ms following the onset of the tone.

returns to normal when treated through thyroxine administration (Goulis et al., 1998).

5.14.4 Objective Measures of Temporal Synchrony

With regard to auditory neurons, temporal synchrony can be referred to as the ability of several neurons to fire simultaneously in response to a broadband stimulus. The integrity of the click-evoked ABR relies heavily on the synchronous firings of several auditory neurons. The technique of ABR described in Chapter 4 can be used as a measure of temporal synchrony. For this purpose, the ABR can be elicited using high-level stimuli, such as 70 and 80 dB normal hearing level (nHL), and the absolute and interpeak latencies, amplitudes, and morphology of the waveforms can be analyzed. It is best to record two waveforms at each presentation level using rarefaction and condensation clicks due to differences in resulting waveform morphology across individuals (Rawool, 1998b, 2007; Rawool & Zerlin, 1988). Relatively higher click repetition rates (e. g., 30 clicks/s) that can increase the sensitivity of the ABR (reviewed in Rawool, 2007) without compromising the integrity of the waveforms are recommended for evoking the response. An example of ABR waveforms showing poor and good synchrony from two different individuals is given in ▶ Fig. 5.33.

Fig. 5.28 Example of normal reflex maintenance at 500 and 1000 Hz. The stimulus levels are 10 dB above the reflex threshold levels established at each stimulus frequency. The traces show good maintenance of the reflex or no decay over the period of 10 seconds.

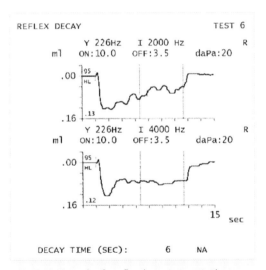

Fig. 5.29 Example of a reflex decay pattern. In the top trace, the reflex amplitude drops by 50% at 6 seconds, indicating the lack of maintenance. For a tonal frequency of 2000 Hz, this pattern is apparent in many normal-hearing subjects. However, a similar decay pattern for tonal frequencies of 500 and 1000 Hz is suggestive of pathology within the acoustic reflex pathway.

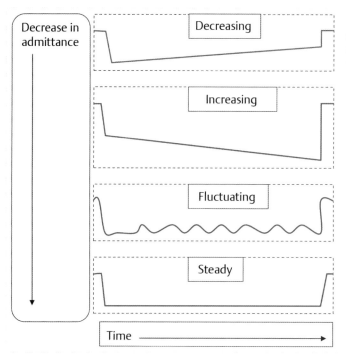

Fig. 5.30 Schematic of acoustic reflex sustainability (decay) patterns in response to 1000 clicks (adapted from Rawool, 1996c).

ABR latency measures can show up to 100% sensitivity in detecting acoustic neuromas larger than 3.0 cm and up to 83.1% sensitivity in detecting tumors 1.0 cm or smaller. ABR waveform morphology is abnormal in 100% of tumors larger than 2.0 cm and in 76.5% of tumors 1.0 cm or smaller (Chandrasekhar, Brackmann, & Devgan, 1995). An increase in stimulus rates can improve the sensitivity of ABR in detecting tumors (Tanaka, Komatsuzaki, & Hentona, 1996). ABR latencies are prolonged in the presence of other pathological conditions involving the auditory nerve and brainstem, including diabetes (Al-Azzawi & Mirza, 2004) and multiple sclerosis (Matas, Matas, Oliveira, & Gonçalves, 2010).

5.14.5 Objective Measures of Gap Detection

Gap Detection Using the Auditory Brainstem Response

When a stimulus is presented to the ear with a gap, the trailing marker evokes an ABR similar to the usual ABR with larger amplitudes for larger gap durations. The gap detection threshold can then be recorded by varying the duration of the gap until the ABR becomes undetectable. The smallest gap duration that yields a detectable ABR is the gap detection threshold for that ABR. Average behavioral gap detection thresholds for gaps in a low pass filtered noise (filter cutoff of 7 kHz) are 2.9 ms for young adults. ABR gap detection thresholds for the same noise are significantly lower with average thresholds of 2.4 ms. There is also a moderate correlation between the ABR and behavioral thresholds among young adults. ABR gap detection thresholds of 3-month-old infants appear to be similar to those of normal-hearing young adults (Werner, Folsom, Mancl, & Syapin, 2001).

Gap Detection Using Late Auditory Evoked Potentials

N1-P2 waveforms can be recorded in response to gaps in a broadband noise in normal-hearing young adults. The responses are apparent for gap durations of 2 ms above behavioral gap detection thresholds (BGDTs). Gaps that are below BGDT do not generally evoke an electrophysiological response. N1-P2 waveform amplitudes increase with increasing gap duration (Palmer & Musiek, 2013).

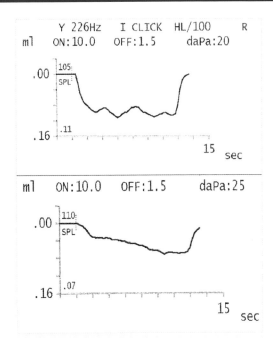

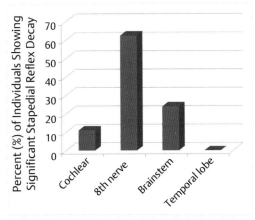

Fig. 5.32 Percentage of individuals showing significant stapedial reflex decay across various sites of pathology (based on Antonelli, Bellotto, & Grandori, 1987).

Fig. 5.31 Examples of reflex temporal maintenance patterns obtained using clicks presented at 100 clicks/s over a period of 10 seconds. The first tracing is an example of a modulating or fluctuating pattern that is apparent in about 30% of normal-hearing individuals. The second trace is a pattern showing the increasing strength of the reflex. Such a pattern is apparent in approximately 10% of normal-hearing young adults and may be indicative of tough ears that are less prone to noise-induced hearing loss.

Gap Detection Using Magnetoencephalography

The middle latency evoked field (gamma response) can be elicited to continuous stimuli and stimuli with gaps. A transient response can be derived as the difference wave between the response to gap stimuli and continuous stimuli with the same duration. The response increases with the increase in gap duration and with the duration of the leading marker and is correlated with behavioral gap detection measures (Rupp, Gutschalk, Uppenkamp, & Scherg, 2004).

5.14.6 Duration Discrimination Using Mismatch Negativity

Mismatch negativity (MMN) can be recorded by using deviant stimuli varying in duration when

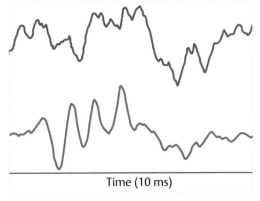

Time (10 ms)

Fig. 5.33 Auditory brainstem response (ABR) waveforms from two young women obtained with condensation clicks at 60 dB normal hearing level (NHL). Better temporal synchrony is apparent in the bottom waveform, as indicated by sharper peaks.

compared to standard stimuli. For example, the standard stimulus can be a 100 ms white noise burst, and deviant stimuli can be either shorter (e.g., 90 ms) or longer (e.g., 110 ms) than the standard stimulus. As shown in ▸ Fig. 5.34, the amplitude of the MMN response increases with the increase in the differences in duration of the standard and deviant stimuli except when the deviant is extremely short in duration (e.g., 1 ms).

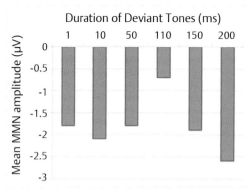

Fig. 5.34 Mean mismatch negativity (MMN) amplitudes (µV) as a function of duration of deviant tones in the presence of standard tones with a duration of 100 ms (based on Jaramillo, Paavilainen, & Näätänen, 2000).

Gap Duration Discrimination Using Mismatch Negativity

MMN can be reliably elicited using standard gap durations of 120 ms, along with deviant gap durations of 20 ms (Kujala, Kallio, Tervaniemi, & Näätänen, 2001).

5.14.7 Temporal Pattern Discrimination Using Magnetoencephalography

MMN can be recorded during passive, distracted listening in most individuals in response to deviant tones occurring at various positions within a tonal pattern when compared to standard tone patterns of four tones. Similar responses can be elicited in fewer individuals when the number of tones in the tonal complex is increased to six tones, suggesting a limit on the short-term auditory storage capacity (Boh, Herlholz, Lappe, & Pantev, 2011).

5.14.8 Correlations between Behavioral and Objective Temporal Processing Measures

Often there is a correlation between behavioral and objective measures of temporal processing. For example, performance on the backward masking task is related to the syllable-evoked brainstem response. Some children with learning impairments have poor backward masking thresholds along with neurophysiological timing deficits in

both transient and sustained brainstem responses to the speech syllable /da/ (Johnson, Nicol, Zecker, & Kraus, 2007). The amplitude of the N1a and N1b component of the AEPs is significantly correlated with the duration of the voice onset time in consonant-vowel syllables and in nonspeech analogs of the voice onset time (Zaehle, Jancke, & Meyer, 2007).

5.15 Physiology of Temporal Processing

The performance on most of the temporal processing tasks discussed above relies on speedy and precise temporal coding of acoustic stimuli within the auditory system. An important factor in determining the temporal processing speed is neural conduction time, which is determined by several factors, including synaptic efficiency, the number and integrity of neurons, axons, and dendrites, and the integrity of myelin sheaths. The preciseness of coding is partially determined by the ability of several neurons to fire simultaneously or with precise interaural delays (e.g., coding of interaural time difference; see Chapter 6). In addition, temporal order judgments or temporal pattern discriminations rely heavily on the integrity of the auditory cortex. As previously mentioned, temporal lobe damage results in impairment in the performance of these tasks.

5.15.1 Inner Hair Cell Synapses

To allow accurate temporal coding of auditory stimuli, the release of neurotransmitters has to be well synchronized with onset and offset of even very brief auditory stimuli. The cochlear hair cell afferent synapses have unique cellular and molecular properties to achieve this goal. The transmitting zone of the hair cell is characterized by an electron-dense structure called the synaptic body or ribbon, known as the hair cell ribbon synapse. Most of these synapses are anchored to the plasma membrane of the inner hair cell (Nouvian, Beutner, Parsons, & Moser, 2006). Each inner hair cell can have between 5 and 20 ribbon synapses with the unbranched peripheral axons of cochlear ganglion neurons (Moser, Predoehl, & Starr, 2013).

Dysfunction of the hair cell ribbon synapses, or auditory synaptopathy, has a negative impact on the neural encoding of acoustic temporal cues. The genetic variants of these synaptopathies include alterations of vesicular glutamate uptake, presynaptic calcium (Ca^{2+}) influx, and synaptic vesicular replenishment. Synaptopathies can be acquired as a result of noise exposure, which can lead to excessive presynaptic release of glutamate, and aging (Moser, Predoehl, & Starr, 2013).

5.15.2 Myelin Integrity

Intact myelin plays an important role in maintaining normal temporal processing speed. For example, Rasminsky and Sears (1972) noted an average internodal conduction time of 19.7 ± 4.6 SD ms in normal ventral root fibers of rats. When the ventral roots were demyelinated by focal application of diphtheria toxin, the intermodal conduction time varied from 26 to more than 600 ms. Due to the slow speed, conduction of impulses in demyelinated fibers can be blocked to a second stimulus if the stimulus occurs in very close proximity to the first stimulus. Repetitive stimulation of demyelinated fibers causes a progressive increase in internodal conduction time, leading to intermittent or total conduction block at the demyelinated internodes. The wide variation in internodal conduction time in demyelinated nerve fibers also can lead to temporal dispersion of impulses in a given nerve or tract, leading to temporal asynchrony. As an example in humans, maximal finger-tapping speed requires high-frequency action potential bursts and is associated with myelin integrity. Both myelin integrity and maximum finger-tapping speed have similar quadratic trajectories, reaching a peak at 39 years of age and declining with an accelerating trajectory thereafter (Bartzokis et al., 2010).

One of the factors contributing to age-related slowing in the cognitive processing speed appears to be myelin breakdown (Lu et al., 2013). Loss of myelin sheaths, along with oligodendrocyte death, is apparent in multiple sclerosis (MS). Some demyelinated axons may rebuild their membranes, whereas others do not, resulting in a temporary or permanent impairment in signal conduction in MS. Loss of myelin can also make axons more vulnerable to damage, leading to impaired axonal integrity and cumulative loss of axons, culminating in irreversible neurologic deficits. For these reasons, myelin repair is considered an important area of research in MS (Kocsis & Waxman, 2007). Reduced auditory processing speed has been documented in some individuals with MS (Matas, Matas, Oliveira, & Gonçalves, 2010; Saberi, Hatamian, Nemati, & Banan, 2012) and older adults through the recording of prolonged latencies of AEPs, especially in response to stimuli presented at high rates (reviewed in Rawool, 2007). Auditory nerve conduction abnormalities have also been noted in some patients with Guillain-Barré syndrome (Nelson, Gilmore, & Massey, 1988; Schiff, Cracco, & Cracco, 1985;), which is characterized by axonal demyelination (Vucic, Kiernan, & Cornblath, 2009).

5.15.3 Temporal Coding within Nerve Tracts

The timing of action potentials is important in coding temporal information. The temporal code is maintained with a phase-locked response of some auditory nerve fibers where the onset of an action potential is locked or synchronized with a particular cycle or phase of the stimulus. Phase locking preserves timing information in both low-frequency sounds and the slower amplitude envelopes of high-frequency carriers. It is more precise for stimuli presented at slower rates (Lu & Wang, 2004).

The relative timing of action potentials traveling through sequential synapses is well preserved in spiral ganglion neurons and auditory brainstem nuclei through special adaptations. At the membrane level, low-threshold, voltage-gated potassium channels and relatively fast-acting transmitter-gated channels allow rapid and precise action potentials. At the neuronal level, some nerve terminals are massive, and there are several functional synaptic release sites for each axon terminal, allowing the release of large amounts of excitatory neurotransmitters. For example, the calyx of Held is a large glutamatergic terminal of the bushy cell in the ventral cochlear nucleus that forms a synapse with a neuron in the medial nucleus of the trapezoid body. It includes approximately 100 donut-like assemblies, each containing approximately 800 synaptic vesicles, 6 to 9 mitochondria, and 5 to 9 active zones (Wimmer, Horstmann, Groh, & Kuner, 2006).

In addition, some large axonal terminals innervate the soma of neurons instead of dendrites, thereby minimizing the slowing caused by dendritic innervations. In the presence of dendritic innervation, the convergence of many axonal inputs ensures faster neural conduction.

Excitatory postsynaptic potentials (EPSPs) in auditory neurons are brief, or precise, which allows accommodation of rapid transmission of stimuli and minimizes any temporal distortions or asynchronies as impulses are transmitted through various synapses. The brief duration of EPSPs is accomplished by having brief excitatory postsynaptic currents (EPSCs). The presence of glutamate and glutamate receptors mediate fast excitatory transmission in the cochlea and auditory brainstem neurons. During repetitive stimulation, *N*-methyl-*d*-aspartate (NMDA) receptors may contribute to a small plateau potential (Trussell, 1999).

Marked synaptic depression is apparent in response to stimuli presented at very high rates in EPSCs in some neurons; it may be due to a reduction in transmitter release in some cases (von Gersdorff, Schneggenburger, Weis, & Neher, 1997). The neural correlate of forward masking is also apparent in the responses of auditory nerve fibers in the form of a depression in responses to a probe stimulus immediately following another stimulus (Harris & Dallos 1979).

5.16 Future Trends

Systematically collected data on normal-hearing individuals and individuals with various structural and functional anomalies within the auditory system will be available for all the objective and behavioral temporal processing tasks in the future. It will also become easier to obtain evoked potential measures with the availability of more affordable and efficient technologies. As an example, see the website for Emotiv Systems (San Francisco, CA; http://www.emotiv.com/), which sells the Emotive EPOC multichannel, portable system for recording contextual EEG. Advances in similar technologies will allow objective assessment of various temporal processes without any active responses from the listener. Such technologies may allow accurate separation of attentional and memory deficits from APDs.

5.17 Review Questions

1. Discuss different ways of measuring temporal resolution and the effect of poor temporal resolution on speech perception.
2. Review temporal asynchrony and its effect on speech perception.
3. Describe the temporal separation (sequential stream segregation) task and its significance for speech perception in noisy or complex environments.
4. Describe temporal ordering and masking and how these tasks are related to speech perception.
5. Describe temporal maintenance or decay procedures for measuring temporal maintenance, and the potential impact of poor temporal maintenance.
6. What is temporal integration or summation? How can you measure temporal summation of loudness at suprathreshold levels?
7. Define the precedence effect and its relation to speech perception in the presence of a competing message.
8. Describe the potential role of acoustic reflex testing in assessing temporal processing.
9. Describe the potential role of auditory evoked potentials in assessing temporal processing.
10. How is temporal processing coded within the auditory system?

References

[1] Al-Azzawi, L. M., & Mirza, K. B. (2004). The usefulness of the brainstem auditory evoked potential in the early diagnosis of cranial nerve neuropathy associated with diabetes mellitus. Electromyography and Clinical Neurophysiology, 44(7), 387–394.

[2] Alcántara, J. I., Cope, T. E., Cope, W., & Weisblatt, E. J. (2012). Auditory temporal-envelope processing in high-functioning children with autism spectrum disorder. Neuropsychologia, 50(7), 1235–1251.

[3] Antonelli, A. R., Bellotto, R., & Grandori, F. (1987). Audiologic diagnosis of central versus eighth nerve and cochlear auditory impairment. Audiology, 26(4), 209–226.

[4] Bacon, S. P., & Gleitman, R. M. (1992). Modulation detection in subjects with relatively flat hearing losses. Journal of Speech and Hearing Research, 35(3), 642–653.

[5] Bacon, S. P., & Viemeister, N. F. (1985). Temporal modulation transfer functions in normal-hearing and hearing-impaired listeners. Audiology, 24(2), 117–134.

[6] Bamiou, D. E., Musiek, F. E., Stow, I., et al. (2006). Auditory temporal processing deficits in patients with insular stroke. Neurology, 67(4), 614–619.

[7] Bartzokis, G., Lu, P. H., Tingus, K., et al. (2010). Lifespan trajectory of myelin integrity and maximum motor speed. Neurobiology and Aging, 31(9), 1554–1562.

[8] Baru, A., & Karaseva, T. (1972). The brain and hearing: Hearing disturbances associated with local brain lesions. New York: Consultation Bureau.

[9] Beattie, R. C., & Rochverger, I. (2001). Normative behavioral thresholds for short tone-bursts. Journal of the American Academy of Audiology, 12(9), 453–461.

[10] Berwanger, D., Wittmann, M., von Steinbüchel, N., & von Suchodoletz, W. (2004). Measurement of temporal-order judgment in children. Acta Neurobiologieae Experimentalis (Warsawz), 64(3), 387–394.

[11] Blackwell, K. L., Oyler, R. F., & Seyfried, D. N. (1991). A clinical comparison of Grason Stadler insert earphones and TDH-50 P standard earphones. Ear and Hearing, 12(5), 361–362.

[12] Bochner, J. H., Snell, K. B., & MacKenzie, D. J. (1988). Duration discrimination of speech and tonal complex stimuli by normally hearing and hearing-impaired listeners. Journal of the Acoustical Society of America, 84(2), 493–500.

[13] Boh, B., Herholz, S. C., Lappe, C., & Pantev, C. (2011). Processing of complex auditory patterns in musicians and nonmusicians. PLoS ONE, 6(7), e21458.

[14] Brännström, K. J., & Lantz, J. (2010). Interaural attenuation for Sennheiser HDA 200 circumaural earphones. International Journal of Audiology, 49(6), 467–471.

[15] Buus, S., Florentine, M., & Poulsen, T. (1999). Temporal integration of loudness in listeners with hearing losses of primarily cochlear origin. Journal of the Acoustical Society of America, 105(6), 3464–3480.

[16] Cacace, A. T., Margolis, R. H., & Relkin, E. M. (1991). Threshold and suprathreshold temporal integration effects in the crossed and uncrossed human acoustic stapedius reflex. Journal of the Acoustical Society of America, 89(3), 1255–1261.

[17] Callan, D. E., Lasky, R. E., & Fowler, C. G. (1999). Neural networks applied to retrocochlear diagnosis. Journal of Speech, Language, and Hearing Research, 42(2), 287–299.

[18] Carhart, R. (1957). Clinical determination of abnormal auditory adaptation. American Medical Association Archives of Otolaryngology, 65(1), 32–39.

[19] Carlyon, R. P., Buus, S., & Florentine, M. (1990). Temporal integration of trains of tone pulses by normal and by cochlearly impaired listeners. Journal of the Acoustical Society of America, 87(1), 260–268.

[20] Chandrasekhar, S. S., Brackmann, D. E., & Devgan, K. K. (1995). Utility of auditory brainstem response audiometry in diagnosis of acoustic neuromas. American Journal of Otology, 16(1), 63–67.

[21] Chermak, G. D., & Lee, J. (2005). Comparison of children's performance on four tests of temporal resolution. Journal of the American Academy of Audiology, 16(8), 554–563.

[22] Chung, D. Y. (1982). Temporal integration: Its relationship with noise-induced hearing loss. Scandinavian Audiology, 11(3), 153–157.

[23] Costello, M. R., & McGee, T. M. (1967). Language impairment associated with bilateral abnormal auditory adaptation. In A. B. Graham (Ed.), Sensorineural hearing processes and disorders. Boston: Little, Brown.

[24] Cranford, J. L., & Romereim, B. (1992). Precedence effect and speech understanding in elderly listeners. Journal of the American Academy of Audiology, 3(6), 405–409.

[25] Danaher, E. M., Wilson, M.P., & Pickett, J. M. (1978). Backward and forward masking in listeners with severe sensorineural hearing loss. Audiology, 17(4), 324–338.

[26] Darling, R. M., & Price, L. L. (1989). Temporal summation of repetitive click stimuli. Ear and Hearing, 10(3), 173–177.

[27] Desloge, J. G., Reed, C. M., Braida, L. D., Perez, Z. D., & Delhorne, L. A. (2011). Temporal masking functions for listeners with real and simulated hearing loss. Journal of the Acoustical Society of America, 130(2), 915–932.

[28] Dorman, M. F., Raphael, L.J., & Isenberg, D. (1980). Acoustic cues for a fricative and affricate contrast in word-final position. Journal of Phonetics, 4, 397–406.

[29] Dorman, M. F., Raphael, L. J., & Liberman, A. M. (1979). Some experiments on the sound of silence in phonetic perception. Journal of the Acoustical Society of America, 65(6), 1518–1532.

[30] Dreschler, W. A., & Plomp, R. (1985). Relations between psychophysical data and speech perception for hearing-impaired subjects. 2. Journal of the Acoustical Society of America, 78(4), 1261–1270.

[31] Dubno, J. R., Horwitz, A. R., & Ahlstrom, J. B. (2003). Recovery from prior stimulation: Masking of speech by interrupted noise for younger and older adults with normal hearing. Journal of the Acoustical Society of America, 113(4, Pt. 1), 2084–2094.

[32] Efron, R. (1963). Temporal perception, aphasia and déjà vu. Brain, 86, 403–424.

[33] Elfenbein, J. L., Small, A. M., & Davis, J. M. (1993). Developmental patterns of duration discrimination. Journal of Speech and Hearing Research, 36(4), 842–849.

[34] Elliott, L. L. (1962). Backward and forward masking of probe tones of different frequencies. Journal of the Acoustical Society of America, 34, 1116–111.

[35] Elliott, L. L. (1971). Backward and forward masking. Audiology, 10, 65–76.

[36] Espinoza-Varas, B., & Watson, C. S. (1986). Temporal discrimination for single components of nonspeech auditory patterns. Journal of the Acoustical Society of America, 80(6), 1685–1694.

[37] Feng, Y., Yin, S., Kiefte, M., & Wang, J. (2010). Temporal resolution in regions of normal hearing and speech perception in noise for adults with sloping high-frequency hearing loss. Ear and Hearing, 31(1), 115–125.

[38] Fielding, E. D., & Rawool, V. W. (2002). Acoustic reflex thresholds at varying click rates in children. International Journal of Pediatric Otorhinolaryngology, 63(3), 243–252.

[39] Fink, M., Churan, J., & Wittmann, M. (2005). Assessment of auditory temporal-order thresholds: A comparison of different measurement procedures and the influences of age and gender. Restorative Neurology and Neuroscience, 23(5-6), 281–296.

[40] Fink, M., Ulbrich, P., Churan, J., & Wittmann, M. (2006). Stimulus-dependent processing of temporal order. Behavioural Processes, 71(2-3), 344–352.

[41] Fitzgibbons, P. J., & Gordon-Salant, S. (1987). Minimum stimulus levels for temporal gap resolution in listeners with sensorineural hearing loss. Journal of the Acoustical Society of America, 81(5), 1542–1545.

[42] Fitzgibbons, P. J., & Gordon-Salant, S. (1994). Age effects on measures of auditory duration discrimination. Journal of Speech and Hearing Research, 37(3), 662–670.

[43] Fitzgibbons, P. J., & Wightman, F. L. (1982). Gap detection in normal and hearing-impaired listeners. Journal of the Acoustical Society of America, 72(3), 761–765.

[44] Florentine, M., Fastl, H., & Buus, S. (1988). Temporal integration in normal hearing, cochlear impairment, and impairment simulated by masking. Journal of the Acoustical Society of America, 84(1), 195–203.

[45] Fuente, A., & McPherson, B. (2007). Central auditory processing effects induced by solvent exposure. International Journal of Occupational Medicine and Environmental Health, 20(3), 271–279.

[46] Fuente, A., McPherson, B., & Cardemil, F. (2013). Xylene-induced auditory dysfunction in humans. Ear and Hearing, 34(5), 651–660.

[47] Gardner, M. B. (1968). Historical background of the Haas and-or precedence effect. Journal of the Acoustical Society of America, 43(6), 1243–1248.

[48] Garner, W. R. (1947). Auditory thresholds of short tones as a function of repetition rates. Journal of the Acoustical Society of America, 19, 600–608.

[49] Glasberg, B. R., & Moore, B. C. (1989). Psychoacoustic abilities of subjects with unilateral and bilateral cochlear hearing impairments and their relationship to the ability to understand speech. Scandinavian Audiology. Supplementum, 32, 1–25.

[50] Glasberg, B. R., Moore, B. C. J., & Bacon, S. P. (1987). Gap detection and masking in hearing-impaired and normal-hearing subjects. Journal of the Acoustical Society of America, 81 (5), 1546–1555.

[51] Goswami, U., Wang, H. L. S., Cruz, A., Fosker, T., Mead, N., & Huss, M. (2011). Language-universal sensory deficits in developmental dyslexia: English, Spanish, and Chinese. Journal of Cognitive Neuroscience, 23(2), 325–337.

[52] Goulis, D. G., Tsimpiris, N., Delaroudis, S., et al. (1998). Stapedial reflex: A biological index found to be abnormal in clinical and subclinical hypothyroidism. Thyroid, 8(7), 583–587.

[53] Grant, K. W., Summers, V., & Leek, M. R. (1998). Modulation rate detection and discrimination by normal-hearing and hearing-impaired listeners. Journal of the Acoustical Society of America, 104(2, Pt. 1), 1051–1060.

[54] Green, D. S. (1978). Tone decay. In J. Katz (Ed.) Handbook of clinical audiology (2nd ed., pp. 188-200). Baltimore: Williams & Wilkins.

[55] Grose, J. H., & Hall, J. W. III. (1996). Cochlear hearing loss and the processing of modulation: Effects of temporal asynchrony. Journal of the Acoustical Society of America, 100(1), 519–527.

[56] Grose, J. H., Hall, J. W. III, & Buss, E. (2001). Gap duration discrimination in listeners with cochlear hearing loss: Effects of gap and marker duration, frequency separation, and mode of presentation. Journal of the Association for Research in Otolaryngology, 2(4), 388–398.

[57] Grose, J. H., Hall, J. W. III, & Buss, E. (2004). Duration discrimination in listeners with cochlear hearing loss: Effects of stimulus type and frequency. Journal of Speech, Language, and Hearing Research, 47(1), 5–12.

[58] Güçlü, B., Sevinc, E., & Canbeyli, R. (2011). Duration discrimination by musicians and nonmusicians. Psychological Reports, 108(3), 675–687.

[59] Hall, J. W., & Fernandes, M. A. (1983). Temporal integration, frequency resolution, and off-frequency listening in normal-hearing and cochlear-impaired listeners. Journal of the Acoustical Society of America, 74(4), 1172–1177.

[60] Hall, J. W. III, Grose, J. H., Buss, E., & Hatch, D. R. (1998). Temporal analysis and stimulus fluctuation in listeners with normal and impaired hearing. Journal of Speech, Language, and Hearing Research, 41(2), 340–354.

[61] Han, M. W., Ahn, J. H., Kang, J. K., et al. (2011). Central auditory processing impairment in patients with temporal lobe epilepsy. Epilepsy and Behavior, 20(2), 370–374.

[62] Harris, D. M., & Dallos, P. (1979). Forward masking of auditory nerve fiber responses. Journal of Neurophysiology, 42 (4), 1083–1107.

[63] Hartley, D. E. H., & Moore, D. R. (2002). Auditory processing efficiency deficits in children with developmental language impairments. Journal of the Acoustical Society of America, 112(6), 2962–2966.

[64] He, S., Buss, E., & Hall, J. W. III. (2010). Monaural temporal integration and temporally selective listening in children and adults. Journal of the Acoustical Society of America, 127 (6), 3643–3653.

[65] Heinrich, A., Alain, C., & Schneider, B. A. (2004). Within- and between-channel gap detection in the human auditory cortex. Neuroreport, 15(13), 2051–2056.

[66] Hellström, A., & Rammsayer, T. H. (2004). Effects of time-order, interstimulus interval, and feedback in duration discrimination of noise bursts in the 50- and 1000-ms ranges. Acta Psychologica (Amsterdam), 116(1), 1–20.

[67] Hess, B. A., Blumsack, J. T., Ross, M. E., & Brock, R. E. (2012). Performance at different stimulus intensities with the with-in- and across-channel adaptive tests of temporal resolution. International Journal of Audiology, 51(12), 900–905.

[68] Himpel, S., Banaschewski, T., Grüttner, A., et al. (2009). Duration discrimination in the range of milliseconds and seconds in children with ADHD and their unaffected siblings. Psychological Medicine, 39(10), 1745–1751.

[69] Hirsh, I. J. (1959). Auditory perception of temporal order. Journal of the Acoustical Society of America, 31, 759–767.

[70] Huss, M., & Moore, B. C. J. (2003). Tone decay for hearing-impaired listeners with and without dead regions in the cochlea. Journal of the Acoustical Society of America, 114(6, Pt. 1), 3283–3294.

[71] Irwin, R. J., & Purdy, S. C. (1982). The minimum detectable duration of auditory signals for normal and hearing-impaired listeners. Journal of the Acoustical Society of America, 71(4), 967–974.

[72] Jaramillo, M., Paavilainen, P., & Näätänen, R. (2000). Mismatch negativity and behavioural discrimination in humans as a function of the magnitude of change in sound duration. Neuroscience Letters, 290(2), 101–104.

[73] Jensen, J. K., & Neff, D. L. (1993). Development of basic auditory discrimination in preschool children. Psychological Science, 4, 104–107.

[74] Jerger, J., & Jerger, S. (1975). A simplified tone decay test. Archives in Otolaryngology, 101(7), 403–407.

[75] Johnsen, N. J., & Terkildsen, K. (1980). The normal middle ear reflex thresholds towards white noise and acoustic clicks in young adults. Scandinavian Audiology, 9(3), 131–135.

[76] Johnson, K. L., Nicol, T. G., Zecker, S. G., & Kraus, N. (2007). Auditory brainstem correlates of perceptual timing deficits. Journal of Cognitive Neuroscience, 19(3), 376–385.

[77] Karnath, H. O., Zimmer, U., & Lewald, J. (2002). Impaired perception of temporal order in auditory extinction. Neuropsychologia, 40(12), 1977–1982.

[78] Keith, R. W. (2000). Random gap detection test. St. Louis, MO: Auditec.

[79] Kidd, G. Jr., Mason, C. R., & Feth, L. L. (1984). Temporal integration of forward masking in listeners having sensorineural hearing loss. Journal of the Acoustical Society of America, 75 (3), 937–944.

[80] King, W. M., Lombardino, L. J., Crandell, C. C., & Leonard, C. M. (2003). Comorbid auditory processing disorder in developmental dyslexia. Ear and Hearing, 24(5), 448–456.

[81] Kocsis, J. D., & Waxman, S. G. (2007). Schwann cells and their precursors for repair of central nervous system myelin. Brain, 130(Pt 8), 1978–1980.

[82] Kujala, T., Kallio, J., Tervaniemi, M., & Näätänen, R. (2001). The mismatch negativity as an index of temporal processing in audition. Clinical Neurophysiology, 112(9), 1712–1719.

[83] Leigh-Paffenroth, E. D., & Elangovan, S. (2011). Temporal processing in low-frequency channels: Effects of age and hearing loss in middle-aged listeners. Journal of the American Academy of Audiology, 22(7), 393–404.

[84] Lister, J. J., Roberts, R. A., Krause, J. C., Debiase, D., & Carlson, H. (2011). An adaptive clinical test of temporal resolution: Within-channel and across-channel gap detection. International Journal of Audiology, 50(6), 375–384.

[85] Lister, J. J., Roberts, R. A., & Lister, F. L. (2011). An adaptive clinical test of temporal resolution: Age effects. International Journal of Audiology, 50(6), 367–374.

[86] Lorenzi, C., Simpson, M. I., Millman, R. E., et al. (2001). Second-order modulation detection thresholds for pure-tone and narrow-band noise carriers. Journal of the Acoustical Society of America, 110(5, Pt. 1), 2470–2478.

[87] Lu, P. H., Lee, G. J., Tishler, T. A., Meghpara, M., Thompson, P. M., & Bartzokis, G. (2013). Myelin breakdown mediates age-related slowing in cognitive processing speed in healthy elderly men. Brain and Cognition, 81(1), 131–138.

[88] Lu, T., & Wang, X. (2004). Information content of auditory cortical responses to time-varying acoustic stimuli. Journal of Neurophysiology, 91(1), 301–313.

[89] Lukose, R., Brown, K., Barber, C. M., & Kulesza, R. J., Jr. (2013). Quantification of the stapedial reflex reveals delayed responses in autism. Autism Research, 6(5), 344–353.

[90] Mackersie, C. L. (2003). Talker separation and sequential stream segregation in listeners with hearing loss: Patterns associated with talker gender. Journal of Speech, Language, and Hearing Research, 46(4), 912–918.

[91] Mackersie, C. L., Prida, T. L., & Stiles, D. (2001). The role of sequential stream segregation and frequency selectivity in the perception of simultaneous sentences by listeners with sensorineural hearing loss. Journal of Speech, Language, and Hearing Research, 44(1), 19–28.

[92] Matas, C. G., Matas, S.L., Oliveira, C. R., & Gonçalves, I. C. (2010). Auditory evoked potentials and multiple sclerosis. Arquivos Neuro-Ppsiquiatria, 68(4), 528–534.

[93] McCrosky, R., & Keith, R. W. (1996). Auditory fusion test: Revised. St. Louis, MO: Auditec.

[94] McCroskey, R. L., & Kidder, H. C. (1980). Auditory fusion among learning disabled, reading disabled, and normal children. Journal of Learning Disabilities, 13(2), 69–76.

[95] Miller, G. A. (1948). The perception of short bursts of noise. Journal of the Acoustical Society of America, 20, 160–170.

[96] Moller, A. R. (1962). Acoustic reflex in man. Journal of the Acoustical Society of America, 34, 1524–1534.

[97] Moore, B. C. J., Glasberg, B. R., Donaldson, E., McPherson, T., & Plack, C. J. (1989). Detection of temporal gaps in sinusoids by normally hearing and hearing-impaired subjects. Journal of the Acoustical Society of America, 85(3), 1266–1275.

[98] Moore, B. C., & Gockel, H. E. (2012). Properties of auditory stream formation. Philosophical Transactions of the Royal Society of London B: Biological Sciences, 367 (1591), 919–931.

[99] Moser, T., Predoehl, F., & Starr, A. (2013). Review of hair cell synapse defects in sensorineural hearing impairment. Otology and Neurotology, 34(6), 995–1004.

[100] Mukari, S. Z., Umat, C., & Othman, N. I. (2010). Effects of age and working memory capacity on pitch pattern sequence test and dichotic listening. Audiology and Neuro-otology, 15 (5), 303–310.

[101] Muluk, N. B., Yalçinkaya, F., & Keith, R. W. (2011). Random gap detection test and random gap detection test-expanded: Results in children with previous language delay in early childhood. Auris Nasus Larynx, 38(1), 6–13.

[102] Munro, K. J., & Contractor, A. (2010). Inter-aural attenuation with insert earphones. International Journal of Audiology, 49(10), 799–801.

[103] Musiek, F. E. (1994). Frequency (pitch) and duration pattern tests. Journal of the American Academy of Audiology, 5(4), 265–268.

[104] Musiek, F. E. (2002). The frequency pattern test: A guide. The Hearing Journal, 55, 58.

[105] Musiek, F. E., Baran, J. A., & Pinheiro, M. L. (1990). Duration pattern recognition in normal subjects and patients with cerebral and cochlear lesions. Audiology, 29(6), 304–313.

[106] Musiek, F. E., & Pinheiro, M. L. (1987). Frequency patterns in cochlear, brainstem, and cerebral lesions. Audiology, 26(2), 79–88.

[107] Musiek, F. E., Shinn, J. B., Jirsa, R., Bamiou, D. E., Baran, J. A., & Zaida, E. (2005). GIN (gaps-in-noise) test performance in subjects with confirmed central auditory nervous system involvement. Ear and Hearing, 26(6), 608–618.

[108] Narne, V. K. (2013). Temporal processing and speech perception in noise by listeners with auditory neuropathy. PLoS ONE, 8(2), e55995.

[109] Nelson, K. R., Gilmore, R. L., & Massey, A. (1988). Acoustic nerve conduction abnormalities in Guillain-Barré syndrome. Neurology, 38(8), 1263–1266.

[110] Noffsinger, D., Wilson, R. H., & Musiek, F. E. (1994). Department of Veterans Affairs compact disc recording for auditory perceptual assessment: Background and introduction. Journal of the American Academy of Audiology, 5(4), 231–235.

[111] Nouvian, R., Beutner, D., Parsons, T. D., & Moser, T. (2006). Structure and function of the hair cell ribbon synapse. Journal of Membrane Biology 209(2-3), 153–165.

[112] Ors, M., Lindgren, M., Blennow, G., Nettelbladt, U., Sahlén, B., & Rosén, I. (2002). Auditory event-related brain potentials in children with specific language impairment. European Journal of Paediatric Neurology, 6(1), 47-62.

[113] Palmer, S. B., & Musiek, F. E. (2013). N1-p2 recordings to gaps in broadband noise. Journal of the American Academy of Audiology, 24(1), 37–45.

[114] Parker, W., & Decker, R. L. (1971). Detection of abnormal auditory threshold adaptation (ATA). Archives of Otolaryngology, 94(1), 1–7.

[115] Pederson, C. B. (1976). Brief tone audiometry. Summary of dissertation submitted to the University of Copenhagen, September 1973. Scandinavian Audiology, 5, 27–33.

[116] Pedersen, C. B., & Salomon, G. (1977). Temporal integration of acoustic energy. Acta Otolaryngologica, 83(5–6), 417–423.

[117] Phillips, D. P., Comeau, M., & Andrus, J. N. (2010). Auditory temporal gap detection in children with and without auditory processing disorder. Journal of the American Academy of Audiology, 21(6), 404–408.

[118] Phillips, D. P., Taylor, T. L., Hall, S. E., Carr, M. M., & Mossop, J. E. (1997). Detection of silent intervals between noises activating different perceptual channels: Some properties of "central" auditory gap detection. Journal of the Acoustical Society of America, 101(6), 3694–3705.

[119] Picton, T. (2013). Hearing in time: Evoked potential studies of temporal processing. Ear and Hearing, 34(4), 385–401.

[120] Pinheiro, M. L., & Ptacek, P. H. (1971). Reversals in the perception of noise and tone patterns. Journal of the Acoustical Society of America, 49(6), 1778–1783.

[121] Pollack, I. (1977). Monaural and between-ear temporal gap detection: 1. Single gaps. Journal of the Acoustical Society of America, 62(4), 955–960.

[122] Prem, G., Shankar, N. S., & Girish, N. (2012). Gaps in noise (GIN) test: Normative data. Amrita Journal of Medicine, 8, 24–27.

[123] Purcell, D. W., John, S. M., Schneider, B. A., & Picton, T. W. (2004). Human temporal auditory acuity as assessed by envelope following responses. Journal of the Acoustical Society of America, 116(6), 3581–3593.

[124] Qiu, W. W., & Stucker, F. J. (1998). Characterization of acoustic reflex latency in normal-hearing subjects. Scandinavian Audiology, 27(1), 43–49.

[125] Rasminsky, M., & Sears, T. A. (1973). Internodal conduction in undissected demyelinated nerve fibres. Journal of Physiology, 227(2), 323–350.

[126] Rawool, V. W. (1995). Ipsilateral acoustic reflex thresholds at varying click rates in humans. Scandinavian Audiology, 24(3), 199–205.

153

[127] Rawool, V. W. (1996a). Click-rate induced facilitation of the acoustic reflex using constant number of pulses. Audiology, 35(4), 171–179.

[128] Rawool, V. W. (1996b). Effect of aging on the click-rate induced facilitation of acoustic reflex thresholds. Journals of Gerontology Series A: Biological Sciences and Medical Sciences, 51(2), B124–B131.

[129] Rawool, V. W. (1996c). Acoustic reflex monitoring during the presentation of 1000 clicks at high repetition rates. Scandinavian Audiology, 25(4), 239–245.

[130] Rawool, V. W. (1998a). Effect of probe frequency and gender on click-rate-induced facilitation of the acoustic reflex thresholds. Scandinavian Audiology, 27(3), 173–177.

[131] Rawool, V. W. (1998b). Effects of click polarity on the brainstem auditory evoked potentials of older men. Audiology, 37(2), 100–108.

[132] Rawool, V. W. (2006a). A temporal processing primer. Part 1. Defining key concepts in temporal processing. Hearing Review, 13(5), 30-34.

[133] Rawool, V. W. (2006b). A temporal processing primer. Part 2. The effects of hearing loss on temporal processing: Looking beyond simple audition. Hearing Review, 13(6), 30-34.

[134] Rawool, V. W. (2007). The aging auditory system: Part 1. Controversy and confusion on slower processing. Hearing Review, 14(7), 14–19.

[135] Rawool, V. W. (2012). Comprehensive audiological, tinnitus, and auditory processing evaluations. In V.W. Rawool (Ed.), Hearing conservation: In occupational, recreational, educational, and home settings. New York: Thieme.

[136] Rawool, V. W. (2013). Temporal processing in the auditory system. In D. Geffner & D. Ross-Swain (Eds.), Auditory processing disorders: Assessment, management, and treatment. San Diego, CA: Plural Publishing.

[137] Rawool, V., & Zerlin, S. (1988). Phase-intensity effects on the ABR. Scandinavian Audiology, 17(2), 117–123.

[138] Roberts, R. A., Koehnke, J., & Besing, J. (2003). Effects of noise and reverberation on the precedence effect in listeners with normal hearing and impaired hearing. American Journal of Audiology, 12(2), 96–105.

[139] Rose, M. M., & Moore, B. C. (1997). Perceptual grouping of tone sequences by normally hearing and hearing-impaired listeners. Journal of the Acoustical Society of America, 102(3), 1768–1778.

[140] Rose, M. M., & Moore, B. C. (2000). Effects of frequency and level on auditory stream segregation. Journal of the Acoustical Society of America, 108(3, Pt. 1), 1209–1214.

[141] Rosenberg, P. E. (1958). Rapid clinical measurement of tone decay. Paper delivered at the annual convention of the American Speech-Language-Hearing Association, New York.

[142] Rosenberg, P. E. (1969). Tone decay. Maico Audiologic Library Series 7, 17–20.

[143] Rupp, A., Gutschalk, A., Uppenkamp, S., & Scherg, M. Middle latency auditory-evoked fields reflect psychoacoustic gap detection thresholds in human listeners. Journal of Neurophysiology, 92(4), 2239–2247.

[144] Saberi, A., Hatamian, H. R., Nemati, S., & Banan, R. (2012). Hearing statement in multiple sclerosis: A case control study using auditory brainstem responses and otoacoustic emissions. Acta Medica Iranica, 50(10), 679–683.

[145] Samelli, A. G., & Schochat, E. (2008). The Gaps-in-Noise test: Gap detection thresholds in normal-hearing young adults. International Journal of Audiology, 47(5), 238–245.

[146] Schiff, J. A., Cracco, R. Q., & Cracco, J. B. (1985). Brainstem auditory evoked potentials in Guillain-Barré syndrome. Neurology, 35(5), 771–773.

[147] Scudder, R. R. (1978). Auditory temporal processing by children with articulation disorders. Unpublished doctoral dissertation, Wichita State University, Wichita, KS.

[148] Shailer, M. J., & Moore, B. C. (1983). Gap detection as a function of frequency, bandwidth, and level. Journal of the Acoustical Society of America, 74(2), 467–473.

[149] Shinn, J. B., Chermak, G. D., & Musiek, F. E. (2009). GIN (gaps-in-noise) performance in the pediatric population. Journal of the American Academy of Audiology, 20(4), 229–238.

[150] Sklare, D. A., & Denenberg, L. J. (1987). Interaural attenuation for tubephone insert earphones. Ear and Hearing, 8(5), 298–300.

[151] Smith, B. L., & Markides, A. (1981). Interaural attenuation for pure tones and speech. British Journal of Audiology, 15(1), 49–54.

[152] Snyder, J. M. (1973). Interaural attenuation characteristics in audiometry. Laryngoscope, 83(11), 1847–1855.

[153] Swisher, L., & Hirsh, I. J. (1972). Brain damage and the ordering of two temporally successive stimuli. Neuropsychologia, 10(2), 137–152.

[154] Tallal, P., & Piercy, M. (1973). Defects of non-verbal auditory perception in children with developmental aphasia. Nature, 241(5390), 468–469.

[155] Tanaka, H., Komatsuzaki, A., & Hentona, H. (1996). Usefulness of auditory brainstem responses at high stimulus rates in the diagnosis of acoustic neuroma. ORL Journal for Oto-Rhino-Laryngology and Its Related Specialties, 58(4), 224–228.

[156] Thompson, M. E., & Abel, S. M. (1992). Indices of hearing in patients with central auditory pathology: 1. Detection and discrimination. Scandinavian Audiology. Supplementum, 35(Suppl. 35), 3–15.

[157] Thomson, J. M., Fryer, B., Maltby, J., & Goswami, U. (2006). Auditory and motor rhythm awareness in adults with dyslexia. Journal of Research in Reading, 29, 334–348.

[158] Thomson, J. M., & Goswami, U. (2008). Rhythmic processing in children with developmental dyslexia: Auditory and motor rhythms link to reading and spelling. Journal of Physiology–Paris, 102(1-3), 120–129.

[159] Trehub, S. E., Schneider, B. A., & Henderson, J. L. (1995). Gap detection in infants, children, and adults. Journal of the Acoustic Society of America, 98(5, Pt. 1), 2532–2541.

[160] Trussell, L. O. (1999). Synaptic mechanisms for coding timing in auditory neurons. Annual Review of Physiology, 61, 477–496.

[161] Turgeon, C., Champoux, F., Lepore, F., Leclerc, S., & Ellemberg, D. (2011). Auditory processing after sport-related concussions. Ear and Hearing, 32(5), 667–670.

[162] Viemeister, N. F. (1979). Temporal modulation transfer functions based upon modulation thresholds. Journal of the Acoustical Society of America, 66(5), 1364–1380.

[163] von Gersdorff, H., Schneggenburger, R., Weis, S., & Neher, E. (1997). Presynaptic depression at a calyx synapse: The small contribution of metabotropic glutamate receptors. Journal of Neuroscience, 17(21), 8137–8146.

[164] Vucic, S., Kiernan, M. C., & Cornblath, D. R. (2009). Guillain-Barré syndrome: An update. Journal of Clinical Neuroscience, 16(6), 733–741.

[165] Warren, R. M., Obusek, C. J., Farmer, R. M., & Warren, R. P. (1969). Auditory sequence: Confusion of patterns other than speech or music. Science, 164(3879), 586–587.

[166] Watson, C. S., & Gengel, R. W. (1969). Signal duration and signal frequency in relation to auditory sesitivity. Journal of the Acoustical Society of America, 46(4), 989–997.

[167] Weihing, J. A, Musiek, F. E., & Shinn, J. B. (2007). The effect of presentation level on the Gaps-In-Noise (GIN) test. Journal of the American Academy of Audiology, 18(2), 141–150.

[168] Werner, L. A., Folsom, R. C., Mancl, L. R., & Syapin, C. L. (2001). Human auditory brainstem response to temporal gaps in noise. Journal of Speech, Language, and Hearing Research, 44(4), 737–750.

[169] Wimmer, V. C., Horstmann, H., Groh, A., & Kuner, T. (2006). Donut-like topology of synaptic vesicles with a central cluster of mitochondria wrapped into membrane protrusions: A novel structure-function module of the adult calyx of Held. Journal of Neuroscience, 26(1), 109–116.

[170] Wittmann, M., Burtscher, A., Fries, W., & von Steinbüchel, N. (2004). Effects of brain-lesion size and location on temporal-order judgment. Neuroreport, 15(15), 2401–2405.

[171] Wojtczak, M., Beim, J. A., Micheyl, C., & Oxenham, A. J. (2013a). Effects of temporal stimulus properties on the perception of across-frequency asynchrony. Journal of the Acoustical Society of America, 133(2), 982–997.

[172] Wojtczak, M., Beim, J. A., Micheyl, C., & Oxenham, A. J. (2013b). Perception of across-frequency asynchrony by listeners with cochlear hearing loss. Journal of the Association for Research in Otolaryngology, 14(4), 573–589.

[173] Wright, B. A., Lombardino, L. J., King, W. M., Puranik, C. S., Leonard, C. M., & Merzenich, M. M. (1997). Deficits in auditory temporal and spectral resolution in language-impaired children. Nature, 387(6629), 176–178.

[174] Yost, W. A., & Soderquist, D. R. (1984). The precedence effect: Revisited. Journal of the Acoustical Society of America, 76(5), 1377–1383.

[175] Zaehle, T., Jancke, L., & Meyer, M. (2007). Electrical brain imaging evidences left auditory cortex involvement in speech and non-speech discrimination based on temporal features. Behavioral and Brain Functions, 3, 63–74.

[176] Zaidan, E., & Baran, J. A. (2013). Gaps-In-Noise (GIN©) test results in children with and without reading disabilities and phonological processing deficits. International Journal of Audiology, 52(2), 113–123.

[177] Zera, J., & Green, D. M. (1993a). Detecting temporal onset and offset asynchrony in multicomponent complexes. Journal of the Acoustical Society of America, 93(2), 1038–1052.

[178] Zera, J., & Green, D. M. (1993b). Detecting temporal asynchrony with asynchronous standards. Journal of the Acoustical Society of America, 93(3), 1571–1579.

[179] Zera, J., & Green, D. M. (1995). Effect of signal component phase on asynchrony discrimination. Journal of the Acoustical Society of America, 98(2, Pt. 1), 817–827.

Chapter 6

Binaural Processing Assessment

6 Binaural Processing Assessment

Halverson (1922) defined listening as being monaural when only one ear is involved in the listening process and as being binaural when both ears are involved. A further distinction was made for binaural listening as being either diotic, when the same stimuli were presented to both ears, or dichotic, when stimuli differing in some aspect (e.g., frequency) were presented to the two ears. Various aspects of binaural processing are discussed in this chapter.

6.1 Disadvantages of Monaural Listening Compared to Binaural Listening

One way to illustrate the importance of binaural listening is to think about listening with just one normal ear. Individuals with unilateral hearing loss miss advantages offered by binaural listening with several potential consequences, which are briefly discussed below to highlight the importance of binaural listening.

6.1.1 Unilateral Hearing Loss

Children with severe unilateral hearing loss have marked difficulty in localizing sounds (Newton, 1983), and they need a significantly higher speech-to-noise ratio while listening in noisy conditions compared to their age-matched peers (Ruscetta, Arjmand, & Pratt, 2005). Children with unilateral hearing loss perform significantly poorly than their normal-hearing peers on horizontal sound localization tasks administered in quiet and in a background of cafeteria noise (Humes, Allen, & Bess, 1980). Besides localization deficits, they have difficulty in recognizing nonsense syllables (Bess, Tharpe, & Gibler, 1986). Speech and language delays are apparent in some children with unilateral hearing loss.

Children with unilateral hearing loss also fail grades at increased rates compared to age-matched peers (Lieu, 2004). A unilateral hearing loss has an adverse effect on some children's performance in school (Oyler, Oyler, & Matkin, 1988). Approximately one third of children with unilateral hearing loss have scholastic or behavioral problems (Brookhouser, Worthington, & Kelly, 1991). Children with unilateral hearing loss are rated significantly poorly in the areas of academics, attention, communication, participation, and behaviors by their teachers when compared to age-matched peers (Dancer, Burl, & Waters, 1995). A report on 406 children from various schools across the United States (mean age 11.5 years) with unilateral hearing loss concluded that 54% needed individualized special education services in addition to audiological support, and 24% were functioning below average relative to their peers (English & Church, 1999).

6.1.2 Monaural Amplification in the Presence of Bilateral Hearing Loss

Binaural processing deficits are also faced by most children who have bilateral hearing loss but choose to wear amplification in only one ear for economic or other reasons (see Chapter 2). In children with bilateral severe or profound hearing loss, unilateral input through one cochlear implant appears to compromise the development of binaural processing. The auditory brainstem and cortical responses evoked by the initial and a second cochlear implant at a later date show significantly more mismatched activity compared to children who receive binaural cochlear implants at the same time. Behavioral responses of children who receive a second cochlear implant after a long period after initial unilateral use suggest that these children cannot process binaural interaural time and level differences in a normal manner (Gordon, Jiwani, & Papsin, 2011).

6.2 Advantages of Binaural Listening

6.2.1 Binaural Summation

Binaural Summation at Threshold

Intensity needed to just barely detect a signal tends to be lower when a person is hearing through both ears compared to when he or she can listen to the signal through only one ear under headphones. The threshold advantage from listening through two ears has been referred to as *binaural summation at threshold* (Hirsh, 1948). The advantage is apparent for a variety of stimuli, including pure tones and noise (Pollack, 1948).

Binaural Summation at Suprathreshold Levels

Binaural summation does not occur just at threshold; it also occurs at suprathreshold levels. Thus, a stimulus that is presented at a given sound pressure level (SPL) tends to sound louder binaurally compared to when it is presented monaurally (Hirsh, 1948). Binaural summation is less than perfect. A binaural sound is less than twice as loud as a monaurally presented sound; that is, the diotic/monaural loudness ratio is less than 2 (Moore & Glasberg, 2007). Binaural summation depends on the procedures used in measuring thresholds and the presentation levels and can range from 6 to 10 dB using the loudness-matching procedure. Binaural summation of loudness is apparent in individuals with bilaterally symmetrical hearing loss (Hawkins, Prosek, Walden, & Montgomery, 1987).

Binaural Loudness Constancy

The amount of binaural loudness summation for speech is significantly less when a speaker is visually present (Epstein & Florentine, 2012), which allows the use of visual cues to compensate for any deficiencies produced by the presence of stimuli in only one ear. This phenomenon is referred to as *binaural loudness constancy* (Epstein & Florentine, 2009).

6.2.2 Binaural Advantage for Differential Sensitivity

Difference Limen for Intensity

Smaller differences in intensity can be detected while listening through both ears when compared to listening to one ear. The ratio of the monaural to binaural difference limen for intensity (DLI) is approximately 1.65 (Jesteadt & Wier, 1977).

Difference Limen for Frequency

Smaller differences in frequency can be detected while listening through both ears when compared to listening to one ear. The ratio of the monaural to binaural difference limen for frequency (DLF) is approximately 1.44 (Jesteadt & Wier, 1977).

6.2.3 Binaural Advantage in Understanding Speech in Background Interference

When listening to speech in the presence of background interference, it is easier to understand the spoken message with two ears when compared to one ear. To document the advantage, the speech recognition thresholds (SRTs) obtained by presenting words or sentences to both ears can be compared to those obtained while presenting the same stimuli to the better ear. When there is a single interfering speaker or noise source, binaural listening improves the SRT by about 2 to 4 dB. When there are two or three interfering sources, the advantage is about 2 to 4 dB for interference by noise or speech-modulated noise and 6 to 7 dB for interference by speech- or time-reversed speech (Hawley, Litovsky, & Culling, 2004).

6.3 Locating Sound Sources

In the real world, the sound images coming to the two ears from a single sound source are slightly different, but these images are compared and often combined together in the central auditory system, which allows us to perceive a fused image and to determine if the sound image is within the head or outside the head and where the sound is located. Accuracy in determining sound location depends on the two ears working together. Cues that are useful in locating the position of the sound source are listed in ▸ Fig. 6.1, and various dimensions involved in sound localization are shown in ▸ Fig. 6.2. Auditory spatial perception can be further modulated through previous related auditory experience, visual cues, and proprioceptive cues (Lackner & Shenker, 1985).

6.3.1 Lateralization

Lateralization refers to the intracranial perception of the image at the ears or at the center of the head or other locations in the head. The phenomenon of lateralization is usually studied by manipulating stimulus parameters presented to the two ears under headphones.

6.3.2 Localization

Localization refers to the extracranial perception of the image somewhere out in the space. The sound image may be perceived as coming from behind or from the front or from the right or left side or from any other angle, as shown in ▶ Fig. 6.2. The phenomenon of localization is usually studied by manipulating stimulus parameters presented from loudspeakers located around the listener. However, sound localization effects can also be simulated under headphones.

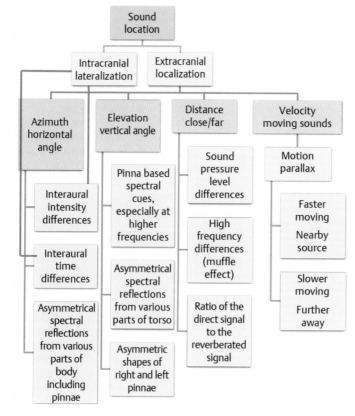

Fig. 6.1 Cues used in lateralization and localization. Note that many of the localization cues can be used to change the perception of the sound image under headphones.

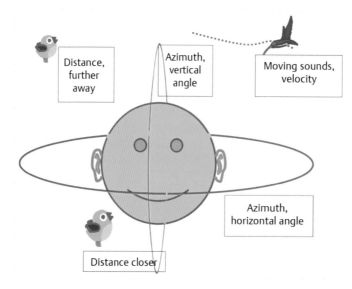

Fig. 6.2 Dimensions of sound localization.

6.3.3 Interaural Intensity Difference

The interaural intensity difference is the difference in intensity between the two ears. For example, if the sound source is on the right side, the intensity of the sound drops slightly by the time it arrives at the left ear. In other words, the sound arriving at the right ear is slightly louder than the one arriving at the left ear, which allows us to realize that the sound is located on the right side. The intensity of the sound reaching the two ears is the same when the sound source is directly in front of or behind the listener, and maximum interaural intensity differences are expected at a 90-degree azimuth or when the sound source is on the right or left side. The importance of the interaural intensity difference in locating a sound can be studied using identification (where is the sound image?) or resolution (interaural intensity difference limen) tasks.

Interaural Intensity Difference Identification

In this test, participants are asked to point to the location of the perceived sound image using a potentiometer while the experimenter changes the interaural intensity difference. Tonal stimuli are lateralized to the right or left ear with an interaural intensity difference of approximately 18 dB. The location of the sound can change with as little as 2 to 6 dB change in interaural intensity difference (Yost, 1981). Interaural intensity difference identification results can be obtained under headphones with a two-channel audiometer by asking the listener to point to the location of the sound image on the head. Initially, the thresholds should be established using 1 dB steps. The presentation level can be adjusted to begin presentations at 0 dB sensation level (SL) in both ears, which in most cases leads to a central perception of the sound image. If the image is not perceived at the center, the interaural intensity should be manipulated until a central image is perceived. After the central image is perceived, further testing can be conducted, as shown in ▶ Fig. 6.3, which displays the results of a 60-year-old woman. The arrows in the figure indicate the location of the perceived sound image related to each interaural intensity difference configuration. Deficits can be seen in terms of asymmetries in the left and right hemifields, inability to perceive a central image and inaccurate perception of images (alloacusis) in the contralateral hemifields. For example, the sound image may be perceived in the right hemifield even though the sensation level is higher in the left ear, or vice versa (Diamond & Bender, 1965).

Interaural Intensity Difference Limen

This is the smallest detectable difference in intensity between the two ears. It can be measured in various ways. Under headphones, as the sound level increases, smaller differences in intensity can be detected at higher sound levels (▶ Fig. 6.4) if the task is to detect that the sound is not a smooth tone due to the roughness in sounds created by the differences in sound intensity between the two ears (Rowland & Tobias, 1967). Normal-hearing individuals usually need about a 0.5 to 3.0 dB difference between the two ears to perceive the interaural intensity difference. Smaller interaural intensity difference limens are expected to lead to more accurate judgment of the sound location and less effort in locating sounds.

6.3.4 Interaural Time Difference

Interaural time difference (ITD) is the difference in the time of arrival of the sound at the two ears. For example, if the sound source is on the right side, the sound arrives earlier at the right ear when compared to the left ear. This ITD can alert the listener that the source of the sound is on the right side. The importance of ITD in locating a sound can be studied using identification (where is the sound image?) or resolution (ITD limen) tasks. Note that there is no difference in arrival time between the two ears when the sound source is directly in front of (0-degree azimuth) or behind (180-degree azimuth) the listener. The maximum difference in arrival time between the two ears is expected when the sound is at a 90-degree azimuth.

Interaural Time or Phase Identification

In this test, the participant is asked to point to the location of the perceived sound image using a potentiometer while the experimenter changes the interaural phase or time difference. With a 0-degree interaural phase difference, the sound is perceived at the center of the head. As the interaural phase difference changes from 0 to 60 degrees, the perceived sound location changes from the center toward one side and continues to change in the

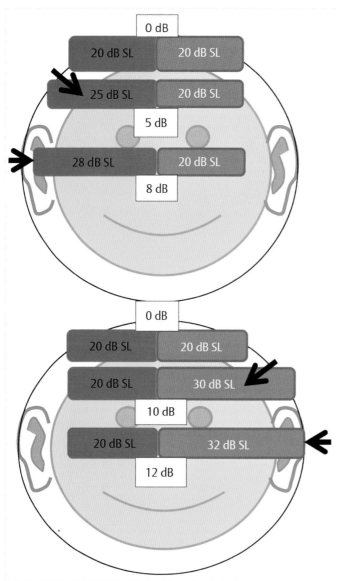

Fig. 6.3 Interaural-level difference test results under headphones from a 60-year-old woman at 4000 Hz with the right ear threshold of 17 dB hearing level (HL) and the left ear threshold at 4 dB HL. The testing began at 20 dB SL in both ears, which generated a sound image at the center of the head. Following this, the presentation level in the left (upper panel) or the right ear (lower panel) was held constant, and the level in the other ear was changed. As seen in the upper panel, an interaural intensity difference of 8 dB caused a shift in the sound image to the right ear. As seen in the lower panel, an interaural intensity difference of 12 dB caused a shift in the sound image to the left ear.

direction of one ear until the image is lateralized to one ear with a phase difference of 90 degree. (Yost, 1981).

Interaural Time Difference Limen or Threshold

This is the smallest detectable difference in sound arrival time between the two ears. In an ITD discrimination task, the test stimulus differs from the standard stimulus in interaural delay (Koehnke, Culotta, Hawley, & Colburn, 1995). For tonal stimuli, ITD thresholds are approximately inversely proportional to the frequency for frequencies ranging from 250 to 700 Hz. The thresholds are smallest for frequencies ranging from 700 to 1000 Hz. Above 1000 Hz, the thresholds increase rapidly and become unmeasurably high above 1400 Hz (Brughera, Dunai, & Hartmann, 2013). However, for narrowband noises or complex tones containing high-frequency information, ITD limens can be measured with thresholds as low as those obtained for tonal stimuli. Listeners appear to use the ITDs available in the slowly fluctuating envelopes of such stimuli (Henning, 1974a,b).

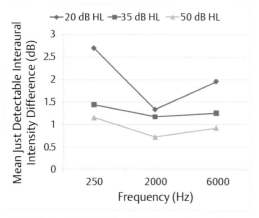

Fig. 6.4 Average just detectable interaural intensity difference (dB) at 250, 2000, and 6000 Hz at three presentation levels (based on Rowland & Tobias, 1969).

6.3.5 Pinna Cues

Horizontal Plane Localization

The localization of high-frequency sounds in the horizontal plane is significantly worse when the various cavities in the pinna are occluded, suggesting that the pinna offers important cues for localization of high-frequency sounds (Musicant & Butler, 1984).

Vertical Plane Localization

Vertical plane localization accuracy rates decrease systematically as more and more of the different cavities in the pinna are filled while leaving the entrance to the ear canal open (Gardner & Gardner, 1973). Accuracy rates also become worse with removal of higher frequencies from the stimulus, suggesting that these frequencies provide the primary pinna-based cues for vertical plane localization (Hebrank & Wright, 1974; Roffler & Butler, 1968). The cavities available within the pinna are relatively small, which is expected to lead to spectral differences only at frequencies higher than about 3 kHz (Algazi, Avendano, & Duda, 2001).

Interaural Pinna Shape Disparity

For stimuli that contain frequencies above 8 to 10 kHz, the asymmetries in the shape of the right and left pinnae may provide some cues for vertical plane localization (Butler, 1969; Middlebrooks, Makous, & Green, 1989).

6.3.6 Spectral Notches

Elevation-dependent notches appear in the spectra recorded at the two ears that extend as low as 700 Hz; such notches can serve as cues for localization in the vertical plane (Algazi et al., 2001).

6.3.7 Torso Reflection Cues

For stimuli containing frequencies up to about 2 to 3 kHz, reflections from the torso can offer cues for sound location, which is more relevant to the vertical plane localization of sounds located away from the midplane (Algazi et al., 2001).

6.3.8 Minimum Audible Angle

One way to examine localization is to determine the smallest difference (angle or difference in azimuth) in location between two sound sources relative to the head that leads to a difference in perceived location. The smallest angle that allows perception of a difference in location is referred to as the minimum audible angle (MAA). For determination of the MAA, the sound sources are located at various angles around the subject, and two stimuli differing in azimuth are presented sequentially. The subject's task is to report if the second tone is to the right or the left of the first tone. The MAA is the smallest separation between the sound sources that allows a correct response from the subject on a set number of trials. The MAA is smallest for frequencies below about 1500 Hz and above 2000 Hz. Thus, between 1500 and 2000 Hz, the location of sound sources is somewhat difficult to determine. The MAA also depends on where the sound sources are located. For horizontal plane localization, when the sound sources are located around the 0-degree azimuth, a slight change in location (1–2 degree) is perceptible; as the sources are moved toward one side of the head, larger and larger changes in location are necessary to perceive a change. When the sources are completely off to one side or facing one ear, the changes are hard to perceive; this is referred to as the *cone of confusion* (Mills, 1958). For broadband signals, the vertical plane MAA is about 4 degrees of the arch for sources located in the median sagittal plane (Perrott & Saberi, 1990), which is less than the 1- to 2-degree accuracy observed during horizontal plane localization. However, for sounds near the 90-degree azimuth, vertical plane localization is more accurate than horizontal plane localization (Makous & Middlebrooks, 1990).

Concurrent Minimum Audible Angle

Instead of presenting two stimuli sequentially as described above, two tones of different frequencies can be presented simultaneously to two loudspeakers separated by a particular angle. The MAA obtained using this procedure is known as the concurrent minimum audible angle (CMAA). The CMAA is the minimum angular separation between the two loudspeakers at which the listener can detect the separation at least 75% of the time. The spatial resolution measured in this way depends on the frequency separation and the azimuth of the sound sources. For smaller frequency separations of about 15 Hz, angular separation between simultaneous sound sources is difficult to perceive (Perrott, 1984).

6.3.9 Distance Perception

Changes in Sound Pressure Level

According to the inverse square law, the sound level decreases by 6 dB with a doubling of the distance from the sound source in an anechoic surrounding (▶ Fig. 6.5). Thus, subjects can use the change in sound level to judge the relative distance of the sound source (Ashmead, LeRoy, & Odom, 1990). The change in intensity that occurs when a subject is walking toward a sound source can serve

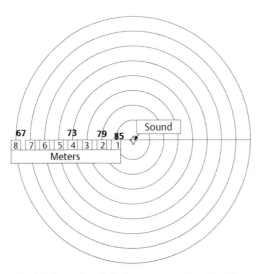

Fig. 6.5 Illustration of the inverse-square law. Doubling of the distance (in meters) away from the sound source results in a 6 dB decrease in the sound pressure level (SPL) in a free field. Adapted from Rawool (2012).

as an absolute cue to distance perception (Ashmead, Davis, & Northington, 1995).

High-Frequency Muffling

High-frequency sounds are attenuated more compared to low-frequency sounds; this causes complex sounds such as speech to be muffled at longer distances. The change in the balance of high- and low-frequency energy at shorter and longer distances serves as a relative cue to distance perception (Coleman, 1968; Little, Mershon, & Cox, 1992).

Ratio of Direct to Reflected Sound

In reverberant environments, the ratio of direct to reflected sound increases as the sound source is moved closer to the listener. This change serves as an absolute cue to distance judgments (Mershon, Ballenger, Little, McMurtry, & Buchanan, 1989; Mershon & Bowers, 1979; Mershon & King, 1975).

6.3.10 Moving Sound Sources

Many cues involved in location of sound sources can be useful in detecting moving sound sources and the direction of their movement. The accuracy of location of moving sound sources can be measured using the minimum audible movement angle (MAMA).

Minimum Audible Movement Angle

The MAMA is the smallest angular distance a moving sound source must travel to be just discriminable from either a stationary sound source or from a source moving in the opposite direction. The subject's task is to determine whether the target signal is moving to the right or the left. For very slow-moving sound sources (velocity 2.8 degree/s) in the horizontal plane, the CMAA is between 2 and 4 degrees for tones varying from 0.8 to 6.4 kHz (Harris & Sergeant, 1971). The MAMA depends on the frequency, velocity, and signal duration. With reference to frequency, the worst performance is in the range of 1.5 to 3.0 kHz. With reference to velocity, the faster the target moves, the greater the MMAA (Perrott & Tucker, 1988). With reference to stimulus duration, for very brief durations, the MMAA is larger. It improves (i.e., becomes smaller) with an increase in stimulus duration up to about 300 to 500 ms (Chandler & Grantham, 1992).

Motion Parallax

The motion parallax is related to the fact that faster moving sound sources are perceived as being closer compared to slower moving sources that are perceived as being farther away. The cues provided by the parallax may be useful in judging the distance of a sound source up to 1.0 ± 1.5 m (3.3–4.9 ft) in the absence of any cues of SPL and reflections (Kim, Suzuki, Takane, & Sone, 2001).

6.3.11 Precedence Effect/Localization Dominance

As noted in Chapter 5, within about 15 to 30 ms, the earlier arriving sound dominates the later arriving sound in determining what we hear. The earlier reflections are integrated with original sounds into a single image. This is referred to as the *precedence effect,* or the principle of the first wavefront. This effect makes localization of sounds easier by suppressing the effects of reflections that arrive at the ears immediately after the original sound. The sound in this case is perceived as being closer to the source generating the leading or earlier arriving sound. This phenomenon is referred to as localization dominance. The accuracy of localization of single words using the precedence effect decreases with the severity of hearing loss (Akeroyd & Guy, 2011). Speech discrimination is generally unaffected by reflections arriving up to about 20 to 30 ms after the original sound. The reflections arriving after the precedence effect time period interfere with speech recognition (Nábělek & Robinette, 1978).

Echo Threshold

The minimal difference between the earlier and later arriving sounds that leads to the perception of two sounds instead of a single fused image is referred to as the *echo threshold.* This threshold is significantly longer for 4- to 5-year-old children (24.3 ms ± 13.6 ms) than adults (15.2 ± 4.9 ms; Litovsky & Godar, 2010).

6.4 Masking-Level Difference

Masking-level difference (MLD) refers to the improvement in perception of a signal in the presence of a masker with manipulation of phase of either the signal or the noise at the two ears. For example, it is easier to detect a signal presented in phase at the two ears in the presence of noise that is presented out of phase at the two ears compared to the condition where both the signal and the noise are presented in phase at both ears (Hirsh, 1948). This is likely to occur because when both the signal and noise are presented in phase to the two ears, the signal and noise images both occur at a central location in the head. When the noise is out of phase, the noise image shifts to the ear that has the 0-degree phase, whereas the image of the in-phase signal remains at the center of the head. This separation of the noise and signal can allow easier detection of the signal when the noise or the signal is out of phase.

6.4.1 S_0N_0 Threshold

A signal can be presented in the presence of noise to the two ears. This is referred to as the S_0N_0 *condition.* The threshold of the signal is determined in the presence of the noise. Let us assume that the threshold is 45 dB hearing level (HL).

6.4.2 S_0N_Π Threshold

In this condition, the noise is presented out of phase at the two ears while keeping the signal in phase. The threshold is reestablished and is found to be 36 dB HL. In this example, the threshold is improved by 9 dB (45 − 36 dB) relative to the S_0N_0 condition. Thus, the MLD is 9 dB.

6.4.3 $S_\Pi N_0$ Threshold

In this condition, the signal is presented out of phase at the two ears, and the noise is presented in phase at the two ears. Let us assume that the signal threshold in this condition is 30 dB HL. Thus, the threshold improved by 15 dB (45 − 30 dB) relative to the S_0N_0 condition. Thus, the MLD is 15 dB.

Some commercially available audiometers allow the measurement of MLD for tonal stimuli. MLDs obtained in one young adult at 125, 250, 500, and 1000 Hz with narrowband noise maskers using an AC40 audiometer (Interacoustics AS, Drejervaenget 8, DK-5610, Assens, Denmark) are shown in ▸ Fig. 6.6. As can be seen, the largest MLDs are obtained at 500 Hz. Thus, in clinical settings, MLD testing is recommended at 500 Hz. ▸ Fig. 6.6 also shows the learning effect apparent on repeat testing for the $S_\Pi N_0$ condition. Thus, some training trials should be administered before obtaining final test results.

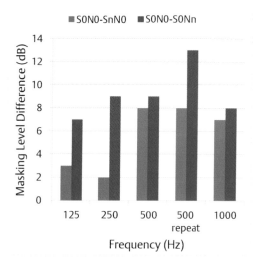

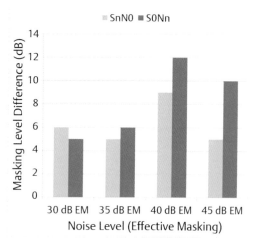

Fig. 6.6 Masking-level differences (MLDs) at various frequencies from a 21-year-old normal-hearing woman. Note the larger MLDs in the $S0N_{\Pi}$ condition. The largest MLDs are obtained at 500 Hz. The MLD test was repeated after 1 week for 500 Hz (500 Hz repeat) and shows an improvement in MLD in the S_0N_n condition.

Fig. 6.7 Masking-level differences (MLDs) at 500 Hz from a 60-year-old woman. The largest MLD was obtained with 40 dB EM.

The noise masker level used during testing should be below the level that can cause acoustic crossover of stimuli to the other ear to ensure that the signal and noise configurations (same phase or antiphase) are maintained at each ear. This level is about 40 dB effective masking (EM) for 500 Hz. ▶ Fig. 6.7 shows MLDs obtained from a 60-year-old woman at four different EM levels. As can be seen, the largest MLDs are apparent at 40 dB EM. Thus, the recommended masker level for evaluating MLD is 40 dB EM. (Note: EM refers to the amount of threshold shift relative to 0 dB HL. For example, 45 dB EM noise shifts all thresholds below 45 dB HL to 45 dB HL. Masking noise on most audiometers is calibrated in EM for easier clinical use.)

6.4.4 Effect of Pathology on Tonal Masking-Level Difference

Abnormal MLDs for tonal stimuli have been reported in patients with multiple sclerosis (MS; Hendler, Squires, & Emmerich, 1990; Noffsinger, Olsen, Carhart, Hart, & Sahagal, 1972; Olsen & Noffsinger, 1976). Children with suspected auditory processing deficits (APDs) can have significantly lower MLDs for tones (Sweetow & Redell, 1978).

6.4.5 Binaural Intelligibility-Level Difference

The binaural intelligibility-level difference (BILD) is the difference between the levels at which a certain percentage of words are repeated correctly for a dichotic condition (S_0N_{Π} or $S_{\Pi}N_0$) and for S_0N_0. Let us assume that the level at which 50% correct word recognition was achieved was 45 dB HL in the S_0N_0 condition. In the S_0N_{Π} condition, the level at which 50% correct recognition was achieved was 40 dB HL. Here, due to the inversion of the noise phase at the two ears, the same amount of speech recognition was possible at a 5 dB lower speech presentation level. The BILD in this example is 5 dB (45 − 40 dB).

MLDs for speech or BILD can be determined by using *Tonal and Speech Materials for Auditory Perceptual Assessment* (U.S. Department of Veterans Affairs, 1998). On this CD, spondee words are recorded after 500 ms of the initiation of a noise burst. In the out-of-phase condition, the spondees are presented out of phase to the two ears, and the noise is presented in phase to the two ears at a level of 65 or 85 dB SPL. The MLD for speech is generally smaller than that obtained for 500 Hz tones.

6.5 Binaural-Level Difference

▶ Fig. 6.8 shows thresholds for 250 Hz tones obtained with monaural presentation, binaural in-phase presentation, and binaural out-of-phase

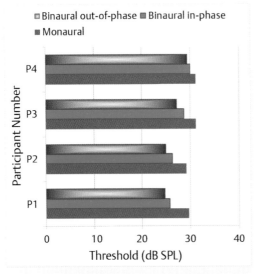

Fig. 6.8 Thresholds (dB SPL) for four participants obtained with monaural and binaural in-phase and out-of-phase 250 Hz tones. The lowest thresholds are apparent in the binaural out-of-phase conditions (based on Diercks & Jeffress, 1962).

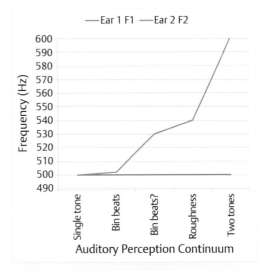

Fig. 6.9 Schematic of the auditory perception continuum as a function of presentation of tones to two ears. With the presentation of the same frequency to two ears, a single tone is perceived. With increased separation of the frequencies (F1, F2) presented to two ears, the perception changes.

presentation. Note that thresholds with binaural presentation are lower than monaural presentation, which shows the binaural summation effect. In addition, thresholds for the out-of-phase condition are better than those for in-phase condition. Thus, binaural thresholds are lower when obtained with signals out of phase at the two ears compared to when they are in phase at the two ears. The difference between these two thresholds is referred to as the binaural-level difference (BLD). It has been suggested that this finding is reminiscent of results of MLD studies where out-of-phase stimuli yield lower thresholds compared to in-phase stimuli in the presence of in-phase noise. Thus, the absolute thresholds obtained during the BLD tasks are really masked thresholds due to internal noise that is somewhat correlated at both ears (Diercks & Jeffress, 1962). The internal noise can occur as a result of continuous spontaneous neural activity (McFadden, 1968).

In individuals with neural presbycusis, the internal noise levels are higher, which leads to significantly larger BLDs compared to younger adults (Novak & Anderson, 1982). As mentioned previously and shown in ▶ Fig. 6.7, MLDs increase with increasing noise levels from 30 to 40 dB EM.

6.6 Binaural Fusion

Even though sounds are produced by the same source, in most instances the arrival time of the sound at two ears is different, and the sound differs in intensity and spectrum at both ears. Regardless, we perceive a single image of the sound. Thus, similar signals reaching the two ears, even though they are not identical, are fused into one image. This is referred to as *binaural fusion*.

6.7 Binaural Beats

When one tone is presented to one ear (f1) and another tone of slightly different frequency (f2) is presented to the other ear, a single fused sound image is perceived with beats. The amount of frequency difference between the two ears ($\Delta f = f2 - f1$) results in various perceptions on a continuum, as shown in ▶ Fig. 6.9. The perception changes from a single image with similar frequencies, to intracranial motion or beats with smaller differences in frequencies between the ears, to roughness, and to perception of different tones in each ear with increasing differences in frequencies at the two ears. The beats are more easily perceptible between 300 and 600 Hz; smaller frequency differences between the two ears are required below

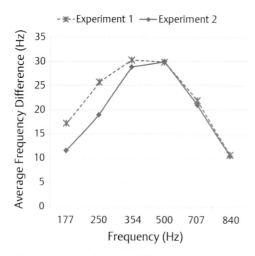

Fig. 6.10 Average frequency differences (Hz) between the two ears at which the perception of beats disappears as a function of the base frequency (based on Licklider, Webster, & Hedlun, 1950). Below the difference, beats are perceived.

and above these frequencies. ▶ Fig. 6.10 shows the average frequency differences (when the differences are changed from smaller to larger) in tones presented at the two ears at which the perception of beats disappears as a function of the base frequency (Licklider, Webster, & Hedlun, 1950). Depending on the stimuli used, all listeners may not perceive beats; when beats are present, the perceptual strength may be relatively weak (Grose, Buss, & Hall, 2012). In some experiments, either the phase or both the phase and amplitude components of a wideband noise are shifted in one ear relative to the other ear by a fixed frequency step (e.g., 5 Hz) to generate the perception of binaural beats. Such wideband noises may generate stronger beat perceptions compared to tonal stimuli (Akeroyd, 2010; Siveke, Ewert, Grothe, & Wiegrebe, 2008).

6.7.1 Effect of Pathology on the Perception of Binaural Beats

Patients with severe aphasia due to a left cerebral aneurysm have difficulty perceiving binaural beats generated by 534 and 540 Hz that are audible to patients with mild aphasia or normal individuals (Barr, Mullin, & Herbert, 1977). Some patients with Parkinson disease may also have difficulty in perceiving binaural beats (Oster, 1973).

6.8 Dichotic Pitch

When two somewhat different noise sources are presented to two ears, under certain conditions, a pitch is perceived, although neither of the sources alone provides any cues to the perceived pitch. The perceived pitch in this case is described as dichotic. Usually the experiment for creating dichotic pitch perception begins with having two similar noise sources, but then a difference in the sources presented at the two ears is created using various procedures. For example, the phase of a narrow band of frequencies can be shifted in one of the ears. When the noise sources at the two ears are the same, the noise is perceived at the center of the head. However, if the phases of a narrow band of frequencies (e.g., 390–410 Hz, center frequency 400 Hz) are shifted in the ongoing noise in one ear, a soft but distinct tone is perceived in the noise.

Other variations of this procedure can create the same perception. For example, the phases of all frequencies in the noise can be shifted except for those within a particular narrow band of frequencies. In one study a complex stimulus consisting of eight simultaneous and continuous pure tones was used (Kubovy, Cutting, & McGuire, 1974). When the phase of one of the tones in one ear was shifted relative to the other ear, the dichotic pitch was perceived. When the phases of only particular tones were shifted in sequence, a melody was perceived that was undetectable by either ear alone. The dichotic pitch can be localized on the left or right side or on both sides (Witton, Hillebrand, Furlong, & Henning, 2012).

6.8.1 Facilitation of the Perception of Dichotic Pitch

Perception of dichotic pitch can be facilitated by meeting the following requirements. The band of frequencies that are shifted or excluded from shifting needs to be relatively narrow. The frequencies that are phase shifted need to be within the range of 200 to 1600 or 2000 Hz. The phase shift needs to be from 90 to 270 degrees. The presentation levels need to be relatively high given that the perceived pitch is relatively soft (Cramer & Huggins, 1958).

Dichotic pitch perception demonstrates the ability of the auditory nervous system to compare the noise presented at the two ears and detect differences within the noise. During dichotic pitch tasks, cortical activation is apparent in the bilateral

Heschl gyri, right planum temporale, and right superior temporal sulcus. Dichotic pitch salience appears to be specifically illustrated in the bilateral Heschl gyri and right planum temporale. The right superior temporal lobe appears to be involved in higher-level processing of pitch. Activation is generally greater in the right temporal lobe (Partanen et al., 2012).

6.8.2 Dichotic Pitch Perception in Dyslexia

Individuals with dyslexia have difficulty perceiving dichotic pitch when compared to average readers, suggesting a deficit in the use of binaural cues to extract sound streams from noisy backgrounds (Dougherty, Cynader, Bjornson, Edgell, & Giaschi, 1998). Individuals with dyslexia with poor dichotic pitch thresholds exhibit greater cortical activity for random noise and lower activity for a dichotic melody. Behavioral performance on phonological reading is correlated to cortical activity generated by dichotic pitch in the right Heschl gyrus and right superior temporal sulcus (Partanen et al., 2012).

6.9 Dichotic Musical Chords

During dichotic listening, contralateral pathways remain dominant (Kimura, 1967). Thus, as shown in ▶ Fig. 6.11, the stimuli presented to each ear first reach contralateral hemispheres. When musical chords are presented to the right ear, the responses first reach the left hemisphere and are then transferred via the corpus callosum to the right hemisphere, where musical stimuli are processed. The transferring process causes a slight delay when compared to the stimuli presented to the left ear. The stimuli presented to the left ear reach the right hemisphere directly, yielding an advantage to the left ear, which is known as the left ear advantage for processing musical chords.

Kimura (1967) presented musical melodies dichotically to listeners and found that the percentage of melodies hummed correctly was higher for melodies presented to the left ear (37%) when compared to those presented to the right ear (23%). Recordings of the magnetoencephalographic (MEG) equivalent of the mismatch negativity (MMN) potential shows that changes in musical chords are coded more distinctly in the right hemisphere than phoneme changes, as indicated by a significantly stronger MMN dipole moment for chord changes than for phoneme changes

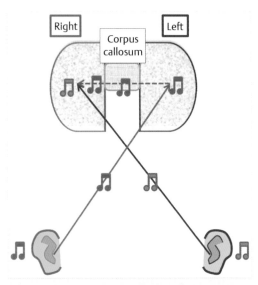

Fig. 6.11 Simplistic model of processing of dichotic musical chords.

(Tervaniemi et al., 1999). The right superior temporal sulcus appears to take a key role in categorical perception of musical chords (Klein & Zattore, 2011). However, the left ear/right hemisphere advantage for musical chords can be modulated by several factors, including the specific content of the musical chords, the specific response tasks, and experience in listening to or playing music. Complex music experiences can engage both auditory cortices in an integrative manner (Tervaniemi, Sannemann, Noyranen, Salonen, & Pihko, 2011).

6.9.1 Clinical Dichotic Musical Chord Test

Tonal and Speech Materials for Auditory Perceptual Assessment (Disc 1.0, U.S. Department of Veterans Affairs, 1998) includes a dichotic chords test. The test includes three tone complexes that meet the definition of musical chords. The listener is presented with a 500 ms dichotic pair of chords; after a 1 second pause, four chords are presented diotically. The listener's task is to mark on a printed form the two chords from the sequence of four that were initially heard during the dichotic presentation. The average performance on this test is approximately 60% correct in each ear when the chords are presented at 70 to 90 dB SPL. The suggested normal cutoff criterion is performance below the 50% level if the listener is forced to take a guess on both chords in each pair. Some listeners may report only the chord heard in one ear due to the difficulty of the task, which can create a highly asymmetric performance (Noffsinger, Martinez, Friedrich, & Wilson, 1994).

6.10 Dichotic Speech Perception

Broadbent (1954) performed several dichotic speech experiments with manipulation of three different stimulus parameters:
- Stimulus materials: Sentences and digits
- Number of digits: Three-pair (six digits) and four-pair (eight digits); fewer errors were present in the three-pair digits conditions.
- Interstimulus interval between each digit pair

Broadbent (1954) also explored performance on three types of binaural recall tasks: free recall, recall in the order of arrival, and directed ear first recall (▶ Fig. 6.12). For the response task that asked participants to repeat the digits in the order of arrival, correct responses improved with an increase in interstimulus intervals from 1.0, 1.5, and 2.0 seconds between each digit pair.

6.10.1 Processing of Dichotic Speech in Auditory Pathways

During monaural processing, the ipsilateral and contralateral pathways are active. However, contralateral pathways are more efficient and elicit larger responses in the hemisphere contralateral to the stimulated ear (Lazzouni, Ross, Voss, &

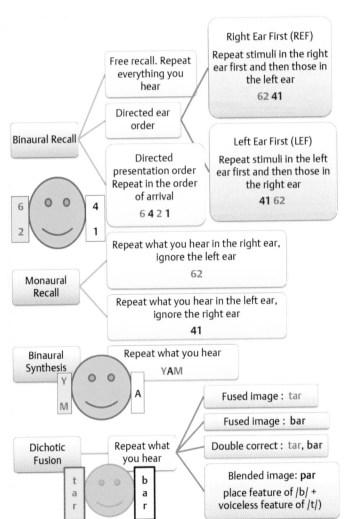

Fig. 6.12 Possible responses during dichotic speech tasks.

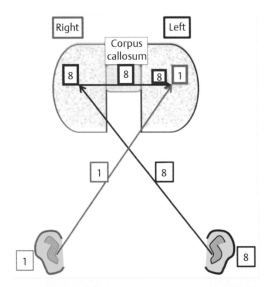

Fig. 6.13 Simplistic model of dichotic digits processing.

Lepore, 2010) because of the larger number of fibers and faster neural conduction rates. During dichotic listening, contralateral pathways remain dominant (Kimura, 1967) with a suppression of the ipsilateral pathways (Lazzouni et al., 2010), which is particularly stronger on the left side (Della Penna et al., 2007). Thus, as shown in ▶ Fig. 6.13, the stimuli presented to each ear first reach contralateral hemispheres. When linguistic stimuli are presented to the left ear, the responses first reach the right hemisphere and are then transferred via the corpus callosum to the dominant left hemisphere. This transfer is necessary for processing linguistic stimuli. The transferring process causes a slight delay of about 25 ms (Ringo, Doty, Demeter, & Simard, 1994) when compared to the stimuli presented to the right ear, which can partially contribute to a left ear deficit. The stimuli presented to the right ear reach the left hemisphere directly, yielding an advantage to the right ear.

The right ear advantage or left ear deficit can be modulated by manipulating attention to the left ear through various means. These include manipulating the level or onset or offset times to give advantage to the left ear and pulling attention to the left ear by beginning part of the stimulus in the left ear first or requesting repetition of stimuli presented to the left ear first. Under such manipulations, the left ear can sometimes yield performance that is equal or superior to the right ear. A laterality score can be calculated for each subject by subtracting left (L) ear scores from the right (R) ear scores, then dividing the difference by the sum of the two scores:

$$\frac{(R - L)}{R + L}$$

6.10.2 Clinical Dichotic Speech Tests

Several tests are available for testing dichotic listening skills. Many different parameters can be adjusted for performing these tests. These include stimuli, onset-offset time at the two ears, and response tasks. Age-maturation effects need to be considered in evaluating each patient's performance for clinical purposes. When the patient is asked to repeat stimuli in both ears, the task is sometimes referred to as a *binaural integration test*. During binaural integration tasks, the patient can be asked to repeat stimuli from both ears, which is referred to as *free recall*, or the patient is asked to repeat stimuli in one ear first and then the other ear, which is referred to as *directed recall*. When the patient is asked to repeat the stimuli in only one ear and ignore the stimuli presented to the other, it is referred to as a *binaural separation task*.

6.10.3 Binaural Recall

Dichotic Digits

Several versions of the dichotic digits tests are available. The stimuli included in a dichotic digits test include numbers from 1 to 10 with the exception of number 7, which has two syllables and thus cannot be approximately aligned with the other stimuli because of its relatively longer duration. The use of digits is especially suitable for individuals who do not have a higher command of English language, such as children and individuals whose first language is not English. Options are available for presenting dichotic digits in one-, two-, three-, and four-pair combinations. Three- or four-pair combinations can make more demands on memory, while the single-digit pair task may be too easy and thus insensitive to auditory processing difficulties.

Effects of age maturation on the right ear advantage on a two-pair dichotic digits test for boys and girls (Kimura, 1963) are shown in ▶ Fig. 6.14. At ages 5 and 6 years, girls significantly outperform boys (Kimura, 1963), but there are no gender differences after the age of 7. At age 5, boys may

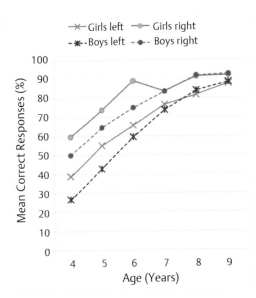

Fig. 6.14 Effects of age maturation on the right ear advantage on a two-pair dichotic digits test for boys and girls. At ages 5 and 6 years, girls significantly outperform boys (based on Kimura, 1963).

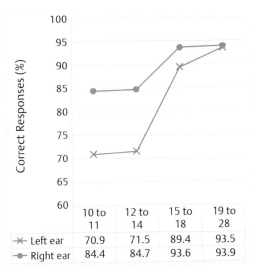

	10 to 11	12 to 14	15 to 18	19 to 28
Left ear	70.9	71.5	89.4	93.5
Right ear	84.4	84.7	93.6	93.9

Fig. 6.15 Normal cutoff criteria (1 standard deviation [SD] below mean) for the two-pair dichotic digits test for age groups from 10 to 28 years (based on Moncrieff & Wilson, 2009).

lag behind girls in establishing left hemisphere dominance for linguistic stimuli (Kimura, 1967). Although a right ear advantage is apparent in 80 to 85% of right-handed individuals, 15 to 20% of right handed individuals can show a left ear advantage or no ear advantage (Moncrieff & Wilson, 2009). In some cases, hemispheric/ear advantage may be difficult to establish due to near-ceiling performance on the dichotic digits test (Kimura, 1967).

Normal cutoff criteria for individuals between the ages of 10 and 28 years (Moncrieff & Wilson, 2009) are shown in ▶ Fig. 6.15. Performance of an adult suspected with attention deficit hyperactivity disorder (ADHD) and APDs in the free recall condition is shown in ▶ Table 6.1 and ▶ Table 6.2. During the first administration (▶ Table 6.1) of the test, a delay in responses was apparent. During the second administration (▶ Table 6.2), the examiner paused the CD after each pair, thus allowing more time for responding. In this case, overall results were improved by allowing more response time. A left ear deficit (score 82%; first digit: 72%, second digit: 92%) is still apparent during the second administration, with more errors on the first digit of the pair presented to the left ear. The results are summarized in ▶ Fig. 6.16. Normal cutoff criterion (1 standard deviation [SD] below average) for this patient is 93.5% in the left ear, as shown in ▶ Fig. 6.15.

Staggered Spondaic Word Test

In the Staggered Spondaic Word (SSW) test, pairs of two-syllable words with equal stress (spondee) on both ears are presented to the ears. As shown in ▶ Fig. 6.17, the first part of the first spondee going to one ear is presented without any competition. The second part of the first spondee and the first part of the second spondee are presented simultaneously to both ears. The last part of the second spondee is presented without competition to the other ear. The ear receiving the first noncompeting stimulus is alternated after each item, thus manipulating attention from the right ear first to the left ear first. Thus, the subject does not have to keep track of the words being presented to the left or right ear. The scores obtained in each condition can be tabulated and graphed for comparison with normative data. SSW normal cutoff values (1 SD below mean) for each age group are shown in ▶ Fig. 6.18 to illustrate age-maturation effects (Katz, 1998). Note the right ear advantage in competing conditions, which is more obvious below 9 years of age. A summary of the results of a 9-year-old girl referred for auditory processing evaluation due to speech and language delays, being easily distracted by background noise, and difficulty following auditory directions is shown in ▶ Fig. 6.19 across the four different listening conditions assessed during SSW, along with normative cutoff

Table 6.1 Responses of an Adult Female Subject with Risk for Attention Deficit Hyperactivity Disorder and Auditory Processing Deficit on the Two-Pair Dichotic Digits Test with Free Recall

	Right Ear				Left Ear					Right Ear				Left Ear			
	First digit		Second digit		First digit		Second digit			First digit		Second digit		First digit		Second digit	
	S	R	S	R	S	R	S	R		S	R	S	R	S	R	S	R
1	4	√	3	√	1	√	6	√	1	10	×	3	×	2	×	9	×
2	3	×	1	×	9	√	10	√	2	10	√	6	√	3	×	8	×
3	9	√	6	√	1	×	5	√	3	10	×	8	√	5	√	1	√
4	2	√	10	√	6	×	8	√	4	6	√	9	√	5	√	8	√
5	4	√	8	√	6	×	9	√	5	1	√	3	√	2	√	5	√
6	9	√	1	√	10	×	2	√	6	5	×	2	√	10	√	1	×
7	2	√	4	√	9	×	10	×	7	3	×	5	√	6	√	9	√
8	1	×	9	×	8	×	6	√	8	8	×	10	×	9	×	1	×
9	2	×	4	√	3	√	9	×	9	4	√	6	√	5	×	2	×
10	1	×	4	×	10	×	5	×	10	10	×	8	√	4	√	5	×
11	2	×	5	√	1	×	3	×	11	4	√	9	√	8	√	2	√
12	4	√	5	√	2	×	6	√	12	5	×	10	×	9	×	2	×
13	3	√	10	√	5	×	6	√	13	1	√	10	√	9	×	3	×
14	4	√	1	×	9	√	5	×	14	5	√	2	√	3	×	8	√
15	4	×	5	√	3	×	8	√	15	10	×	4	√	8	√	1	×
16	9	√	5	√	4	×	1	×	16	6	√	2	√	8	×	10	√
17	4	√	5	√	10	√	2	×	17	8	√	4	√	5	×	3	×
18	9	√	8	√	3	×	4	√	18	3	√	4	√	1	√	2	√
19	9	×	10	√	8	√	5	×	19	3	√	9	√	4	√	5	√
20	8	√	6	√	4	×	1	×	20	9	√	3	√	5	×	4	√
21	6	√	8	×	10	√	2	√	21	10	√	2	√	6	√	4	√
22	9	√	1	√	2	√	8	√	22	8	√	6	√	10	×	4	×
23	6	√	9	√	3	×	1	×	23	5	√	10	√	6	×	4	×
24	1	√	2	√	3	√	9	√	24	3	√	2	√	10	×	6	×
25	5	×	3	×	2	×	1	×	25	10	×	9	×	1	×	3	×

S, stimulus; R, response. Score for the right ear: 73% (first digit 66%, second digit 80%).
Score for the left ear: 45% (first digit 40%, second digit 50%)
U.S. Department of Veterans Affairs, Tonal and Speech Materials for Auditory Perceptual Assessment, Disc 2.0; Tracks 3 and 4 (two-pair digit).

Table 6.2 Responses of an Adult Female Subject with Risk for Attention Deficit Hyperactivity Disorder and Auditory Processing Disorder on the Two-Pair Dichotic Digits Test with Free Recall and Pauses after Each Pair

	Right Ear				Left Ear					Right Ear				Left Ear			
	First digit		Second digit		First digit		Second digit			First digit		Second digit		First digit		Second digit	
	S	R	S	R	S	R	S	R		S	R	S	R	S	R	S	R
1	4	√	3	√	1	√	6	√	1	10	√	3	√	2	√	9	√
2	3	√	1	×	9	√	10	√	2	10	√	6	√	3	√	8	√
3	9	√	6	√	1	√	5	√	3	10	×	8	√	5	√	1	√
4	2	√	10	√	6	√	8	√	4	6	√	9	√	5	×	8	√
5	4	√	8	√	6	×	9	√	5	1	√	3	√	2	×	5	√
6	9	√	1	√	10	×	2	√	6	5	×	2	√	10	×	1	√
7	2	√	4	√	9	√	10	√	7	3	√	5	√	6	√	9	×
8	1	√	9	√	8	√	6	√	8	8	√	10	√	9	√	1	√
9	2	√	4	√	3	√	9	√	9	4	√	6	√	5	×	2	√
10	1	√	4	√	10	√	5	√	10	10	√	8	√	4	√	5	√
11	2	√	5	√	1	√	3	√	11	4	√	9	√	8	√	2	√
12	4	√	5	√	2	√	6	√	12	5	√	10	√	9	×	2	√
13	3	√	10	√	5	√	6	√	13	1	√	10	√	9	×	3	√
14	4	√	1	√	9	√	5	√	14	5	√	2	√	3	√	8	√
15	4	√	5	√	3	√	8	√	15	10	√	4	√	8	√	1	×
16	9	√	5	√	4	√	1	√	16	6	√	2	√	8	√	10	√
17	4	√	5	√	10	√	2	√	17	8	√	4	√	5	×	3	√
18	9	√	8	√	3	√	4	×	18	3	√	4	√	1	√	2	√
19	9	√	10	√	8	×	5	√	19	3	√	9	√	4	√	5	√
20	8	√	6	√	4	×	1	×	20	9	√	3	√	5	√	4	√
21	6	√	8	√	10	√	2	√	21	10	√	2	√	6	√	4	√
22	9	√	1	√	2	×	8	√	22	8	√	6	√	10	√	4	√
23	6	√	9	√	3	×	1	√	23	5	√	10	√	6	√	4	√
24	1	√	2	√	3	×	9	√	24	3	√	2	√	10	√	6	√
25	5	√	3	√	2	√	1	√	25	10	×	9	√	1	√	3	√

S, stimulus; R, response. Score for the right ear: 96% (first digit 94%, second digit 98%).
Score for the left ear: 82% (first digit 72%, second digit 92%)
U.S. Department of Veterans Affairs, Tonal and Speech Materials for Auditory Perceptual Assessment, Disc 2.0; Tracks 3 and 4 (two-pair digit).

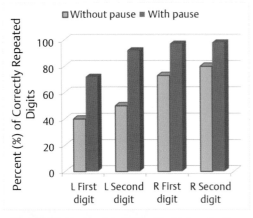

Fig. 6.16 Responses of an adult with risk for attention deficit hyperactivity disorder (ADHD) and auditory processing deficit (APD) on the two-pair dichotic digits test. The performance improved with insertion of a pause after the presentation of each pair, allowing more response time. L, left ear; R, right ear.

values for her age. ▶ Fig. 6.20 shows her performance in the right ear first (SSW REF) and left ear first (SSW LEF) tasks, which illustrates a right ear advantage.

Competing Words Test

The Competing Words (CW) subtest is included in the SCAN-C (Keith, 2000) and SCAN-3 (Keith, 2009ab) test batteries. In this test, monosyllabic word pairs are used with the presentation of one word simultaneously to each ear (e.g., *coat/tent*). In the SCAN-3 (Keith, 2009ab) version of the CW test, the words are digitally compressed as necessary to achieve approximately equal duration at the two ears that is within 3 ms for the free recall word pairs and within 10 ms for the directed recall word pairs (Keith, 2009). The task can be completed either in free recall or directed recall conditions (e.g., after the prompt "Say the word in the right ear first, then say the word in the left ear").

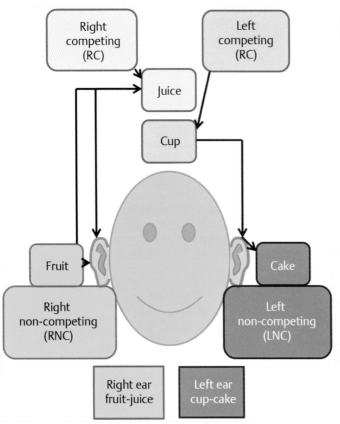

Fig. 6.17 Four conditions of the Staggered Spondaic Word (SSW) test.

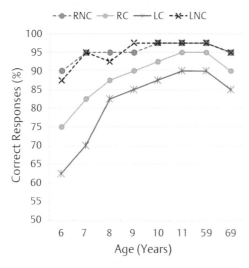

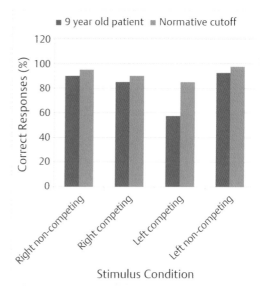

Fig. 6.18 Normal cutoff values (1 SD below mean) across age groups on the SSW test (based on Katz, 1998). LC, left competing; LNC, left noncompeting; RC, right competing; RNC, right noncompeting.

Fig. 6.19 Summary of SSW results of a 9-year-old girl referred for auditory processing evaluation due to speech and language delays, being easily distracted by background noise, and difficulty following auditory directions. Green bars indicate normative cutoff values for the subject's age group.

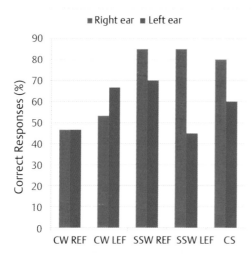

Fig. 6.20 Results of the same 9-year-old girl as in ▶ Fig. 6.19 who was referred for auditory processing evaluation due to speech and language delays, being easily distracted by background noise, and difficulty following auditory directions on three dichotic listening tests. CS, competing sentences; CW, competing words; LEF, left ear first; REF, right ear first; SSW, staggered spondaic words.

A summary of the results of a 9-year-old girl (previously mentioned under the SSW section) referred for auditory processing evaluation due to speech and language delays, being easily distracted

by background noise, and difficulty following auditory directions is shown in ▶ Fig. 6.20. Her responses using the directed recall response task on the CW test are shown for each ear in the right ear first (CW REF) and left ear first (CW LEF) conditions. The performance of this child is in the ninth percentile rank, which indicates an overall borderline performance during dichotic listening. This type of performance can explain her difficulties in listening in noisy surroundings and following auditory directions. She also shows a lack of a right ear advantage in the right ear first task apparent in most normal-hearing right-handed children; only 15% of the children in her age group exhibit a lack of right ear advantage on the right ear first task. The clear right ear advantage shown on other listening conditions (SSW and Competing Sentences) suggests that she may have had difficulties following directions for switching attention to the requested ear on the CW task (Richard, 2007). Normal-hearing children tend to show poorer performance on the CW test compared to the SSW test.

Larsen (1984) used a CW test in which the time interval between each dichotic pair was 660 ms and the intertrial interval was 15 seconds. He calculated a laterality index to determine the left

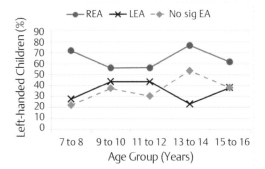

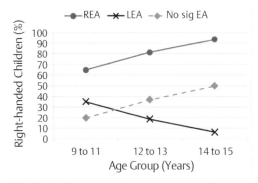

Fig. 6.21 Percentage of left- and right-handed children showing a right ear (REA) or left ear (LEA) advantage based on ear difference scores and those showing no significant ear advantage (based on Larsen, 1984).

versus right ear advantage, which was then used to determine if the left-right asymmetry was significant. His data for left- and right-handed individuals are given in ▶ Fig. 6.21 for various age groups. Among left-handed individuals, 22 to 54% may not show significant ear advantage; among right-handed individuals, 20 to 50% may not show significant ear advantage. The number of individuals displaying a lack of significant ear advantage increases with age. This could be due to improvement in scores, with age leading to ceiling effects that can obscure any ear advantages.

Dichotic Sentence Identification

Each sentence in the Dichotic Sentence Identification (DSI) test contains seven words that are third-order approximations, so that every successive three words form a meaningful phrase (see Chapter 7). For example, the synthetic sentence "Down by the time is real enough" has the phrases "down by the," "by the time," and "the time is." Two synthetic sentences are presented to each ear

simultaneously. The sentences begin and end at around the same time within 100 µsec. The patient is given a list of numbered sentences and is requested to report the two numbers corresponding to the two sentences heard (Fifer, Jerger, Berlin, Tobey, & Campbell, 1983).

6.10.4 Binaural Separation

Competing Sentence Test

The Competing Sentence Test (CST) is one of the subtests included in the SCAN-C and SCAN-3 test battery. In this test, sentences are presented simultaneously to both ears. In the SCAN-3 version of the test, the sentences are digitally compressed to achieve approximately equal duration that is within 10 ms for each pair. The patient is instructed to ignore sentences in one ear and repeat sentences presented to the other ear. In SCAN-C, the responses were recorded as either being correct or incorrect for the entire sentence. For example, if the target sentence is "The apple pie was hot," the expected correct response is the entire sentence, and the correct response received a score of 1. In the SCAN-3 version, scoring is based on repetition of key words. Thus, a score of 1 is awarded for each key word (*apple, pie, was, hot*) for the above sentence, which makes a maximum possible score of 4 for the sentence. The performance of the previously mentioned 9-year-old girl with speech and language delays is shown in ▶ Fig. 6.20 on the SCAN-C version using the whole sentence scoring procedure (CS). Her performance is within normal limits with a 25th percentile rank and shows a right ear advantage.

6.10.5 Dichotic Speech Fusion

Dichotic Consonant-Vowel Pairs

In this test, syllables with consonant-vowel (CV) pairs are presented simultaneously to two ears. The CV pairs include voiced and voiceless stop consonants: /pa/, /ba/, /ta/, /da/, /ka/, and /ga/ (Studdert-Kennedy & Shankweiler, 1970). Because the two syllables often fuse, the patient may report only one syllable instead of two. The mean scores for each ear are usually around 50%, as shown in ▶ Fig. 6.22 (Shinn, Baran, Moncrieff, & Musiek, 2005). When both syllables are repeated, the score is recorded as being double correct. Voiceless syllables are more frequently reported than voiced syllables in simultaneous dichotic voiced and

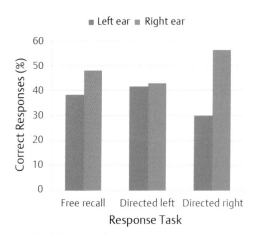

Fig. 6.22 Effects of response mode on the dichotic consonant-vowel (CV) task in young adults (based on Shinn, Baran, Moncrieff, & Musiek, 2005). The figure shows mean scores for each recall condition.

voiceless listening conditions, regardless of the ear receiving the stimuli (Berlin, Lowe-Bell, Cullen, & Thompson, 1973).

Rimol, Eichele, and Hugdahl (2006) noted a right ear advantage when the dichotic pairs consisted of voiced syllables to both ears or unvoiced syllables to both ears or unvoiced syllables to the right ear along with voiced syllables to the left ear. However, a significant left ear advantage emerged when the left ear received the voiceless syllable, while the right ear received the voiced syllable. In this case, because voiceless syllables are longer, the duration of syllables containing voiceless stops (/pa/, /ta/, /ka/) is longer compared to syllables containing voiced stops (/ba/, /da/, /ga/), which might provide longer time for processing voiceless syllables. When the dichotic stimuli lack perfect onset and/ or offset alignment due to duration differences, the ear receiving stimuli with longer durations may yield better scores.

A commercial version of the test is available on the *Tonal and Speech Materials for Auditory Perceptual Assessment* (1992) CD (Noffsinger, Martinez, & Wilson, 1994). The syllables, ranging in duration from 241 to 284 ms, were digitized from one channel of the original Kresge Hearing Institute of the South recordings (Berlin et al., 1973) and subsequently were edited to produce the 30 possible CV pairs. Track 5 on the CD has 30 randomized dichotic CVs with simultaneous onsets. Other randomizations of the 30 dichotic CVs are available with a 90 ms onset lag (Wilson & Leigh, 1996), which allows lags to either right or left ears. The effect of response tasks (free recall vs. directed recall) is shown in ▶ Fig. 6.22. Note a distinct right ear advantage when the subjects are asked to repeat the syllable in the right ear first (Shinn et al., 2005).

Dichotic Rhyme Test

In this test, all stimuli are monosyllabic consonant-vowel-consonant (CVC) words that begin with one of six stop consonants: /b/, /p/, /d/, /t/, /g/, /k/. The words rhyme, differing only with the initial consonant (e.g., *ten/pen, pit/kit*). The response task is a closed task in which patients point to pictures in a set corresponding to the words (Johnson, Sommers, & Weidner, 1977), or they can choose a response from a set of four rhyming words that differ only in the initial consonant. Among right-handed subjects, 85% showed a right ear advantage, 12% showed a left ear advantage, and 3% showed no ear advantage. However, only 49% of the right-handed subjects showed a statistically significant ear advantage, and in 98% of these cases, a right ear advantage was apparent. Among left-handed subjects, only 36% showed a statistically significant ear advantage, and only 30% of these individuals showed a left ear advantage (Wexler & Halwes, 1983). If the patients are asked to repeat what they hear (open response task), the ear advantage on this test tends to be similar in free (repeat any stimuli heard in either ear) or monaural recall (repeat what is heard in one ear and ignore the other ear) conditions, although some individual differences are apparent (Shinn et al., 2005). Split-brain patients due to commissurotomy show a large right ear advantage, marked left ear deficits, and a large ear difference score (Musiek et al., 1989).

6.10.6 Binaural Synthesis

In binaural synthesis tasks, information presented to each ear is not meaningful, but synthesis of the information presented to each ear in the central auditory system allows the perception of meaningful units. Broadbent (1955) showed that if low-pass segments (up to 450 Hz) of speech are presented to one ear, and high-pass segments (2000 Hz and above) are presented to the other ear, a fused image is perceived by most listeners even though the signals are spectrally different in two ears. Top-down processing may be involved in this type of fusion because of the missing segments from 450

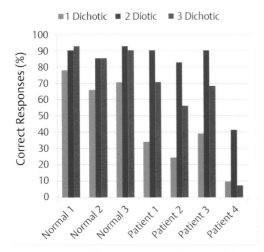

Fig. 6.23 Responses of three normal subjects and four patients on the bisyllabic filtered words following administration in the dichotic, diotic, and dichotic sequence. Note the improvement in dichotic scores during the second administration following the opportunity to listen to the stimuli in the diotic mode except for patient 4 (based on Matzker, 1959).

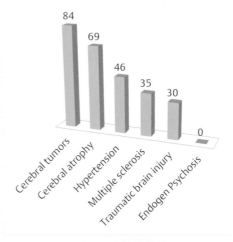

Fig. 6.24 Percentage of individuals showing abnormal results on the bisyllabic filtered words binaural synthesis test (based on Matzker, 1959).

to 2000 Hz, even though the listeners need to hear and decode the low- and high-pass segments.

Bisyllabic Filtered Words Synthesis

In this test, bisyllabic phonetically balanced words are filtered through two bands. The lower frequency pass band (500–800 Hz) is presented to one ear, and the high-frequency pass band (1815 –2500 Hz) is presented to the other. Although information in each of the bands is not meaningful, when presented simultaneously to the two ears, the bisyllabic words can be recognized. Matzker (1959) administered three variations of the test in the following order to several normal-hearing subjects and patients: (1) dichotic (low-frequency band to the right ear and high-frequency band to the left ear), (2) diotic (both bands presented to both ears), and (3) repetition of test 1. The scoring was based on correct recognition of vowels within the words. Most normal-hearing subjects and patients show improvement in dichotic scores after listening to both bands diotically. Sample improvements for three normal subjects and three patients are shown in ▶ Fig. 6.23. As shown in ▶ Fig. 6.24, patients with various lesions have difficulty with synthesis on this task (Matzker, 1959).

Monosyllabic Filtered Words Synthesis

Monosyllabic words reduce the redundancy in the signal and may improve sensitivity of the tests compared to bisyllabic words. In this test, monosyllabic (CVC) words are filtered through two bands. The pass band with lower frequencies (360 –890 Hz) mainly has vowel information. The pass band with higher frequencies (1750–2220 Hz) contains mainly consonant information. Consonants have lower energy compared to vowels. Thus, the center frequency gain in the higher band is raised by 10 dB compared to the low-frequency band. The test consists of three binaural conditions, dichotic A, diotic, and dichotic B, as shown in ▶ Fig. 6.25. To minimize systematic fatigue or learning effects, the test conditions are alternated after every word. So, for example, the first word of the dichotic A list is presented, then the first word of the diotic list is presented, which is followed by the first word of the dichotic B list. This pattern is repeated through the test administration. The test is presented at 30 dB SL. Normal cutoff criteria (1 SD below mean) and results from three patients with temporal lobe (TL) lesions and four patients with brainstem (BS) lesions are shown in ▶ Fig. 6.26 (Smith & Resnick, 1972).

A commercial version of the monosyllabic filtered words synthesis test is available (Department of Veteran Affairs, 1998). In this version, the

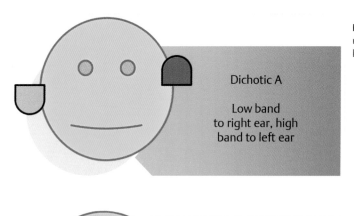

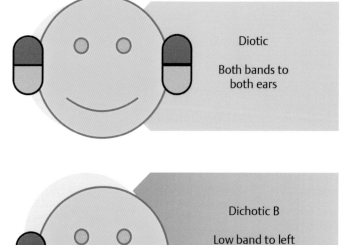

Fig. 6.25 The stimulus configuration used in the Smith and Resnick (1972) binaural synthesis test.

words from the Northwestern University No. 6 lists (Tillman & Carhart, 1966) are low-pass filtered with a 1500 Hz cutoff and high-pass filtered with a 2100 Hz cutoff with 115 dB/octave rejection. The filter cutoffs are based on a preliminary experiment with different filter cutoffs to determine optimal cutoff criteria. When the filtered version is presented monaurally at 35 dB HL, a level that is likely to minimize speech crossover to the other ear, 56.4 monosyllabic words are correctly identified in the low-pass filtered version, and 53% words are correctly identified with the high-pass version. When both versions are presented simultaneously with low pass to one ear and high pass to the other ear at 36 dB HL, 95.2% words are recognized correctly, with a standard deviation of 4.3.

Thus, the normal cutoff criterion for adults for the dichotic version is about 91% (Bornstein, Wilson, & Cambron, 1994). Because of minimal filtering, this particular synthesis test is expected to be less affected by mild or moderate, relatively flat peripheral hearing loss.

Segmented-Alternated Consonant-Vowel-Consonant Words Synthesis

In this test, the consonant segments of a word are presented to one ear, and the vowel segments are presented to the other. The carrier phrase ("Show me") before the word is presented to both ears. Most normal-hearing listeners are able to

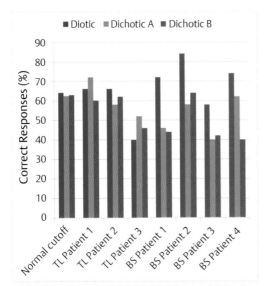

Fig. 6.26 Results of binaural synthesis test based on Smith and Resnick (1972). Normal cutoff criteria represent 1 SD below normal performance. Data are shown from three patients with temporal lobe (TL) lesions and four patients with brainstem (BS) lesions. In the diotic condition, both low- (360–890 Hz) and high- (1750–2220 Hz) frequency pass bands are delivered to both ears. In the dichotic A mode, the high band is delivered to the left ear, and the low band is delivered to the right ear. In the dichotic B condition, the low band is delivered to the left ear, and the high band is delivered to the right ear.

recognize more than 90% of the words at 30 dB HL (mean 95.2%, SD 3.9) while listening to both segments simultaneously (Wilson, 1994).

Rapidly Alternating Sentence Perception

In this procedure, sentence material is switched at periodic intervals between the two ears. Thus, each ear receives alternate bursts of unintelligible speech in a sequential and alternate manner. Normal listeners are able to synthesize the information to create intelligible sentences. Willeford and Billger (1978) used an alternating speech test in which sentence materials were divided in 300 ms segments and switched between ears. The task is fairly simple even for 5-year-old children. The test appears to be sensitive for aging effects, and an age and gender interaction is apparent in older age groups (▶ Fig. 6.27). Older individuals yield significantly poorer scores than younger adults, and older men show significantly poorer scores and a

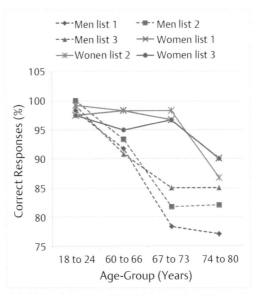

Fig. 6.27 Age and gender effects on the rapidly alternating speech perception test from the Willeford Central Auditory Processing test battery (based on Riensche, Thuman, Lincoln, & Lamb, 1983). The figure shows average scores.

wider range of scores compared to older women (Riensche, Thuman, Lincoln, & Lamb, 1983).

6.11 Spatial Stream Segregation

Most environments are complex, with several sounds occurring at the same time. Most listeners are able to detect, recognize, and continuously track sounds of interests (e.g., speech, music) and differentiate them from other background sounds (e.g., traffic). This ability to track sounds of interest in the presence of complex backgrounds has been referred to as *stream segregation* (Remez & Rubin, 1983) or *auditory scene analysis* (Bregman, 1990). Stream segregation can be measured in several ways and appears to be more efficient with the use of two ears. When target sounds are at a different location than background noises, spatial cues can be used to detect targets. Knowledge of target location improves identification of the sound in both quiet and noisy surroundings where several different background sounds are present (Kidd, Arbogast, Mason, & Gallun, 2005).

Hirsh (1950) determined reception thresholds for spondees by presenting speech and noise under various configurations and noted that thresholds were better when speech was presented on the

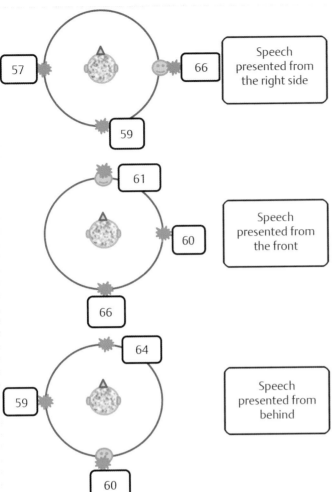

57 · 66 · 59

Speech presented from the right side

61 · 60 · 66

Speech presented from the front

64 · 59 · 60

Speech presented from behind

Fig. 6.28 Spondee reception thresholds (dB SPL) as a function of broadband noise (80 dB SPL) position in an anechoic chamber without fixing the head (based on Hirsh, 1950).

right side and noise was either in the back or on the left side compared to several other configurations (▶ Fig. 6.28). Broadbent (1954) presented speech with speaker 1 at 0-degree azimuth and competing speech with a different speaker at either 0- or 90-degree azimuth. Listeners made more errors when the competing message was at 0-degree azimuth than when the competition was presented at 90-degree azimuth. In the case of 90-degree azimuth, listeners are able to separate the target speaker's voice from the competing speaker's voice by using the differences in the location of the voices; this is referred to as the *spatial advantage*. In one study, Gelfand, Ross, and Miller (1988) presented sentences and a 12-talker babble either in front of the listener or from the right or left side. The speech presentation level was fixed at 70 dB SPL, while the

babble level was varied to find the lowest level or speech recognition threshold (SRT) at which sentences could be recognized 50% of the time. When both speech and babble were presented from front speakers, the babble could be raised only to 72 dB SPL (signal-to-noise [S/N] ratio = −2 dB) to establish the SRT; when the sentences were presented from the side and the babble from the front, the babble could be raised to about 80 dB SPL (S/N ratio = −10 dB) to establish SRT. Similarly, when the speech was in front, and the babble was presented on the side, the babble could be raised to 78 dB SPL (S/N ratio = −8 dB). These results confirm previous findings about easier speech recognition when the target and competing messages are spatially separated.

The spatial advantage noted above can be assessed in clinical settings where a booth, two

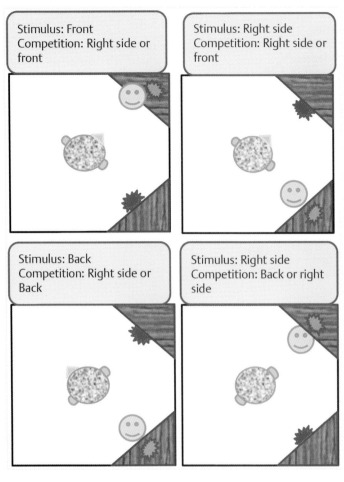

Stimulus: Front
Competition: Right side or front

Stimulus: Right side
Competition: Right side or front

Stimulus: Back
Competition: Right side or Back

Stimulus: Right side
Competition: Back or right side

Fig. 6.29 Examples of various stimulus/competition configurations in a sound booth for assessing stream segregation. Additional configurations are possible by making the listener face or turn his or her back to the other speaker, which will allow target stimuli to be presented on the left side.

loudspeakers, and a two-channel audiometer are available. The signal can be spondee words that are available in audiology clinics for obtaining SRTs. The noise can be speech noise available on audiometers or continuous speech materials available on CDs. ▶ Fig. 6.29 shows various stimulus configurations. A difference score between two configurations gives an idea about the spatial advantage achieved by each client. For example, we obtained a difference score or advantage of 7 dB when spondees were presented on the left side along with 45 dB EM speech noise presented in front of the listener over the condition when both the spondees and the noise were presented from the loudspeaker in front of a normal-hearing listener. When the difference score or spatial advantage is close to zero, the patient may have a deficit in using spatial advantage or a spatial sound-processing disorder (Griffiths, Dean, Woods, Rees, & Green, 2001).

The spatial advantage can also be documented by measuring speech recognition scores (SRSs) at average conversational levels with a 0 dB S/N ratio. For example, when monosyllabic words were presented to a listener at 45 dB HL in the presence of 45 dB EM speech-shaped noise, with both the words and noise located in front of the listener, the word recognition score was 16%, and the phoneme recognition score was 38.67%. When the words were presented on the left side with noise in front of the listener, the word recognition score improved to 72% and the phoneme recognition score to 84%. Thus, the spatial advantage for word recognition was 56% (72% − 16%), and phoneme recognition was 45.33% (84% − 38.67%). If necessary, any spatial processing deficit can be more formally assessed using commercially available tests, such as the Listening in Spatialized Noise −Sentences Test (LISN-S) (Cameron & Dillon, 2009).

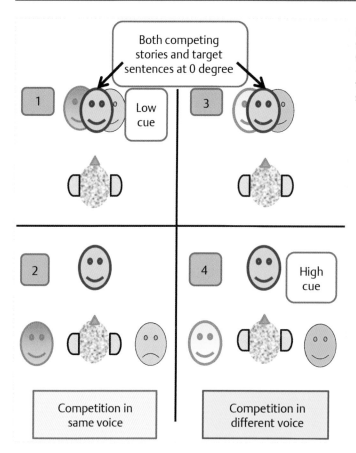

Fig. 6.30 The four stimulus configurations simulated under headphones in the Listening in Spatialized Noise–Sentences Test (LISN-S) for evaluating the ability to segregate speech streams.

6.11.1 Listening in Spatialized Noise–Sentences Test (LISN-S)

The LISN-S, developed by Cameron and Dillon (2009), evaluates auditory segregation skills, or the ability to differentiate auditory signals arriving simultaneously at the two ears and to recognize target signals.

Stimuli

Target sentences are manipulated to appear at 0-degree azimuth in the presence of competing looped children's stories spoken either by the same speaker delivering the target sentences or by different speakers. The competing stories are presented at either 0- or 90-degree azimuth on the right and left side (▶ Fig. 6.30). The listener can use a talker difference advantage when the competing speakers are different or a spatial advantage when the competing stories arrive at the left and right side. Both of these advantages can be used when competing stories appear on the left and right side and are delivered by speakers who are different than the speaker who presents the target sentences. The stimuli are delivered through headphones using a computer.

Stimulus Configurations

A simulated three-dimensional environment is created by presynthesizing speech stimuli with head-related transfer functions (HRTFs). The simulation allows the target voice to always appear in front of the listener. The competing looped children's stories can be either in front of the listener or on the left and right sides. The different configurations are shown in ▶ Fig. 6.30.

Response Task

The listener is expected to repeat the sentence that is perceived as being in front of him or her.

Table 6.3 Listening in Spatialized Noise–Sentences Test: Patterns of Results and Suggested Interpretations

Low Cue SRT	High Cue SRT	Talker Advantage	Spatial Advantage	Total Advantage	Suggested Deficit
Normal	2 SD below mean	Normal	2 SD below mean	2 SD below normal	Spatial processing deficit
1 SD below mean	1 SD below mean	Normal	Normal	Normal	Possible memory deficit; advantage (difference) measures may control for memory deficit and yield normal results
SRTs decline over the test administration					Auditory fatigue or declining attention

Abbreviations: SD, standard deviation; SRT, speech recognition threshold.

Procedure

The level at which 50% of the words in a sentence (SRT) is determined for sentences presented in different configurations, as shown in ▸ Fig. 6.30. The presentation level of competing speech is held at 55 dB SPL. The target sentence presentation begins with 62 dB SPL and is then adjusted adaptively until the SRT is established. The conditions are always presented in a specified order for establishing SRT (conditions 4, 2, 3, and 1; ▸ Fig. 6.30).

Results

Advantage scores based on SRTs established in different conditions and SRTs in the low and high cue conditions are used for test interpretation. More specifically, the following measures are used in interpreting test results:

1. SRT in high cue condition (▸ Fig. 6.30, 4)
2. SRT in low cue condition (▸ Fig. 6.30, 1)
3. Spatial advantage measure: Take the SRT difference in conditions 1 and 2.
4. Talker advantage measure: Take the SRT difference between conditions 1 and 3.
5. Total advantage measure: Take the SRT differences between conditions 1 and 4.

Normative cutoff criteria are used that are built in the software to determine if the results are within normal limits for each of the above measures. The pattern of normal or abnormal results is used to suggest underlying problems, as shown in ▸ Table 6.3.

6.12 Objective Measures

6.12.1 Efferent Suppression of Otoacoustic Emissions through Contralateral Noise

The amplitude of otoacoustic emissions (OAEs) is reduced when noise is presented to the contralateral ear; this reduction is achieved through the activation of medial olivocochlear (MOC) efferent fibers that innervate the cochlea. The amount of suppression of the emissions represents the strength of the MOC reflex. The suppression is almost absent in vestibular neurotomized patients (Giraud et al., 1997). Some children with APDs and associated learning disabilities show less suppression of transient evoked otoacoustic emissions (TEOAEs) compared to gender- and age-matched normal children (Muchnik et al., 2004).

Activation of the MOC systems through contralateral noise improves speech perception, and the improvement is correlated with the amount of suppression of OAEs through contralateral noise (Giraud et al., 1997; Kumar & Vanaja, 2004). In normal-hearing adults, the activation of the MOC is related to phoneme discrimination in noise. Following improvement in phoneme discrimination in noise through training, the MOC activity increases, as is apparent from greater OAE suppression after training (de Boer & Thornton, 2008). Individuals with poor monosyllabic word recognition in noise show significantly less suppression of OAE amplitudes compared to individuals who have better word recognition (Tokgoz-Yilmaz, Kose, Turkyilmaz, & Atay, 2013).

185

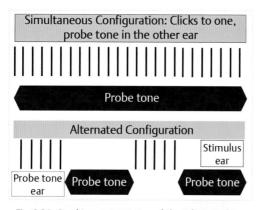

Fig. 6.31 Graphic representation of the "alternated" and "simultaneous" conditions for measuring binaural summation in reflex thresholds.

6.12.2 Binaural Summation in the Middle Ear Stapedial Acoustic Reflex

The binaural summation effect can be measured quickly and reliably using click-evoked acoustic reflex measures. The equipment that can be used to obtain click-evoked reflex thresholds has been described previously (Rawool, 1995, 1996). The polarity of the clicks is condensation, and duration is 100 µs. To check binaural summation, click-evoked contralateral reflex thresholds can be obtained at the click rates of 100/s with two stimulus configurations, as shown in ▶ Fig. 6.31. In the first configuration (alternated or multiplexed stimuli), the presentation of the probe tone is alternated with the presentation of the clicks. The envelope of the multiplexed stimulus is 115 ms. The total rise and fall time of the envelope is 18 ms. Within this period, clicks are presented for 44 ms, and the probe is presented for 53 ms. The clicks are off during the presentation of the probe. Thus, the reflex is measured after the clicks are turned off for a brief period by presenting the probe tone. This is possible because the reflex has a relatively long off latency (see Chapter 5). In the second condition (simultaneous stimuli), the probe tone and the clicks are presented simultaneously (▶ Fig. 6.31). Probe tone frequency can be set at 226 Hz, and the intensity of the probe tone is 85 dB SPL.

Thresholds obtained from 21 women ages 19 to 32 years are shown in ▶ Fig. 6.32. Acoustic reflex thresholds were established for each subject by placing the probe in the left ear and presenting the clicks to the right ear through a button transducer. Reflex thresholds were determined by increasing or decreasing click levels in 5 dB steps. All the data were collected in a quiet room. As can be seen in ▶ Fig. 6.32, normal young adults show a 5 to 20 dB improvement in thresholds in the "simultaneous" configuration over the "alternated" configuration. The average thresholds in the "simultaneous" condition are 86.43 dB peak equivalent sound pressure level (peSPL), and those in the "alternated" condition are 97.38 dB peSPL. The average difference in the two thresholds is 10.95 dB peSPL. This is similar to the 6 to 10 dB binaural summation effect apparent with behavioral loudness-matching procedures (Hawkins et al., 1987). Thus, in the "simultaneous" condition, the probe tone and the click appear to interact, creating an improvement in thresholds. In some older adults, this improvement is absent or less than 5 dB, suggesting a binaural summation deficit.

6.12.3 Objective Documentation of Binaural Beat Perception

Relatively lower base frequencies and lower frequency differences tend to produce more frequent or more robust electrophysiological responses corresponding to the beats. For example, in one study, 100% of the participants yielded the 40 Hz binaural beat steady-state response evoked by tone pairs of 390 and 430 Hz, but only 10% of the participants yielded a response for a higher tone pair of 810 and 850 Hz (Grose & Mamo, 2012). In another study, the amplitudes of beat-evoked oscillations were higher, to 250 Hz compared to 1000 Hz base frequency and to 3 Hz compared to 6 Hz beat frequency (Pratt et al., 2009).

Some studies suggest that the sources of the beat-evoked oscillations are mostly located in the left temporal lobe (e.g., Pratt et al., 2010). However, neuromagnetic responses to binaural beats in Japanese participants suggest that dominant current sources are located in bilateral superior temporal lobes. In addition, in some participants, the

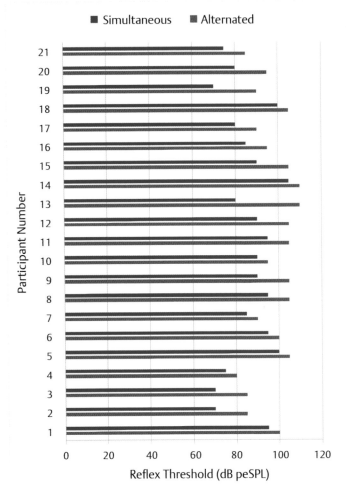

■ Simultaneous ■ Alternated

Participant Number

Reflex Threshold (dB peSPL)

Fig. 6.32 Contralateral acoustic reflex thresholds obtained from 21 women in the "alternated" and "simultaneous" conditions. Note the better or lower thresholds in the "simultaneous" condition.

posterior parietal regions, including superior or inferior parietal lobules, are activated (Karino et al., 2006).

6.12.4 Interaural Time and Intensity Difference Coding in the Auditory Brainstem Response

The amplitude of wave V of the auditory brainstem response (ABR) using rarefaction clicks is largest for clicks that are perceived at the center of the head compared to clicks that are perceived laterally due to interaural intensity or time differences. Similarly, the latency of wave V of the ABR is shortest when interaural time differences are zero compared to when interaural differences cause lateral perception of the stimuli (Riedel & Kollmeier, 2002).

6.12.5 Binaural Level Difference in the Auditory Brainstem Response

This is the difference in ABRs (see Chapter 4) elicited with binaural clicks presented in phase and out of phase at both ears. The latency of the click-evoked ABR depends on a complex interaction between click polarity and intensity. Generally, at high presentation levels, rarefaction clicks yield earlier latencies, and at lower presentation levels, condensation clicks yield earlier latencies. The level at which the polarity reversal occurs is somewhat different for each individual (Rawool & Zerlin, 1988). The concept of dominant or preferred polarity configuration has been developed to address these differences. The condition that elicits earlier latencies for the in-phase condition (binaural rarefaction vs. binaural condensation) is marked as the dominant in-phase condition for

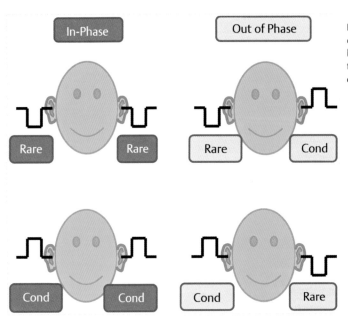

Fig. 6.33 In-phase and out–of-phase configurations used in determining the binaural-level difference in the auditory brainstem response (ABR). Cond, condensation; Rare, rarefaction.

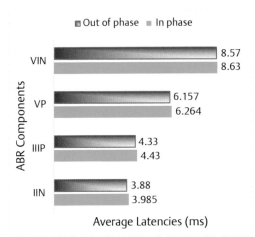

Fig. 6.34 Mean latencies (ms) obtained with dominant or preferred binaural in-phase and out-of-phase click configurations for various components of the auditory brainstem response (ABR) (based on Rawool & Ballachanda, 1990).

each individual. Similarly, the condition that elicits earlier latencies for the out-of-phase condition is marked as the dominant out-of-phase condition for each individual (▶ Fig. 6.33). As noted in Chapter 4, the ABR waveforms are identified as I, II, III, IV, V, and VI. The peaks of these components are recorded by adding the letter P (e.g., IIP), and the troughs following the peaks are noted by adding the letter N (e.g., IIN) to each component. The

latencies for IIN ($p = .049$), IIIP ($p = .012$) and VIN ($p = .044$) of the ABR components are significantly earlier for the dominant, preferred out-of-phase condition compared to the preferred in-phase condition. ▶ Fig. 6.34 shows the mean latencies for these components, along with those for the frequently measured component VP ($p = .099$) (Rawool & Ballachanda, 1990).

6.12.6 Binaural Interaction Component of the Auditory Brainstem Response

ABRs elicited with binaural stimulation yield larger amplitudes than those elicited with monaural stimulation (Jewett, 1970). However, the binaural response tends to be smaller, especially at lower frequencies, when compared to the summation of monaural responses obtained from the left and right ears (predicted binaural, or L + R, response). The waveform obtained with binaural stimulation can be subtracted from the predicted binaural waveform to reveal the binaural interaction component (BIC) (Dobie & Berlin, 1979). Amplitudes of the wave V component of the ABR for the binaural, predicted binaural (L + R), and the BIC in response to 500 Hz tone bursts are shown in ▶ Fig. 6.35 (based on Fowler & Horn, 2012). The predicted binaural wave V is larger in amplitude compared to the wave V obtained by binaural stimulation of the ear. Absence of clearly demonstrable ABR wave

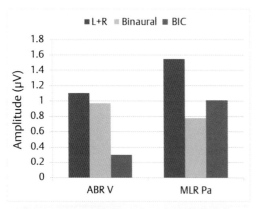

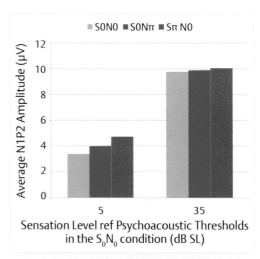

Fig. 6.35 Mean Amplitudes of the wave V component of the auditory brainstem response (ABR) and Pa component of the auditory middle latency response (AMLR) evoked with 500 Hz tone bursts. L + R = Summed response obtained from monaural stimulation of left and right ears. Binaural = Response obtained with binaural stimulation. BIC = (L + R) − Binaural (based on Fowler & Horn, 2012).

Fig. 6.36 Average N1P2 amplitudes evoked with clicks in the presence of 65 dB SPL broadband noise with three configurations (based on Yonovitz, Thompson, & Lozar, 1979).

V binaural interaction component in children may be suggestive of an APD with a sensitivity and specificity of up to 76% (Delb, Strauss, Hohenberg, & Plinkert, 2003).

6.12.7 Binaural Interaction Component of the Auditory Middle Latency Response

The binaural interaction component of the auditory middle latency response (AMLR) can be studied using the same procedure described previously under the ABR section. Amplitudes of the Pa component of the AMLR for the binaural, predicted binaural (L + R), and BIC in response to 500 Hz tone bursts are shown in ▶ Fig. 6.35. The predicted binaural Pa is larger in amplitude compared to the Pa obtained by binaural stimulation (Fowler & Horn, 2012). Among individuals with symmetric auditory sensitivity but asymmetrical ability in recognizing speech, the NaPa amplitudes of the binaural interaction component of the AMLR are significantly correlated with performance on the MLD task (Leigh-Paffenroth, Roup, & Noe, 2011).

6.12.8 Masking-Level Differences in the Late Auditory Evoked Response

As shown in ▶ Fig. 6.36, N1P2 amplitudes of the late auditory response evoked with clicks

presented at 5 and 35 dB sensation levels are larger in the out-of-phase configurations ($S_\pi N_0$ or $N_0 S_\pi$) when compared to in-phase ($S_0 N_0$) configurations (Yonovitz, Thompson, & Lozar, 1979), which is similar to the improvements apparent in the psychoacoustic MLD procedures.

6.12.9 Masking-Level Differences in Auditory Evoked Magnetoencephalography

The amplitudes of N1 m response in both right and left hemispheres are significantly larger and latencies significantly shorter for the $S_\pi N_0$ configuration when compared to those obtained in the $S_0 N_0$ configuration. The difference is greater at 250 Hz when compared to 1000 and 4000 Hz (Sasaki et al., 2005).

6.13 Binaural Measures in the Presence of Hearing Loss

During binaural processing tests, it is important to ensure that the signal is audible in each ear and that the signals reaching the ears are at equal sensation levels. Not using equal sensation levels can lead to artificial ear advantages or deficits and therefore wrong conclusions. For example, ▶ Fig. 6.3 shows the interaural intensity (or level) difference (IID) of a listener with thresholds of

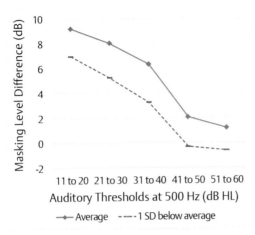

Fig. 6.37 Effect of hearing loss on the masking-level difference (MLD). The figure shows average MLDs and values 1 SD below average at 500 Hz in the presence of an 80 dB SPL broadband noise masker as a function of auditory sensitivity at 500 Hz (based on Jerger, Brown, & Smith, 1984).

4 dB HL in the left ear and 17 dB HL in the right. Thus, when calculating IIDs, sensation levels at each ear should be used. Absolute IIDs will lead to wrong conclusions about significant asymmetries in the left and right hemifields. Binaural processing deficits have been noted in some individuals with hearing loss (Leigh-Paffenroth et al., 2011). Some tests show a systematic effect of hearing loss. As an example, ▶ Fig. 6.37 shows the effect of symmetric hearing loss at 500 Hz on the MLD established at 500 Hz in the presence of an 80 dB SPL broadband noise masker (Jerger, Brown, & Smith, 1984).

6.14 Physiology of Binaural Processing

Depending on the expected response task, binaural auditory processing requires ongoing comparison of information arriving at the two ears (e.g., dichotic pitch, MLD), fusion of information arriving at the two ears (localization, binaural fusion), or separation of information arriving at the two ears (talker on the right side, noise on the left side). A complex interaction of the following three factors appears to allow the human auditory system to process information arriving at the two ears efficiently.

6.14.1 Bilateral Representation of Signals Arriving at Each Ear

Neural impulses arriving at each of the cochlear nuclei travel to both the superior olivary complexes through afferent pathways. Thus, stimulation of each ear is generally represented bilaterally at the superior olivary complexes and all other higher levels in the auditory system. In addition, there are dedicated brainstem pathways for processing low- and high-frequency information. This allows more accurate processing of ITD cues, which rely on low-frequency information, and interaural intensity difference cues, which rely on high-frequency information. The medial superior olive (MSO) has a relatively high number of neurons with lower characteristic frequencies and also appears to be specialized in processing ITD information (Goldberg & Brown, 1969; Yin & Chan, 1990). The lateral superior olive has a relative overrepresentation of high-frequency neurons, which are important for processing interaural-intensity differences (Tollin, 2003). This high- versus low-frequency separation is maintained throughout the higher auditory pathways via tonotopic organization in humans (De Martino et al., 2013).

6.14.2 Interhemispheric Communication

The auditory cortices in each hemisphere communicate with each other through the corpus callosum (▶ Fig. 6.38). During periods of auditory exposure, callosal connections between auditory cortices modulate neuronal activity through excitatory inputs (Carrasco et al., 2013). Interhemispheric communication across the corpus callosum may be involved in enhancing or suppressing the binaural signals used during dichotic tasks, such as MLD (Wack et al., 2012). The corpus callosum also may enhance dynamic and flexible interactions between bottom-up and top-down factors involved in processing dichotic stimuli (Westerhausen & Hugdahl, 2008).

6.14.3 Efferent Pathways

Several efferent connections exist in the auditory system that allow communication between the highest level in the auditory cortex and the lowest level at the cochlea. An example of the efferent connections is the efferent projection from the

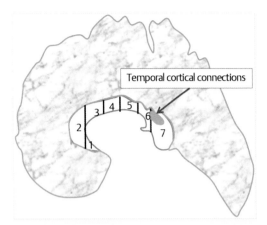

Temporal cortical connections

Fig. 6.38 Corpus callosum with various sections: 1. rostrum, 2. genu, 3. rostral body, 4. anterior midbody, 5. posterior midbody, 6. isthmus, 7. splenium. Temporal cortical connections between the two hemispheres occur in the isthmus and splenium areas (purple). The depiction of temporal cortical connections is based on a functional magnetic resonance imaging mapping study conducted by Fabri and Polonara (2013).

superior olivary complex to the cochlea known as the olivocochlear bundle or system (see Chapter 1). This system has two branches. The thin unmyelinated lateral olivocochlear fibers innervate afferent auditory nerve fibers under inner hair cells, and the thick myelinated medial olivocochlear fibers innervate the outer hair cells (Guinan, 2006). Activation of the olivocochlear bundle changes cochlear responses and suppresses auditory nerve fiber responses to sounds presented in a quiet background (Ruben & Sekula, 1960). It also enhances auditory nerve responses to sounds presented in a noisy background (Kawase, Delgutte, & Liberman, 1993).

The difference in OAE amplitudes obtained without and with noise reveals suppression due to the olivocochlear reflex and is used as a measure of olivocochlear reflex strength (Chéry-Croze, Moulin, Collet, & Morgon, 1994). The sound localization performance of individuals with a stronger olivocochlear reflex strength is less affected by background noise, suggesting that the activation of the medial olivocochlear system by noise helps to counteract the effects of background noise on neural representations of direction-dependent spectral features that assist in localizing sounds (Andéol et al., 2011). As mentioned previously, activation of the medial olivocochlear systems through contralateral noise improves

speech perception; the improvement is correlated with suppression of OAEs through contralateral noise (Kumar & Vanaja, 2004).

6.15 Pathologies that Can Lead to Binaural Processing Deficits

Structural or functional deficits in any of the areas involved in binaural processing can be expected to lead to deficits in binaural processing. Thus, unilateral, bilateral, and central lesions, as well as lesions in the pathways or commissures that link the right and left sides and efferent pathways, may lead to degraded performance on binaural processing tasks. Some examples of lesions leading to binaural processing deficits are reviewed below.

6.15.1 Central Pontine Lesions

Lesions in the central pontine involving the trapezoid body may lead to deficits in localizing sounds and detecting sound movements (Griffiths et al., 1997).

6.15.2 Caudal Pontine Lesions

Some individuals with minor caudal pontine lesions show deficits in lateralization tasks. The deficits may involve perceiving stimuli at the center of the head regardless of interaural time or level differences, or they can be lateralized to just one side of the head. Individuals with major caudal pontine lesions perceive most stimuli at the center of the head and exhibit difficulties in lateralizing stimuli (Furst et al., 2000).

6.15.3 Unilateral Inferior Colliculus Lesion

Champoux et al. (2007) reported the results of binaural auditory processing tasks in the presence of a very circumscribed lesion of the right inferior colliculus in a 12-year-old boy. His sound source localization in the horizontal plane was impaired, with marked impairment in the left hemifield contralateral to the right lesioned side. He showed a significantly deficient performance on the duration pattern task using both a verbal and a humming response. He also showed poor speech recognition in the left ear when either words or speech babble was presented simultaneously to the right ear.

6.15.4 Left Hemisphere Dysfunction

Individuals with focal left hemisphere brain damage show deficits in using interaural intensity and interaural time difference cues for locating sounds, especially in the right hemifield, under headphones (Spierer, Bellmann-Thiran, Maeder, Murray, & Clarke, 2009). Left hemisphere damage may also lead to deficits on binaural fusion tasks (Baran, Bothfeldt, & Musiek, 2004). Some adults with left mesial temporal sclerosis (LMTS) due to left temporal lobe epilepsy show significantly poor performance on the dichotic digits test in both ears when compared to normal adults. Other adults with left hemisphere damage may show a significant right ear deficit with relatively good performance in the left ear (Baran et al., 2004; Rocha, Miziara, Manreza, & Schochat, 2010).

6.15.5 Right Hemisphere Dysfunction

Individuals with focal damage to the right hemisphere can show deficits in using interaural time difference cues for locating sounds in both hemifields with many perceptual shifting errors across the midline (alloacusis) under headphones. There is a significant association between right temporal lobe lesions and impairment on lateralization tasks (Spierer et al., 2009).

6.15.6 Corpus Callosal Lesions

Acallosal listeners are less accurate in localizing sounds occurring at midline and at other points in the auditory field than matched listeners (Poirier, Miljours, Lassonde, & Lepore, 1993). A significant leftward bias in localization is noted in some listeners with partial or total section of the corpus callosum (Hausmann, Corballis, Fabri, Paggi, & Lewald, 2005). Adults born with agenesis of the corpus callosum have difficulty in localizing moving sound targets (Lessard, Lepore, Villemagne, & Lassonde, 2002). Right-handed patients with surgical sectioning of the corpus callosum have difficulty in repeating verbal stimuli presented to the left ear during dichotic listening tasks (Milner, Taylor, & Sperry, 1968; Musiek et al., 1989; Musiek & Wilson, 1979; Musiek, Wilson, & Pinheiro, 1979). More specifically, splenial lesions in the corpus callosum can lead to significant left ear deficits without improvement in left ear performance even after directing attention to the left ear (Pollmann, Maertens, von Cramon, Lepsien, & Hugdahl, 2002).

6.16 Functional Effects of Binaural Processing Deficits

Difficulties in accurately processing binaural stimuli can lead to difficulties in accurately localizing sounds in quiet and noisy surroundings. These difficulties can further lead to deficits in understanding speech in noisy surroundings. Children with binaural processing deficits may have difficulty understanding their teachers or classmates. Binaural processing deficits have been noted in children with ADHD (see Chapter 13) or with language-related impairments, including dyslexia (see Chapter 14).

6.17 Future Trends

Systematically collected data on normal individuals and individuals with various structural and functional anomalies within the auditory system will be available for various tests that are listed in ▶ Table 6.4 and ▶ Table 6.5. Advances in virtual auditory display technologies will improve the ability to represent complex sound environments under headphones. It will also become easier to obtain evoked potential measures with the availability of more affordable and efficient technologies. As an example, see the website http://www. emotiv.com/, which sells the Emotive EPOC multi-channel, portable system for recording contextual EEG. Advances in similar technologies will allow objective assessment of various binaural processes using speech and nonspeech stimuli without any active responses from the listener; such technologies will allow accurate separation of attentional and memory deficits from APDs.

6.18 Review Questions

1. What are the advantages of binaural listening over monaural listening?
2. Describe the various cues that are useful in localizing sound sources.
3. Describe various dichotic nonspeech measures, including precedence effect, binaural beats, binaural-level difference, masking-level difference, dichotic pitch, and dichotic musical chords. What types of abnormal results may be apparent on these tests?

Table 6.4 Recommended Behavioral Tests for Assessing Binaural Processing

Process	Purpose	Results	Results Suggesting Deficit
Interaural intensity difference lateralization	To assess the ability to make use of interaural intensity cues	Is image perceived at the center with appropriate manipulation of levels at the two ears?	Failure to perceive a fused central image
		Does a sufficient increase in intensity at one ear cause a shift in the sound image in the correct hemifield?	The image that should be perceived in the left hemisphere due to higher sensation levels in the left ear is perceived in the right hemifield and vice versa. Failure to lateralize the image: the image is always perceived in the center of the head.
Masking level difference at 500 Hz in the presence of a 40 dB EM narrowband noise masker centered on 500 Hz	To assess the ability to make use of differences in interaural phase cues in tonal and narrowband noise signals	Does the threshold in the $S_\pi N_0$ condition improve sufficiently over that obtained in the $S_0 N_0$ condition?	There may be no improvement or minimal improvement in thresholds in the $S_\pi N_0$ condition compared to that obtained in the $S_0 N_0$ condition.
Binaural recall with two-pair dichotic digits	To assess the ability to recall stimuli presented simultaneously to both ears	Free recall. Directed right ear first and left ear first recall. Percentage of correct scores: right ear first digit, right ear second digit, left ear first digit, left ear second digit	Left and/or right ear deficit may be apparent.
Binaural separation (SCAN-3 competing sentences)	To assess the ability to separate and recall stimuli presented to one ear in the presence of simultaneously presented stimuli to the other ear	Percentage of correct scores, right ear, left ear	Left and/or right ear deficit may be apparent. Combination of stimuli presented to the two ears may be recalled, suggesting an inability to separate the speech streams occurring at the two ears.
Binaural synthesis (VA CD; NU-6 lists low-pass filtered with a 1500 Hz cutoff and high-pass filtered with a 2100 Hz cutoff with 115 dB/octave rejection	To assess the ability to combine low- and high-frequency information presented to each ear for meaningful interpretation of words	Percentage correct scores: 1. Low pass to left ear and high pass to right ear 2. High pass to left ear and low pass to right ear	Scores may be poorer in one or both stimulus configurations, suggesting difficulty with binaural synthesis of spectral information.
Binaural synthesis with segmented alternated CVC words (VA CD)	To assess the ability to combine alternating CVC information to two ears for meaningful interpretation of words	Percentage of correct scores: 1. Consonant to the left ear and vowels to the right ear 2. Vowels to the left ear and consonants to the right ear	Scores may be poorer in one or both stimulus configurations, suggesting difficulty with binaural synthesis of phonemic units.

Table 6.4 continued

Process	Purpose	Results	Results Suggesting Deficit
Spatial stream segregation	To assess the ability to take advantage of spatial separation of spondees and competing stimuli to improve spondee recognition in a sound booth	SRT in free field with 1. Target and competing stimuli at 0-degree azimuth 2. Target at 90-degree azimuth and competing stimuli at 0-degree azimuth 3. The improvement (difference) in SRTs in condition 2 over condition 1	Failure of SRT to improve with spatial separation of target and competing stimuli
Spatial processing with LISN-S	To assess the ability to take advantage of spatial separation and talker differences to improve target recognition with simulated conditions under headphones	Sentence recognition thresholds in various stimulus configurations	Failure to improve SRT in the presence of talker or spatial advantage (see ▶ Table 6.3)

Abbreviations: CVC, consonant-vowel-consonant; EM, effective masking; LISN-S, Listening in Spatialized Noise–Sentences Test; NU-6, Northwestern University Auditory Test No. 6; SRT, speech recognition threshold; VA CD. U.S. Department of Veterans Affairs. Tonal and Speech Materials for Auditory Perceptual Assessment, 1998, computer disc.

Table 6.5 Recommended Objective Tests for Assessing Binaural Processing

Process	Purpose	Results	Results Suggesting Deficit
Efferent suppression of OAEs through contralateral noise	To assess the integrity of the MOC efferent fibers innervating the cochlea or the strength of the MOC reflex	The difference in the OAE amplitudes with and without contralateral noise	No differences or minimal differences in the amplitudes of the OAEs with and without contralateral noise, suggesting a deficit in MOC function
Binaural summation of the acoustic reflex	To assess the binaural summation effect within the acoustic reflex pathway	The difference in contralateral reflex thresholds elicited with multiplexed/alternated presentation of probe tones and clicks and those obtained with simultaneous presentation of probe tones and clicks	No difference or difference less than 5 dB between the two conditions

Abbreviations: MOC, medial olivocochlear; OAE, otoacoustic emission.

4. Describe the various categories of dichotic speech tests. What types of abnormal results may be apparent on these tests?
5. Discuss the spatial advantage in the context of recognizing speech in the presence of background noise. What is a spatial sound-processing disorder? Describe the purpose, procedure, and interpretation of the Listening in Spatialized Noise test.
6. Discuss three factors that allow efficient processing of information arriving at both ears in the human auditory system.
7. What procedures can be used to measure the medial olivocochlear efferent suppression effect?
8. Describe objective procedures for measuring binaural summation, binaural-level difference, and masking-level differences.
9. Discuss procedures for measuring the binaural interaction component in the auditory brainstem response and auditory middle latency response.
10. Review some pathological conditions that can lead to binaural processing deficits, and list the potential functional impact of binaural processing deficits.

References

[1] Akeroyd, M. A. (2010). A binaural beat constructed from a noise (L). Journal of the Acoustical Society of America, 128 (6), 3301–3304.

[2] Akeroyd, M. A., & Guy, F. H. (2011). The effect of hearing impairment on localization dominance for single-word stimuli. Journal of the Acoustical Society of America, 130(1), 312–323.

[3] Algazi. V. R., Avendano. C., & Duda, R. O. (2001). Elevation localization and head-related transfer function analysis at low frequencies. Journal of the Acoustical Society of America, 109(3), 1110–1122.

[4] Andéol, G., Guillaume, A., Micheyl, C., Savel, S., Pellieux, L., & Moulin, A. (2011). Auditory efferents facilitate sound localization in noise in humans. Journal of Neuroscience, 31(18), 6759–6763.

[5] Ashmead, D. H., Davis, D. L., & Northington, A. (1995). Contribution of listeners' approaching motion to auditory distance perception. Journal of Experimental Psychology: Human Perception and Performance, 21(2), 239–256.

[6] Ashmead, D. H., LeRoy, D., & Odom, R. D. (1990). Perception of the relative distances of nearby sound sources. Perception and Psychophysics, 47(4), 326–331.

[7] Baran, J. A., Bothfeldt, R. W., & Musiek, F. E. (2004). Central auditory deficits associated with compromise of the primary auditory cortex. Journal of the American Academy of Audiology, 15(2), 106–116.

[8] Barr, D. F., Mullin, T. A., & Herbert, P. S. (1970). Application of binaural beat phenomenon with aphasic patients. Archives of Otolaryngology, 103(4), 192–194.

[9] Berlin, C. I., Lowe-Bell, S. S., Cullen, J. K., Jr., & Thompson, C. L. (1973). Dichotic speech perception: An interpretation of right-ear advantage and temporal offset effects. Journal of the Acoustical Society of America, 53(3), 699–709.

[10] Bess, F. H., Tharpe, A. M., & Gibler, A. M. (1986). Auditory performance of children with unilateral sensorineural hearing loss. Ear and Hearing, 7(1), 20–26.

[11] Bornstein, S. P., Wilson, R. H., & Cambron, N. K. (1994). Low- and high-pass filtered Northwestern University Auditory Test No. 6 for monaural and binaural evaluation. Journal of the American Academy of Audiology, 5(4), 259–264.

[12] Bregman, A. S. (1990). Auditory scene analysis: The perceptual organization of sound. Cambridge, MA: MIT Press.

[13] Broadbent, D. E. (1954). The role of auditory localization in attention and memory span. Journal of Experimental Psychology, 47(3), 191–196.

[14] Broadbent, D. E. (1955). A note on binaural fusion. Quarterly Journal of Experimental Psychology, 7, 46–47.

[15] Brookhouser, P. E., Worthington, D. W., & Kelly, W. J. (1991). Unilateral hearing loss in children. Laryngoscope, 101(12, Pt. 1), 1264–1272.

[16] Brughera, A., Dunai, L., & Hartmann, W. M. (2013). Human interaural time difference thresholds for sine tones: The high-frequency limit. Journal of the Acoustical Society of America, 133(5), 2839–2855.

[17] Butler, R. A. (1969). Monaural and binaural localization of noise bursts vertically in the median sagittal plane. Journal of Audiology Research, 9, 230–235.

[18] Cameron, S., & Dillon, H. (2009). Listening in Spatialized Noise–Sentences Test (LiSN-S) (Version 1.014) (computer software). Murten, Switzerland: Phonak Communications.

[19] Carrasco, A., Brown, T. A., Kok, M. A., Chabot, N., Kral, A., & Lomber, S. G. (2013). Influence of core auditory cortical areas on acoustically evoked activity in contralateral primary auditory cortex. Journal of Neuroscience, 33(2), 776–789.

[20] Champoux, F., Paiement, P., Mercier, C., Lepore, F., Lassonde, M., & Gagné, J. P. (2007). Auditory processing in a patient with a unilateral lesion of the inferior colliculus. European Journal of Neuroscience, 25(1), 291–297.

[21] Chandler, D. W., & Grantham, D. W. (1992). Minimum audible movement angle in the horizontal plane as a function of stimulus frequency and bandwidth, source azimuth, and velocity. Journal of the Acoustical Society of America, 91(3), 1624–1636.

[22] Chéry-Croze, S., Moulin, A., Collet, L., & Morgon, A. (1994). Is the test of medial efferent system function a relevant investigation in tinnitus? British Journal of Audiology, 28(1), 13–25.

[23] Coleman, P. D. (1968). Dual role of frequency spectrum in determination of auditory distance. Journal of the Acoustical Society of America, 44(2), 631–632.

[24] Cramer, E. M., & Huggins, W. H. (1958). Creation of pitch through binaural interaction. Journal of the Acoustical Society of America, 30, 413–417.

[25] Dancer, J., Burl, N. T., & Waters, S. (1995). Effects of unilateral hearing loss on teacher responses to the SIFTER: Screening Instrument for Targeting Educational Risk. American Annals of the Deaf, 140(3), 291–294.

[26] de Boer, J., & Thornton, A. R. (2008). Neural correlates of perceptual learning in the auditory brainstem: Efferent activity predicts and reflects improvement at a speech-in-noise discrimination task. Journal of Neuroscience, 28(19), 4929–4937.

[27] Delb, W., Strauss, D. J., Hohenberg, G., & Plinkert, P. K. (2003). The binaural interaction component (BIC) in children with central auditory processing disorders (CAPD). International Journal of Audiology, 42(7), 401–412.

[28] Della Penna, S., Brancucci, A., Babiloni, C., et al. (2007). Lateralization of dichotic speech stimuli is based on specific auditory pathway interactions: Neuromagnetic evidence. Cerebral Cortex, 17(10), 2303–2311.

[29] De Martino, F., Moerel, M., van de Moortele, P. F., et al. (2013). Spatial organization of frequency preference and selectivity in the human inferior colliculus. Nature Communications, 4, 1386.

[30] Diamond, S. P., & Bender, M. B. (1965). On auditory extinction and alloacusis. Transactions of the American Neurological Association, 90, 154–157.

[31] Diercks, K. J., & Jeffress, L. A. (1962). Interaural phase and the absolute threshold for tone. Journal of the Acoustical Society of America, 34(7), 981–984.

[32] Dobie, R. A., & Berlin, C. I. (1979). Binaural interaction in brainstem-evoked responses. Archives of Otolaryngology, 105(7), 391–398.

[33] Dougherty, R. F., Cynader, M. S., Bjornson, B. H., Edgell, D., & Giaschi, D. E. (1998). Dichotic pitch: A new stimulus distinguishes normal and dyslexic auditory function. Neuroreport, 9, 3001–3005. Retrieved from http://journals.lww.com/neuroreport/ Abstract/1998/09140.

[34] English, K., & Church, G. (1999). Unilateral hearing loss in children: An update for the 1990s. Language, Speech, and Hearing Services in Schools, 30, 26–31.

[35] Epstein, M., & Florentine, M. (2009). Binaural loudness summation for speech and tones presented via earphones and loudspeakers. Ear and Hearing, 30(2), 234–237.

[36] Epstein, M., & Florentine, M. (2012). Binaural loudness summation for speech presented via earphones and loudspeaker with and without visual cues. Journal of the Acoustical Society of America, 131(5), 3981–3988.

[37] Fabri, M., & Polonara, G. (2013). Functional topography of human corpus callosum: An fMRI mapping study. Neural Plasticity, 15, 1-15. Retrieved from http://www.hindawi.com/journals/np/2013/251308/.

[38] Fifer, R. C., Jerger, J. F., Berlin, C. I., Tobey, E. A., & Campbell, J. C. (1983). Development of a dichotic sentence identification test for hearing-impaired adults. Ear and Hearing, 4(6), 300–305.

[39] Fowler, C. G., & Horn, J. H. (2012). Frequency dependence of binaural interaction in the auditory brainstem and middle latency responses. American Journal of Audiology, 21(2), 190–198.

[40] Furst, M., Aharonson, V., Levine, R. A., et al. (2000). Sound lateralization and interaural discrimination: Effects of brainstem infarcts and multiple sclerosis lesions. Hearing Research, 143(1-2), 29–42.

[41] Gardner, M. B., & Gardner, R. S. (1973). Problem of localization in the median plane: effect of pinnae cavity occlusion. Journal of the Acoustical Society of America, 53(2), 400–408.

[42] Gelfand, S. A., Ross, L., & Miller, S. (1988). Sentence reception in noise from one versus two sources: Effects of aging and hearing loss. Journal of the Acoustical Society of Ericaca, 83(1), 248–256.

[43] Giraud, A. L., Garnier, S., Micheyl, C., Lina, G., Chays, A., & Chéry-Croze, S. (1997). Auditory efferents involved in speech-in-noise intelligibility. Neuroreport, 8(7), 1779–1783.

[44] Goldberg, J. M., & Brown, P. B. (1969). Response of binaural neurons of dog superior olivary complex to dichotic tonal stimuli: Some physiological mechanisms of sound localization. Journal of Neurophysiology, 32(4), 613–636.

[45] Gordon, K. A., Jiwani, S., & Papsin, B. C. (2011). What is the optimal timing for bilateral cochlear implantation in children? Cochlear Implants International, 12(Suppl. 2), S8–S14.

[46] Griffiths, T. D., Bates, D., Rees, A., Witton, C., Gholkar, A., & Green, G. G. (1997). Sound movement detection deficit due to a brainstem lesion. Journal of Neurology, Neurosurgery, and Psychiatry, 62(5), 522–526.

[47] Griffiths, T. D., Dean, J. L., Woods, W., Rees, A., Green, G. G. R. (2001). The Newcastle Auditory Battery (NAB): A temporal and spatial test battery for use on adult naïve subjects. Hearing Research, 154(1-2), 165–169.

[48] Grose, J. H., Buss, E., & Hall, J. W. III. (2012). Binaural beat salience. Hearing Research, 285(1–2), 40–45.

[49] Grose, J. H., & Mamo, S. K. (2012). Electrophysiological measurement of binaural beats: effects of primary tone frequency and observer age. Ear and Hearing, 33(2), 187–194.

[50] Guinan, J. J., Jr. (2006). Olivocochlear efferents: Anatomy, physiology, function, and the measurement of efferent effects in humans. Ear and Hearing, 27(6), 589–607.

[51] Halverson, H. M. (1922). Binaural localization of tones as dependent upon differences of phase and intensity. American Journal of Psychology, 33(2), 178–212.

[52] Harris, J. D., & Sergeant, R. L. (1971). Monaural-binaural minimum audible angles for a moving sound source. Journal of Speech and Hearing Research, 14(3), 618–629.

[53] Hausmann, M., Corballis, M. C., Fabri, M., Paggi, A., & Lewald, J. (2005). Sound lateralization in subjects with callosotomy, callosal agenesis, or hemispherectomy. Brain Research. Cognitive Brain Research, 25(2), 537–546.

[54] Hawkins, D. B., Prosek, R. A., Walden, B. E., & Montgomery, A. A. (1987). Binaural loudness summation in the hearing impaired. Journal of Speech and Hearing Research, 30(1), 37–43.

[55] Hawley, M. L., Litovsky, R. Y., & Culling, J. F. (2004). The benefit of binaural hearing in a cocktail party: Effect of location and type of interferer. Journal of the Acoustical Society of America, 115(2), 833–843.

[56] Hebrank, J., & Wright, D. (1974). Spectral cues used in the localization of sound sources on the median plane. Journal of the Acoustical Society of America, 56(6), 1829–1834.

[57] Hendler, T., Squires, N. K., & Emmerich, D. S. (1990). Psychophysical measures of central auditory dysfunction in multiple sclerosis: Neurophysiological and neuroanatomical correlates. Ear and Hearing, 11(6), 403–416.

[58] Henning, G. B. (1974a). Detectability of interaural delay in high-frequency complex waveforms. Journal of the Acoustical Society of America, 55(1), 84–90.

[59] Henning, G. B. (1974b). Lateralization and the binaural masking-level difference. Journal of the Acoustical Society of America, 55(6), 1259–1262.

[60] Hirsh, I. J. (1948). The influence of interaural phase on interaural summation and inhibition. Journal of the Acoustical Society of America, 20, 536–544.

[61] Hirsh, I. J. (1950). The relation between localization and intelligibility. Journal of the Acoustical Society of America, 22, 196–200.

[62] Humes, L. E., Allen, S. K., & Bess, F. H. (1980). Horizontal sound localization skills of unilaterally hearing-impaired children. Audiology, 19(6), 508–518.

[63] Jerger, J., Brown, D., & Smith, S. (1984). Effect of peripheral hearing loss on the masking level difference. Archives of Otolaryngology, 110(5), 290–296.

[64] Jesteadt, W., & Wier, C. (1977). Comparison of monaural and binaural discrimination of intensity and frequency. Journal of the Acoustical Society of America, 61(6), 1599–1603.

[65] Jewett, D. L. (1970). Volume-conducted potentials in response to auditory stimuli as detected by averaging in the cat. Electroencephalography and Clinical Neurophysiology, 28(6), 609–618.

[66] Johnson, J. P., Sommers, R. K., & Weidner, W. E. (1977). Dichotic ear preference in aphasia. Journal of Speech and Hearing Research, 20(1), 116–129.

[67] Karino, S., Yumoto, M., Itoh, K., et al. (2006). Neuromagnetic responses to binaural beat in human cerebral cortex. Journal of Neurophysiology, 96(4), 1927–1938.

[68] Katz, J. (1998). SSW test manual (5th ed.). Vancouver, WA: Precision Acoustics.

[69] Kawase, T., Delgutte, B., & Liberman, M. C. (1993). Antimasking effects of the olivocochlear reflex: II. Enhancement of auditory-nerve response to masked tones. Journal of Neurophysiology, 70(6), 2533–2549.

[70] Keith, R. W. (2009a). SCAN-3 for adolescents and adults: Test for auditory processing disorders. San Antonio, TX: Pearson.

[71] Keith, R. W. (2009b). SCAN-3: C tests for auditory processing disorders for children. San Antonio, TX: Pearson.

[72] Keith, R. W. (2000). SCAN-C: Test for auditory processing disorders in children-revised. San Antonio, TX: Psychological Corporation.

[73] Kidd, G., Jr., Arbogast, T. L., Mason, C. R., & Gallun, F. J. (2005). The advantage of knowing where to listen. Journal of the Acoustical Society of America, 118(6), 3804–3815.

[74] Kim, H.-Y., Suzuki, Y., Takane, S., & Sone, T. (2001). Control of auditory distance perception based on the auditory parallax model. Applied Acoustics, 62, 245–270.

[75] Kimura, D. (1963). Speech lateralization in young children as determined by an auditory test. Journal of Comparative and Physiological Psychology, 56, 899–902.

[76] Kimura, D. (1967). Functional asymmetry of the brain in dichotic listening. Cortex, 3, 163–178.

[77] Klein, M. E., & Zatorre, R. J. (2011). A role for the right superior temporal sulcus in categorical perception of musical chords. Neuropsychologia, 49(5), 878–887.

[78] Koehnke, J., Culotta, C. P., Hawley, M. L., & Colburn, H. S. (1995). Effects of reference interaural time and intensity differences on binaural performance in listeners with normal and impaired hearing. Ear nnd Hearing, 116(4), 331–353.

[79] Kubovy M., Cutting J. E., & McGuire R. M. (1974). Hearing with the third ear: Dichotic perception of a melody without monaural familiarity cues. Science, 186(4160), 272-274.

[80] Kumar, U. A., & Vanaja, C. S. (2004). Functioning of olivocochlear bundle and speech perception in noise. Ear and Hearing, 25(2), 142–146.

[81] Lackner, J. R., & Shenker, B. (1985). Proprioceptive influences on auditory and visual spatial localization. Journal of Neuroscience, 5(3), 579–583.

[82] Larsen, S. (1984). Developmental changes in the pattern of ear asymmetry as revealed by a dichotic listening task. Cortex, 20(1), 5–17.

[83] Lazzouni, L., Ross, B., Voss, P., & Lepore, F. (2010). Neuromagnetic auditory steady-state responses to amplitude modulated sounds following dichotic or monaural presentation. Clinical Neurophysiology, 121(2), 200–207.

[84] Leigh-Paffenroth, E. D., Roup, C. M., & Noe, C. M. (2011). Behavioral and electrophysiologic binaural processing in persons with symmetric hearing loss. Journal of the American Academy of Audiology, 22(3), 181–193, quiz 194–195.

[85] Lessard, N., Lepore, F., Villemagne, J., & Lassonde, M. (2002). Sound localization in callosal agenesis and early callosotomy subjects: Brain reorganization and/or compensatory strategies. Brain, 125(Pt. 5), 1039–1053.

[86] Licklider, J. C. R., Webster, J. C., & Hedlun, J. M. (1950). On the frequency limits of binaural beats. Journal of the Acoustical Society of America, 22(4), 468–473.

[87] Lieu, J. E. (2004). Speech-language and educational consequences of unilateral hearing loss in children. Archives of Otolaryngology–Head and Neck Surgery, 130(5), 524–530.

[88] Litovsky, R. Y., & Godar, S. P. (2010). Difference in precedence effect between children and adults signifies development of sound localization abilities in complex listening tasks. Journal of the Acoustical Society of America, 128(4), 1979–1991.

[89] Little, A. D., Mershon, D. H., & Cox, P. H. (1992). Spectral content as a cue to perceived auditory distance. Perception, 21(3), 405–416.

[90] Makous, J. C., & Middlebrooks, J. C. (1990). Two-dimensional sound localization by human listeners. Journal of the Acoustical Society of America, 87(5), 2188–2200.

[91] Matzker, J. (1959). Two new methods for the assessment of central auditory functions in cases of brain disease. Annals of Otology, Rhinology, and Laryngology, 68, 1185–1197.

[92] McFadden, D. (1968). Masking-level differences determined with and without interaural disparities in masker intensity. Journal of the Acoustical Society of America, 44(1), 212–223.

[93] Mershon, D. H., Ballenger, W. L., Little, A. D., McMurtry, P. L., & Buchanan, J. L. (1989). Effects of room reflectance and background noise on perceived auditory distance. Perception, 18(3), 403–416.

[94] Mershon, D. H., & Bowers, J. N. (1979). Absolute and relative cues for the auditory perception of egocentric distance. Perception, 8(3), 311–322.

[95] Mershon, D. H., & King, E. (1975). Intensity and reverberation as factors in the auditory perception of egocentric distance. Perception and Psychophysics, 18, 409–415.

[96] Middlebrooks, J. C., Makous, J. C., & Green, D. M. (1989). Directional sensitivity of sound-pressure levels in the human ear canal. Journal of the Acoustical Society of America, 86(1), 89–108.

[97] Mills, A. W. (1958). On the minimum audible angle. Journal of the Acoustical Society of America, 30, 237–246.

[98] Milner, B., Taylor, L., & Sperry, R. W. (1968). Lateralized suppression of dichotically presented digits after commissural section in man. Science, 161(3837), 184–186.

[99] Moncrieff, D, W,, & Wilson, R. H. (2009). Recognition of randomly presented one-, two-, and three-pair dichotic digits by children and young adults. Journal of the American Academy of Audiology, 20(1), 58–70.

[100] Moore, B. C., & Glasberg, B. R. (2007). Modeling binaural loudness. The Journal of the Acoustical Society of America, 121(3), 1604-1612.

[101] Muchnik, C., Ari-Even Roth, D., Othman-Jebara, R., Putter-Katz, H., Shabtai, E. L., & Hildesheimer, M. (2004). Reduced medial olivocochlear bundle system function in children with auditory processing disorders. Audiology and Neurootology, 9(2), 107–114.

[102] Musicant, A. D., & Butler, R. A. (1984). The influence of pinnae-based spectral cues on sound localization. Journal of the Acoustical Society of America, 75(4), 1195–1200.

[103] Musiek, F. E., Kurdziel-Schwan, S., Kibbe, K. S., Gollegly, K. M., Baran, J. A., & Rintelmann, W. F. (1989). The dichotic rhyme task: Results in split-brain patients. Ear and Hearing, 10(1), 33–39.

[104] Musiek, F. E., & Wilson, D. H. (1979). SSW and dichotic digit results pre- and post-commissurotomy: A case report. Journal of Speech and Hearing Disorders, 44(4), 528–533.

[105] Musiek, F. E., Wilson, D. H., & Pinheiro, M. L. (1979). Audiological manifestations in "split brain" patients. Journal of the American Audiology Society, 5(1), 25–29.

[106] Nábělek, A. K., & Robinette, L. (1978). Influence of the precedence effect on word identification by normally hearing and hearing-impaired subjects. Journal of the Acoustical Society of America, 63(1), 187–194.

[107] Newton, V. E. (1983). Sound localisation in children with a severe unilateral hearing loss. Audiology, 22(2), 189–198.

[108] Noffsinger, D., Martinez, C. D., Friedrich, B. W., & Wilson, R. H. (1994). Dichotic listening to musical chords: Background and preliminary data. Journal of the American Academy of Audiology, 5(4), 243–247.

[109] Noffsinger, D., Martinez, C. D., & Wilson, R. H. (1994). Dichotic listening to speech: Background and preliminary data for digits, sentences, and nonsense syllables. Journal of the American Academy of Audiology, 5(4), 248–254.

[110] Noffsinger, D., Olsen, W. O., Carhart, R., Hart, C. W., & Sahgal, V. (1972). Auditory and vestibular aberrations in multiple sclerosis. Acta Otolaryngologica, 303(Suppl.), 1–63

[111] Novak, R. E., & Anderson, C. V. (1982). Differentiation of types of presbycusis using the masking-level difference. Journal Speech and Hearing Research, 25(4), 504–508.

[112] Olsen, W. O., & Noffsinger, D. (1976). Masking level differences for cochlear and brain stem lesions. Annals of Otology, Rhinology, and Laryngology, 85(6, Pt. 1), 820–825.

[113] Oster, G. (1973). Auditory beats in the brain. Scientific American, 229(4), 94–102.

[114] Oyler, R. F., Olyler, A. L., & Matkin, N. D. (1988). Unilateral hearing loss: Demographics and educational impact. Language, Speech, and Hearing Services in Schools, 19, 201–210.

[115] Partanen, M., Fitzpatrick, K., Mädler, B., Edgell, D., Bjornson, B., & Giaschi, D. (2012). Cortical basis for dichotic pitch perception in developmental dyslexia. Brain & Language, 123, 104–112.

[116] Perrott, D. R. (1984). Concurrent minimum audible angle: A re-examination of the concept of auditory spatial acuity. Journal of the Acoustical Society of America, 75(4), 1201–1206.

[117] Perrott, D. R., & Saberi, K. (1990). Minimum audible angle thresholds for sources varying in both elevation and azimuth. Journal of the Acoustical Society of America, 87(4), 1728–1731.

[118] Perrott, D. R., & Tucker, J. (1988). Minimum audible movement angle as a function of signal frequency and the velocity of the source. Journal of the Acoustical Society of America, 83(4), 1522–1527.

[119] Poirier, P., Miljours, S., Lassonde, M., & Lepore, F. (1993). Sound localization in acallosal human listeners. Brain, 116 (Pt. 1), 53–69.

[120] Pollack, I. (1948). Monaural and binaural threshold sensitivity for tones and white noise. Journal of the Acoustical Society of America, 20, 52–57.

[121] Pollmann, S., Maertens, M., von Cramon, D. Y., Lepsien, J., & Hugdahl, K. (2002). Dichotic listening in patients with splenial and nonsplenial callosal lesions. Neuropsychology, 16 (1), 56–64.

[122] Pratt, H., Starr, A., Michalewski, H. J., Dimitrijevic, A., Bleich, N., & Mittelman, N. (2010). A comparison of auditory evoked potentials to acoustic beats and to binaural beats. Hearing Research, 262(1–2), 34–44.

[123] Rawool, V. W. (1995). Ipsilateral acoustic reflex thresholds at varying click rates in humans. Scandinavian Audiology, 24(3), 199–205.

[124] Rawool, V. W. (1996). Effect of aging on the click-rate induced facilitation of acoustic reflex thresholds. Journals of Gerontolgoy Series A: Biological Sciences and Medical Sciences, 51(2), B124–B131.

[125] Rawool, V. W. (2012). Documenting hazardous noise levels and exposures. In V. W. Rawool (Ed.), Hearing conservation: In occupational, recreational, educational, and home settings. New York: Thieme.

[126] Rawool, V. W., & Ballachanda, B. B. (1990). Homo- and antiphasic stimulation in ABR. Scandinavian Audiology, 19(1), 9–15.

[127] Rawool, V., & Zerlin, S. (1988). Phase-intensity effects on the ABR. Scandinavian Audiology, 17(2), 117–123.

[128] Riensche, L. L., Thuman, P. R., Lincoln, K. L., & Lamb, L. E. (1983). Age effects on performance on the Willeford Central Auditory Processing Test Battery. Journal of Auditory Research, 23, 131–135.

[129] Remez, R. E., & Rubin, P. E. (1983). The stream of speech. Scandinavian Journal of Psychology, 24(1), 63–66.

[130] Richard, G. J. (2007). Cognitive-communicative and language factors associated with (central) auditory processing disorder: A speech-language pathology perspective. In G. D. Chermak & F. E. Musiek (Eds.), Handbook of (central) auditory processing disorder: Comprehensive intervention (Volume. 1, pp. 397–415). San Diego, CA: Plural Publishing.

[131] Riedel, H., & Kollmeier, B. (2002). Auditory brain stem responses evoked by lateralized clicks: Is lateralization extracted in the human brain stem? Hearing Research, 163(1–2), 12–26.

[132] Rimol, L. M., Eichele, T., & Hugdahl, K. (2006). The effect of voice-onset-time on dichotic listening with consonant-vowel syllables. Neuropsychologia, 44(2), 191–196.

[133] Ringo, J. L., Doty, R. W., Demeter, S., & Simard, P. Y. (1994). Time is of the essence: A conjecture that hemispheric specialization arises from interhemispheric conduction delay. Cerebral Cortex, 4(4), 331-343.

[134] Rocha, C. N., Miziara, C. S., Manreza, M. L., & Schochat, E. (2010). Electrophysiological and auditory behavioral evaluation of individuals with left temporal lobe epilepsy. Arquivos de Neuro-Psiquiatria, 68(1), 18–24.

[135] Roffler, S. K., & Butler, R. A. (1968). Factors that influence the localization of sound in the vertical plane. Journal of the Acoustical Society of America, 43(6), 1255–1259.

[136] Rowland, R. C., & Tobias, J. V. (1967). Interaural intensity difference limen. Washington, DC: Federal Aviation Administration, Office of Aviation Medicine.

[137] Ruben, R. J., & Sekula, J. (1960). Inhibition of central auditory response. Science, 131(3394), 163.

[138] Ruscetta, M. N., Arjmand, E. M., & Pratt, S. R. (2005). Speech recognition abilities in noise for children with severe-to-profound unilateral hearing impairment. International Journal of Pediatric Otorhinolaryngology, 69(6), 771–779.

[139] Sasaki, T., Kawase, T., Nakasato, N., et al. (2005). Neuromagnetic evaluation of binaural unmasking. Neuroimage, 25(3), 684–689.

[140] Shinn, J. B., Baran, J. A., Moncrieff, D. W., & Musiek, F. E. (2005). Differential attention effects on dichotic listening. Journal of the American Academy of Audiology, 16(4), 205–218.

[141] Siveke, I., Ewert, S. D., Grothe, B., & Wiegrebe, L. (2008). Psychophysical and physiological evidence for fast binaural processing. Journal of Neuroscience, 28(9), 2043–2052.

[142] Smith, B. B., & Resnick, D. M. (1972). An auditory test for assessing brain stem integrity: Preliminary report. Laryngoscope, 82(3), 414–424.

[143] Spierer, L., Bellmann-Thiran, A., Maeder, P., Murray, M. M., & Clarke, S. (2009). Hemispheric competence for auditory spatial representation. Brain, 132(Pt. 7), 1953–1966.

[144] Studdert⌐Kennedy, M., Shankweiler, D., & Schulman, S. (1970). Opposed effects of a delayed channel on perception of dichotically and monotically presented CV syllables. The Journal of the Acoustical Society of America, 48(2B), 599-602.

[145] Sweetow, R. W., & Reddell, R. C. (1978). The use of masking level differences in the identification of children with perceptual problems. Ear and Hearing, 4(2), 52–56.

[146] Tervaniemi, M., Kujala, A., Alho, K., Virtanen, J., Ilmoniemi, R. J., & Näätänen, R. (1999). Functional specialization of the human auditory cortex in processing phonetic and musical sounds: A magnetoencephalographic (MEG) study. Neuroimage, 9(3), 330–336.

[147] Tervaniemi, M., Sannemann, C., Noyranen, M., Salonen, J., & Pihko, E. (2011). Importance of the left auditory areas in chord discrimination in music experts as demonstrated by MEG. European Journal of Neuroscience, 34(3), 517–523.

[148] Tillman, T. W., & Carhart, R. (1966). An expanded test for speech discrimination utilizing CNC monosyllabic words: Northwestern University auditory test no. 6. (Tech. Rep. SAM-TR-66–55). Brooks AFB, TX: USAF School of Aerospace Medicine.

[149] Tokgoz-Yilmaz, S., Kose, S. K., Turkyilmaz, M. D., & Atay, G. (2013). The role of the medial olivocochlear system in the complaints of understanding speech in noisy environments by individuals with normal hearing. Auris Nasus Larynx, 40 (6), 521–524.

[150] Tollin, D. J. (2003). The lateral superior olive: A functional role in sound source localization. Neuroscientist, 9(2), 127–143.

[151] U.S. Department of Veterans Affairs. (1998). Tonal and speech materials for auditory perceptual assessment (compact disc 2.0). Mountain Home, TN: VA Medical Center.

[152] Wack, D. S., Cox, J. L., Schirda, C. V., et al. (2012). Functional anatomy of the masking level difference: An fMRI study. PLoS ONE, 7(7), e41263.

[153] Westerhausen, R., & Hugdahl, K. (2008). The corpus callosum in dichotic listening studies of hemispheric asymmetry: A review of clinical and experimental evidence. Neuroscience and Biobehavioral Reviews, 32(5), 1044–1054.

[154] Wexler, B. E., & Halwes, T. (1983). Increasing the power of dichotic methods: The fused rhymed words test. Neuropsychologia, 21(1), 59–66.

[155] Willeford, J. A., & Billger, J. M. (1978). Auditory perception in children with learning disabilities. In J. Katz (Ed.), Handbook of clinical audiology (2nd ed., pp. 410–425). Baltimore, MD: Williams & Wilkins.

[156] Wilson, R. H. (1994). Word recognition with segmented-alternated CVC words: Compact disc trials. Journal of the American Academy of Audiology, 5(4), 255–258.

[157] Wilson, R. H., & Leigh, E. D. (1996). Identification performance by right- and left-handed listeners on dichotic CV materials. Journal of the American Academy of Audiology, 7(1), 1–6.

[158] Witton, C., Hillebrand, A., Furlong, P. L. & Henning, G. B. (2012). A novel binaural pitch elicited by phase-modulated noise: MEG and psychophysical 0bservations. Cerebral Cortex, 22, 1271–1281.

[159] Yin, T. C., & Chan, J. C. (1990). Interaural time sensitivity in medial superior olive of cat. J Neurophysiol, 64(2), 465–488.

[160] Yonovitz, A., Thompson, C. L., & Lozar, J. (1979). Masking level differences: Auditory evoked responses with homophasic and antiphasic signal and noise. Journal of Speech and Hearing Research, 22(2), 403–411.

[161] Yost, W. A. (1981). Lateralization position of sinusoids presented with interaural intensive and temporal differences. Journal of the Acoustical Society of America, 70, 397–409.

Chapter 7

Assessment of the Processing of Monaural Low-Redundancy Speech

7 Assessment of the Processing of Monaural Low-Redundancy Speech

In real-life situations, the spoken message is often degraded because of background noise and reverberant environments or because a speaker talks softly, rapidly, or from a distance. The ability of a listener to process speech can be assessed by using low-redundancy speech stimuli. Various aspects of recognition of low redundancy or degraded speech are covered in this chapter.

7.1 Variables Affecting the Results of Speech Recognition Tests

As noted in Chapter 3, outcomes of speech recognition testing are affected by several variables:
- Test environment (quiet, sound booth, etc.)
- Calibration of test equipment used in delivering the materials
- Recorded versus monitored live-voice presentation
- Male versus female speakers
- Specific test or speech material used
- Use of partial (e.g., 25 words) or full word (e.g., 50 words) list. Extreme scores such as 0 to 10% or 90 to 100% tend to be more stable as shown in Fig. 3.30 even with the use of partial word lists (e.g., 25 words). However, as noted in Chapter 3, full word lists (e.g., 50 words) can improve reliability when the scores are in the middle range.
- Presentation level: With increasing presentation levels, speech recognition performance improves to a certain point. A decrease in speech intelligibility can occur when levels are increased above 80 dB sound pressure level (SPL; French & Steinberg, 1947; Studebaker, Sherbecoe, McDaniel, & Gwaltney, 1999).
- Closed versus open response task
- Nonsense versus meaningful materials
- Use of sentence, word, or phoneme scoring

All of these factors can have an effect on the results of modified speech tests. Some of the above variables can be easily controlled: the test environment, use of properly calibrated equipment, and recorded presentation, for instance. Administering recorded speech materials in a sound booth through a two-channel audiometer allows proper control of presentation levels and any extraneous noise that is not part of the test materials. Although more time consuming, the use of full word lists (e.g., if a list has 50 words, presenting all 50 words before computing a score) and phoneme scoring (see ▶ Table 7.1) allows for more valid and reliable estimates of speech recognition ability (Cherry & Rubinstein, 2005). Phoneme scoring also minimizes the influence of language skills (Boothroyd, 1968).

Presentation levels should be adjusted based on the purpose of testing. If the purpose is to find speech recognition skills at average conversational speech levels, the presentation level should be around 45 dB hearing level (HL). If the purpose is to find the best possible speech recognition ability, then the level should be adjusted to allow maximum audibility and clarity of the signal. Such adjustment is more important for individuals with hearing loss.

7.2 Intrinsic Redundancy in the Auditory System

The spoken message reaching the ear elicits neural impulses that travel through the central auditory pathways, which contain a high level of redundancy in the form of several neurons, bilateral (double) representation, multiple interneural connections, afferent, efferent, and commissural connections, and connections with associated areas. This is referred to as *intrinsic redundancy*. The intrinsic redundancy allows corrections of degradation in spoken messages (▶ Table 7.2, row 2; Teatini, 1970).

7.3 Extrinsic Redundancy in Speech

Everyday conversational speech has a great amount of redundancy that may be as high as 50%. In other words, speech has many elements, including spectral and temporal information (gaps, tempo, rhythm, and duration), than are unnecessary to convey a message. This has been referred to as *extrinsic redundancy* (Teatini, 1970). For example, the sentence "I bought a pair of shoes" can still be understood if several elements are missing, including the last *s* in *shoes* or *b* in *bought* or the entire

Table 7.1 Written Responses of a Normal-Hearing Listener to NU-6 List 3A Presented at 45 dB HL in the Left Ear in the Presence of Ipsilateral Noise of 45 dB EM

	Stimulus	Response	Word Score	Phoneme Score
1	Base	Peace	0	1
2	Mess	Moose	0	2
3	Cause	Pass	0	0
4	Mop	No	0	0
5	Good	Goo	0	2
6	Luck	Need	0	0
7	Walk	Walk	1	3
8	Youth	Loose	0	1
9	Pain	Pan	0	2
10	Date	Dear	0	1
11	Pearl	Boy	0	0
12	Search	Search	1	3
13	Ditch	Dish	0	2
14	Talk	Don't	0	0
15	Ring	Rain	0	1
16	Germ	Jar	0	1
17	Life	Love	0	1
18	Team	Two	0	1
19	Lid	You've	0	0
20	Pole	Boot	0	0
21	Rode	Lope	0	1
22	Shall	Shell	0	2
23	Late	Need	0	0
24	Cheek	Cheap	0	2
25	Beg	No Response	0	0
	Total score		2/25 = 8%	26/75 = 34.67%

Abbreviations: EM, effective masking; HL, hearing level; NU-6, Northwestern University Auditory Test No. 6.

word *pair*. When words are used as stimuli, the knowledge of phonological rules offers extrinsic redundancy. For meaningful sentence materials, additional extrinsic redundancy exists in the form of syntactic rules and semantic context.

7.4 Low-Redundancy Speech Tests

A spoken message can be degraded in the temporal dimension if someone speaks at a very fast rate, in the spectral dimension because of background noise, or in the amplitude dimension when a person speaks very softly. Such modifications reduce the extrinsic redundancies in the spoken message.

7.4.1 Use of Low-Redundancy Speech Tests in Identifying Processing Deficits

When individuals with normal auditory processing capabilities are presented with normal speech materials, they can understand most of the material (► Table 7.2, row 1). This is also true for individuals with auditory processing deficits (APDs; ► Table 7.2, row 3). Extrinsic redundancy in the speech material allows them to recognize most of the material. When the speech material is degraded, the extrinsic redundancy in the materials is reduced or minimized. When this material is presented to normal-hearing individuals, they can use the intrinsic redundancies within the central nervous system to compensate for the reduced extrinsic redundancy, which allows for accurate recognition of most of the material (► Table 7.2, row 2). However, when degraded material is presented to individuals with APDs, they have difficulty recognizing the material due to reduced intrinsic redundancy within their auditory systems, in addition to the reduced extrinsic redundancy in the degraded speech (► Table 7.2, row 4). Low-redundancy speech tests such as filtered words have been used in the past to improve the sensitivity of speech audiometry in detecting lesions within the central auditory system (Bocca, Calearo, & Cassinari, 1954). Modified speech tests have been shown to be sensitive to temporal lobe and other lesions (Korsan-Bengtsen, 1973). These tests are currently recommended for evaluation of central auditory deficits (American Academy of Audiology, 2010). Speech can be degraded or modified in the spectral, temporal, or amplitude domains.

7.5 Spectral Modifications of Speech

Spectral modifications involve filtering the speech, smearing the spectrum, or using noise-vocoded speech as explained below.

Table 7.2 Effect of Intrinsic and Extrinsic Redundancy on Speech Recognition

Extrinsic Redundancy (Redundancy of Spoken Message)	Intrinsic Redundancy (Redundancy within the Central Auditory System)	Speech Recognition Performance
Normal	Normal	Good
Low redundancy	Normal	Relatively good; fair with greater message degradation
Normal	Reduced due to structural or functional deficits in the system	Good
Low redundancy	Reduced due to structural or functional deficits in the system	Poor

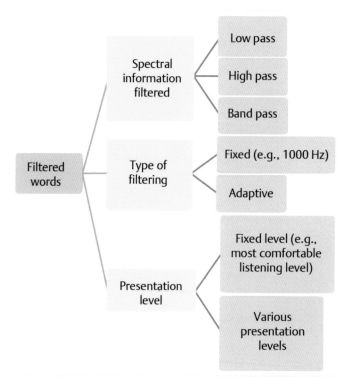

Fig. 7.1 Variations in conducting filtered word testing.

7.5.1 Filtered Speech

Filtered speech is created by spectral filtering of some elements of speech. The speech can be filtered by setting a filter cutoff frequency or frequencies and determining filter slopes. Filtered speech testing can be conducted in several different ways (▶ Fig. 7.1), and the outcomes vary depending on the procedure used. Information from the words can be filtered using low-pass, high-pass, or band pass filters. The most frequently used procedure is low-pass filtered words. Recognition of filtered speech is partially dependent on the ability to fill in the missing spectral information.

Bocca, Calearo, Cassinari, and Migliavacca (1955) filtered bisyllabic words through a low-pass filter with 1000 Hz cutoff frequency. They found that many patients with temporal lobe pathology perform poorly on the filtered words task. Their results on undistorted (normal) and filtered word tests for patients with right and left temporal lobe pathologies are shown in ▶ Fig. 7.2 and ▶ Fig. 7.3. The following patterns are apparent from these figures:

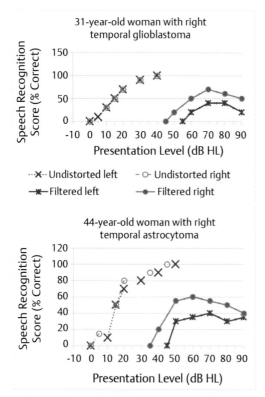

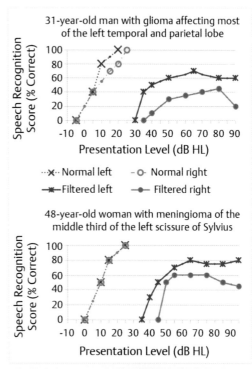

Fig. 7.2 Normal (undistorted) and low-pass (1000 Hz) filtered word test results from adults with right temporal lobe pathologies. Normal-hearing individuals yield relatively symmetric scores ranging from 60 to 80% on the filtered words task (based on Bocca, Calearo, Cassinari, & Migliavacca, 1955).

Fig. 7.3 Normal (undistorted) and low-pass (1000 Hz) filtered word test results from adults with left temporal lobe pathologies. Normal-hearing individuals yield relatively symmetric scores ranging from 60 to 80% on the filtered words task (based on Bocca et al., 1955).

1. Patients with temporal lobe pathologies yield normal speech recognition functions on undistorted speech tasks.
2. Much higher presentation levels are necessary to achieve 50% recognition for filtered word tests when compared to unfiltered word tests. Thus, the speech recognition thresholds for filtered word tests are higher than those for unfiltered words. In some cases, 50% recognition may not be achieved.
3. The performance on filtered words tasks is worse in the ear contralateral to the temporal lobe pathology when compared to the ear ipsilateral to the lesion. The difference appears even at high presentation levels where acoustic crosstalk is possible.

Bornstein, Wilson, and Cambron (1994) evaluated monosyllabic word recognition performance on the Northwestern University Auditory Test No. 6 (NU-6) at 70 dB SPL using four low-pass (800, 1200, 1500, and 1700 Hz) and four high-pass (1700, 2100, 2500, and 3000 Hz) cutoff frequencies in adults. With the increase in low-pass cutoff frequency from 800 to 1700 Hz, mean word recognition scores improved from 30 to 88% correct. With a decrease in the high-pass cutoff frequency from 3000 to 1700 Hz, the performance improved from 35 to 91% correct. The conditions that yielded 70 to 80% correct performance were 1500 Hz low-pass cutoff and 2100 Hz high-pass cutoff.

Other investigators have suggested use of an adaptive filter cutoff instead of fixed filter cutoffs to determine the cutoff that yields a specific recognition score (e.g., 66% correct). As expected, age has an effect on performance on filtered word tests. ▶ Fig. 7.4 shows the mean low-pass filter cutoff frequencies that yield 50.0 and 70.7% performance on the Northwestern University Children's Perception of Speech (NU-CHIPS) test at 60 dB HL

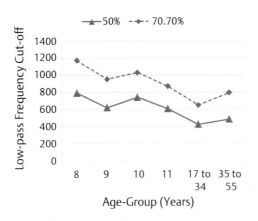

Fig. 7.4 Mean low-pass filter cutoff frequencies across different age groups that yield 50.0 and 70.7% performance for Northwestern University Children's Perception of Speech (NU-CHIPS) stimuli presented at 60 dB hearing level (HL) with a closed-set response task (based on O'Beirne, McGaffin, & Richard, 2012).

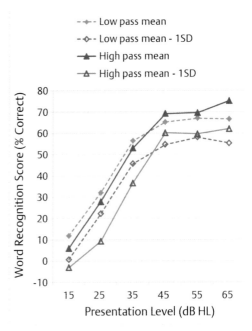

Fig. 7.5 Word recognition scores of normal-hearing adults with the low-pass (1500 Hz) and high-pass (2100 Hz) filtered cutoff versions of the Northwestern University Auditory Test No. 6 (NU-6) across different presentation levels (based on Bornstein, Wilson, & Cambron, 1994).

across different ages using a closed-set response task. More spectral content is necessary to achieve higher speech recognition scores across all age groups. Eight-year-old children need significantly higher low-pass cutoff frequencies than 11-year-olds to yield 70.7% performance. In addition, more spectral content appears to be necessary in the oldest age group (35 to 55 years) compared to the 17 to 34 years age group (O'Beirne, McGaffin, & Rickard, 2012).

Low-pass (1500 Hz cutoff) and high-pass (2100 Hz) filtered cutoff versions of the NU-6 are available on the *Tonal and Speech Materials for Auditory Perceptual Assessment* CD (Noffsinger, Wilson, & Musiek, 1994; U.S. Department of Veterans Affairs, 1992). The average performance of normal adults on this test at different presentation levels is shown in ▶ Fig. 7.5. As expected, performance improves with an increase in presentation levels up to about 45 dB HL (Bornstein et al., 1994). Beyond 45 dB HL, acoustic crossover to the other ear can be expected with the use of supra-aural earphones.

Farrer and Keith (1981) administered low-pass filtered versions of the Phonetically Balanced Kindergarten (PBK) words at 50 dB HL with a filter rejection rate of 18 dB/octave with filter cutoffs of 500, 750, and 1000 Hz to children with auditory-based learning disabilities and their age-matched normal-hearing peers. Children in both groups scored in the range of 92 to 100% on the unfiltered version of the test. Children with learning disabilities performed significantly worse on the filtered versions of the test (▶ Fig. 7.6). The versions with the 1000 Hz filter cutoff showed the least amount of overlap in the distribution among the two groups. Thus, the filter cutoff frequency used in the SCAN-C versions is 1000 Hz (Keith, 2000).

The SCAN-3 tests also include a filtered monosyllabic words test. The words are low-pass filtered at 750 Hz with a filter cutoff of 30 dB/octave. Two practice items and 20 filtered words are presented to each ear. This particular version of the filtered words test does not appear to be able to discriminate between individuals with APDs and normal-hearing individuals (Keith, 2009). Most individuals between the ages of 13 and 50 years obtain a score of about 75% correct on this test.

7.5.2 Spectrally Smeared Speech

One feature of cochlear hearing loss is reduced frequency selectivity. Attempts have been made to simulate reduced frequency selectivity by smearing the speech spectra. The smearing is designed to evoke excitation patterns in a normal ear similar

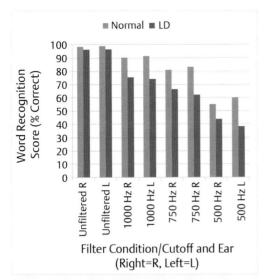

Fig. 7.6 Mean word recognition performance on the Phonetically Balanced Kindergarten (PBK) word list in unfiltered and low-pass filtered conditions in children with learning disabilities (LD) and age-matched normal peers (based on Farrer & Keith, 1981).

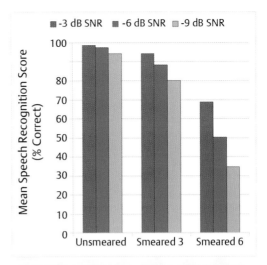

Fig. 7.7 Mean speech recognition scores at decreasing signal-to-noise (single male talker) ratios (SNRs) as a function of spectral smearing. Smeared 3: broadening of auditory filter by 3; mild smearing. Smeared 6: broadening of auditory filter by 6; moderate smearing (based on Baer & Moore, 1994).

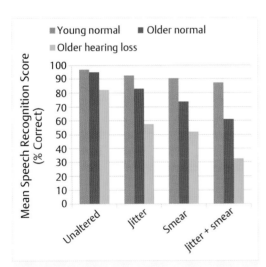

Fig. 7.8 Effect of temporal jitter, spectral smear, and a combination of the two distortions on speech recognition performance of young and older adults with normal hearing and older adults with hearing loss (based on Smith, Pichora-Fuller, Wilson, & MacDonald, 2012).

to those evoked in ears with hearing loss using normal speech. Spectrally smeared sentences are highly intelligible to normal-hearing listeners even if the smearing is designed to simulate auditory

filters that are 6 times broader than normal. However, the intelligibility of spectrally smeared sentences in a speech-shaped noise decreases with a decrease in the signal-to-noise ratio (Baer & Moore, 1992). Similar results are apparent when the masker is a single interfering male talker instead of speech-shaped noise (▶ Fig. 7.7; Baer & Moore, 1994). Smearing of low-frequency components (0–1.2 kHz) has a more detrimental effect on speech recognition when compared to the smearing of high-frequency components (1.2–7.0 kHz) in speech (MacDonald, Pichora-Fuller, & Schneider, 2010). Some individuals with APDs, including those with auditory neuropathy, can have poor frequency resolution or pitch discrimination abilities (Zeng, Kong, Michalewski, & Starr, 2005). Such individuals may show poor recognition of spectrally smeared speech compared to age-matched peers. ▶ Fig. 7.8 shows the performance of young normal adults and older adults with normal hearing and hearing loss on spectrally smeared NU-6 monosyllabic words (Smith, Pichora-Fuller, Wilson, & MacDonald, 2012).

7.5.3 Noise-Vocoded Speech

In this case, the speech spectrum is divided into two or more frequency bands, and the amplitude envelope is extracted from each of the frequency bands by half-wave rectification and low-pass filtering. Various cutoff frequencies can be used for low-pass filtering, including 16, 50, 160, and 500 Hz, for extracting the temporal envelope. The temporal envelope is then used to modulate white noise, which is spectrally limited by the same band pass filters used in dividing the original speech spectrum. All bands are then recombined. Stated differently, spectral information in speech is removed in specific frequency bands and is replaced by a band-limited noise. The resulting speech consists of preserved amplitude and temporal cues but reduced spectral information (Shannon, Zeng, Kamath, Wygonski, & Ekelid, 1995). The intelligibility of noise-vocoded speech increases systematically with the increase in the number of frequency channels used in the vocoding. Speech remains fully intelligible with 16 bands (Peelle, Gross, & Davis, 2013), but relatively high speech recognition is possible with only three time-varying bands of noise representing the temporal envelope of speech containing only rudimentary spectral information (Shannon et al., 1995). This shows that as long as the dynamic temporal rhythm of speech is available in spectrally degraded speech, adults can recognize the speech most likely due to the enhanced synchronization of neuronal oscillations to the overall speech envelope (Peelle et al., 2013).

Children in the age range of 5 to 7 years have significantly more difficulty in recognizing noise-vocoded speech and need more spectral details for decoding such speech. Part of this deficit appears to be related to difficulty in making full use of available sensory information, and part of it is related to immaturity in the linguistic and cognitive domains (Eisenberg, Shannon, Martinez, Wygonski, & Boothroyd, 2000).

7.6 Temporally Degraded Speech

Investigators have used a variety of approaches to alter speech in the temporal dimension.

7.6.1 Interrupted Speech

In this case, the speech is intermittently greatly attenuated so that it becomes inaudible or appears turned off at intervals. Comprehension of interrupted speech requires the ability to fill in the missing or removed segments (closure). Three variables can be manipulated in generating interrupted speech samples: the frequency or number of interruptions/s, the degree of regularity of interruption, and the speech-time fraction or the proportion of time the speech is on in the sample. When the speech time fraction is about 50%, interruptions are periodic and occur more than 100 times/s, monosyllabic words can be easily recognized. When interruptions are less than 1/s, the word or the final or initial phoneme of the word can be missed, which decreases speech recognition performance. If the average duration of a monosyllabic word is 0.6 second, the speech fraction time is 50%, and the interruptions occur at a rate of 5/s, the listener gets on an average three glimpses of the words. For most of the words, three glimpses allow one glimpse at each phoneme, which is sufficient to allow almost 100% intelligibility (Miller & Licklider, 1950). Lexical difficulty of words has an important impact on the recognition of interrupted speech. Less acoustic information is necessary for lexically easy words than hard words to obtain a similar degree of word recognition performance (Wang & Humes, 2010). Interrupted speech with 7 interruptions/s appears to be very sensitive to cerebellopontine angle tumors and also has fair sensitivity to brainstem and cortical lesions (▸ Fig. 7.9; Karlsson & Rosenhall, 1995). About 50% of workers exposed to ototoxic materials, including solvents and jet fuel, have shown abnormal performance on interrupted speech tasks (Odkvist, Arlinger, Edling, Larsby, & Bergholtz, 1987), while a few patients with a closed head injury have difficulty recognizing interrupted speech (Bergemalm & Lyxell, 2005).

7.6.2 Speech Interrupted by Noise

In speech interrupted by noise, instead of intermittent attenuation, continuous speech is masked intermittently by using an interrupted masking noise. The intelligibility of monosyllabic words in this situation depends on the signal-to-noise ratio, the frequency of interruptions, the regularity of interruptions, and noise or speech-time fraction. When the speech fraction is 50%, and the signal-to-noise ratio is between 9 and −18 dB, maximum (95–75%) recognition is apparent with an interruption frequency of 10/s for regularly spaced bursts of noise. Thus, when there are 10 bursts/s, the listeners are able to get sufficient glimpses of every word to allow correct recognition of the words. With lower or higher frequencies of interruptions per second, speech recognition is lower for signal-to-noise ratios between 0 and −18 dB (Miller & Licklider, 1950). As shown in ▸ Fig. 7.10,

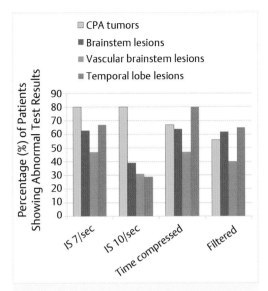

Fig. 7.9 Percentage of patients showing abnormal performance (2 standard deviations [SD] below normal peers) on modified sentence tests with four key words for different sites of lesions. Interrupted speech (IS) was presented with 7 and 10/s interruptions. For 7 interruptions/s, the speech signal was on for 70 ms between interruptions; for 10 interruptions/s, the speech signal was on for 50 ms between interruptions. For time-compressed speech, the words occurred at approximately 290 words/min. For filtered versions, the speech was filtered through three band pass filters with a width of one-third octave band and center frequencies of 0.5, 0.64, and 0.8 kHz (based on Karlsson & Rosenhall, 1995). CPA, cerebellopontine angle.

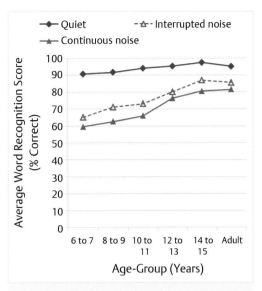

Fig. 7.10 Average recognition (percentage correct) of monosyllabic words (NU-CHIPS) presented at 30 dB HL in quiet and continuous and interrupted speech-shaped noise at 0 dB signal-to-noise ratio. The interrupted noise was on 50% of the time (based on Stuart, 2005).

the performance of young children is more negatively affected by interrupted noise than adults and improves with age (Stuart, 2005). Patients with demyelinating lesions, such as multiple sclerosis (MS), show impairment in recognizing speech in interrupted masking noise (Rappaport et al., 1994).

7.6.3 Speech Alternating with Noise

In this case, silent intervals in the interrupted speech are filled with noise. Thus, the speech and noise alternate in time. This allows an estimation of any backward or forward effects of masking noise on speech. Like speech interrupted by noise, maximum recognition is apparent at 10 interruptions/s, with a speech fraction of 50%. When interruptions are more than 10 or 15/s, speech recognition performance becomes poorer with

increasing signal-to-noise ratios. When speech is interrupted about 10 to 15 times/s, the speech is intelligible, but the interruptions are obvious. When a somewhat more intense noise is introduced in these gaps or silent intervals, the speech begins to appear as though it is continuous or uninterrupted or more natural. This has been referred to as the "picket fence" effect because a landscape appears continuous behind the pickets, even though the pickets interrupt the view at regular intervals (Miller & Licklider, 1950).

7.6.4 Rapid Speech

Asking someone to speak at a relatively rapid rate produces this type of speech. TV and radio news announcers often speak at relatively faster rates. Some individuals process speech at a slower rate and thus may have difficulty in processing rapid speech. Fast speaking rates can increase phoneme recognition errors by about 30% compared to normal speech, with more errors apparent in recognizing the place of articulation feature (Meyer, Jürgens, Wesker, Brand, & Kollmeier, 2010).

Calearo and Lazzaroni (1957) used three procedures to present sentences at faster speaking rates: asking a speaker with abilities to speak at very fast rates to present the stimuli, recording speech and

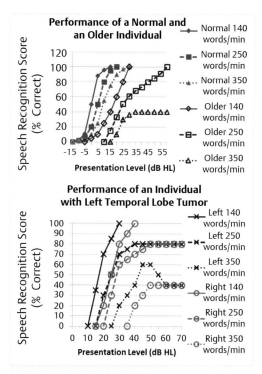

Fig. 7.11 Speech recognition performance for sentences presented at a normal speaking rate of 150 words/min and two faster rates (based on Calearo & Lazzaroni, 1957).

interrupted speech. Thus, comprehension requires closure, or the ability to fill in missing elements. However, in this case the remaining elements are moved closer together. Therefore, the time available for filling in the missing elements is shorter than that which is available during the comprehension of interrupted speech. Time-compressed speech sounds like rapid speech, and, as can be expected, individuals with slower processing speed have more difficulty in recognizing time-compressed speech.

The amount of time compression is often described by the compression rate (e.g., 40%), which refers to the duration of temporal segments removed from the original signal (100%). For example, to achieve 40% compression, 18 ms segments can be discarded, while 27 ms segments can be retained at regular intervals Thus, 40% of the speech is removed, and 60% is retained. At higher compression rate, less speech is retained. This results in the original sample being of shorter duration at higher rates. For example, an uncompressed phrase (0% compressions) of 1070 ms will be about 625 ms in duration with a compression rate of 45%, 385 ms with a compression rate of 65%, and 253 ms with a compression rate of 75% (Wilson, Preece, Salamon, Sperry, & Bornstein, 1994).

Some investigators have used time-expanded or slower speech in addition to time-compressed or faster speech with different criteria for describing rates of speech. For example, McCroskey and Thompson (1973) described the rate variations as follows: rate 1 60% (6.8 syllables/s), rate 2 80% (5 syllables/s), rate 3 100% or normal (3.6 syllables/s), rate 4 140% (2.9 syllables/s), rate 5 180% (2.3 syllables/s).

Several investigators have confirmed the sensitivity of time-compressed speech to central processing deficits. At the rate of 60% compression, individuals with diffused temporal lobe lesions show poorer performance than normal-hearing individuals (Kurdziel, Noffsinger, & Olsen, 1976). Older individuals also have more difficulty in recognizing time-compressed speech even in the presence of normal hearing. Practice in listening to faster speech can minimize age-related difficulty in understanding time-compressed speech (Gordon-Salant & Friedman, 2011).

Time-compressed monosyllabic words are available on *Tonal and Speech Materials for Auditory Perceptual Assessment* (U.S. Department of Veterans Affairs, 1998). The test includes NU-6 monosyllabic words that are compressed at two compression rates, 45 and 65%. ► Fig. 7.12 shows

rotating the magnetic tape at various speeds, and using a special procedure to accelerate speech without any alteration of frequency. They noted no significant difference in speech recognition performance across these three types of temporal speed manipulations. They assessed the performance of normal-hearing individuals, older individuals, and individuals with temporal lobe pathologies. Both older individuals and individuals with temporal lobe pathologies showed degraded performance with an increase in speaking rates from 150 to 350 words/min (► Fig. 7.11). The authors noted that older individuals and individuals with pathologies in the central auditory system suffer from a slower processing speed and that superimposition of fast speech on the existing central delay leads to a marked impairment in speech recognition.

7.6.5 Time-Compressed Speech

In time-compressed speech, tiny segments are removed from the spoken message (words or sentences), as done during the generation of

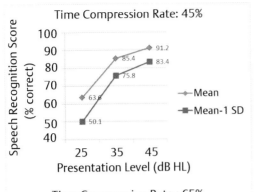

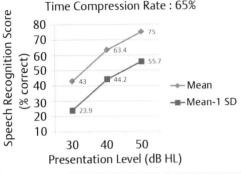

Time Compression Rate: 45%

Time Compression Rate : 65%

Fig. 7.12 Performance of young adults on the recognition of Northwestern University Auditory Test Number 6 (NU-6) words time compressed at the rate of 45 and 65% (based on Wilson, Preece, Salamon, Sperry, & Bornstein, 1994).

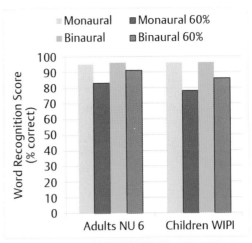

Fig. 7.13 Average word recognition performance of adults on the Northwestern University Auditory Test Number 6 (NU-6) test and children on the Word Intelligibility by Picture Identification (WIPI) test at 0 and 60% time-compression rates in monaural and binaural conditions (based on Bornstein, 1994). The word presentation level was 50 dB SPL in all conditions.

the performance of normal-hearing adults at different presentation levels on this test during monaural listening conditions (Wilson et al., 1994). Note that at the 65% compressions rate, the performance is poorer with greater variability than at the 45% compression rate. Binaural listening allows near-normal performance (91%) on NU-6 words at the 65% time-compression rate in young normal-hearing adults. At the same compression rate, children's performance also improves, from 78% during monaural listening to 86% during binaural listening, on the Word Intelligibility by Picture Identification (WIPI) test, which is a closed-response listening task (▶ Fig. 7.13; Bornstein, 1994).

McCroskey (1984) developed the Wichita Auditory Processing Test (WAPT), which includes time-altered sentences at the ratios of 100% (uncompressed), 200% (expanded), 70% (compressed), and 130% (expanded). Ten sentences are presented at each rate, and the child is expected to point to the appropriate picture. Normative data are provided for different age groups at each of the compression

rates. Time-compressed sentences are available on a test developed by Keith (2002) that is designed for children between the ages of 6 and 11 years. The sentences are compressed at the rate of 40 and 60%. Uncompressed sentences are available for practice and for obtaining baseline scores. An updated version of this test comprising 20 sentences time compressed at the rate of 60% is included in the supplementary tests provided in the SCAN-3 test battery. The scoring of items is based on key words within each sentence. Individuals with APDs show significantly poor performance on this test compared to their age-matched peers (Keith, 2009).

7.6.6 Reverberant Speech

Many listening environments, such as classrooms and places of worship, are reverberant. Reverberation results in temporal waveform distortion due to the smearing of the original signal by reflections of the original signal from surrounding surfaces. Individuals with temporal processing difficulties may have increased difficulty in understanding reverberant speech. Phoneme identification scores determined with the use of nonsense syllables (vowel-consonant-vowel [VCV]) in reverberant conditions improve with age up to 13 years, when the performance becomes similar to

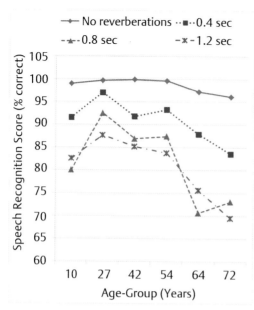

Fig. 7.14 Monaural speech recognition performance at 70 dB sound pressure level (SPL) across various age groups in different reverberation conditions (based on Nábělek & Robinson, 1982).

that of adults. An increase in reverberation time worsens the performance. Binaural listening improves performance over monaural listening in reverberant conditions (Neuman & Hochberg, 1983). ▶ Fig. 7.14 shows the performances of children and adults in various age groups on the Modified Rhyme Test (MRT; Bell, Kreul, & Nixon, 1972; Kreul et al., 1968) across different reverberation times in monaural listening conditions at 70 dB SPL. Adults in the 27-years age group appear to have better performance than children and older adults (Nábělek & Robinson, 1982).

7.6.7 Temporally Jittered Speech

In this case, the sequence of amplitude values in the sound file is changed by shifting them slightly earlier or later in the sequence. This type of speech attempts to simulate neural asynchrony, or the inability of auditory neurons to fire in a synchronous manner to a single phase of the stimuli, referred to as *phase locking* (Miranda & Pichora-Fuller, 2002). Temporal jittering distorts the fine structure of the speech signal with almost no alternation of spectral or amplitude envelope characteristics. Speech recognition performance of young adults for temporally jittered (at frequencies below 1.2 kHz) speech in noise is similar to that of older adults for

normal speech in noise (Pichora-Fuller, Schneider, MacDonald, Pass, & Brown, 2007). Temporally jittered speech may be sensitive to temporal processing deficits in populations such as individuals with auditory neuropathy. ▶ Fig. 7.8 shows the performance of young normal-hearing adults and older adults with normal hearing and hearing loss on temporally jittered NU-6 monosyllabic words (Smith et al., 2012).

7.6.8 Speech with Temporal Asynchrony

The pattern of energy in different frequency regions in normal speech is precisely timed with the periodic action of the vocal folds or the fundamental frequency of the speaker's voice. Temporal asynchrony in speech can be created by misaligning some frequency bands (e.g., 12.5–100 ms) in the temporal domain compared to other frequency bands. Healy and Bacon (2002) suggested that reverberation times for low frequencies can be longer than high-frequency sounds given that low-frequency sounds are absorbed less efficiently. Thus, low-frequency components can persist longer in a reverberant field than high-frequency components, which can make the indirect signals asynchronous. This suggests that poor tolerance for temporal asynchrony in some individuals can contribute to difficulty in perceiving speech in reverberant environments. Healy and Bacon (2002) used a speech recognition task requiring across-frequency integration of temporal speech information. Temporal asynchrony was created by misalignments of some frequency bands ranging from 12.5 to 100 ms. Even when information was synchronous across frequency, some individuals with hearing loss performed more poorly than those with normal hearing. In addition, the performance of individuals with hearing loss showed steeper deterioration as a function of asynchrony than normal-hearing individuals.

7.7 Speech Mixed with Other Competing Signals

When speech is mixed with other competing signals, the temporal waveform of the speech signal can get masked by other signals, and some individuals may have difficulty in separating the source signal from the background noise. Several tests are available for assessing speech recognition in the

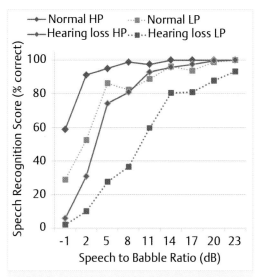

Fig. 7.15 Average speech recognition scores across various speech-to-babble ratios for Speech Perception in Noise (SPIN) sentences with high predictability (HP) and low predictability (LP) in the presence of a fixed babble level of 80 dB SPL (based on Wilson & McArdle, 2012).

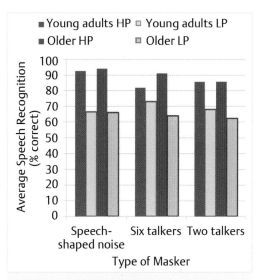

Fig. 7.16 The effect of different maskers on the Speech Perception in Noise (SPIN) test among normal listeners Based on Desjardins & Doherty, (2012). Note that for the six-talker masker, the difference in speech recognition between highly predictable (HP) words and words with low predictability (LP) is smaller for younger adults when compared to other types of maskers.

presence of competing signals. Some of the available tests are discussed below.

7.7.1 Speech Perception in Noise

In the revised Speech Perception in Noise (SPIN) test, multitalker babble is used as the masker. Listeners are expected to repeat the last word in the sentence. Half of the sentences allow prediction of the last word due to syntactic, semantic, and prosodic cues. For example, in the sentence "Let's decide by tossing a coin," the target word *coin* is highly predictable. The target words in the remaining half of the sentences are not predictable. For example, the word *coin* in the sentence "Jane has a problem with the coin" is not predictable (Bilger, 1984; Bilger, Nuetzel, Rabinowitz, & Rzeczkowski, 1984; Kalikow, Stevens, & Elliott, 1977). With a 0 dB signal-to-babble ratio, 11-year old children perform better than 9-year-olds, and 15- to 17-year-olds perform better than 11- and 13-year-olds on the high-predictability words of the SPIN test (Elliott, 1979). Individuals with normal hearing and hearing loss show better performance on the high-predictability words compared to low-predictability words at lower signal-to-babble ratios (▶ Fig. 7.15; Wilson & McArdle, 2012). ▶ Fig. 7.15 illustrates three variables that have an

impact on speech recognition performance: level of redundancy or predictability in the speech material, speech-to-masker ratio, and any peripheral hearing loss. ▶ Fig. 7.16 shows the effect of another variable (type of masker) on the SPIN test among normal listeners (Desjardins & Doherty, 2013). Note that for the six-talker masker, the difference in speech recognition between highly predictable (HP) words and words with low predictability (LP) is smaller for younger adults when compared to other types of maskers.

Masking effects determined using traditional masking noises (e.g., wide band) are referred to as *energetic masking,* which reflects the limits of cochlear processing (Fletcher, 1940). Depending on the type of target speech stimuli, maskers composed of two or three different speakers can increase the difficulty in recognizing target speech due to the target–masker similarity. This has been referred to as *informational* or *perceptual masking* (Carhart, Tillman, & Greetis, 1969), which reduces the listener's ability to segregate the speech target from the speech masker. Informational maskers may be more sensitive to deficits or immaturity in central auditory processes when compared to energetic maskers. A difference in the performance obtained with energetic masking noise and information speech maskers can provide an estimate of the ability of the central auditory system to segregate two speech streams. The performance of children between the ages of 11 and 13 years on a consonant identification task in the presence of speech-shaped noise is like that of adults. However, when a two-talker masker (female talkers with no silent pauses longer than 300 ms) is used instead of speech-shaped noise, children in the same age group perform significantly worse than adults (Bonino, Leibold, & Buss, 2013). Semantically meaningful competition may be more effective in differentiating children with APDs from normal age-matched peers compared to white noise or backward speech (Cherry & Kruger, 1983).

7.7.2 SCAN Auditory Figure-Ground Test

The SCAN-C (Keith, 2000) test battery includes a speech test with monosyllabic words in the presence of competing multitalker babble. The test is referred to as subtest 2 Auditory Figure-Ground. The recording includes monosyllabic words that are 8 dB louder than the multitalker speech babble. Two practice words and 20 test words are presented to each ear. The listener is expected to repeat each word. A revised version of the Auditory Figure-Ground test is available in the SCAN-3 test battery. The test is available for administration with 0, +8, and +12 dB signal-to-babble ratios. Significant differences between individuals with APDs and age-matched peers have been reported at all three signal-to-babble ratios. In addition, listeners with APDs show a significantly higher right ear advantage compared to their age-matched peers when the test is conducted using either the +8 or +12 dB signal-to-babble ratios (Keith, 2009).

7.7.3 MAPA Monaural Selective Auditory Attention Test (MSAAT)

The Multiple Auditory Processing Assessment (MAPA) test battery is described in Chapter 4. The target stimuli included in the MSAAT test are the monosyllabic words from the WIPI test (Ross & Lerman, 1971). The competing background is an interesting story about dinosaurs. The interstimulus interval between words is varied around 10 seconds to allow the target words to coincide with speech and not with pauses within the competition. Both the target words and the story are spoken by the same talker with a signal-to-

competition ratio of 0 dB. Twenty-five words are presented to each ear. Norms for children between the ages of 4 and 9 years using a closed-response picture identification task are available for the original version of the test, the Selective Auditory Attention Test. The competing message condition is administered only if the scores in quiet on the same test are 88% or higher. The test has high interlist and intertest reliability (Cherry, 1980). Cherry (1992) obtained data from 325 children from three groups: children with normal educational achievements, those with learning disabilities, and those with questionable educational achievements. As shown in ▶ Fig. 7.17, children with a learning disability performed significantly worse on this test than those with questionable educational achievements, and those with questionable achievements performed significantly worse than children with normal achievements (Cherry, 1992). The performance of left and right ears does not differ on this test. Scores on the word list that is administered first tend to be poorer than the lists that are administered later, suggesting learning effects following the first presentation but not during later presentations. To control for the learning effect, the test can be initially administered with diotic presentation, which yields a higher score than that which is achieved following monotic presentations (Cherry & Rubinstein, 2006). The norms for children ages 8 to 12 years and adults are included in the MAPA test manual.

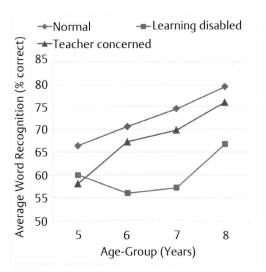

Fig. 7.17 Average performance of children with normal and questionable (teacher concerned) achievement and those with learning disabilities on the Selective Auditory Attention Test (SAAT) (based on Cherry, 1992).

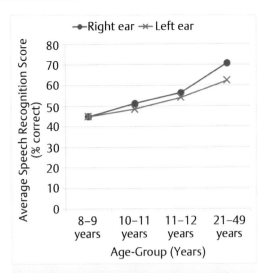

Fig. 7.18 Average speech recognition scores on the Multiple Auditory Processing Assessment (MAPA) SAAT test across various age groups (based on Schow, Seikel, Brockett, & Whitaker, 2007).

Average speech recognition scores across various age groups on this test are shown in ▶ Fig. 7.18 (Schow, Seikel, Brockett, & Whitaker, 2007).

7.7.4 MAPA Speech in Noise for Children and Adults (MAPA SINCA)

The target words in this test are from the PBK word list. The competition is a four-speaker babble. The words are presented at varying signal-to-babble ratios until the ratio decreases to 0 dB. It is recommended for screening monaural listening capabilities along with the MSAAT test. It is also recommended only as a supplementary test due to low test–retest reliability (Schow et al., 2007).

7.7.5 Synthetic Sentence Identification with Ipsilateral Competing Message (SSI-ICM)

Each sentence in this test contains seven words that are third-order approximations, so that every successive three words form a meaningful phrase. For example, in the sentence "Go change your car color is red," the following phrases are meaningful: "Go change your," "change your car," and "your car color." All of the words included in the test are from a pool of the 1000 most common words in the Thorndike and Lorge (1944) word lists. The third-order approximations in the sentences are created by first generating second-order approximations. For creation of second-order approximations, a word was first selected randomly from the common pool. This word was then provided to an individual who was asked to select another word from the common pool that could logically follow the first word in a declarative or imperative sentence. The second word was then provided to a third individual with the same instruction for selecting the next word. For the construction of third-word approximations, one of the randomly selected word pairs used in the second-order sentences was provided to an individual who was instructed to choose a third word from the common pool that could logically follow the two words. Next, the last two of these three words were provided to another individual who supplied the next word. The process was repeated until the synthetic sentence had seven words (Speaks & Jerger, 1965). The listener's task is to identify the spoken sentence from a printed numbered list of 10 sentences by saying aloud the number that corresponds to the sentence. Thus, the listener needs to have sufficient reading skills. When unsure, the listener is encouraged to guess. A score of 10% is assigned to each correctly identified sentence.

The sentences can be presented monaurally with a competing message consisting of a narration regarding the events in the life of pioneer Davy Crockett presented to the same ear. This task is referred to as Synthetic Sentence Identification with Ipsilateral Competing Message (SSI-ICM). The competing message and the synthetic sentences are recorded by the same talker. The signal-to-message ratio is varied from + 10 to −30 dB in 10 dB steps. The performance of normal-hearing individuals with these varying ratios varies from 100 to 20%. Some patients with intra-axial brainstem lesions (Jerger & Jerger, 1974), eighth nerve lesions, and temporal lobe lesions (Jerger & Jerger, 1975) show abnormally poor performance on the SSI-ICM task. In patients with eighth nerve lesions, the performance is poor in the ear ipsilateral to the site of the lesion, whereas in brainstem lesions, the performance tends to be poor in the contralateral ear. Patients with temporal lobe lesions can have poor performance in both ears (Jerger & Jerger, 1975). As shown in ▶ Fig. 7.19, individuals with chronic alcoholism perform significantly worse in both ears compared to age-matched peers. In ▶ Fig. 7.19, the differences are more obvious at message-to-competition ratios from 0 to −20 dB (Spitzer & Ventry, 1980).

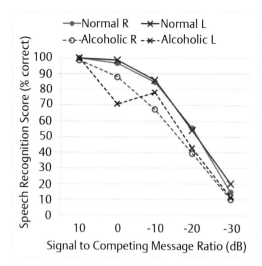

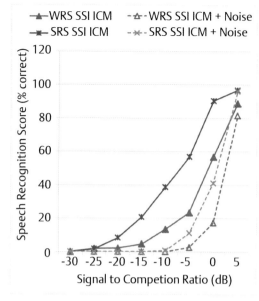

Fig. 7.19 Performance of individuals with chronic alcoholism and age-matched peers on the Synthetic Sentence Identification with Ipsilateral Competing Message (SSI-ICM) test in the right (R) and left (L) ears (based on Spitzer & Ventry, 1980).

Fig. 7.20 Average right ear scores of young normal adults on the SSI-ICM test with and without speech-shaped noise added to the competing message. The targets are presented at 50 dB sensation level (SL) (1000 Hz). Word recognition score (WRS): percentage of correctly repeated words. Sentence recognition score (SRS): prediction of percentage of correctly identified sentences based on correct identification of at least one word in the sentence (based on Martin & Mussell, 1979).

Some listeners report guessing the correct sentences based on the identification of one or more words in the sentence, and the guessing improves with practice. The pauses in the competing message allow easier recognition of some of the target words. If speech noise is mixed with the competing message at a message-to-noise ratio of −6 dB, the scores become poorer. ▶ Fig. 7.20 shows word recognition scores and predicted sentence recognition scores based on the recognition of one of the words on the SSI-ICM with and without speech-shaped noise added to the competing message. As is apparent, the addition of speech-shaped noise degrades the performance at least partially due to the inability to hear during the pauses in the competing message (Martin & Mussell, 1979). If this modification of the SSI-ICM is used, the performance is near the floor below the 0 dB message-to-competition ratio. Thus, only message-to-competition ratios of 0 and 5 should be used in clinical settings.

Large intrasubject variability has been noted in the initial trials of the SSI test with cafeteria noise as the masker. It may be possible to control the variability by presenting at least three practice trials under difficult listening conditions at the beginning of each test session and by including

at least 30 sentences in each test session (Dubno & Dirks, 1983). Specifically, for the AUDiTEC (Maplewood, MO) version of the SSI-ICM with the original competing message, the following recommendations have been made to minimize learning effects and improve reliability:

1. Young adults should receive at least one practice word list, and older adults should receive at least three practice lists before initiating testing.
2. Only lists A, C, D, E, G, and I should be used for comparing different listening conditions, such as left versus right ear.
3. The performance of several lists should be averaged to obtain a more stable test score (Feeney & Hallowell, 2000).

Speech perception in the presence of a competing signal during binaural listening conditions is discussed in Chapter 6.

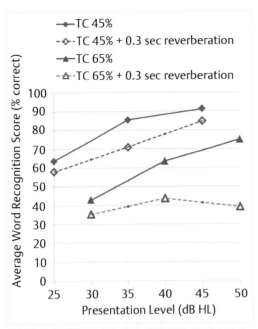

Fig. 7.21 Performance of normal-hearing young adults on the recognition of NU-6 words time compressed (TC) at the rate of 45 and 65% with and without 0.3-second reverberation (based on Wilson, Preece, Salamon, Sperry, & Bornstein, 1994).

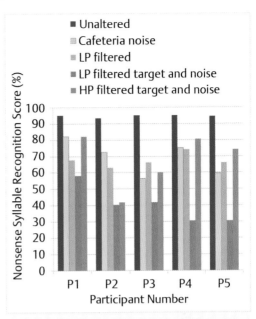

Fig. 7.22 Right ear performance of five normal-hearing young adults on the Nonsense Syllables test at 50 dB HL in five test conditions. LP, low-pass filtered with a cutoff frequency of 1 kHz; HP, high-pass filtered with a cutoff frequency of 500 Hz. The filter slope is 24 dB/octave for all filtered conditions. In all noise conditions, the noise is cafeteria noise, and the signal-to-noise ratio is 11 dB (based on Rawool, 2012).

7.8 Combined Speech Modifications

In many investigations, the combined use of different modifications such as reverberation and noise has been examined because some degradation can occur in combination in natural settings. As an example, ▶ Fig. 7.21 shows the effect of the combination of time compression and reverberation on word recognition. In this case, performance becomes worse when reverberation is added to time-compressed speech (Wilson et al., 1994). ▶ Fig. 7.8 shows that the combination of temporal jitter and spectral smearing leads to further deterioration of speech recognition performance compared to temporal jitter and spectral smear alone (Smith et al., 2012). Another example is given in ▶ Fig. 7.22. In this case, the right ear performance is best in the unaltered condition on the Nonsense Syllables Test (NST; Resnick, Dubno, Hoffnung, & Levitt, 1975) and worst when low-pass filtering and noisy background are combined. More specifically, when both the syllables and cafeteria noise

are filtered through a low-pass filter with cutoff frequency of 1000 Hz and a filter slope of 24 dB/octave, the performance is worst compared to other conditions (Rawool, 2012).

7.9 Objective Measures of Speech Perception

Several procedures have been used to measure speech perception objectively in quiet and degraded listening conditions. Some of these measures are discussed below.

7.9.1 Speech-evoked Auditory Brainstem Response in Competing Sounds

Speech-evoked auditory brainstem response (ABR) has been used to get an estimate of speech perception in quiet and in the presence of competing

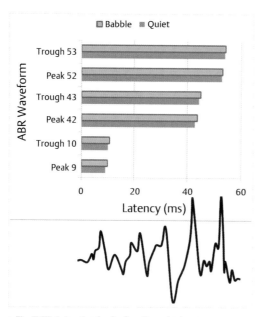

Fig. 7.23 Latencies (ms) of auditory brainstem responses (ABRs) evoked by 170 ms /da/ syllable, including 120 ms steady-state vowel, in children (age 8–13 years) in quiet and in six-talker babble with a signal-to-noise ratio of 10 dB. Peaks and troughs are named based on their approximate average latencies (based on Hornickel, Knowles, & Kraus, 2012). An idealized response waveform is shown below the graph.

sounds. An idealized waveform obtained by using the syllable /da/ with a duration of 170 ms including the 120 ms vowel is shown in ▶ Fig. 7.23. The waveform includes an onset response with a peak (wave V) at around 9 ms (P9) and trough at around 10 ms (T10) and the peaks and troughs following the glottal pulse of the stimulus at approximately every 10 ms. In the graph, latencies are shown only for the peaks and troughs that can be reliably obtained in the presence of the competing six-talker babble. Responses in babble are characterized by significantly delayed latencies and smaller amplitudes compared to those in noise (Hornickel, Knowles, & Kraus, 2012). The response appears to be mature by the age of 5 years in children (Johnson, Nicol, Zecker, & Kraus, 2008). Test–retest reliability for speech-evoked ABR is good in children (Hornickel et al., 2012) and young adults (Song, Nicol, & Kraus, 2011). During monaural presentation, the responses from right ear stimulation are more robust and show earlier latencies when compared to those yielded by stimulating the left ear (Hornickel, Skoe, & Kraus, 2009).

7.9.2 Speech-evoked Auditory Brainstem Response and Self-perceived Speech Perception in Noise

A shorter 40 ms /d/ without the accompanying vowel can be used to elicit the ABR. Such stimuli elicit a strong wave V with some neural processing delay in response to the onset of the stimulus, which has a positive peak (V) and a negative trough (A). The response also has a trough (labeled O) at the offset of the stimulus. The response is analyzed using various parameters:

1. Onset latency for wave V: The time between the onset of the stimulus and the peak of wave V
2. Offset latency: The time between the offset of the stimulus and the stimulus offset trough of O
3. Onset slope: The slope between the onset peak V and its trough A, which provides a measure of the sharpness of wave V
4. Stimulus-to-response correlation (STRr): This is obtained by cross-correlating the aligned stimulus and response waveforms to obtain a measure of overall neural fidelity and response morphology. The right ear speech-evoked brainstem response using the 40 ms /da/ syllable presented at 80.3 dB SPL through insert earphones is related to self-perception of the ability to perceive speech in noise. More specifically, the offset latency (O) and the STRr variables are related to self-perceived speech perception in noise (Anderson, Parbery-Clark, White-Schwoch, & Kraus, 2013).

7.9.3 P1-N1-P2 Complex

The examination of the P1-N1-P2 complex allows the examination of thalamocortical structures of the auditory pathway. When the complex is generated passively in response to the syllable /ba/ presented at 65 dB SPL, in the presence of 68 dB SPL maskers, N1 amplitudes are significantly smaller in the presence of four-talker babble when compared to speech-shaped continuous noise, suggesting more effective masking in the presence of informational maskers (Billings, Bennett, Molis, & Leek, 2011). The N1 component appears to be sensitive to the position of the consonant in the utterance (first position: consonant-vowel [CV], middle position: CVC), voice onset time of consonants, and noise masking (Dimitrijevic, Pratt, & Starr, 2012).

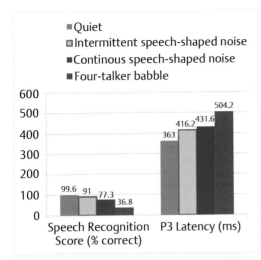

Fig. 7.24 Latencies of the P300 responses with right ear presentation of /da/ (deviant, 20%) and /ba/ (standard, 80%) at a level of 65 dB SPL in quiet and in the presence of various maskers at 68 dB SPL. For the behavioral speech recognition task, low context sentences each with five key words were presented at 65 dB SPL to the right ear (based on Bennett, Billings, Molis, & Leek, (2012).

7.9.4 Speech-evoked P300 and Word Recognition in Competing Backgrounds

Latencies of the P300 response elicited by presenting /da/ (rare, 20%) and /ba/ (frequent, 80%) stimuli to the right ear at 65 dB SPL in the presence of four-talker speech babble are significantly longer when compared to those obtained in the presence of an interrupted or continuous speech-shaped masker presented at 68 dB SPL (► Fig. 7.24). P300 latencies are significantly correlated with speech recognition in noise using a sentence-in-noise task at similar presentation levels and signal-to-noise ratios (−3 dB). More specifically, longer P300 latencies are associated with poorer word recognition (Bennett et al., 2012).

7.9.5 Speech Coding Due to Phase Locking in the Theta Range

Time-frequency analysis of single trials in response to standard speech stimuli (/ba/) with /da/ and /bi/ as deviant stimuli shows that the mismatch negativity (MMN) results from phase synchronization of oscillations in the theta (θ)range (4–7 Hz), with less synchronization apparent in children than

adults. The MMN appears to result from phase resetting in the theta frequency band rather than an increase in the power in the same band (Bishop & Hardiman, 2010; Bishop, Hardiman, & Barry, 2011). The M100 response elicited using magnetoencephalography (MEG) also reveals that in the presence of speech-shaped noise, low-frequency auditory cortical oscillations are consistently synchronized to the slow temporal modulations of speech even when the speech-to-noise ratio is relatively poor. The reliable synchronization is maintained through intensity contrast gain control and adaptive processing of temporal modulations at different time scales corresponding to the neural delta (δ) and theta (θ) bands. This allows the formation of nearly noise-invariant neural representation of the speech prosody in the auditory cortex. The precision of this cortical entrainment or synchronization to speech can provide a neural correlate of how well a listener can understand speech in noise (Ding & Simon, 2013).

7.10 Physiology of Speech Perception

The spectral and temporal characteristics of speech are coded in various ways through the central auditory pathways. The frequency characteristics of speech stimuli are coded through tonotopic organization, where certain areas are more responsive to certain frequencies. For example, in the cochlea, high frequencies cause maximal activation in the basal areas, whereas lower frequencies cause maximum activation in the apical regions. Auditory nerve fibers attached at the base of the inner hair cells in the cochlea follow this tonotopic organization, so that fibers at the base of the cochlea are tuned to higher frequencies, and those at the apical regions have lower characteristic frequencies. The tonotopic organization continues through various levels, including the cochlear nuclei and the auditory cortex. The temporal characteristics of stimuli are partially tracked through the phase-locked response of auditory neurons.

The production of syllables is marked by cyclical movements of speech articulators, along with vocal cord movements; these cyclical movements dominate the temporal envelope of the speech with a frequency of 4 to 8 Hz. Neuroimaging studies, including electroencephalography (EEG) and MEG, show that ongoing cortical oscillations are phase locked to the low-frequency information in the speech envelope. The adaptation of one quasi-periodic system, such as the intrinsic neural oscillations, to match the phase of another quasi-periodic system, such as speech modulations, is referred to as *synchronization* or *entrainment.* Such entrainment can enhance sensitivity to important acoustic cues in speech (Peelle & Davis, 2012). Neuronal oscillations occurring in other distinct frequency bands may be relevant to speech perception. More specifically, phonetic features with a duration of 20 to 50 ms may be associated with gamma (γ, > 50 Hz) and beta (β, 15–30 Hz) oscillations, syllables and words with mean durations up to 250 ms may be associated with theta (4–8 Hz) oscillations, and sequences of syllables and words embedded within a prosodic phrase with mean durations ranging from 500 to 2000 ms may be associated with delta oscillations (< 3 Hz; Ghitza, 2011). Nested endogenous neural oscillations across these frequency bands may enhance activity in response to target stimuli and suppress activity for background competition (Horton, D'Zmura, & Srinivasan, 2013).

A meta-analysis of 10 studies suggests activation of several cortical areas during the perception of degraded speech, including bilateral posterior middle temporal gyri (MTG), anterior superior temporal sulci (STS), anterior insulae, and anterior supplementary motor area (pre-SMA). The activation of anterior insulae suggests the use of general cognitive or executive resources in speech perception. During the perception of degraded speech, there may be an increased involvement of areas governing speech production, such as the pre-SMA and bilateral anterior STS areas (Adank, 2012). Studies using transmagnetic stimulation (TMS) also suggest that motor areas related to speech production play an important role in speech perception. During speech perception tasks, an increase in excitability of speech production motor areas is apparent (Murakami, Ugawa, & Ziemann, 2013). Involvement of speech production areas is expected when the response task involves repetition of the speech stimulus by the listener, and the verbal repetition response task may enhance speech perception.

7.11 Future Trends

In the future, carefully collected normative data will be available on many of the modified speech versions across different age groups (▶ Fig. 7.25). Such data collection will carefully control acoustic crosstalk by presenting stimuli and any competing messages at levels below those where the stimuli or competing messages can cross over to the other side. When the task involves speech recognition, scoring for all speech stimuli will be based on both phoneme and word scoring. This will improve the test–retest reliability rate because of an increase in the number of scored items, as shown in ▶ Table 7.1. In addition, this type of scoring will allow the identification of specific types of errors and confusions that vary depending on the type of speech modification (Winn, Chatterjee, & Idsardi, 2013) or masker (Phatak & Allen, 2007; Phatak, Lovitt, & Allen, 2008). For example, speech-shaped masking noise has more impact on the recognition of the /b/ versus /p/ contrast, whereas low-pass filtering of speech has more impact on the /d/ versus /t/ contrast (Winn et al., 2013). Furthermore, routine use of computerized scoring will improve scoring and error pattern analyses.

EEG traces in response to syllables varying in voice onset time are unique and allow decoding of what the listener was listening to when the voice onset time is adjusted to allow a clear perception of voiced or voiceless contrasts. In addition, the native language of the listeners can be decoded on the basis of EEG data evoked with speech stimuli with accuracy above 80% (Brandmeyer, Farquhar, McQueen, & Desain, 2013). Further refinement of such techniques will allow quick assessment of the accuracy and efficiency of auditory processing of speech stimuli.

7.12 Review Questions

1. List various factors that can affect the outcome of speech recognition testing.
2. Differentiate between intrinsic and extrinsic redundancy in the context of monaural modified speech assessment.
3. How can low-redundancy speech tests aid in identifying auditory processing deficits?
4. List and discuss spectral degradations of speech stimuli. What is the effect of central pathologies on the perception of filtered speech?
5. List and discuss various temporal alterations of speech stimuli.
6. What are the effects of central auditory pathologies on the perception of temporally degraded speech stimuli?
7. Discuss the effect of hearing loss on temporally degraded speech perception.
8. List and discuss the variables that contribute to speech recognition performance in the

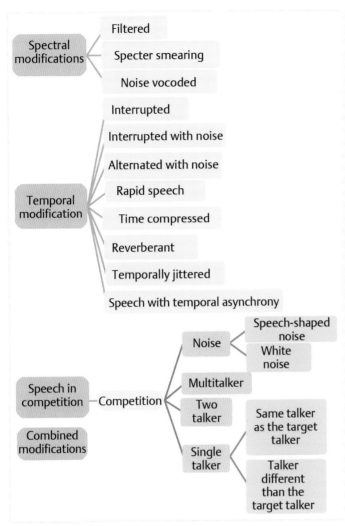

Fig. 7.25 Examples of low-redundancy speech stimuli. The length of the speech stimuli can vary from phonemes, syllables, words, phrases, sentences, and paragraphs.

presence of background competition. Review some commercial tests that allow measurement of speech recognition in the presence of competing sounds.

9. Review potential objective measures for assessing the perception of degraded speech.

10. Discuss potential future trends in the assessment of monaural speech perception.

References

[1] Adank, P. (2012). The neural bases of difficult speech comprehension and speech production: Two Activation Likelihood Estimation (ALE) meta-analyses. Brain and Language, 122(1), 42–54.

[2] American Academy of Audiology. (2010). Clinical practice guidelines: Diagnosis, treatment and management of children and adults with central auditory processing disorder (Guidelines). Retrieved from www.audiology.org/resources/documentlibrary/Documents/CAPD%20Guidelines%208–2010.pdf.

[3] Anderson, S., Parbery-Clark, A., White-Schwoch, T., & Kraus, N. (2013). Auditory brainstem response to complex sounds predicts self-reported speech-in-noise performance. Journal of Speech, Language, and Hearing Research, 56(1), 31–43.

[4] Baer, T., & Moore, B. C. J. (1993). Effects of spectral smearing on the intelligibility of sentences in noise. Journal of the Acoustical Society of America, 94(3), 1229–1241.

[5] Baer, T., & Moore, B. C. J. (1994). Effects of spectral smearing on the intelligibility of sentences in the presence of interfering speech. Journal of the Acoustical Society of America, 95 (4), 2277–2280.

[6] Bell, D. W., Kreul, E. J., & Nixon, J. C. (1972). Reliability of the modified rhyme test for hearing. Journal of Speech and Hearing Research, 15(2), 287–295.

[7] Bennett, K. O., Billings, C. J., Molis, M. R., & Leek, M. R. (2012). Neural encoding and perception of speech signals in informational masking. Ear and Hearing, 33(2), 231–238.

[8] Bergemalm, P. O., & Lyxell, B. (2005). Appearances are deceptive? Long-term cognitive and central auditory sequelae from closed head injury. International Journal of Audiology, 44(1), 39–49.

[9] Bilger, R. C. (1984). Speech recognition test development. ASHA Reports,14, 2–15.

[10] Bilger, R. C., Nuetzel, J. M., Rabinowitz, W. M., & Rzeczkowski, C. (1984). Standardization of a test of speech perception in noise. Journal of Speech and Hearing Research, 27(1), 32–48.

[11] Billings, C. J., Bennett, K. O., Molis, M. R., & Leek, M. R. (2011). Cortical encoding of signals in noise: Effects of stimulus type and recording paradigm. Ear and Hearing, 32(1), 53–60.

[12] Bishop, D. V. M., & Hardiman, M. J. (2010). Measurement of mismatch negativity in individuals: A study using single-trial analysis. Psychophysiology, 47(4), 697–705.

[13] Bishop, D. V. M., Hardiman, M. J., & Barry, J. G. (2011). Is auditory discrimination mature by middle childhood? A study using time-frequency analysis of mismatch responses from 7 years to adulthood. Developmental Science, 14(2), 402–416.

[14] Bocca, E., Calearo, C., & Cassinari, V. (1954). A new method for testing hearing in temporal lobe tumours: Preliminary report. Acta Otolaryngologica, 44(3), 219–221.

[15] Bocca, E., Calearo, C., Cassinari, V., & Migliavacca, F. (1955). Testing "cortical" hearing in temporal lobe tumours. Acta Otolaryngologica, 45(4), 289–304.

[16] Bonino, A. Y., Leibold, L. J., & Buss, E. (2013). Release from perceptual masking for children and adults: Benefit of a carrier phrase. Ear and Hearing, 34(1), 3–14.

[17] Boothroyd, A. (1968). Developments in speech audiometry. Sound, 2, 3–10.

[18] Bornstein, S. P. (1994). Time compression and release from masking in adults and children. Journal of the American Academy of Audiology, 5(2), 89–98.

[19] Bornstein, S. P., Wilson, R. H., & Cambron, N. K. (1994). Low- and high-pass filtered Northwestern University Auditory Test No. 6 for monaural and binaural evaluation. Journal of the American Academy of Audiology, 5(4), 259–264.

[20] Brandmeyer, A., Farquhar, J. D. R., McQueen, J. M., & Desain, P. W. M. (2013). Decoding speech perception by native and non-native speakers using single-trial electrophysiological data. PLoS ONE, 8(7), e68261.

[21] Calearo, C., & Lazzaroni, A. (1957). Speech intelligibility in relation to the speed of the message. Laryngoscope, 67(5), 410–419.

[22] Carhart, R., Tillman, T. W., & Greetis, E. S. (1969). Perceptual masking in multiple sound backgrounds. Journal of the Acoustical Society of America, 45(3), 694–703.

[23] Cherry, R. (1980). Selective Auditory Attention Test (SAAT). St. Louis, MO: Auditec.

[24] Cherry, R. (1992). Screening and evaluation of central auditory processing disorders in young children. In J. Katz, N. Stecker, & D. Henderson (Eds.), Central auditory processing: A transdisciplinary view (pp. 129–140). St. Louis, MO: Mosby Year Book.

[25] Cherry, R. S., & Kruger, B. (1983). Selective auditory attention abilities of learning disabled and normal achieving children. Journal of Learning Disabilities, 16(4), 202–205.

[26] Cherry, R., & Rubinstein, A. (2005). A comparison of two approaches to assessment of speech recognition ability in single cases. Journal of the American Academy of Audiology, 16(1), 54–62, quiz 63–64.

[27] Cherry, R., & Rubinstein, A. (2006). Comparing monotic and diotic selective auditory attention abilities in children. Language, Speech, and Hearing Services in Schools, 37(2), 137–142.

[28] Desjardins, J. L., & Doherty, K. A. (2013). Age-related changes in listening effort for various types of masker noises. Ear and Hearing, 34(3), 261–272.

[29] Dimitrijevic, A., Pratt, H., & Starr, A. (2013). Auditory cortical activity in normal hearing subjects to consonant vowels presented in quiet and in noise. Clinical Neurophysiology, 124(6), 1204–1215.

[30] Ding, N., & Simon, J. Z. (2013). Adaptive temporal encoding leads to a background-insensitive cortical representation of speech. Journal of Neuroscience, 33(13), 5728–5735.

[31] Dubno, J. R., & Dirks, D. D. (1983). Suggestions for optimizing reliability with the synthetic sentence identification test. Journal of Speech and Hearing Disorders, 48(1), 98–103.

[32] Eisenberg, L. S., Shannon, R. V., Martinez, A. S., Wygonski, J., & Boothroyd, A. (2000). Speech recognition with reduced spectral cues as a function of age. Journal of the Acoustical Society of America, 107(5, Pt. 1), 2704–2710.

[33] Elliott, L. L. (1979). Performance of children aged 9 to 17 years on a test of speech intelligibility in noise using sentence material with controlled word predictability. Journal of the Acoustical Society of America, 66(3), 651–653.

[34] Farrer, S. M., & Keith, R. W. (1981). Filtered word testing in the assessment of children's central auditory abilities. Ear and Hearing, 2(6), 267–269.

[35] Feeney, M. P., & Hallowell, B. (2000). Practice and list effects on the synthetic sentence identification test in young and elderly listeners. Journal of Speech, Language, and Hearing Research, 43(5), 1160–1167.

[36] Fletcher, H. (1940). Auditory patterns. Reviews of Modern Physics, 12, 47–65.

[37] French, N. R., & Steinberg, J. C. (1947). Factors governing the intelligibility of speech sounds. Journal of the Acoustical Society of America, 19, 90–119.

[38] Ghitza, O. (2011). Linking speech perception and neurophysiology: Speech decoding guided by cascaded oscillators locked to the input rhythm. Frontiers in Psychology, 2, 130.

[39] Gordon-Salant, S., & Friedman, S. A. (2011). Recognition of rapid speech by blind and sighted older adults. Journal of Speech, Language, and Hearing Research, 54(2), 622–631.

[40] Healy, E. W., & Bacon, S. P. (2002). Across-frequency comparison of temporal speech information by listeners with normal and impaired hearing. Journal of Speech, Language, and Hearing Research, 45(6), 1262–1275.

[41] Hornickel, J., Knowles, E., & Kraus, N. (2012). Test-retest consistency of speech-evoked auditory brainstem responses in typically-developing children. Hearing Research, 284(1–2), 52–58.

[42] Hornickel, J., Skoe, E., & Kraus, N. (2009). Subcortical laterality of speech encoding. Audiology and Neurootology, 14(3), 198–207.

[43] Horton, C., D'Zmura, M., & Srinivasan, R. (2013). Suppression of competing speech through entrainment of cortical oscillations. Journal of Neurophysiology, 109(12), 3082–3093.

[44] Jerger, J., & Jerger, S. (1974). Auditory findings in brain stem disorders. Archives of Otolaryngology, 99(5), 342–350.

[45] Jerger, J., & Jerger, S. (1975). Clinical validity of central auditory tests. Scandinavian Audiology, 4, 147–163.

[46] Johnson, K. L., Nicol, T., Zecker, S. G., & Kraus, N. (2008). Developmental plasticity in the human auditory brainstem. The Journal of Neuroscience, 28(15), 4000–4007.

[47] Kalikow, D. N., Stevens, K. N., & Elliott, L. L. (1977). Development of a test of speech intelligibility in noise using sen-

tence materials with controlled word predictability. Journal of the Acoustical Society of America, 61(5), 1337–1351.

[48] Karlsson, A. K., & Rosenhall, U. (1995). Clinical application of distorted speech audiometry. Scandinavian Audiology, 24(3), 155–160.

[49] Keith, R. W. (2000). SCAN-C: Tests for auditory processing disorders in children—Revised. San Antonio, TX: Psychological Corp.

[50] Keith, R. W. (2002). Time-Compressed Sentence Test: Examiner's manual. St. Louis, MO: Auditec.

[51] Keith, R. W. (2009). SCAN-3 for adolescents and adults: Tests for auditory processing disorders. San Antonio, TX: Pearson.

[52] Korsan-Bengtsen, M. (1973). Distorted speech audiometry: A methodological and clinical study. Acta Otolaryngologica (Supplementum), 310, 1–75.

[53] Kreul, E. J., Nixon, J. C., Kryter, K. D., Bell, D. W., Lang, J. S., & Schubert, E. D. (1968). A proposed clinical test of speech discrimination. Journal of Speech and Hearing Research, 11, 536–552.

[54] Kurdziel, S., Noffsinger, D., & Olsen, W. (1976). Performance by cortical lesion patients on 40 and 60% time-compressed materials. Journal of the American Audiology Society, 2(1), 3–7.

[55] MacDonald, E. N., Pichora-Fuller, M. K., & Schneider, B. A. (2010). Effects on speech intelligibility of temporal jittering and spectral smearing of the high-frequency components of speech. Hearing Research, 261(1–2), 63–66.

[56] Martin, F. N., & Mussell, S. A. (1979). The influence of pauses in the competing signal on synthetic sentence identification scores. Journal of Speech and Hearing Disorders, 44(3), 282–292.

[57] McCroskey, R. (1984). Wichita Auditory Processing Test: User's manual. Tulsa, OK: Modern Education Corp.

[58] McCroskey, R. L., & Thompson, N. W. (1973). Comprehension of rate-controlled speech by children with learning problems. Journal of Learning Disabilities, 6(10), 621–627.

[59] Meyer, B. T., Jürgens, T., Wesker, T., Brand, T., & Kollmeier, B. (2010). Human phoneme recognition depending on speech-intrinsic variability. Journal of the Acoustical Society of America, 128(5), 3126–3141.

[60] Miller, G. A., & Licklider, J. C. R. (1950). The intelligibility of interrupted speech. Journal of the Acoustical Society of America, 22(2), 167–173.

[61] Miranda, T. T., & Pichora-Fuller, M. K. (2002). Temporally jittered speech produces performance intensity, phonetically balanced rollover in young normal-hearing listeners. Journal of the American Academy of Audiology, 13(1), 50–58.

[62] Murakami, T., Ugawa, Y., & Ziemann, U. (2013). Utility of TMS to understand the neurobiology of speech. Frontiers in Psychology, 4, 446.

[63] Nábělek, A. K., & Robinson, P. K. (1982). Monaural and binaural speech perception in reverberation for listeners of various ages. Journal of the Acoustical Society of America, 71(5), 1242–1248.

[64] Neuman, A. C., & Hochberg, I. (1983). Children's perception of speech in reverberation. Journal of the Acoustical Society of America, 73(6), 2145–2149.

[65] Noffsinger, D., Wilson, R. H., & Musiek, F. E. (1994). Department of Veterans Affairs compact disc recording for auditory perceptual assessment: Background and introduction. Journal of the American Academy of Audiology, 5(4), 231–235.

[66] O'Beirne, G. A., McGaffin, A. J., & Rickard, N. A. (2012). Development of an adaptive low-pass filtered speech test for the identification of auditory processing disorders. International Journal of Pediatric Otorhinolaryngology, 76(6), 777–782.

[67] Odkvist, L. M., Arlinger, S. D., Edling, C., Larsby, B., & Bergholtz, L. M. (1987). Audiological and vestibulo-oculomotor findings in workers exposed to solvents and jet fuel. Scandinavian Audiology, 16(2), 75–81.

[68] Peelle, J. E., & Davis, M. H. (2012). Neural oscillations carry speech rhythm through to comprehension. Frontiers in Psychology, 3, 320.

[69] Peelle, J. E., Gross, J., & Davis, M. H. (2013). Phase-locked responses to speech in human auditory cortex are enhanced during comprehension. Cerebral Cortex, 23(6), 1378–1387.

[70] Phatak, S. A., & Allen, J. B. (2007). Consonant and vowel confusions in speech-weighted noise. Journal of the Acoustical Society of America, 121(4), 2312–2326.

[71] Phatak, S. A., Lovitt, A., & Allen, J. B. (2008). Consonant confusions in white noise. Journal of the Acoustical Society of America, 124(2), 1220–1233.

[72] Pichora-Fuller, M. K., Schneider, B. A., MacDonald, E., Pass, H. E., & Brown, S. (2007). Temporal jitter disrupts speech intelligibility: A simulation of auditory aging. Hearing Research, 223(1–2), 114–121.

[73] Rappaport, J. M., Gulliver, J. M., Phillips, D. P., Van Dorpe, R. A., Maxner, C. E., & Bhan, V. (1994). Auditory temporal resolution in multiple sclerosis. Journal of Otolaryngology, 23(5), 307–324.

[74] Rawool, V. W. (2012). Simulated high frequency hearing impairment in noise and low frequency noise attenuation. Hearing Review, 19(1), 32–39.

[75] Resnick, S. B., Dubno, J. R., Hoffnung, S., & Levitt, H. (1975). Phoneme errors on a nonsense syllable test. Journal of the Acoustical Society of America, 58(Suppl. 1), 114.

[76] Ross, M., & Lerman, J. (1971). Word intelligibility by picture identification. Pittsburgh, PA: Stanwix House.

[77] Schow, R. L., Seikel, J. A., Brockett, J. E., & Whitaker, M. M. (2007). Multiple Auditory Processing Assessment (MAPA): Test manual 1.0, version. St. Louis, MO: Auditec.

[78] Shannon, R. V., Zeng, F.-G., Kamath, V., Wygonski, J., & Ekelid, M. (1995). Speech recognition with primarily temporal cues. Science, 270(5234), 303–304.

[79] Smith, S. L., Pichora-Fuller, M. K., Wilson, R. H., & MacDonald, E. N. (2012). Word recognition for temporally and spectrally distorted materials: The effects of age and hearing loss. Ear and Hearing, 33(3), 349–366.

[80] Song, J. H., Nicol, T., & Kraus, N. (2011). Test-retest reliability of the speech-evoked auditory brainstem response. Clinical Neurophysiology, 122(2), 346–355.

[81] Speaks, C., & Jerger, J. (1965). Method for measurement of speech identification. Journal of Speech and Hearing Research, 8, 185–194.

[82] Spitzer, J. B., & Ventry, I. M. (1980). Central auditory dysfunction among chronic alcoholics. Archives of Otolaryngology, 106(4), 224–229.

[83] Stuart, A. (2005). Development of auditory temporal resolution in school-age children revealed by word recognition in continuous and interrupted noise. Ear and Hearing, 26(1), 78–88.

[84] Studebaker, G. A., Sherbecoe, R. L., McDaniel, D. M., & Gwaltney, C. A. (1999). Monosyllabic word recognition at higher-than-normal speech and noise levels. Journal of the Acoustical Society of America, 105(4), 2431–2444.

[85] Teatini, G. P. (1970). Sensitized Speech Tests (SST): Results in normal subjects. In C. Rojskjaer (Ed.), Speech audiometry. (pp. 37–43). Second Danavox Symposium, Odense, Denmark.

[86] Thorndike, E. L., & Lorge, I. (1944). The teachers word book of 30,000 Words. New York: Bureau of Publications, Teachers College, Columbia University.

223

[87] U.S. Department of Veterans Affairs. (1998). Tonal and speech materials for auditory perceptual assessment (compact disc 2.0). Mountain Home, TN: VA Medical Center.

[88] Wang, X., & Humes, L. E. (2010). Factors influencing recognition of interrupted speech. Journal of the Acoustical Society of America, 128(4), 2100–2111.

[89] Wilson, R. H., McArdle R. (2012). Speech-in-noise measures: Variable versus fixed speech and noise levels. International Journal of Audiology, 51(9), 708–712.

[90] Wilson, R. H., Preece, J. P., Salamon, D. L., Sperry, J. L., & Bornstein, S. P. (1994). Effects of time compression and time compression plus reverberation on the intelligibility of Northwestern University Auditory Test No. 6. Journal of the American Academy of Audiology, 5(4), 269–277.

[91] Winn, M. B., Chatterjee, M., & Idsardi, W. J. (2013). Roles of voice onset time and F0 in stop consonant voicing perception: Effects of masking noise and low-pass filtering. Journal of Speech, Language, and Hearing Research, 56(4), 1097–1107.

[92] Zeng, F. G., Kong, Y. Y., Michalewski, H. J., & Starr, A. (2005). Perceptual consequences of disrupted auditory nerve activity. Journal of Neurophysiology, 93(6), 3050–3063.

Chapter 8

Intervention for Auditory Processing Deficits

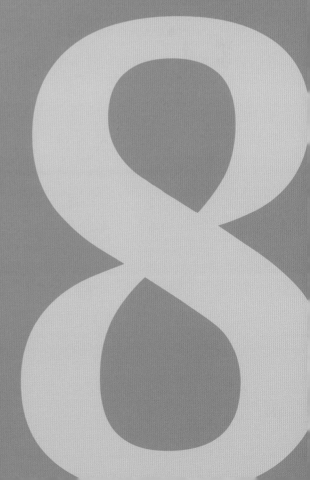

8 Intervention for Auditory Processing Deficits

The term *intervention* refers to actions taken to improve a situation, specifically a medical disorder, including treatment and management. The term *treatment* can refer to any specific procedure used to prevent, remediate, or ameliorate a deficit (American Academy of Audiology, 2010). The term *management* can be used to describe compensatory approaches (e.g., strategies and technologies) used to reduce the impact of deficits in real-life settings until the deficit is remediated or to compensate for any residual deficits following treatment. This chapter provides an overview of the various intervention strategies that can be used for individuals with auditory processing deficits.

8.1 Intervention

The intervention plan for any individual diagnosed with an auditory processing deficit (APD) can initially include both treatment and management approaches based on the identified deficits through the diagnostic procedures or based on the client's specific concerns in real-life situations. The approach should be individualized to meet the specific needs of the client. A multidisciplinary team should be involved in planning and providing intervention for clients with comorbid conditions, such as attention deficit hyperactivity disorder (ADHD; see Chapter 13), language or speech impairment, and reading deficits (see Chapter 14). The constitution of the multidisciplinary team will vary depending on the identified comorbid condition(s). Examples of professionals who may be included in the multidisciplinary team are speech language pathologists, reading specialists, learning disability specialists, neurologists, and psychologists. The intervention techniques can be classified as bottom-up (▶ Fig. 8.1) and top-down (▶ Fig. 8.2) strategies.

8.2 Bottom-Up Strategies

Bottom-up strategies (▶ Fig. 8.1) are designed to improve the perception of sounds.

8.2.1 Acoustic Environment

Effect of Poor Acoustic Environment on Language and Academic Achievements

Studies have shown that poor or noisier acoustic environments can negatively affect language and reading performance and other behaviors important for learning, such as sustained attention. Students attempting to learn in poor acoustic environments show greater susceptibility to induced helplessness.

One study examined the effect of noise on children's prereading skills in a child care center that was not located near any major external noise sources (Maxwell & Evans, 2000). The noise in the classrooms was a result of poor acoustical design. Ninety children in the age range of 4 to 5 years

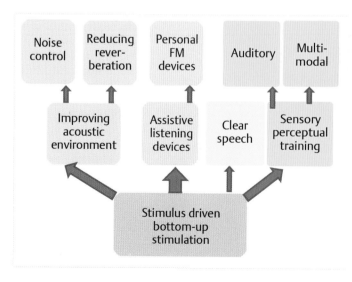

Fig. 8.1 Components of bottom-up intervention for auditory processing deficits.

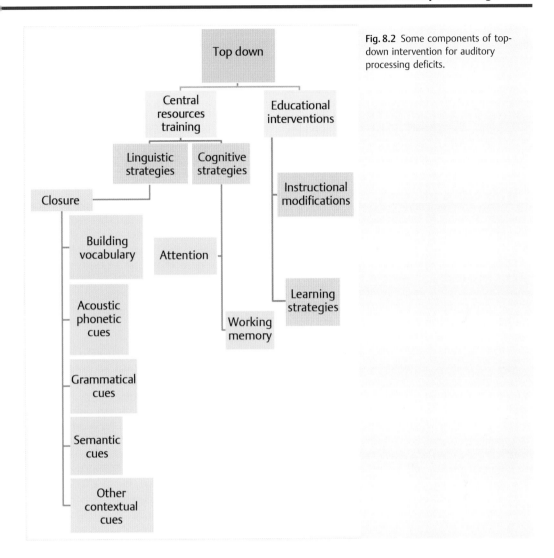

Fig. 8.2 Some components of top-down intervention for auditory processing deficits.

were tested on cognitive measures of prereading skills and were rated by classroom teachers on their comprehension and use of language. The testing and ratings were conducted in year 1, before the installation of sound-absorbent panels in the classroom ceilings and in year 2 following the installation, which reduced the noise in the classroom by 5 dB. In the quieter condition, children scored higher than their noisier cohort on the letter/number/word recognition measures and received higher rating on comprehension and use of language. Children in the quieter classroom were also less susceptible than those in the noisy classroom to induced helplessness. To test for the susceptibility to induced helplessness, children were first given an unsolvable jigsaw puzzle consisting of five geometric shapes. The children were then presented with another moderately difficult but solvable puzzle and were allowed to work on it for a maximum of 4 minutes. Children in the noisier classroom took a longer time to solve the second puzzle than those in the quiet room, suggesting greater susceptibility to induced helplessness (Maxwell & Evans, 2000). Similarly, school-aged children who have poor speech perception skills due to chronic noise exposure show poor reading skills (Evans & Maxwell, 1997). The negative correlation between background noise levels and reading comprehension remains significant after controlling for the effects of poverty rates on achievement (Ronsse & Wang, 2010).

Both chronic and acute exposure to noise inside and outside the classroom is negatively correlated with children's learning and performance on standardized assessment tests after controlling for socioeconomic status. For noise outside the classroom, individual noisy events have the most negative impact, whereas for noise inside the classroom, the background noise has a significant negative impact. The performance of children with special educational needs on verbal tasks appears to be more negatively affected by classroom babble compared to the performance of their normal-hearing peers (Shield & Dockrell, 2008a,b).

Poor classroom acoustics, including longer reverberation time, can have a negative impact on the development of auditory-verbal skills that are necessary for reading. In one study, the effects of classroom reverberation were analyzed in elementary school children from 21 classrooms with reverberation times ranging from 0.49 to 1.11 seconds (Klatte, Hellbrück, Seidel, & Leistner, 2010). Repeated measurements of performance were carried out in the children's regular classrooms and in control classrooms with shorter reverberation or better acoustics. Children from classrooms with a reverberation time longer than 1 second performed worse on a phonological processing task than children from classrooms with a reverberation time less than 0.6 second. The children from highly reverberant classrooms noted a higher burden of indoor noise and perceived the relations to their peers and teachers and their achievement motivation less positively when compared to children from classrooms with a shorter reverberation time (Klatte et al., 2010).

Besides background noise levels and reverberation time, a metric that may be useful in determining the impact of acoustic conditions on speech perception in classroom is the distortion of frequency-smoothed magnitude (DFSM; Shinn-Cunningham, Kopco & Martin, 2005). The DFSM is generated by averaging the absolute differences between the reverberant signal and a corresponding "pseudo-anechoic" signal, which is free of all room reflections in each one-third octave band. A shorter path from the source to the receiver, sources directly facing the receiver, and less reverberation generate a lower DFSM value. Lower DFSM values can lead to better sound source localization ability. They also generally lead to higher language scores (Ronsse & Wang, 2013).

ANSI/ASA (2010) Acoustical Guideline for Classrooms

The American National Standards Institute/Acoustical Society of America (ANSI/ASA S12.60–2010/Part 1) standard has specified 35 dB(A) and 55 dB(C) as the maximum 1-hour averaged A-weighted and C-weighted steady background noise level in unoccupied and furnished core learning spaces (e.g., classrooms, instructional pods, group instruction rooms, conference rooms, libraries, speech clinics, offices used for educational purposes, and music rooms used for instruction, practice, and performance) with volumes equal to or less than 20,000 square feet. For core learning areas with volumes greater than 20,000 square feet and all ancillary (e.g., corridors, cafeterias, gymnasia, and indoor swimming pools) learning areas, the specified maximum noise levels are 40 dB(A) and 60 dB(C). The 35 dB(A) maximum noise criterion is based on the assumption of a minimum speech level of 50 dB and a need of at least a + 15 dB speech-to-noise ratio to ensure that the noise levels will not impede learning in the classroom.

The ANSI (ANSI/ASA S12.60–2010/Part 1) standard has also specified maximum reverberation times for sound pressure levels in octave bands with midband frequencies of 500, 1000, and 2000 Hz. These are 0.6 second for core learning areas with volumes less than 10,000 sq ft and 0.7 second for areas with volumes in the range of 10,000 to 20,000 sq ft. These criteria apply for unoccupied and furnished spaces. For occupied classrooms, the reverberation times are expected to be 0.1 or 0.2 second. Both the noise and reverberation criteria need to be applied simultaneously to achieve a speech-to-noise ratio of at least + 15 dB. The standard also specifies noise isolation design requirements.

In general, noise and reverberation in classrooms and other learning spaces should be minimized to ensure good access to auditory information presented in such spaces to all students, including those with hearing loss. The annex B and annex C of the ANSI/ASA S12.60–2010/Part 1 standard include useful design guidelines for controlling noise and reverberation in classrooms and other learning spaces. Although excessive reverberation can impede speech recognition, excessive sound absorption treatments can reduce beneficial early sound reflections leading to a rapid decrease in sound levels that can negatively impact speech recognition for students who are sitting away from the talker. Thus, a proper balance is necessary in applying acoustic treatments to address reverberation.

Annex F of the ANSI (2010) standard addresses concerns about indoor air quality (IAQ) and multiple chemical sensitivity (MCS) issues that can lead some schools to remove all porous materials from the classroom and/or from the ventilation supply ducts, which compromises the benefits these materials can offer for reducing noise. Based on available literature and other sources, the standard states that there is little or no conflict between the applications of the standard for classroom acoustics and IAQ and MCS issues provided absorptive materials are properly selected and maintained. For example, if tennis ball halves are used on chair legs to minimize shuffling noise, these should be periodically cleaned and replaced given that the ball halves can develop an active fungal growth. A better method for reducing chair-shuffling noise is to use neoprene chair leg tips.

Recommendations of the Oticon Foundation of New Zealand (2002)

The Oticon Foundation in New Zealand (2002) has made several specific recommendations for improving classroom acoustics, some of which are listed here:

- In classrooms where group work is dominant, an acoustic/absorptive ceiling is preferred. All new primary classrooms should be designed with absorptive ceilings.
- If retrofitting ceilings with acoustic tiles is necessary, classrooms with high or vaulted ceilings should be retrofitted first.
- In purchasing computers or any electronics, equipment with the lowest noise ratings should be ordered.
- It is important to find out the noise levels of any heating or air conditioning systems that are going to be installed so that the noise generated by these systems will not lead to an increase in noise levels that is beyond what is specified by established standards.
- A solid floor construction is recommended to minimize the drumming associated with light timber-framed construction. In addition, two layers of particleboard or a concrete slab is recommended instead of just one layer.
- A double stud wall is recommended between a restroom and instructional space. The two walls should be structurally separated, and the piping should be attached to the restroom side only.
- Teacher training and in-service should provide information about the importance of a good acoustic environment for learning and for minimizing vocal strain.
- School staff and administrators should be aware of the risks of noise entering the classroom from outside. For example, noisy activities such as lawn mowing can be scheduled outside the school hours.

Renovation of Existing Classrooms

It should be noted that classroom designers may be tempted to design creative spaces that look different than the usual plain classroom design. However, creative designs (e.g., ceilings that are not parallel to the floor) can increase the number of hard surfaces in the classroom and can compromise acoustic comfort, audibility, and sleep routines in preschool classrooms (Maxwell & Evans, 2000). College classrooms can also be noisy, and students seated in the back of large classrooms may have more difficulty understanding instructors than those seated in the front of classrooms. Reduction of background noise levels is recommended for such classrooms (Hodgson, 2002).

8.2.2 Assistive Listening Devices

Many individuals with APDs have difficulty understanding speech in noisy environments or when the teacher is not at a close distance. A child who cannot understand the teacher may show poor academic performance due to the APD. Use of assistive listening devices such as frequency modulation (FM) systems can deliver a clean speech signal to the listener's ears in the presence of noisy or reverberant environments or when the talker is not closer to the listener. The FM device includes a microphone that is attached to a transmitter and is positioned near the speaker's (e.g., classroom teacher's) mouth. The device also includes a receiving unit that is positioned near the listener and is coupled to the listener's ear. The signal from the speaker is sent via radio signals to the receiving unit near the listener. The signal transmitted to the listener's ears is free from noise and reverberation in the listener's environment. It is also presented at a comfortable listening level regardless of the distance of the speaker from the listener. Use of the device can continue until the individual can benefit from direct auditory training and can function well in difficult listening environments. Some individuals such as older adults with peripheral hearing loss in addition to central auditory deficits may have to continue to use the device in difficult listening environments, such as places of worship, movie theaters, and noisy work environments.

Sound Field FM Systems

In sound field FM systems, the sound picked up from the teacher's microphone is relayed to several loudspeakers placed at various locations in the classroom. Such systems can improve the performance of children on several tasks. For example, in one study the performance of children who were identified as being at risk through the use of the Screening Instrument for Targeting Educational Risk (SIFTER; Anderson, 1989) was compared before and after installation of sound field amplification systems in their classrooms. A large proportion of these children showed an improvement in their listening behaviors according to their responses on the Children's Auditory Processing Performance Scale (CHAPPS, Smoski et al., 1992) after the installation of sound field systems (McSporran, Butterworth, & Rowson, 1997). The learning and listening behaviors of 9th- and 12th-grade children with learning disabilities improve with the use of the sound field FM systems. The main benefit reported by the teachers is their ability to get and maintain children's attention (DiSarno, Schowalter, & Grassa, 2002). The speed with which directions are followed can improve with the use of sound field systems in children with ADHD and those with emotional or behavioral problems (Maag & Anderson, 2006, 2007). College students also report improvement in listening and understanding their professors while using sound field amplification systems (Woodford, Tomkowski, & Lawrence, 1998).

Limitations of Sound Field Systems

Although some clinicians have suggested the use of sound field amplification instead of personal FM units, with the idea of improving listening for all students, sound field amplification can increase overall classroom sound levels, potentially leading to uncomfortable listening levels and the spread of sound to adjacent classrooms, which can interfere with the learning of students in the adjacent rooms. Thus, sound field amplification systems should not be routinely installed in typical small classrooms. In addition, personal FM systems are largely immune to reverberation compared to sound field systems (Acoustical Society of America, 2003).

Personal FM Devices

Personal FM devices are preferred over sound field FM devices. Modern miniaturized personal FM devices, such as the Phonak EduLink (Stäfa, Switzerland), are compact and lightweight. The EduLink's microphone and transmitter are ultra-lightweight and thus offer maximum comfort to the wearer. The microphone is designed to pick up the speech signal relatively free from noise. The receiver can be hung over the ear, with the end of the receiver tube in the concha and the battery door behind the pinna. The EduLink earpiece is minimally visible. It does not occlude the ear, which allows the wearer access to other environmental sounds (classmates' speech) without removing the device.

In one randomized control study, 23 children ages 6 to 11 years with reading delays received a 6-week trial of personal FM systems (Purdy, Smart, Baily, & Sharma, 2009). A significant improvement was noted in teacher ratings and children's ratings of classroom listening for difficult situations in the FM treatment group but not in the matched control group of 23 children. In another study, after 1 year of use of an FM system, children with dyslexia showed improvement in their phonological awareness and reading skills, and their subcortical responses to sounds became less variable or more robust. A matched control group without FM devices did not show similar effects (Hornickel, Zecker, Bradlow, & Kraus, 2012). Children can also be fitted with FM devices for both home and school use. With use of an FM device during one school year, children with APDs showed improved speech perception in noisy environments and significant academic and psychosocial benefits compared to a matched control group. After prolonged use of the FM device, the improvement in speech perception was evident even in the absence of the use of the FM device (Johnston, John, Kreisman, Hall, & Crandell, 2009).

8.2.3 Clear Speech

Clear speech is produced by full, clear, and accurate production of all phonemes in each word, deliberate pauses as appropriate to minimize slurring of words together, and stress on adjectives, verbs, and nouns (Picheny, Durlach, & Braida, 1985). In clear speech, word endings are not dropped (Schum, 1997). Although with some effort clear speech can be produced without slowing the speaking rate (Krause & Braida, 2002), when compared to conversational speech, clear speech is generally characterized by a slower speaking rate due to insertion of pauses between words and lengthening of durations of individual sounds.

In addition, the articulation contact pressure is greater for some phonemes (Searl & Evitts, 2013). In conversational speech, when stops occur in the final position of a word, the associated bursts are often not released, whereas these are frequently released in clear speech. Vowels are frequently modified or reduced in conversational speech; in clear speech, vowels are modified to a lesser degree (Picheny, Durlach, & Braida, 1986). Elements in the 1000 to 3000 Hz range tend to be louder in clear speech. In addition, low-frequency modulations have greater depth (Krause & Braida, 2004), which can make it easy to detect modulations.

Children with APDs need some training to overcome a deficit. However, even after training, some residual deficits may remain in some children. Use of clear speech by speech-language pathologists, caregivers, parents, and teachers can allow a child with an APD better opportunities to access the spoken message, which can lead to easier acquisition of speech, language, reading, and learning skills. Greater difficulty in the production of novel words for words presented at faster speaking rates has been noted in children with specific language impairments when compared to age-matched controls (Ellis Weismer, & Hesketh, 1996). Use of clear speech may allow more processing time due to the inherent slower speaking rate during clear speech production reported in most studies. Clear speech is known to improve speech perception in noise in children with and without learning disabilities (Bradlow, Kraus, & Hayes, 2003). When new nonwords are taught to young children (9–11 years old) in quiet or noisy conditions, children who are trained in quiet environments produce the word forms more accurately than those who are trained in noise. Training using clear speech results in more accurate word form productions than that conducted using plain or conversational speech in both quiet and noisy conditions. Training using clear speech in noise and conversational speech in quiet elicits similar outcomes. It appears that use of clear speech can enhance expressive vocabulary in children in both quiet and noisy environments (Riley & McGregor, 2012). The advantage of clear speech over conversational speech in improving speech intelligibility is more obvious in environments with higher noise levels and reverberation (Payton, Uchanski, & Braida, 1994). Both native and nonnative talkers can benefit from the use of clear speech while communicating with each other (Smiljanić & Bradlow, 2011).

Training in Producing Clear Speech

Most talkers may not be able to improve the clarity of their speech significantly with minimal instructions (Gagné, Masterson, Munhall, Bilida, & Querengesser, 1994), and there is considerable variation among talkers in the amount of speech vowel intelligibility benefit that can be achieved as a result of the use of clear speech compared to conversational speech (Ferguson, 2012). Variations in instructions on how to produce clear speech can lead to variation in the amount of improvement in speech intelligibility. There is some individual variability in terms of the types of instructions that elicit the clearest or most intelligible speech from each speaker. Thus, determination of the most effective instructions for each speaker may be important for maximizing intelligibility (Lam & Tjaden, 2013). Teachers, parents, and caregivers may benefit from training in producing clear speech. Formal training is based on three stages: formal instruction on clear speech, guided training in producing clear speech, and real-world practice (Tye-Murray & Witt, 1997). The following suggestions for providing training in using clear speech are based on those provided by Caissie and Tranquilla (2010).

Formal Instruction

During formal instruction, trainees can be informed about the advantages of clear speech for individuals with APDs and the benefits to the talkers, including easier conversations and less need for repeating the messages. The trainees can be presented with taped examples of clear and conversational speech in quiet and varying noise backgrounds. Such examples are available at websites such as http://acoustics.org/pressroom/httpdocs/145th/clr-spch-tab.htm from the press room website of The Acoustical Society of America. A handout describing the procedure for producing clear speech with an emphasis on clear pronunciation of each of the speech sounds, the use of pauses to minimize two words running together, and accurate acoustic stress on key words should be provided to the trainees. Written examples of clear and conversational speech can also be provided. Such information is readily available at websites such as http://www.betterhearing.org/hearingpedia/counseling-articles-tips/clear-speech from the Better Hearing Institute.

Guided Learning

During guided learning, trainees can be asked to circle key words and mark natural pause occurrences on a list of short sentences. The sentence materials can be selected based on the age and interests of the individuals. The trainees can then be asked to read the sentences using clear speech, and feedback can be provided about the clarity of speech. Alternatively, trainees can be asked to record their speech and complete a self-evaluation to see if there is scope for improving the clarity of the recorded samples. The clinician and the trainees can then converse with each other on a specific topic using clear speech. The clinician can provide feedback on the clarity of speech as necessary.

Real-World Practice

In this stage, trainees are asked to speak clearly with an individual with APD. They should note that the communication exchange may be slower with the use of clear speech, but the talker may not have to repeat instructions as often as required during conversational speech. Use of clear speech should be encouraged especially in noisy or reverberant conditions or when the listener and talker are not closer together.

The benefit of training in producing clear speech appears to be dependent on the motivation of the talkers to produce clear speech and the amount of practice devoted to production of clear speech (Caissie et al., 2005).

8.2.4 Sensory Training

In most cases of APDs, direct sensory training should be focused on improving the perceptual ability of the auditory system. However, in cases where the deficit is apparent across various sensory modalities, including auditory and visual modalities (e.g., temporal processing deficit), multimodal training may enhance auditory perception. In some cases, the use of visual stimuli during the training task may interfere with auditory processing learning. In such cases, initial training should focus on auditory stimuli without accompanying visual stimuli.

Auditory Training

Auditory training is designed to improve the perception of auditory stimuli. The improved auditory perception, referred to as *perceptual learning,* can be accompanied by changes in the relevant parts of the neural systems. Perceptual learning can occur during passive listening through the repetitive presentation of stimuli, such as jingles associated with advertisements presented on TV or radio. Training designed to address specific deficits may lead to more efficient perceptual learning.

Deficit-Specific Training

The most efficient way to offer auditory training is to provide it based on the specific deficits noted following an assessment battery (see Chapters 4 to 7). Different groups of neural substrates may be involved in processing different dimensions of auditory stimuli, including temporal, spectral, amplitude, binaural, and interaural dimensions. Thus, training to address each specific deficit can activate different neural substrates and may make new connections among different neurons or make the existing connections stronger. This is similar to exercising different body muscles by performing different activities, such as running and swimming.

8.2.5 Mechanisms of Perceptual Learning

Perceptual learning is the process of improving perception. Goldstone (1998) discussed four mechanisms of perceptual learning (▶ Fig. 8.3): stimulus imprinting, differentiation, unitization, and attentional weighting.

Stimulus Imprinting

Repeated exposure to stimuli or specific features of stimuli can stimulate the development of specialized internalized detectors, or receptors. The form of the detector is shaped by the imprinting stimulus. These specialized detectors can enhance the speed, accuracy, and ease with which the imprinting stimuli are processed.

Whole Stimulus Imprinting

Each exposure to a word can lead to an internalized trace of that stimulus. If the same word is heard repeatedly, more traces are left, and the word is recognized more easily because more relevant traces can be retrieved, and the time required for retrieval is reduced. Thus, words that occur with a high frequency in a language are easier to understand compared to infrequently occurring words.

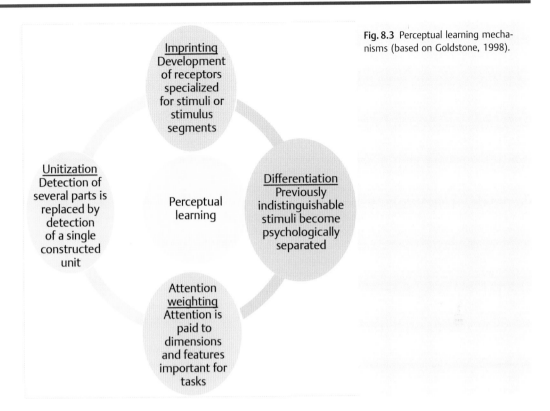

Fig. 8.3 Perceptual learning mechanisms (based on Goldstone, 1998).

Feature Imprinting

If a stimulus part (e.g., gap duration of 100 ms) is important, is varied independently of other parts (e.g., gap markers of 1000 Hz tone pips), and is presented frequently, listeners may develop specialized detectors for detecting the standard gap duration. If the same standard gap is then presented with gap markers of different frequency (e.g., 4000 Hz tone pips), listeners can still efficiently discriminate between the standard gap of 100 ms from gaps varying slightly in duration (Karmarkar & Buonomano, 2003; Wright, Buonomano, Mahncke, & Merzenich, 1997). In this example, the feature of 100 ms gap duration is imprinted.

Topological Imprinting

In this case, environmental regularities that span across a set of stimuli can be internalized. For example, the tonotopic arrangement of frequencies is apparent through the various levels of the auditory system and assists in identification of stimulus frequency. The feature of loudness is internalized across frequencies so that regardless of the frequency of the sound, the sound can be identified as being loud or soft.

Differentiation

This is a core mechanism of perceptual learning by which percepts become increasingly differentiated from each other and allows differentiation of percepts that were originally perceived as being the same.

Differentiation of Whole Stimuli

In this case, whole stimuli that appeared the same before training become distinguishable after training. For example, a patient may confuse the word *bad* with the word *dad* before training. After training, the words become clearly distinguishable. Such differentiation is enhanced by training in which the trained words are presented by various speakers of different genders and different ages.

Psychophysical Differentiation

An example of this type of differentiation is training a participant to perceive very small differences in frequencies or to perceive very small gaps in two stimuli. Normal-hearing listeners can develop hyperacuity after training. The hyperacuity can be explained by various mechanisms. It could develop due to a larger brain area devoted to the tasks compared to other tasks. For example, owl monkeys trained in frequency discrimination tasks develop larger cortical representations for the trained frequencies than do control owl monkeys. Another possible mechanism is that the tuning of the neurons devoted to certain frequencies may become sharper (Recanzone, Schreiner, & Merzenich, 1993). Another possible mechanism for improved acuity is a reduction in internal noise. Children may perform poorly when compared to young adults due to elevated internal noise levels. For example, the neural representation of intensity may be unstable or variable in children when compared to adults, which may lead to poorer intensity discrimination thresholds in children (Buss, Hall, & Grose, 2006, 2009). Auditory training can reduce internal noise levels, leading to improvement in frequency discrimination (Jones, Moore, Amitay, & Shub, 2013).

Unitization

Unitization integrates several parts into single wholes. Thus, a task that previously required detection of several parts can be completed by detecting a single unit. Parts tend to be unitized if they co-occur frequently and the co-occurring parts require a similar response. For example, if the individual sounds in *cell phone* are heard frequently together, it is perceived as a whole word and not separate sounds. Such unitization can minimize the cognitive resources required in perceiving stimuli.

Attentional Weighting

Perceptual performance on different tasks and environments can improve by enhancing the attention paid to perceptual dimensions and features that are important (e.g., voice onset time in speech stimuli) and by decreasing attention to irrelevant dimensions and features (background noise). In this description, feature is a unique stimulus element, such as 40 ms or low-frequency noise. Examples of dimensions are duration and frequency, which include a set of features.

One way to evaluate the influence of attention on perceptual learning is to present physically identical tones in three intervals to listeners. The listeners can then be instructed to select the interval that is either different in pitch or different in loudness to direct their attention to either the frequency or intensity dimension of stimuli. Random

feedback can be provided to listeners about their response being "correct" on one third of the trials. After this type of listening practice, frequency and intensity discrimination can improve even though the stimuli during the training do not differ in either frequency or intensity. No such improvements were apparent in a control groups of listeners who did not receive any training (Halliday, Moore, Taylor, & Amitay, 2011). The degree of improvement can be similar to that apparent in listeners who receive an adaptive type of training to improve frequency discrimination where frequency of the comparison stimulus is changed relative to that of the standard tone depending on a listener's response (Amitay, Irwin, & Moore, 2006). If two groups of monolingual listeners are presented with words in a non-native language, the group who is instructed to attend to consonants shows posttraining improvement in consonant perception. The group of listeners instructed to attend to vowels do not show similar improvements in consonant perception (Pederson & Guion-Anderson, 2010). Such results show that direction of attention through instructions to specific stimulus features can improve the perception of that feature. Some tasks, such as the Test of Attention in Listening (TAIL), which measures reaction time during temporal and spectral processing of auditory stimuli, may be useful in identifying and separating the contribution of different components of attention to auditory perception (Zhang, Barry, Moore, & Amitay, 2012).

8.2.6 Principles for Efficient Auditory Training

It is important to consider the specific needs of each patient. Individual patients may be affected differently by their specific auditory processing difficulties. For example, a classroom teacher who has an APD may struggle to understand a student sitting at a distance in a noisy classroom. A retired older individual may struggle to enjoy television or music. Training should be designed with consideration to how the specific deficits uncovered during testing may affect participation in regular life activities and how the deficits can be addressed to meet the specific needs of the patient.

Stimuli

Stimuli should be designed to address each deficit discovered through the assessment process. For speech stimuli, the stimuli should include the smallest phonemic units and, as necessary, larger units, including sentences and paragraphs. If deficits are known for differentiating specific phonemes, the practice should focus on these phonemes. The practice stimuli should be large in number and should be spoken by various speakers, including male and female talkers, across younger and older age spans. In some cases, specific stimuli, such as the spoken words of a significant family member, should be incorporated in the background of noises typically occurring in the patient's household.

Whenever possible, it is important to maintain stimulus novelty. Novel stimuli can challenge the brain and force it to work in new ways through remodeling of existing circuits and building new pathways for processing information.

Procedure

Training can begin with easier stimuli and processes to ensure success. However, it can rapidly proceed to more difficult processes and stimuli, as exposure to and training at more difficult levels can lead to faster learning for easier stimuli and processes.

The stimulus presentation should be adjusted in such a way that the task is challenging enough to minimize boredom, but it should not be so difficult that it is discouraging or frustrating. Performance should be maintained in such a way that the response accuracy is between 50 and 80%. If the performance is below 50%, the stimuli should be changed to make the perception easier; if the performance is closer to 80%, the stimuli should be changed to make the perception more difficult. Deficit-specific training sessions can be conducted in parallel to each other, which can be helpful in minimizing boredom and can simultaneously improve performance on various tasks. During adaptive training tasks, some listeners can learn the adaptive strategy and improve their performance by guessing. For such listeners, constant (non-adaptive) stimulus trials should be interspersed to ensure that their performance is actually improving on the specific task. Although some transfer of training can occur on untrained tasks, greater improvements have been reported on tasks that are similar to those used during testing (Barcroft et al., 2011).

Feedback

When the participant is performing very poorly, use of feedback can be detrimental, as the listener is told that he or she is wrong as often as he or she is informed that the response is correct. Once the listener becomes more comfortable with the task and begins to perform better, feedback may be helpful. Also, not all listeners can use feedback to improve their performance effectively (Campbell & Small, 1963). If feedback is provided, it should be given immediately after the response to each stimulus. In the presence of incorrect responses, the correct response should be modeled.

Reinforcement

Some form of reinforcement should be built into the training session to ensure continuous practice with the task. During live training tasks, verbal reinforcements can often be sufficient for children.

Training Duration

Training duration should be based on achievement of optimum possible performance within a session and across sessions to maximize the benefit and effectiveness of training. Participants who take an extended rest break early while learning a keyboard melody showed the largest improvement in performance compared to those who took a break later during practice or those who did not take any break (Duke, Allen, Cash, & Simmons, 2009). The rest periods can provide time for consolidation of the neurophysiological processes involved in the trained task and can improve the possibility of generalization to untrained tasks and visual modality. For example, training on an auditory discrimination task can improve both auditory and visual discrimination performance after a rest period, and the consolidation effect is larger with a rest period of 24 hours compared to a rest period of 5 minutes (Bratzke, Schröter, & Ulrich, 2013). Continuous accumulation of improvement over days on auditory discrimination tasks may require some critical training duration per day, which may be dependent on the particular skill that is being trained. For example, improvements in gap-detection discrimination can occur with 360 training trials per day, whereas more daily trials may be needed to improve frequency discrimination (Wright & Sabin, 2007).

With extensive training beyond the achievement of optimal performance, performance can deteriorate. The worsening of performance may be related to overstimulation of the specific neural circuits used in performing the task (Huyck & Wright, 2013). An example of initial improvement

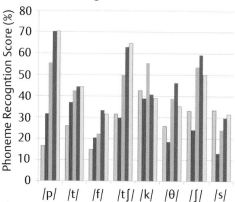

- Simulated high frequency loss no AE
- Simulated high frequency loss with AE (pretraining)
- Post training 15 minutes
- Post training 30 minutes
- Post training 45 minutes

Fig. 8.4 Effect of duration of auditory training on normal listeners with simulated high-frequency hearing loss with and without audibility extender (AE) and after training with AE. In most cases, maximum improvement in phoneme recognition is apparent with 15 or 30 minutes of training. Additional training can degrade performance due to fatigue or motivation factors, as apparent for /θ/ and /ʃ/ (based on Korhonen & Kuk, 2008).

and later deterioration of performance with auditory training designed to improve phoneme recognition with a linear frequency transposition technique is shown in ▶ Fig. 8.4. The linear frequency transposition technique referred to as audibility extender (AE) is designed to improve audibility of high-frequency sounds in the presence of severe to profound high-frequency hearing loss. The technique captures a selected region of high-frequency spectrum and lowers the frequency of that spectrum. The lowered portion of the signal is then mixed with the original unprocessed signal. ▶ Fig. 8.4 shows the performance of normal-hearing listeners with simulated high-frequency loss and with AE after training. Depending on the particular phoneme, maximum performance is apparent after 15 or 30 minutes after training. In some cases, the (/k/, /θ/, /s/) performance deteriorates after additional training (Korhonen & Kuk, 2008), probably because of fatigue or reduced motivation.

Some investigators have used specific criteria to determine if the training should continue. For example, the following criteria can be used to determine if training should continue:

1. Low-level achievement: The performance is lower than the 20th percentile performance of age-matched peers.
2. Unstable performance: The performance in one of the last two training sessions is below that of the previous session.
3. Maximum possible achievement not reached: The performance is showing continuous improvement without any plateau (Schäffler, Sonntag, Hartnegg, & Fischer, 2004).

8.2.7 Auditory Training in the Presence of Hearing Loss

Before providing auditory training to individuals with hearing loss who also have APDs, it is important that an attempt is made to provide maximum audibility through the use of the technology that is most suitable for the particular patient (Kuk & Keenan, 2010). Also, if real ear measures are not performed for hearing aid fittings, unexpected notches can remain in the frequency response that can produce artificial difficulties in processing some of the speech sounds.

8.2.8 Generalization

The ultimate goal of auditory training is to improve the function of the client in real-life situations where processing of various sounds, including speech, is required. For special populations such as children with comorbid language impairment or dyslexia or attention deficits, auditory training can bring improvements in language, reading, and attention skills. In this context, skills obtained during auditory training can be expected to generalize or have a positive impact on language acquisition, reading skills, and auditory attention skills.

Generalization of Auditory Training to Language and Reading Skills

Improvement on training for auditory tasks such as frequency discrimination, intensity discrimination, and gap detection can transfer to language-related skill and improve spelling skills in children who make spelling errors due to APDs (Schäffler et al., 2004). In another study, a 3-hour intervention game designed for improving phonological awareness enhanced reading skills and neural processing accuracy (Lovio, Halttunen, Lyytinen, Näätänen, & Kujala, 2012).

Another study demonstrated that training incorporating auditory-visual sequences of nonlinguistic stimuli that closely imitate skills required during reading without the semantic processing required during reading can improve reading skills of children with reading difficulties. In this study, children were given feedback on the accuracy of their performance during training trials. Such training can also enhance the auditory mismatch negativity response, suggesting plastic changes within the auditory system accompanying improvements in reading skills (Kujala et al., 2001).

Generalization of the Benefit of Auditory Training to the Cognitive Domain

The benefit of training designed to enhance the perception of auditory stimuli along with auditory-visual stimuli can transfer to the cognitive domain. In one study, older adults were trained with the use of the Brain Fitness (BF) video game (PositScience.com, Posit Science Corp., San Francisco, CA), which, like training software, focuses on adaptive learning. Following the training, participants' everyday problem-solving and reasoning skills were found to be enhanced without any specific training for these abilities. Such findings suggest that auditory perceptual training may be a good strategy for minimizing cognitive aging (Strenziok et al., 2014). In another study, similar training showed significant improvements in memory, whereas no improvements in memory were apparent in active or no-contact control groups (Mahncke et al., 2006).

Generalization of the Benefit of Modified Speech Training to Duration Discrimination

A somewhat reverse effect is also possible, where training using modified speech stimuli can improve duration discrimination ability for tonal stimuli (Agnew, Dorn, & Eden, 2004). In this study, the speech modification involved time expansion and amplification of the most rapidly changing aspects of speech stimuli to improve their salience. The modified speech was embedded in computer games. During training, the speech rate and volume of the consonant vowel (CV) syllables were adaptively moved toward those found in normal speech (Tallal et al., 1996).

Generalization from Trained to Untrained Nonlinguistic Stimuli and Features

At a more basic level, generalization can occur from one trained stimulus to another untrained stimulus. For example, frequency discrimination can be improved with training by using a stimulus frequency of 1000 Hz and other stimuli differing slightly around 1000 Hz (e.g., 1002 or 1004 Hz). The improvement in discrimination can generalize to other untrained frequencies, such as 4000 Hz, and to the untrained ear. In some cases, the generalization can be complete in the sense that the same degree of improvement is apparent for untrained stimuli when compared to that apparent for trained stimuli. In other cases, the improvement is partial, so that the improvement for trained stimuli is greater than that apparent for untrained stimuli. There can also be individual variability in the degree of generalization (Delhommeau, Micheyl, & Jouvent, 2005; Delhommeau, Micheyl, Jouvent, & Collet, 2002). Generalization of frequency discrimination skills to untrained stimuli may depend on the type of stimuli used during training (Demany & Semal, 2002) and may be reflected in steeper slopes or faster learning during training of untrained stimuli.

Generalization may not occur for certain stimulus features, such as gap duration, suggesting the need for specific training for target gap durations. Gap duration discrimination thresholds can improve in many participants when they are expected to discriminate between a standard gap of 100 ms marked by short 1 kHz tone pips and a comparison gap. There is some individual variability in the amount of improvement, and the improvement can generalize to a similar 100 ms gap that is marked by tones of different frequencies, such as 4 or 3.75 kHz. However, the learning does not always transfer to a different standard gap duration of 50, 200, or 500 ms (Karmarkar & Buonomano, 2003; Wright et al., 1997). Similarly, the minimum gap that can be detected between narrowband noises of different frequencies improves with training but does not generalize to gaps between untrained stimulus pairs (Avivi-Reich, Arnott, Tavares, & Schneider, 2013).

Generalization of Auditory Perceptual Learning to Visual Modality

Some investigators have demonstrated that gap duration discrimination can generalize to visual modality, thus showing cross-modal transfer (Bratzke, Seifried, & Ulrich, 2012).

Assessment of Generalization

The extent of generalization to untrained stimuli can be assessed using various stimulus and training paradigms, as shown in ▶ Fig. 8.5. The addition of a control group of participants who undergo testing but do not receive any training can allow an estimate of the amount of training that can occur as a result of testing.

8.2.9 Music Training

The processing of music and speech requires similar sensory processing, or bottom-up skills, such as encoding of pitch, rhythm, and different auditory streams (▶ Fig. 8.6). With reference to rhythm, there is a strong association between music and word stress perception in adults who reported that they had normal hearing (Hausen, Torppa, Salmela, Vainio, & Särkämö, 2013). In addition, similar top-bottom skills are required, including recognizing syntactic violations in music or spoken language, holding and manipulating auditory percepts in working memory, and selectively attending to relevant auditory percepts among a background of several auditory stimuli (reviewed in Shahin, 2011).

Musicians show better speech recognition in noise than nonmusicians (Parbery-Clark et al., 2009). The mismatch negativity response to pure tones, music, and speech occurs earlier in musicians than nonmusicians (Nikjeh, Lister, & Frisch, 2009), and its amplitude is larger in musicians compared to nonmusicians when participants are asked to pay attention to speech stimuli (Tervaniemi et al., 2009).

Persons with congenital amusia, a musical disorder that appears mainly as a defect in processing pitch, but also encompasses musical memory and recognition, tend to have subtle deficits in speech processing that are reflected in below-average phonological awareness (Jones, Lucker, Zalewski, Brewer, & Drayna, 2009), difficulties in recognizing emotions through prosodic variations (Thompson, Marin, & Stewart, 2012), and poor speech intonation perception (Patel, Wong, Foxton, Lochy, & Peretz, 2008).

When allowed to sing along with an auditory model while learning novel songs, patients with aphasia (the loss of ability to process speech) can repeat and recall more words than when they are allowed to speak in unison with an auditory model (Racette, Bard, & Peretz, 2006). Longitudinal studies in which children are assigned to either a music or other training group suggest that music training enhances speech-processing skills in the presence of background interference. For example, in one study performed over a duration of 2 years, 8-year-old children were arbitrarily assigned to either music or painting training. Their ability to extract nonwords from a continuous flow of non-sense syllables was evaluated before and after training. The performance on this task was similar in the two groups before training. After training, only the group with music training showed improvement in their speech segregation skills (François, Chobert, Besson, & Schön, 2012). In another similar study, improvement in preattentive processing of syllabic duration and voice onset time, as reflected in greater amplitude of the mismatch negativity response, was found after 12 months of training in only the group with music training (Chobert, François, Velay, & Besson, 2012).

In summary, current evidence suggests that skills acquired through musical training may transfer to and thus improve speech perception, especially under degraded listening conditions, such as the presence of background noise or reverberation, possibly due to a shared auditory neural network and generalization of bottom-up and top-down processing skills. The ability of music to improve central auditory fitness is considered similar to the ability of exercise to improve physical fitness (Kraus & Chandrasekaran, 2010). Thus, musical training may serve as an important tool for improving listening abilities of individuals with APDs.

Caution about Music Training

Just as excessive physical exercise can lead to physical injury, overexposure to loud music can lead to injury to the ear or hearing loss. Musicians are considered at risk for hearing loss depending on several factors, including the type of instrument played, the loudness of the instrument, and the hours of exposure to music. Rawool (2012) has provided a review of these factors and strategies for minimizing hearing loss. In providing music lessons or during music practice, it is important to

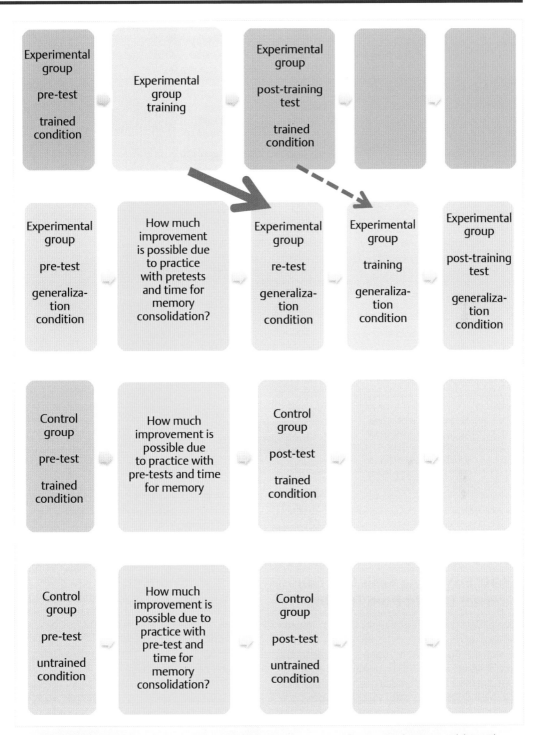

Fig. 8.5 Methods for assessment of generalization of training. Blue arrows indicate generalization possibilities. The dotted arrow indicates that generalization may be demonstrated during training on the generalization conditions by rapid learning, as suggested by reduced training time or steeper learning curves. The control group does not receive training.

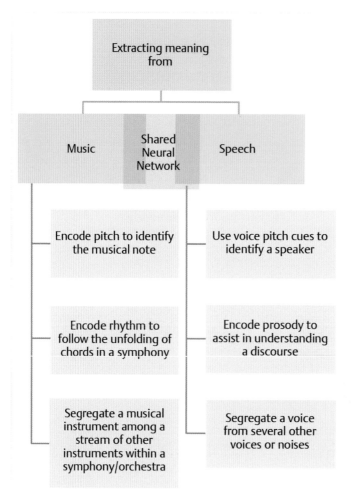

Fig. 8.6 Common aspects of processing music and speech.

keep the loudness of the music well within safe levels, or below 85 dB(A).

8.2.10 Enhancing Skills that Can Augment Benefit from Training

If the patient has some attributes that can impede learning, addressing these attributes can improve the benefit drawn from training. For example, some children with ADHD can show impulsive response behavior during training, which is indicated by a high false-alarm rate. In false alarms, also referred to as commission errors, the participant indicates the presence of a stimulus in the absence of stimulus presentation. The false-alarm rate of children on a task involving the detection of tones in the presence of contralateral noise can be reduced through adaptive training with visual feedback on performance (Gray, Miller, & Evans, 2012).

There is considerable variability in the attentiveness of children with ADHD. Thus, some children with ADHD may benefit from training that is designed to ignore distracting sounds, in addition to training to improve focus on sounds that are of significance, such as teacher's voice. In this case, in addition to focusing on the teacher's voice, the child is expected to ignore other distracting stimuli occurring in the classroom. Some children with ADHD may benefit from training designed to improve their ability to use other cognitive resources, such as sustained auditory attention or auditory vigilance.

8.3 Top-Down Training

As shown in ▶ Fig. 8.2, improving cognitive, and linguistic skills can help children process auditory stimuli.

8.3.1 Attention

Auditory vigilance or sustained auditory attention refers to the ability to sustain attention to auditory stimuli over a relatively long period of time. When normal-hearing listeners listen to lectures, they are able to attend to and understand the key points of the lecture. Individuals with APDs may have difficulty in attending to a lecture over an entire class period due to the difficulties they face in processing auditory stimuli. Improvement in auditory vigilance skill can enhance their auditory attention skills or allow them to attend a variety of lectures through the day without excessive fatigue. Selective attention is specifically important in understanding speech in noisy surroundings, and both ignoring the background noise and focusing attention on the speech signal can enhance speech recognition in noise.

Attention is important during auditory training activities. If a child is not attending to the auditory stimuli that are delivered to him or her during perceptual training sessions, the training may not be as effective as when the child is paying attention. During auditory training, various techniques can be used to ensure that maximum attention is devoted to the delivered stimuli. For example, the child may be required to indicate readiness by saying "ready" or by raising his or her hand, or in computer-based training, by clicking on yes or no on screen. Reinforcements for correct responses can also enhance attention.

Some computer-based interventions that are designed to improve listening and language skills can enhance neural mechanisms of selective auditory attention that may be deficient in some children, including those with specific language impairment (Stevens, Fanning, Coch, Sanders, & Neville, 2008). In this particular intervention, the training involved paying attention to several auditory stimuli. Although training using auditory stimuli is likely to be more beneficial for children with APDs, attention can also be enhanced using visual stimuli and may be beneficial in the presence of comorbid deficits, including reading difficulties.

Relatively short duration training using visual stimuli can lead to improvement in behavioral and neural measures of attention in typically developing preschoolers, and the benefits of training can generalize to measures of nonverbal intelligence (Rueda, Rothbart, McCandliss, Saccomanno, & Posner, 2005). Adolescents with dyslexia show greater benefits from a 10-week writing intervention if they first receive 10 weeks of training designed to enhance their attention skills (Chenault, Thomson, Abbott, & Berninger, 2006). Visual attention therapy programs that stress various aspects of arousal, activation, and vigilance have been noted to be effective in improving attention and reading comprehension in children with reading deficits. In this case, five attention-enhancing programs involving perceptual accuracy, visual efficiency, visual search, visual scan, and visual span were used (Solan, Shelley-Tremblay, Ficarra, Silverman, & Larson, 2003). Computerized programs such as Computerized Progressive Attentional Training (CPAT) are available for improving attention. The CPAT program includes four sets of tasks that are designed to improve sustained attention, selective attention, orientation of attention, and executive attention. Following training with the program, parents of young children with ADHD report a significant reduction in inattentiveness, and the benefits of training generalize to reading comprehension and passage-copying skills (Shalev, Tsal, & Mevorach, 2007).

8.3.2 Working Memory

Working memory is the ability to store and manipulate information temporarily. For example, during a working memory task, the child may be presented with three numbers and a little later is asked to repeat the numbers in reverse order. Thus, the child has to remember the numbers and manipulate the order of the numbers. Various other procedures are used for assessing working memory, as shown in ▶ Fig. 8.7, ▶ Fig. 8.8, and ▶ Fig. 8.9. In many of these procedures, the number of units that can be accurately stored and manipulated in the memory and the reaction time are recorded as a variation of task difficulty. The tasks can be made harder in various ways, including by increasing the length of the stimuli and the interstimulus time interval.

Working Memory Model

A proposed model of working memory has three or four major components (▶ Fig. 8.10). A key component is the executive function, which is an attentionally limited control system that integrates feedback from the auditory-articulatory phonological loop and the vision-based visuospatial sketch pad. The executive system assists in the manipulation of stimuli that are temporarily stored on the visuospatial sketch pad or within the phonological

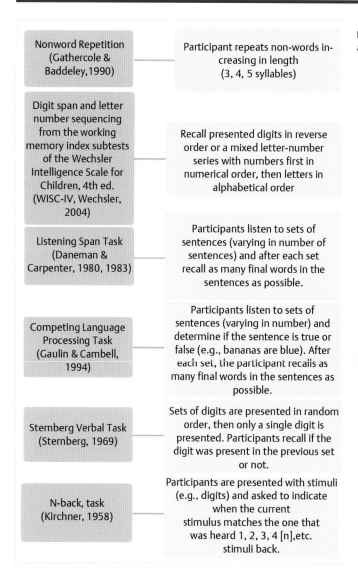

Nonword Repetition (Gathercole & Baddeley, 1990)	Participant repeats non-words increasing in length (3, 4, 5 syllables)
Digit span and letter number sequencing from the working memory index subtests of the Wechsler Intelligence Scale for Children, 4th ed. (WISC-IV, Wechsler, 2004)	Recall presented digits in reverse order or a mixed letter-number series with numbers first in numerical order, then letters in alphabetical order
Listening Span Task (Daneman & Carpenter, 1980, 1983)	Participants listen to sets of sentences (varying in number of sentences) and after each set recall as many final words in the sentences as possible.
Competing Language Processing Task (Gaulin & Cambell, 1994)	Participants listen to sets of sentences (varying in number) and determine if the sentence is true or false (e.g., bananas are blue). After each set, the participant recalls as many final words in the sentences as possible.
Sternberg Verbal Task (Sternberg, 1969)	Sets of digits are presented in random order, then only a single digit is presented. Participants recall if the digit was present in the previous set or not.
N-back, task (Kirchner, 1958)	Participants are presented with stimuli (e.g., digits) and asked to indicate when the current stimulus matches the one that was heard 1, 2, 3, 4 [n], etc. stimuli back.

Fig. 8.7 Examples of tools used for assessing auditory working memory.

loop. The phonological loop has two subcomponents. There is a temporary storage component, which holds memory traces over a brief period during which the traces can decay unless refreshed by a second subcomponent involving subvocal rehearsal. For those items that can be named, subvocal rehearsal is used in preventing the decay of items in the visuospatial store or sketch pad (Baddeley, 2003; Baddeley & Hitch, 1974). Through subvocal rehearsals, the items can be stored in the long-term memory and be used for understanding spoken messages and visual gestures, as well as for learning language and reading skills.

As shown in ▶ Fig. 8.10, in children with visual impairments or blindness, tactile input (e.g.,

feeling of lip movements or vocal cord vibrations) may have an important role in language comprehension and braille reading (Cohen, Scherzer, Viau, Voss, & Lepore, 2011). In children with hearing loss or APDs, kinesthetic input provided by articulatory structures may play an important role in the subvocal rehearsal component of the phonological loop of working memory, especially for visually presented stimuli. In children who are deaf and blind or have both visual and auditory processing deficits, both tactile and kinesthetic input may have a prominent role.

Although a complex neural network, including the cerebellum, is involved in working memory, the phonological loop is expected to recruit

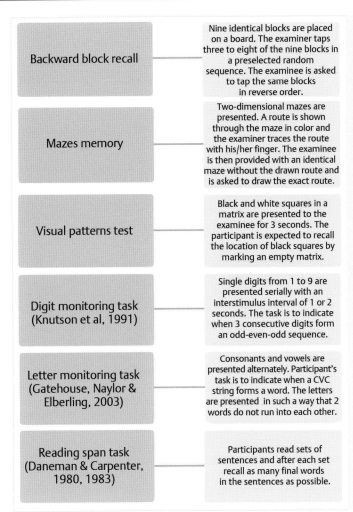

Fig. 8.8 Examples of tools used for assessing visuospatial working memory.

Task	Description
Backward block recall	Nine identical blocks are placed on a board. The examiner taps three to eight of the nine blocks in a preselected random sequence. The examinee is asked to tap the same blocks in reverse order.
Mazes memory	Two-dimensional mazes are presented. A route is shown through the maze in color and the examiner traces the route with his/her finger. The examinee is then provided with an identical maze without the drawn route and is asked to draw the exact route.
Visual patterns test	Black and white squares in a matrix are presented to the examinee for 3 seconds. The participant is expected to recall the location of black squares by marking an empty matrix.
Digit monitoring task (Knutson et al, 1991)	Single digits from 1 to 9 are presented serially with an interstimulus interval of 1 or 2 seconds. The task is to indicate when 3 consecutive digits form an odd-even-odd sequence.
Letter monitoring task (Gatehouse, Naylor & Elberling, 2003)	Consonants and vowels are presented alternately. Participant's task is to indicate when a CVC string forms a word. The letters are presented in such a way that 2 words do not run into each other.
Reading span task (Daneman & Carpenter, 1980, 1983)	Participants read sets of sentences and after each set recall as many final words in the sentences as possible.

regions primarily in the language-dominant left hemisphere, including the temperoparietal region and the Broca's area. The visuospatial sketch pad is expected to activate the related regions predominantly in the right hemisphere, including the frontoparietal and occipital cortices (Smith & Jonides, 1997; Smith, Jonides, & Koeppe, 1996). The central executive function is mostly mediated by the prefrontal cortex (Kane & Engle, 2002; Smith & Jonides, 1998). More specifically, verbal content activates the left midlateral prefrontal cortex, and spatial content activates the caudal superior frontal sulcus (Nee et al., 2013). Two concurrent verbal and spatial working memory tasks may be coordinated by the dorsal lateral prefrontal cortex (D'Esposito et al., 1995).

During working memory tasks, electroencephalographic (EEG) rhythms appear distributed over several brain regions. The amplitudes of the theta (θ) rhythm in the frontal lobe increase during the manipulation of items in short-term memory. The amplitude of the alpha (α) rhythm in the temporal areas during auditory working memory tasks and parietal areas during verbal working memory tasks increases during both the storage and manipulation periods. Phase synchronization analyses suggest that the task-relevant brain areas are coordinated by local (auditory or visuospatial) alpha synchronization during the memory storage buffer stage, by distant theta synchronization for central executive function, and by coupling of the theta and alpha rhythms for interfunctional integration (Kawasaki, Kitajo, & Yamaguchi, 2010). Thus, synchronization of oscillatory phases between two different brain regions may have an important role in working memory (Fell & Axmacher, 2011). The central executive may dynamically control which memory units should be synchronized for

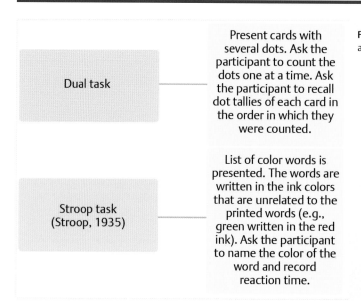

Present cards with several dots. Ask the participant to count the dots one at a time. Ask the participant to recall dot tallies of each card in the order in which they were counted.

List of color words is presented. The words are written in the ink colors that are unrelated to the printed words (e.g., green written in the red ink). Ask the participant to name the color of the word and record reaction time.

Fig. 8.9 Examples of tools used to assess executive working memory.

processing and which units should be out of phase, thus putting the encoded memory for those units on standby for later processing as necessary (Chik, 2013).

Deficient Working Memory

Many individuals with APDs have difficulty understanding speech in degraded listening environments. The ability to recognize speech in noisy backgrounds is related to working memory. Hearing-impaired individuals with poor working memory have more difficulty in recognizing speech in complex noisy backgrounds than those with better working memory (Gatehouse, Naylor, & Elberling, 2003; Lunner & Sundewall-Thorén, 2007). Listeners with better working memory capacity find listening in noise less effortful than individuals with lower working memory capacity (Rudner, Lunner, Behrens, Thorén, & Rönnberg, 2012).

In children with APDs, the auditory input part of the working memory model (▶ Fig. 8.10) is deficient, which may disrupt accurate and consistent subvocal rehearsal, thereby leading to deficits in working memory, which in turn could lead to language and/or reading deficits. A weak to moderate correlation has been reported between the short-term and working memory components of the Test of Auditory Perceptual Skills–Revised (TAPS-R) test results and the dichotic digits and pitch pattern sequence test scores (Wilson et al., 2011). Auditory memory deficits can occur in 73.4% of children who are considered at risk for APDs

(Yathiraj & Maggu, 2013). Children with specific language impairments suffer from working memory deficits possibly due to impairment in the phonological storage component of the loop. More specifically, they show deficits in the ability to hear and repeat back nonwords (Gathercole & Baddeley, 1990; Montgomery, 2003). Some children with language impairments can show deficits in the central executive function in addition to the phonological loop (Pickering & Gathercole, 2004). About two thirds of the children with very poor working memory have difficulty with reading and mathematics. One third of the children with very poor working memory need additional classroom support (Alloway, Gathercole, Kirkwood, & Elliott, 2009).

Verbal and visuospatial memory deficits have been noted in patients with aphasia and associated left hemisphere lesions (Kasselimi et al., 2013). Children who have aphasia or apraxia cannot perform subvocal rehearsals due to impairments in the speech-motor system, which impedes their working memory (Caplan & Waters, 1995; Martins & Ortiz, 2009). Children with reading disabilities show reduced verbal working memory (Kibby & Cohen, 2008). Deficient working memory has been noted in approximately one third of children with ADHD (Coghill, Seth, & Matthews, 2013). In children who have comorbid deficits (e.g., attention deficit and reading disabilities), more than one component of the working memory circuit may be deficient (Kibby & Cohen, 2008). Children with general learning difficulties, including difficulties

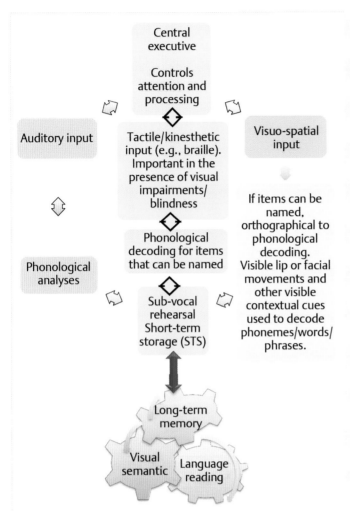

Fig. 8.10 Working memory model and the connection of working memory to language and reading skills (adapted from Baddley, 2003, and Baddley & Hicks, 1974).

with literacy and mathematics, perform poorly in all components of working memory (Pickering & Gathercole, 2004).

Training to Improve Working Memory

Several strategies can be used to allow children to continue to learn language, reading, and other skills in the presence of poor working memory, as outlined in ▶ Fig. 8.11. In addition, several procedures can be used to improve working memory, depending on the component that is deficient, as shown in ▶ Fig. 8.12. Efficient training appears to be successful in improving working memory at least in some individuals. For example, preterm-born preschoolers with very low birth weight benefit from a computerized working memory training program that is offered over 5 weeks, with a training period of 10 to 15 minutes daily except for weekends (Grunewaldt, Løhaugen, Austeng, Brubakk, & Skranes, 2013). Adolescents with extremely low birth weights also show improvement in working memory following computerized training, and the improvement is maintained for at least 6 months (Løhaugen et al., 2011).

The success of computerized training programs may depend on the types of stimuli and tasks included in the program and the specific population undergoing training. For example, the Cogmed RoboMemo (Cogmed RM from Pearson Education Inc., New York, NY) computerized training program can improve verbal and nonverbal working memory storage but may not generalize to other domains of functions, such as manipulation of stimulus items stored in the memory (Chacko

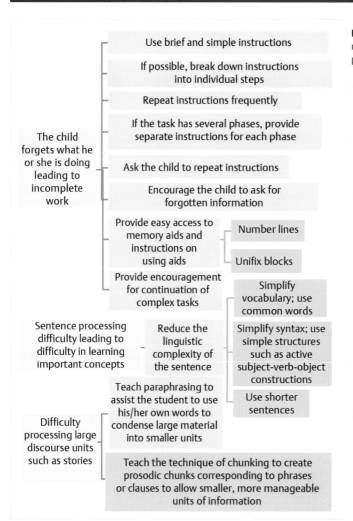

Fig. 8.11 Management strategies for reducing working memory loads in the presence of working memory deficits.

The child forgets what he or she is doing leading to incomplete work
- Use brief and simple instructions
- If possible, break down instructions into individual steps
- Repeat instructions frequently
- If the task has several phases, provide separate instructions for each phase
- Ask the child to repeat instructions
- Encourage the child to ask for forgotten information
- Provide easy access to memory aids and instructions on using aids
  - Number lines
  - Unifix blocks
- Provide encouragement for continuation of complex tasks

Sentence processing difficulty leading to difficulty in learning important concepts
- Reduce the linguistic complexity of the sentence
  - Simplify vocabulary; use common words
  - Simplify syntax; use simple structures such as active subject-verb-object constructions
  - Use shorter sentences

Difficulty processing large discourse units such as stories
- Teach paraphrasing to assist the student to use his/her own words to condense large material into smaller units
- Teach the technique of chunking to create prosodic chunks corresponding to phrases or clauses to allow smaller, more manageable units of information

et al., 2013) or classroom activities that tax working memory (Dunning, Holmes, & Gathercole, 2013). Other studies have suggested that the training program improves processing speed in children with ADHD, and the training effect may be accompanied by long-lasting improvement in reading in children (Egeland, Aarlien, & Saunes, 2013). The Cogmed RM computerized training program appears to be focused on improving visuospatial working memory perhaps because visuospatial deficits can be addressed more easily with computers compared to auditory working memory training. Inclusion of auditory working memory exercises in the training program may minimize learning or language delays in children with working memory deficits.

Working memory deficits following traumatic brain injury can be addressed using computerized working memory training. Structured and intensive computerized working memory training can improve cognitive function with related improvement in occupational performance and overall health in patients with acquired traumatic brain injuries (Lundqvist, Grundström, Samuelsson, & Rönnberg, 2010). A systematic review similarly suggests that persons with stroke may benefit from specific executive function training and may learn compensatory strategies to minimize the functional consequences of deficient executive function (Poulin, Korner-Bitensky, Dawson, & Bherer, 2012). Some of the compensatory strategies that may be useful are task-specific checklists and the Neuropage (Hersh & Treadgold, 1994) cueing system. With Neuropage, the pager sends electronic prompts to complete self-selected tasks, such as taking medications, watering plants, and

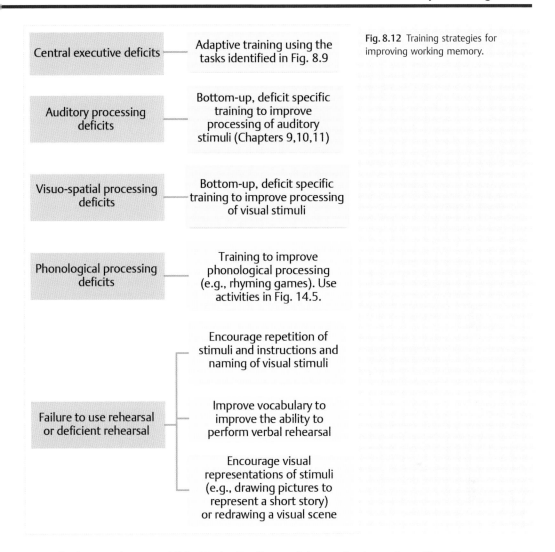

Fig. 8.12 Training strategies for improving working memory.

remembering appointments (Fish, Manly, Emslie, Evans, & Wilson, 2008). In addition to providing direct reminders, the paging system can trigger a process of goal monitoring that bridges the gap between intention and action (Fish, Manly, & Wilson, 2008). In cases of more severe memory impairments, the use of a wearable camera such as Microsoft's SenseCam or Google glasses may allow the automatic capture of daily events that can be watched by the patient later to refresh and consolidate the memory (Berry et al., 2007), although the legality of all such recordings is questionable.

Cognitive plasticity is apparent over a relatively large older age span and can be used to improve working memory deficits in older adults. Training for improving all three components of working memory—visuospatial, verbal, and executive—for 9 sessions distributed over a period of 3 weeks in adults ranging in age from 65 to 95 years can lead to significant improvements in all three areas. In addition, the improvements appear to transfer to a fluid intelligence task, and the training outcomes remain stable for a period of at least 9 months (Zinke et al., 2014). Depending on the specific tasks used in training, younger adults may show greater improvement in working memory compared to older adults (Heinzel et al., 2014). Audio-based personal memory aids can be helpful in improving the memory of auditory stimuli that occur over a long duration, such as lectures and seminars. Such memory prostheses record audio and contextual information and provide different retrieval tools to improve the accuracy and completeness of recall (Hayes et al., 2004; Vemuri, Schmandt, Bender, Tellex, & Lassey, 2004), although the legality of some of the recordings is questionable.

Transcranial Direct Current Stimulation (tDCS)

If transcranial direct current stimulation (tDCS) is applied during completion of the n-back working memory task (▶ Fig. 8.7), significantly greater improvement is apparent on the digit span forward task, compared with tDCS applied while at rest and sham tDCS during the n-back task. Similar improvements are not apparent with the digit span backward tasks (Andrews, Hoy, Enticott, Daskalakis, & Fitzgerald, 2011). Adults over the age of 65 years appear to benefit from 10 sessions of computer-assisted cognitive training combined with tDCS of the bilateral prefrontal cortex, as indicated by significant improvement in verbal working memory, with the effect lasting for at least 4 weeks following training (Park, Seo, Kim, & Ko, 2014).

The effect of tDCS depends on the polarity of the electrode. Anodal polarization generally increases cortical excitability, and cathodal polarization decreases it. The effect may also depend on the duration, the specific areas selected for receiving stimulation, and the particular tasks employed during stimulation. For example, anodal tDCS of the left dorsolateral prefrontal cortex can lead to faster reaction times for naming of pictures at the end of stimulation in young healthy adults, while cathodal tDCS has no effect (Fertonani, Rosini, Cotelli, Rossini, & Miniussi, 2010). In one study, working memory performance on a 3(n)-back task improved only after 20 minutes of stimulation to the left prefrontal cortex, with further improvement apparent after 30 minutes of stimulation (Ohn et al., 2008). In another study, 15-minute bilateral cathodal or anodal stimulation during a visual Sternberg task over two frontolateral (F3 and F4) locations did not improve performance and resulted in slower reaction times possibly due to interference with the oscillatory EEG activity, such as theta (Marshall, Molle, Siebner, & Born, 2005). Application of the tDCS over other areas, such as the cerebellum, can impair the practice-dependent proficiency increase in verbal working memory (Ferruci et al., 2008). Brain lesions can occur at high current densities and longer durations possibly because of burning of brain tissue. The size of lesions increases linearly with charge density (Liebetanz et al., 2009). Thus, caution is necessary in using higher tDCS in children (Kessler et al., 2013).

Self-Regulation through Real-Time Functional Magnetic Resonance Imaging

Some studies have reported the use of real-time functional magnetic resonance imaging (fMRI) techniques to allow listeners to control localized brain activation. More specifically, the real-time fMRI technique locates a region of interest using high spatial resolution and provides the blood oxygenation level–dependent (BOLD) signal in the region of interest in real time to guide participants in self-regulating brain activation. In one study, the real-time fMRI technique was used to train subjects to increase the activation significantly in the left dorsolateral prefrontal cortex (DLPFC), which is linked to verbal working memory (Zhang, Yao, Zhang, Long, & Zhao, 2013). No such increase in DLPFC activation was apparent in the control group that received sham feedback/training. The increased activation was accompanied by a significantly larger improvement in the digit span tasks following training in the experimental group when compared to that apparent in the control group. These preliminary findings suggest that working memory performance can be improved through learned regulation of activation in associated brain regions using real-time fMRI. For regular clinical applications, optimal timing, delay and presentation of feedback, use of conscious strategies to maximize benefit from feedback, long-term effectiveness, and cost-effectiveness of the techniques need to be evaluated (Weiskopf, 2012). Further studies are necessary to investigate if increased activation in certain areas is accompanied by decreased activation of other areas that may be important for tasks, such as reading.

8.3.3 Auditory Closure

Auditory closure refers to the ability to fill in missing elements in a message by making use of available cues. To achieve closure, several cues can be used by the listener, including syntactic, semantic, and contextual cues. For example, in the sentence "I went to the mall for __opping," most listeners can easily fill in the missing *sh* based on vocabulary, world knowledge, and semantic cues. Similarly, in the sentence "While climbing down the stairs, __ dropped her toy," the missing word *she* is predictable based on syntactic cues. If a parent is showing a picture to a child and says that the fish is swimming in the ocean, and the child fails to hear the word *fish,* based on contextual cues of where the ocean is and the fact that there is nothing else in the ocean, the child will be able to guess that the parent was talking about the fish.

Assessment of Closure

Filtered or interrupted speech (see Chapter 7) can be used to assess spectral or temporal closure skills. A more common way to assess closure skills is to determine the ability to recognize speech in noise. Masking effects determined using traditional broadband masking noises are referred to as *energetic masking,* which reflects the limits of cochlear processing (Fletcher, 1940). Depending on the type of target speech stimuli, maskers comprising of two or three different talkers can increase the difficulty in recognizing target speech due to the target–masker similarity. This *informational* or *perceptual masking* (Carhart, Tillman, & Greetis, 1969) reduces the listener's ability to segregate the speech target from the speech masker.

Speech Perception in Noise

In the revised Speech Perception in Noise (SPIN) test, multitalker babble is used as the masker. Listeners are expected to repeat the last word in the sentence. Half of the sentences allow prediction of the last word due to syntactic, semantic, and prosodic cues. For example, in the sentence "Let's decide by tossing a coin," the target word *coin* is highly predictable. The target words in the remaining half of the sentences are not predictable. For example, the word *coin* in the sentence "Jane has a problem with the coin" is not predictable (Bilger, 1984; Bilger, Nuetzel, Rabinowitz, & Rzeczkowski, 1984; Kalikow, Stevens, & Elliott, 1977). With a 0 dB signal-to-babble ratio, 11-year-old children perform better than 9-year-olds, and 15- to 17-year-olds perform better than 11- to 13-year-olds

on the high-predictability words of the SPIN test (Elliott, 1979). Individuals with normal hearing and hearing loss show better performance on the high-predictability words compared to low-predictability words at lower signal-to-babble ratios (Wilson & McArdle, 2012). Similar difficulty on both high- and low-predictability sentences suggests deficient closure skills or difficulty in making use of available linguistic cues to predict words.

Critical Signal-to-Noise Ratio

To determine the critical signal-to-noise ratio, the softest levels at which 50% of speech can be recognized is determined by adaptively varying the signal-to-noise ratio. The masker level is usually fixed, while the speech level is varied adaptively, which leads to variation in the signal-to-noise ratio. For example, if the masker level is fixed at 50 dB effective masking (EM), most listeners can repeat half of the presented spondee words at a presentation level of 50 dB hearing level (HL). In this case, the critical signal-to-noise ratio is 0 dB. However, if a listener needs the spondee levels to be 60 dB HL to recognize 50% of the spondee words correctly in the presence of 50 dB EM, then the critical signal-to-noise ratio is 10 dB. The critical signal-to-noise ratio can be determined by using sentences that provide more linguistic cues to fill in missing segments. One factor contributing to the need for higher signal-to-noise ratios for understanding 50% of sentences is poor closure skills. Thus, the measure of critical signal-to-noise ratio can be used to determine closure skills by presenting sentences that have high predictability.

Visual Analog of the Auditory Critical Sentence-to-Noise Ratio Measure

In this case, sentences are presented visually in red letters on a white background, and black bars are used for occluding or masking the visually accessible text, as shown in ▶ Fig. 8.13. The exact position

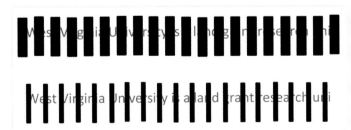

Fig. 8.13 Example of the types of masking used in the Text Reception Threshold test. The percentage of unmasked test is 50% in the top panel and 75% in the bottom panel.

of the black bars is varied randomly to minimize the possibility of occluding the same letters during each presentation. At the beginning of each trial, the bar pattern is presented on a computer screen, and the text of each sentence appears behind the bars in a word-by-word fashion. After the presentation of the last word of the sentence, the sentence remains visible on the screen for 3.5 seconds (Zekveld, George, Kramer, Goverts, & Houtgast, 2007) or 0.5 second (Besser, Zekveld, Kramer, Rönnberg, & Festen, 2012). The percentage of unmasked or visible text is varied adaptively from 28 to 70% with steps of 6% to determine the percentage needed to correctly recognize 50% of a sentence. There is a significant practice effect on the test during the first six repetitions of the test (Zekveld et al., 2007). In individuals with normal hearing, the mean values of unmasking needed to get 50% correct in sentence reading vary from 53.6% (Zekveld, Kramer, Vlaming, & Houtgast, 2008) to 58.2% (George et al., 2007). Performance on this test is associated with speech recognition ability in fluctuating nonspeech maskers (Besser et al., 2012; George et al., 2007). As can be predicted, the performance on this closure task is related to language proficiency (Goverts et al., 2011).

Improving Closure Skills

A key part of good closure skills is excellent vocabulary and word knowledge.

Building Vocabulary

If a child does not have good vocabulary, several strategies can be used to improve vocabulary and word knowledge. Some of these strategies (Christ & Wang, 2010) are outlined below:
1. Provide purposeful exposure to new words: Purposeful exposure to new words can be provided by asking the child to read aloud short paragraphs or read short paragraphs that contain the new words within a rich context. Illustrations of the new words or introduction of the new words through computer media with animation as necessary can enhance the acquisition of new words and related concepts. If the words are drawn from classroom textbooks, the acquisition of these words can enhance learning ability.
2. Intentionally teach word meanings: Ask the child specific questions after asking him or her to read aloud materials or after reading the materials to the child. The questions should be designed to prompt the child to think about the new words and concepts.

3. Teach strategies to acquire new vocabulary through modeling the thought process involved in finding the meaning of new words, guiding the child to follow the model, then providing the necessary practice. Because a child is expected to acquire a large amount of vocabulary in a relatively short amount of time, he or she needs to learn to master new words and concepts independently.
4. Offer opportunities to use new words in a variety of contexts: The child can be asked to retell what he or she has read, draw a picture of the word and related concepts, or role play in an activity that requires the use of the newly mastered vocabulary. Engaging activities can motivate a child to learn new words and maintain the child's interest.

Direct Activities for Improving Closure Skills

Most activities for improving closure skills involve practice in filling missing elements in sentences. The missing element can be a phoneme, a syllable, a word, two or more words, or a phrase. If a child has difficulty completing a sentence, the child is provided with cues or prompts to complete the sentence. The cues can be in the form of pointing attention to a specific part of the sentence. For example, in the sentence "While climbing down the stairs, __ dropped her toy," the child's attention can be drawn to the word *her.* Other types of questions may prompt the child to think about the context. For example, the child can be asked "Where do we go to shop for clothes?" for completing the sentence "I went to the mall for __opping." Tasks that are used for assessing closure can also be used for improving closure skills.

In selecting materials for closure skill training, the age and interests of the listener must be considered to maintain motivation. For example, for younger children, auditory closure fun deck cards are available from Super Duper (Super Duper Publications, Greenville, SC) publications. Older children and adults can do crossword puzzles to improve closure. Games such as Wheel of Fortune or applications such as sentence, language, and story builder may enhance closure skills.

8.4 Computerized Training

Many computerized training programs are currently being marketed that claim to improve bottom-up and top-down processing of auditory and

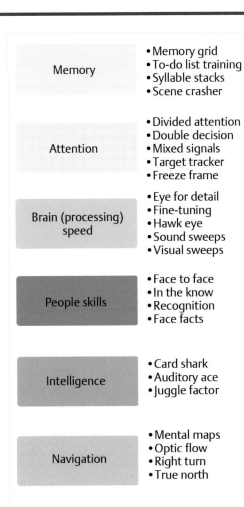

visual stimuli. Examples of some of these training programs are provided below. The descriptions here are based on the information and demonstrations provided at the websites of companies that market the training programs. Most of the training programs automatically generate reports to allow educators, parents, and other professionals to track the progress of the participant. Readers are encouraged to visit the websites to get more information, including any evidence of efficiency.

8.4.1 BrainHQ

BrainHQ training programs from Posit Science are designed to improve the overall function of the brain and involve both auditory and visual modalities. The targeted brain functions and associated exercises are shown in ▶ Fig. 8.14. The types of auditory stimuli dispersed through the program

are shown in ▶ Fig. 8.15. Brief descriptions of examples of exercises are presented below.

Memory Exercises

In the exercise titled Syllable Stacks, the participant listens to a series of syllables, then repeats them in the presented order. The difficulty of the task is varied by changing the number of syllables to be recalled, the duration of the syllables, the speed with which syllables are presented, and the distracting buttons that do not represent any of the presented syllables.

Attention Exercises

Divided Attention

In this exercise, the listener is shown two shapes on the screen and is asked to press the left arrow

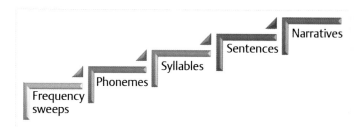

Fig. 8.15 Auditory stimuli dispersed in the BrainHQ training programs with potential for improving auditory processing skills.

key when the two meet specified criteria. For example, the listener might be asked to press the left arrow key when the two shapes are the same shape or color and the right arrow key when they are not, even if the two shapes have something else in common (e.g., both shapes may be circles of two different colors). The difficulty is varied by adding more complex instructions and increasing the speed with which the images appear on the screen.

Mixed Signals

This exercise is based on the Stroop (1935) task explained in Fig. 8.9. It is designed to challenge the brain to focus on desired information in the presence of competing information. Participants are required to listen to a number, letter, color, or other piece of information while looking at similar competing information. If the auditorily presented information matches the visual information in a specific way, the listener is expected to hit the space bar. If not, the listener is expected to refrain from hitting the space bar. For example, *aaiaa* may appear on the computer screen, and the participant is required to hit the space bar if what he or she hears matches the middle letter. In this case, the listener will hit the bar only when he or she hears *i*. If the listener hears any other letter, he or she is supposed to refrain from hitting the bar.

Brain Speed Exercises

Fine Tuning

In this case, the participant is expected to discriminate between two syllables that sound alike, such as *bo* and *do*. One of the distinguishing characteristics of the phonemes /b/ and /d/ is that they differ in the onset frequency of the second formant. The selected syllables are harder to differentiate, especially under degraded listening conditions. Differentiation of such sounds requires synchronous onset and offset firing of neurons tuned to

specific frequencies. The exercises in fine tuning are designed to help neurons to turn on and off at appropriate times to allow the clear perception of the sounds. The syllables are synthesized to make them more easily distinguishable at the beginning of the exercise, and, depending on the listener's response, the speed is increased to represent average conversational speech and to push neurons to respond more quickly. Such exercises may reduce the perception of people mumbling that is experienced by individuals with APDs.

Sound Sweeps

This task involves pitch pattern perception. Participants are presented with frequency sweeps and are expected to determine if the sweeps are moving upward or downward. The difficulty of the task is varied by changing the frequency of the sounds and by increasing the speed with which the two sounds occur one after the other. With practice, the task may lead to less backward masking (see Chapter 6).

People Skills Exercises

In the exercise titled "In the Know," listeners are presented with paragraphs of information, then asked to answer questions based on that information. The difficulty of the task is varied by increasing the length of the paragraphs, increasing the speed with which sentences are spoken, and shortening the intersentence time intervals.

Intelligence Exercises

Auditory Ace

This task is based on the n-back working memory assessment procedure (▶ Fig. 8.7). The participant listens to information about cards. The information is presented one card at a time. The response task involves a decision about whether the current card information matches the card information presented a specific number of steps back in the sequence. For example, in the first, easier level, the participant must decide if the current card information matches the information on the preceding card. In later levels, participants decide if the current card information matches the information presented further back (two or three cards back) in the sequence. The difficulty of the task is increased by increasing the number of sequences presented on each trial and the amount of information included on each card. In addition, the card information is presented at increasingly faster rates.

Navigation Exercises

These exercises are designed to improve visuospatial skills.

8.4.2 Fast ForWord Language Version 2

This software from Scientific Learning Corp. (Oakland, CA) is designed to improve listening accuracy, phonological awareness, and language structures to minimize learning or reading difficulties.

Areas Targeted to Improve Brain Functioning

- Processing and discrimination of auditory and linguistic stimuli, including phonemes, words, and sentences
- Sequencing skills for accurate reception and expression of correct word order in simple and complex sentences
- Working and long-term memory
- Ability to focus and selective attention

Components Incorporated to Maximize Neural Plasticity

Frequency and Intensity

The participant is expected to complete sets of exercises at relatively high frequency and in a relatively short period.

Adaptivity

The difficulty of the training exercises is modified in an adaptive manner based on the responses of the participant to keep the learning task challenging but not too frustrating.

Simultaneous Development

Major cognitive and reading skills are targeted simultaneously to produce long-lasting improvements.

Timely Motivation

Correct responses are reinforced to maximize motivation.

Example of Exercises

Sky Gym

Students differentiate between sweep sounds to improve sequencing skills, sound processing, and working memory.

Robo-Dog

Students hear a word and identify the matching picture to improve listening accuracy and word recognition skills.

Ele-Bot

Students build language comprehension skills as they determine which illustrations correctly match the spoken sentence.

8.4.3 HearBuilder

HearBuilder from Super Duper Publications is designed to provide systematic instruction in following directions, phonological awareness, sequencing, and auditory memory. Four separate software programs are available for each of these areas that allow flexibility in using the software in the classroom, media center, computer lab, and at home.

Following Directions

This module is designed to teach children to follow increasingly difficult oral directions in five areas:
- Basic directions (e.g., Click on the small red car.)
- Sequential directions: (e.g., First, set the temperature to cold; next, set the shape to square and then click start.)
- Quantitative and spatial directions (e.g., Choose three of the red trucks.)
- Temporal directions (e.g., Before you put a guitar in the box, put the robot in the box.)
- Conditional directions (e.g., If a robot is in the box, put the box on the truck.)

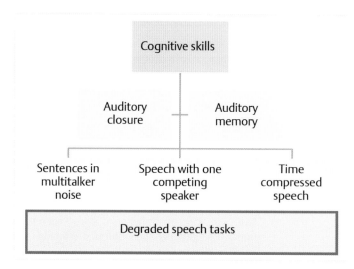

Fig. 8.16 Example of combining training in bottom-up and top-down processing incorporated in the LACE program (based on Neurotone, Inc., Redwood City, CA).

Phonological Awareness

This module includes exercises for nine phonological awareness skills: sentence segmentation, syllable blending, syllable segmentation, rhyming, phoneme blending, phoneme segmentation and identification, phoneme deletion, phoneme addition, and phoneme manipulation.

Auditory Memory

The auditory memory activities are designed to improve memory for numbers, words, details, and "wh" (who, what, when, where, and why) information. Additional activities involve auditory closure skills. Tips are included for improving auditory memory.

Sequencing

The sequencing module includes exercises for sequencing stories or instructions. The sequencing can be completed by using a combination of pictures, text, and audio, or pictures and audio, text and audio, or pictures and text.

8.4.4 Listening and Communication Enhancement (LACE)

This software from Neurotone Inc. (Redwood City, CA) is designed to improve speech perception in difficult listening situations, such as noise in the background, rapidly speaking talkers, and multiple talkers. The program incorporates both top-down and bottom-up training (▶ Fig. 8.16). Both perceptual and neurophysiological changes have been demonstrated following the use of LACE. Such studies demonstrate that short-term auditory training improves the neural representation of cues that are important for listening to speech in noisy conditions (Song, Skoe, Banai, & Kraus, 2012).

8.4.5 Advantages of Computerized Training

There are several advantages to computerized training, including the following:
- Computerized training allows users to decide when and how long training is conducted.
- Many programs automatically track the progress of learners and allow professionals access to review the progress so that appropriate changes in intervention can be made as necessary.
- Greater flexibility is possible in manipulating stimuli acoustically than is possible through live-voice presentations.
- Computer programs allow presentation of more stimuli in a relatively short amount of time than is possible through live presentations.
- Computer programs make training more interesting through the use of animation and video games.
- Computerized training offers motivating verbal and visual reinforcement for each correct response.

8.4.6 Potential Disadvantages of Computerized Training for Auditory Processing Deficits

There are several potential disadvantages associated with computerized auditory training for individuals with APDs:

- Visual stimuli that are inherent in computerized training programs may interfere with the development of auditory processing skills in some children.
- Depending on the particular training program, some participants may show improved performance only on the trained tasks with limited or no generalization to real-life functions (Owen et al., 2010).
- Some older adults may be uncomfortable using computers, which can negatively affect outcomes.
- Some participants may prefer live interactions with a professional, leading to better motivation, better compliance with training tasks, and thus better learning.

8.4.7 Cautions about Computerized or Video Game –Based Training

Although action video games can help dyslexic children read better (Franceschini et al., 2013), the violence that is often part of action video games can increase the risk of aggressive behavior in some children (Anderson & Dill, 2000). This is especially true for those who are at higher risk for aggressive tendencies, including those with ADHD. In addition, violent action games may make children less sensitive to the pain and suffering of others and more fearful of the world around them. Thus, video games should be carefully analyzed before using them for training children.

For individuals between the ages of 5 and 21 years, total screen time, including TV, computer, and mobile electronic devices (e.g., handheld video games and cell phones), should be limited to 2 hours daily due to the association between extended screen time and increased risks for low school performance, overweight, and violent behavior. For children between the ages of 2 and 5 years, total screen time should be limited to 1 hour daily. Television viewing is discouraged for children younger than 2 years of age (American Academy of Pediatrics, 2001; Massachusetts Health Quality Partners, 2012). Limiting the availability of electronic entertainment and communication devices in children's bedrooms and discouraging nighttime use has been recommended to promote sleep and to reduce childhood obesity (Chahal, Fung, Kuhle, & Veugelers, 2013). Thus, computerized training should be offered on a limited basis, and the use should be restricted to daytime.

8.5 Ensuring Compliance with Training

There are some limits to perceptual learning, or more specifically, auditory training, as shown in ▶ Fig. 8.17. One limit may be imposed by poor compliance with the training protocol. In programs where the training attempts to address multiple cognitive or sensory processing issues, compliance with home-based computerized or video training may not be optimum. Making the process more entertaining through games may be helpful in improving compliance (Sweetow & Sabes, 2010). Too much training beyond the point at which maximum performance is possible (▶ Fig. 8.4) can reduce compliance on training for other specific deficit tasks. Training that is not individualized can also reduce compliance. For example, in the presence of a sensory deficit and good cognition, training that tries to address both sensory and cognitive deficits may become discouraging and boring to listeners. When cognition is very good, training should focus on sensory deficits or the use of bottom-up strategies.

8.6 Future Trends

Several future trends are likely to aid improvement in memory (▶ Fig. 8.18) that could lead to consolidation of perceptual learning. At the whole brain level, memories can be reinforced during sleep. For example, in one study, participants first learned to produce two melodies in time with moving visual symbols (Antony, Gobel, O'Hare, Reber, & Paller, 2012). One of the melodies was then presented covertly during an afternoon nap. The memory consolidation effect was better for the melody that was presented during the nap without disrupting sleep, as confirmed by EEG. Sensory habituation due to continuous exposure to stimuli may limit the extent to which reactivation of learning is promoted during sleep (Oudiette & Paller, 2013).

Investigators are attempting to reinforce sleep features, such as slow waves and spindles, to indirectly reactivate memories. Methods that could

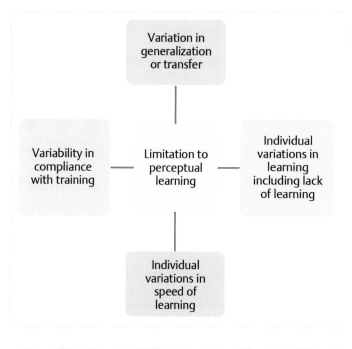

Fig. 8.17 Potential limitations to perceptual learning.

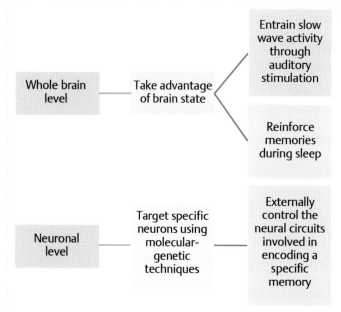

Fig. 8.18 Future trends in improving hippocampus-dependent memories that may improve perceptual learning.

reinforce the key sleep features include transcranial magnetic stimulation and acoustic stimulation (reviewed in Spiers & Bendor, 2014). Acoustic stimulation administered at 0.8 Hz may be one of the less invasive ways to entrain slow wave activity (Ngo, Claussen, Born, & Mölle, 2013). A current limitation to this approach is that the stimulation delays sleep onset and could lead to sleep deprivation when the participant is required to wake up at a specific time because of job or school requirements.

Optogenetics combines techniques from optics and genetics to modulate and monitor the activities of individual neurons or specific groups of neurons in living tissue. In the future, memory improvement may be possible through optogenetic stimulation. A specific memory appears to be encoded by a sparse population of neurons that can be tagged during learning for subsequent identification and stimulation. Activation of the specific ensemble of hippocampal neurons that contribute to a specific memory engram can lead to recall of that memory in rats (Liu et al., 2012).

More computerized training programs and further refinement of current software is likely in the future. In addition, programs that combine listening skills and physical movement (e.g., tap to the beat) may be available with feedback on accuracy of the response using wearable technologies.

For children with comorbid reading deficits, practice in writing some responses to speech stimuli may lead to faster improvements in reading and writing compared to typing a response or using a computer mouse.

For older adults who do not wish to use computers, training programs that rely on CDs or DVDs and live training will continue to be useful. Such programs may also be useful for young children. The live training offers active human interaction that may enhance listening skills in a different manner than what is achievable through the use of computers, videotapes, or audiotapes. In one study, 9-month-old American infants easily learned phonemes and words in Mandarin Chinese when they were given an opportunity to interact with a Chinese speaker (Kuhl, Tsao, & Liu, 2003). The same ease in learning the sounds was not apparent if the same sounds were delivered by television or audiotapes with no opportunities for interaction.

The effectiveness of any training programs is highly dependent on the skill, experience, and creativity of clinicians implementing them. Skilled implementation is likely to lead to improvements in a relatively short period. Student clinicians must practice such skills on patients or through simulation of APDs by presenting the stimuli at softer levels.

8.7 Review Questions

1. Discuss the effects of poor acoustic environment on language and academic achievements. Review the key elements of the American National Standards Institute/ Acoustical Society of America (ANSI/ASA, 2010) guidelines for classroom acoustics. List some strategies for improving classroom acoustics.

2. How can frequency modulation (FM) systems improve listening skills and learning? Why are personal FM systems preferred over sound field FM systems?

3. What are some characteristics of clear speech? How can you train teachers to produce clear speech?

4. What is perceptual learning? Discuss the key mechanisms of perceptual learning. What are some limits to perceptual learning? How can you improve compliance with training protocols?

5. Discuss the key principles for providing efficient auditory training. What are some possible generalization effects of auditory training? How can you assess generalization?

6. What strategies can be used to improve attention?

7. What is working memory? Describe the connection between working memory and auditory processing deficits. What strategies can be used to improve working memory? Discuss future trends related to improvement of hippocampus-dependent memory.

8. Describe procedures for assessing closure skills. How can you improve closure skills?

9. What are some common elements of music and speech perception? What are some potential effects of music training on speech perception? What precautions are necessary during music training?

10. Explore and compare some computerized training programs that could improve auditory perception. Discuss the potential advantages and disadvantages of computerized training. What precautions are necessary in using computerized training programs with children?

References

[1] Acoustical Society of America (ASA). (2003). Position on the use of sound amplification in the classroom. Retrieved from http://asa.aip.org/amplification.pdf.

[2] Agnew, J. A., Dorn, C., & Eden, G. F. (2004). Effect of intensive training on auditory processing and reading skills. Brain and Language, 88(1), 21–25.

[3] Alloway, T. P., Gathercole, S. E., Kirkwood, H., & Elliott, J. (2009). The cognitive and behavioral characteristics of children with low working memory. Child Development, 80(2), 606–621.

[4] American Academy of Audiology (AAA). (2010). American Academy of Audiology clinical practice guidelines: Diagnosis, treatment and management of children and adults with central auditory processing disorder. Retrieved October 28, 2013, from http://www.audiology.org/resources/documentlibrary/Documents/CAPD%20Guidelines%208–2010.pdf.

[5] American Academy of Pediatrics. Committee on Public Education. (2001). American Academy of Pediatrics: Children, adolescents, and television. Pediatrics, 107(2), 423–426.

[6] American National Standards Institute (ANSI). (2010). Acoustical performance criteria, design requirements, and guideline for schools: ANSI/ASA S12.60–2010/Part1. New York: Author.

[7] Amitay, S., Irwin, A., & Moore, D. R. (2006). Discrimination learning induced by training with identical stimuli. Nature Neuroscience, 9(11), 1446–1448.

[8] Anderson, C. A., & Dill, K. E. (2000). Video games and aggressive thoughts, feelings, and behavior in the laboratory and in life. Journal of Personality and Social Psychology, 78(4), 772–790.

[9] Anderson, K. (1989) Screening instrument for targeting educational risk (SIFTER) in children with identified hearing loss. Tampa, FL: Educational Audiology Association (previously by Pro-Ed and Interstate Publishers and Printers). Now available at www.sifteranderson.com.

[10] Andrews, S. C., Hoy, K. E., Enticott, P. G., Daskalakis, Z. J., & Fitzgerald, P. B. (2011). Improving working memory: The effect of combining cognitive activity and anodal transcranial direct current stimulation to the left dorsolateral prefrontal cortex. Brain Stimulation, 4(2), 84–89.

[11] Antony, J. W., Gobel, E. W., O'Hare, J. K., Reber, P. J., & Paller, K. A. (2012). Cued memory reactivation during sleep influences skill learning. Nature Neuroscience, 15(8), 1114–1116.

[12] Avivi-Reich, M., Arnott, S., Tavares, T., & Schneider, B. (2013). The influence of auditory training on measures of temporal resolution in younger and older adults (Abstract). In Proceedings of Meetings on Acoustics (Vol. 19, No. 1, p. 050063). Acoustical Society of America. Retrieved from http://scitation.aip.org.

[13] Baddeley, A. (2003). Working memory and language: An overview. Journal of Communication Disorders, 36(3), 189–208.

[14] Baddeley, A. D., & Hitch, G. J. (1974). Working memory. In G. A. Bower (Ed.), Recent advances in learning and motivation (Vol. 8, pp. 47–90). New York: Academic Press.

[15] Barcroft, J., Sommers, M. S., Tye-Murray, N., Mauzé, E., Schroy, C., & Spehar, B. (2011). Tailoring auditory training to patient needs with single and multiple talkers: Transfer-appropriate gains on a four-choice discrimination test. International Journal of Audiology, 50(11), 802–808.

[16] Berry, E., Kapur, N., Williams, L., et al. (2007). The use of a wearable camera, SenseCam, as a pictorial diary to improve autobiographical memory in a patient with limbic encephalitis: A preliminary report. Neuropsychological Rehabilitation, 17(4-5), 582–601.

[17] Besser, J., Zekveld, A. A., Kramer, S. E., Rönnberg, J., & Festen, J. M. (2012). New measures of masked text recognition in relation to speech-in-noise perception and their associations with age and cognitive abilities. Journal of Speech, Language, and Hearing Research, 55(1), 194–209.

[18] Bilger, R. C. (1984). Speech recognition test development. ASHA Reports, 14, 2–15.

[19] Bilger, R. C., Nuetzel, J. M., Rabinowitz, W. M., & Rzeczkowski, C. (1984). Standardization of a test of speech perception in noise. Journal of Speech and Hearing Research, 27(1), 32–48.

[20] Bradlow, A. R., Kraus, N., & Hayes, E. (2003). Speaking clearly for children with learning disabilities: Sentence perception in noise. Journal of Speech, Language, and Hearing Research, 46(1), 80–97.

[21] Bratzke, D., Schröter, H., & Ulrich, R. (2014). The role of consolidation for perceptual learning in temporal discrimination within and across modalities. Acta Psychologica, 147, 75-79.

[22] Bratzke, D., Seifried, T., & Ulrich, R. (2012). Perceptual learning in temporal discrimination: Asymmetric cross-modal transfer from audition to vision. Experimental Brain Research, 221(2), 205–210.

[23] Buss, E., Hall, J. W. III, & Grose, J. H. (2006). Development and the role of internal noise in detection and discrimination thresholds with narrow band stimuli. Journal of the Acoustical Society of America, 120(5, Pt. 1), 2777–2788.

[24] Buss, E., Hall, J. W. III, & Grose, J. H. (2009). Psychometric functions for pure tone intensity discrimination: Slope differences in school-aged children and adults. Journal of the Acoustical Society of America, 125(2), 1050–1058.

[25] Caissie, R., Campbell, M. M., Frenette, W. L., Scott, L., Howell, I., & Roy, A. (2005). Clear speech for adults with a hearing loss: Does intervention with communication partners make a difference? Journal of the American Academy of Audiology, 16(3), 157–171.

[26] Caissie, R., & Tranquilla, M. (2010). Enhancing conversational fluency: Training conversation partners in the use of clear speech and other strategies. Seminars in Hearing, 31(2), 95–103.

[27] Campbell, R. A., & Small, A. M. (1963). Effect of practice and feedback on frequency discrimination. Journal of the Acoustical Society of America, 35, 1511–1514.

[28] Caplan, D., & Waters, G. S. (1995). On the nature of the phonological output planning processes involved in verbal rehearsal: Evidence from aphasia. Brain and Language, 48(2), 191–220.

[29] Carhart, R., Tillman, T. W., & Greetis, E. S. (1969). Perceptual masking in multiple sound backgrounds. Journal of the Acoustical Society of America, 45(3), 694–703.

[30] Chacko, A., Bedard, A. C., Marks, D. J., Feirsen, N., Uderman, J. Z., Chimiklis, A., ... & Ramon, M. (2014). A randomized clinical trial of Cogmed working memory training in school-age children with ADHD: A replication in a diverse sample using a control condition. Journal of Child Psychology and Psychiatry, 55, 247-255.

[31] Chahal, H., Fung, C., Kuhle, S., & Veugelers, P. J. (2013). Availability and night-time use of electronic entertainment and communication devices are associated with short sleep duration and obesity among Canadian children. Pediatric Obesity, 8(1), 42–51.

[32] Chenault, B., Thomson, J., Abbott, R. D., & Berninger, V. W. (2006). Effects of prior attention training on child dyslexics' response to composition instruction. Developmental Neuropsychology, 29(1), 243–260.

[33] Chik, D. (2013). Theta-alpha cross-frequency synchronization facilitates working memory control: A modeling study. Springerplus, 2(14), 1-10. Retrieved from http://link.springer.com/article/10.1186/2193-1801-2-14/fulltext.html.

[34] Chobert, J., François, C., Velay, J.-L., & Besson, M. (2014). Twelve months of active musical training in 8- to 10-year-old children enhances the preattentive processing of syllabic duration and voice onset time. Cerebral Cortex, 24(4), 956-967.

[35] Christ, T., & Wang, X. C. (2010). Bridging the vocabulary gap: What the research tells us about vocabulary instruction in early childhood. Young Children, 65(4), 84–91.

[36] Coghill, D. R., Seth, S., & Matthews, K. (2013). A comprehensive assessment of memory, delay aversion, timing, inhibition, decision making and variability in attention deficit hy-

peractivity disorder: Advancing beyond the three-pathway models. Psychological Medicine, 31, 1–13.

[37] Cohen, H., Scherzer, P., Viau, R, Voss, P., & Lepore, F. (2011). Working memory for braille is shaped by experience. Communicative and Integrative Biology, 4(2), 227–229.

[38] Daneman, M., & Carpenter, P. A. (1980). Individual differences in working memory and reading. Journal of Verbal Learning and Verbal Behavior, 19, 450–466.

[39] Daneman, M., & Carpenter, P. (1983). Individual differences in integrating information between and within sentences. Journal of Experimental Psychology: Learning, Memory, and Cognition, 9, 561–584.

[40] Delhommeau, K., Micheyl, C., & Jouvent, R. (2005). Generalization of frequency discrimination learning across frequencies and ears: Implications for underlying neural mechanisms in humans. Journal of the Association for Research in Otolaryngology, 6(2), 171–179.

[41] Delhommeau, K., Micheyl, C., Jouvent, R., & Collet, L. (2002). Transfer of learning across durations and ears in auditory frequency discrimination. Perception and Psychophysics, 64(3), 426–436.

[42] Demany, L., & Semal, C. (2002). Learning to perceive pitch differences. Journal of the Acoustical Society of America, 111(3), 1377–1388.

[43] D'Esposito, M., Detre, J. A., Alsop, D. C., Shin, R. K., Atlas, S., & Grossman, M. (1995). The neural basis of the central executive system of working memory. Nature, 378(6554), 279–281.

[44] DiSarno, N., Schowalter, M., & Grassa, P. (2002). Classroom amplification to enhance student performance. Teaching Exceptional Children, (July/August), 20–26.

[45] Duke, R. A., Allen, S. E., Cash, C. D., & Simmons, A. L. (2009). Effects of early and late rest breaks during training on overnight memory consolidation of a keyboard melody. Annals of the New York Academy of Sciences, 1169, 169–172.

[46] Dunning, D. L., Holmes, J., & Gathercole, S. E. (2013). Does working memory training lead to generalized improvements in children with low working memory? A randomized controlled trial. Developmental Science, 16(6), 915–925.

[47] Egeland, J., Aarlien, A. K., & Saunes, B.-K. (2013). Few effects of far transfer of working memory training in ADHD: A randomized controlled trial. PLoS ONE, 8(10), e75660.

[48] Elliott, L. L. (1979). Performance of children aged 9 to 17 years on a test of speech intelligibility in noise using sentence material with controlled word predictability. Journal of the Acoustical Society of America, 66(3), 651–653.

[49] Ellis Weismer, S., & Hesketh, L. J. (1996). Lexical learning by children with specific language impairment: Effects of linguistic input presented at varying speaking rates. Journal of Speech and Hearing Research, 39(1), 177–190.

[50] Evans, G. W., & Maxwell, L. (1997). Chronic noise exposure and reading deficits: The mediating effects of language acquisition. Environment and Behavior, 29(5), 638–656.

[51] Fell, J., & Axmacher, N. (2011). The role of phase synchronization in memory processes. Nature Reviews Neuroscience, 12(2), 105–118.

[52] Ferguson, S. H. (2012). Talker differences in clear and conversational speech: Vowel intelligibility for older adults with hearing loss. Journal of Speech, Language, and Hearing Research, 55(3), 779–790.

[53] Ferrucci, R., Marceglia, S., Vergari, M., et al. (2008). Cerebellar transcranial direct current stimulation impairs the practice-dependent proficiency increase in working memory. Journal of Cognitive Neuroscience, 20(9), 1687–1697.

[54] Fertonani, A., Rosini, S., Cotelli, M., Rossini, P. M., & Miniussi, C. (2010). Naming facilitation induced by transcranial direct current stimulation. Behavioural Brain Research, 208(2), 311–318.

[55] Fish, J., Manly, T., Emslie, H., Evans, J. J., & Wilson, B. A. (2008). Compensatory strategies for acquired disorders of memory and planning: Differential effects of a paging system for patients with brain injury of traumatic versus cerebrovascular aetiology. Journal of Neurology, Neurosurgery, and Psychiatry, 79(8), 930–935.

[56] Fish, J.,, Manly, T., & Wilson, B. A. (2008). Long-term compensatory treatment of organizational deficits in a patient with bilateral frontal lobe damage. Journal of the International Neuropsychology Society, 14(1), 154–163.

[57] Fletcher, H. (1940). Auditory patterns. Reviews of Modern Physics, 12, 47–65.

[58] Franceschini, S., Gori, S., Ruffino, M., Viola, S., Molteni, M., & Facoetti, A. (2013). Action video games make dyslexic children read better. Current Biology, 23(6), 462–466.

[59] François, C., Chobert, J., Besson, M., & Schön, D. (2013). Music training for the development of speech segmentation. Cerebral Cortex, 23(9), 2038–2043.

[60] Gagne, J. P., Masterson, V. M., Munhall, K. G., Bilida, N., & Querengesser, C. (1994). Across talker variability in auditory, visual, and audiovisual speech intelligibility for conversational and clear speech. Journal of Korean Academy of Rehabilitative Audiology, 127, 135–158.

[61] Gatehouse, S., Naylor, G., & Elberling, C. (2003). Benefits from hearing aids in relation to the interaction between the user and the environment. International Journal of Audiology, 42 (Suppl. 1), S77–S85.

[62] Gathercole, S. E., & Baddeley, A. D. (1990). Phonological memory deficits in language disordered children: Is there a causal connection? Journal of Memory and Language, 29, 336–360.

[63] Gaulin, C. A., & Campbell, T. F. (1994). Procedure for assessing verbal working memory in normal school-age children: Some preliminary data. Perceptual and Motor Skills, 79(1, Pt. 1), 55–64.

[64] George, E. L. J., Zekveld, A. A., Kramer, S. E., Goverts, S. T., Festen, J. M., & Houtgast, T. (2007). Auditory and nonauditory factors affecting speech reception in noise by older listeners. Journal of the Acoustical Society of America, 121(4), 2362–2375.

[65] Goldstone, R. L. (1998). Perceptual learning. Annual Review of Psychology, 49(1), 585-612.

[66] Goverts, S. T., Huysmans, E., Kramer, S. E., de Groot, A. M., & Houtgast, T. (2011). On the use of the distortion-sensitivity approach in examining the role of linguistic abilities in speech understanding in noise. Journal of Speech, Language, and Hearing Research, 54(6), 1702–1708.

[67] Gray, L., Miller, B. S., & Evans, S. W. (2012). Training children with ADHD to minimize impulsivity in auditory contralateral masking. International Journal of Pediatric Otorhinolaryngology, 76(4), 483–487.

[68] Grunewaldt, K. H., Løhaugen, G. C., Austeng, D., Brubakk, A. M., & Skranes, J. (2013). Working memory training improves cognitive function in VLBW preschoolers. Pediatrics, 131(3), e747–e754.

[69] Halliday, L. F., Moore, D. R., Taylor, J. L., & Amitay, S. (2011). Dimension-specific attention directs learning and listening on auditory training tasks. Attention, Perception, and Psychophysics, 73(5), 1329–1335.

[70] Hausen, M., Torppa, R., Salmela, V. R., Vainio, M., & Särkämö, T. (2013). Music and speech prosody: A common rhythm. Frontiers in Psychology, 4, 566:1-16.

[71] Hayes, G. R., Patel, S. N., Truong, K. N., et al. (2004). The personal audio loop: Designing a ubiquitous audio-based memory aid. In Proceedings of the Mobile HCI 2004: The 6th International Symposium on Mobile Human-Computer Interaction (pp. 168–179). Berlin/Heidelberg: Springer.

[72] Heinzel, S., Schulte, S., Onken, J., et al. (2014). Working memory training improvements and gains in non-trained cognitive tasks in young and older adults. Neuropsychology, Development, and Cognition. Section B, Aging, Neuropsychology, and Cognition, 21(2), 146–173.

[73] Hersh, N. A., & Treadgold, L. G. (1994). NeuroPage: The rehabilitation of memory dysfunction by prosthetic memory and cueing. NeuroRehabilitation, 4(3), 187–197.

[74] Hodgson, M. (2002). Rating, ranking, and understanding acoustical quality in university classrooms. Journal of the Acoustical Society of America, 112(2), 568–575.

[75] Hornickel, J., Zecker, S. G., Bradlow, A. R., & Kraus, N. (2012). Assistive listening devices drive neuroplasticity in children with dyslexia. Proceedings of the National Academy of Sciences of the United States of America, 109(41), 16731–16736.

[76] Huyck, J. J., & Wright, B. A. (2013). Learning, worsening, and generalization in response to auditory perceptual training during adolescence. Journal of the Acoustical Society of America, 134(2), 1172–1182.

[77] Johnston, K. N., John, A. B., Kreisman, N. V., Hall, J. W. III, & Crandell, C. C. (2009). Multiple benefits of personal FM system use by children with auditory processing disorder (APD). International Journal of Audiology, 48(6), 371–383.

[78] Jones, J. L., Lucker, J., Zalewski, C., Brewer, C., & Drayna, D. (2009). Phonological processing in adults with deficits in musical pitch recognition. Journal of Communication Disorders, 42(3), 226–234.

[79] Jones, P. R., Moore, D. R., Amitay, S., & Shub, D. E. (2013). Reduction of internal noise in auditory perceptual learning. Journal of the Acoustical Society of America, 133(2), 970–981.

[80] Kalikow, D. N., Stevens, K. N., & Elliott, L. L. (1977). Development of a test of speech intelligibility in noise using sentence materials with controlled word predictability. Journal of the Acoustical Society of America, 61(5), 1337–1351.

[81] Kane, M. J., & Engle, R. W. (2002). The role of prefrontal cortex in working-memory capacity, executive attention, and general fluid intelligence: An individual-differences perspective. Psychonomic Bulletin and Review, 9(4), 637–671.

[82] Karmarkar, U. R., & Buonomano, D. V. (2003). Temporal specificity of perceptual learning in an auditory discrimination task. Learning and Memory, 10(2), 141–147.

[83] Kasselimis, D. S., Simos, P. G., Economou, A., Peppas, C., Evdokimidis, I., & Potagas, C. (2013). Are memory deficits dependent on the presence of aphasia in left brain damaged patients? Neuropsychologia, 51, 1773-1776.

[84] Kawasaki, M., Kitajo, K., & Yamaguchi, Y. (2010). Dynamic links between theta executive functions and alpha storage buffers in auditory and visual working memory. European Journal of Neuroscience, 31(9), 1683–1689.

[85] Kessler, S. K., Minhas, P., Woods, A. J., Rosen, A., Gorman, C., & Bikson, M. (2013). Dosage considerations for transcranial direct current stimulation in children: A computational modeling study. PLoS ONE, 8(9), e76112.

[86] Kibby, M. Y., & Cohen, M. J. (2008). Memory functioning in children with reading disabilities and/or attention deficit/hyperactivity disorder: A clinical investigation of their working memory and long-term memory functioning. Child Neuropsychology, 14(6), 525–546.

[87] Kirchner, W. K. (1958). Age differences in short-term retention of rapidly changing information. Journal of Experimental Psychology, 55(4), 352–358.

[88] Klatte, M., Hellbrück, J., Seidel, J., & Leistner, P. (2010). Effects of classroom acoustics on performance and well-being in elementary school children: A field study. Environment and Behavior, 42(5), 659–692.

[89] Knutson, J. F., Schartz, H. A., Gantz, B. J., Tyler, R. S., Hinrichs, J. V., & Woodworth, G. (1991). Psychological change following 18 months of cochlear implant use. Annals of Otology, Rhinology, and Laryngology, 100(11), 877–882.

[90] Korhonen, P., & Kuk, F. (2008). Use of linear frequency transposition in simulated hearing loss. Journal of the American Academy of Audiology, 19(8), 639–650.

[91] Krause, J. C., & Braida, L. D. (2002). Investigating alternative forms of clear speech: The effects of speaking rate and speaking mode on intelligibility. Journal of the Acoustical Society of America, 112(5, Pt. 1), 2165–2172.

[92] Krause, J. C., & Braida, L. D. (2004). Acoustic properties of naturally produced clear speech at normal speaking rates. Journal of the Acoustical Society of America, 115(1), 362–378.

[93] Kraus, N., & Chandrasekaran, B. (2010). Music training for the development of auditory skills. Nature Reviews Neuroscience, 11(8), 599–605.

[94] Kuhl, P. K., Tsao, F. M., & Liu, H. M. (2003). Foreign-language experience in infancy: Effects of short-term exposure and social interaction on phonetic learning. Proceedings of the National Academy of Sciences of the United States of America, 100(15), 9096–9101.

[95] Kujala, T., Karma, K., Ceponiene, R., et al. (2001). Plastic neural changes and reading improvement caused by audiovisual training in reading-impaired children. Proceedings of the National Academy of Sciences of the United States of America, 98(18), 10509–10514.

[96] Kuk, F., & Keenan, D. (2010). Frequency transposition: Training is only half the story. Hearing Review, 17(12), 38–46.

[97] Lam, J., & Tjaden, K. (2013). Intelligibility of clear speech: Effect of instruction. Journal of Speech, Language, and Hearing Research, 56(5), 1429–1440.

[98] Liebetanz, D., Koch, R., Mayenfels, S., König, F., Paulus, W., & Nitsche, M. A. (2009). Safety limits of cathodal transcranial direct current stimulation in rats. Clinical Neurophysiology, 120(6), 1161–1167.

[99] Liu, X., Ramirez, S., Pang, P. T., et al. (2012). Optogenetic stimulation of a hippocampal engram activates fear memory recall. Nature, 484(7394), 381–385.

[100] Løhaugen, G. C., Antonsen, I., Håberg, A., et al. (2011). Computerized working memory training improves function in adolescents born at extremely low birth weight. Journal of Pediatrics, 158(4), 555–561, e4.

[101] Lovio, R., Halttunen, A., Lyytinen, H., Näätänen, R., & Kujala, T. (2012). Reading skill and neural processing accuracy improvement after a 3-hour intervention in preschoolers with difficulties in reading-related skills. Brain Research, 1448, 42–55.

[102] Lundqvist, A., Grundström, K., Samuelsson, K., & Rönnberg, J. (2010). Computerized training of working memory in a group of patients suffering from acquired brain injury. Brain Injury, 24(10), 1173–1183.

[103] Lunner, T., & Sundewall-Thorén, E. (2007). Interactions between cognition, compression, and listening conditions: Effects on speech-in-noise performance in a two-channel hearing aid. Journal of the American Academy of Audiology, 18(7), 604–617.

[104] Maag, J. W., & Anderson, J. M. (2006). Effects of sound-field amplification to increase compliance of students with emotional and behavior disorders. Behavioral Disorders, 31(4), 378–393.

[105] Maag, J. W., & Anderson, J. M. (2007). Sound-field amplification to increase compliance to directions in students with ADHD. Behavioral Disorders, 32(4), 238–254.

[106] Mahncke, H. W., Connor, B. B., Appelman, J., et al. (2006). Memory enhancement in healthy older adults using a brain plasticity-based training program: A randomized, controlled study. Proceedings of the National Academy of Sciences of the United States of America, 103(33), 12523–12528.

[107] Marshall, L., Mölle, M., Siebner, H. R., & Born, J. (2005). Bifrontal transcranial direct current stimulation slows reaction time in a working memory task. BMC Neuroscience, 6(1), 23.

[108] Martins, F. C., & Ortiz, K. Z. (2009). The relationship between working memory and apraxia of speech. Arquivos de Neuro-Psiquiatria, 67(3B), 843–848.

[109] Massachusetts Health Quality Partners (MHQP). (2012). 2012/13 Pediatric routine preventive care recommendations. Retrieved November 17, 2013, from http://www.mhqp.org/guidelines/pedPreventive/pedGuidelines.asp?nav=041114.

[110] Maxwell, L., & Evans, G. W. (2000). The effects of noise on pre-school children's pre-reading skills. Journal of Environmental Psychology, 20(1), 91–98.

[111] McSporran, E., Butterworth, Y., & Rowson, V. J. (1997). Sound field amplification and listening behaviour in the classroom. British Educational Research Journal, 23, 81–96.

[112] Montgomery, J. W. (2003). Working memory and comprehension in children with specific language impairment: What we know so far. Journal of Communication Disorders, 36(3), 221–231.

[113] Nee, D. E., Brown, J. W., Askren, M. K., et al. (2013). A meta-analysis of executive components of working memory. Cerebral Cortex, 23(2), 264–282.

[114] Ngo, H. V., Claussen, J. C., Born, J., & Mölle, M. (2013). Induction of slow oscillations by rhythmic acoustic stimulation. Journal of Sleep Research, 22(1), 22–31.

[115] Nikjeh, D. A., Lister, J. J., & Frisch, S. A. (2009). Preattentive cortical-evoked responses to pure tones, harmonic tones, and speech: Influence of music training. Ear and Hearing, 30(4), 432–446.

[116] Ohn, S. H., Park, C. I., Yoo, W. K., et al. (2008). Time-dependent effect of transcranial direct current stimulation on the enhancement of working memory. NeuroReport, 19(1), 43–47.

[117] Oticon Foundation in New Zealand. (2002). Classroom acoustics: A New Zealand perspective. Retrieved November 3, 2011, from http://download.contentx.ch/160/new%20zeeland.pdf.

[118] Oudiette, D., & Paller, K. A. (2013). Upgrading the sleeping brain with targeted memory reactivation. Trends in Cognitive Sciences, 17(3), 142–149.

[119] Owen, A. M., Hampshire, A., Grahn, J. A., et al. (2010). Putting brain training to the test. Nature, 465(7299), 775–778.

[120] Parbery-Clark, A., Skoe, E., Lam, C., & Kraus, N. (2009). Musician enhancement for speech-in-noise. Ear and Hearing, 30(6), 653–661.

[121] Park, S. H., Seo, J. H., Kim, Y. H., & Ko, M. H. (2014). Long-term effects of transcranial direct current stimulation combined with computer-assisted cognitive training in healthy older adults. NeuroReport, 25(2), 122–126.

[122] Patel, A. D., Wong, M., Foxton, J., Lochy, A., & Peretz, I. (2008). Speech intonation perception deficits in musical tone deafness (congenital amusia). Music Perception, 25, 357–368.

[123] Payton, K. L., Uchanski, R. M., & Braida, L. D. (1994). Intelligibility of conversational and clear speech in noise and reverberation for listeners with normal and impaired hearing. Journal of the Acoustical Society of America, 95(3), 1581–1592.

[124] Pederson, E., & Guion-Anderson, S. (2010). Orienting attention during phonetic training facilitates learning. Journal of the Acoustical Society of America, 127(2), EL54–EL59.

[125] Picheny, M. A., Durlach, N. I., & Braida, L. D. (1985). Speaking clearly for the hard of hearing: 1. Intelligibility differences between clear and conversational speech. Journal of Speech and Hearing Research, 28(1), 96–103.

[126] Picheny, M. A., Durlach, N. I., & Braida, L. D. (1986). Speaking clearly for the hard of hearing: 2. Acoustic characteristics of clear and conversational speech. Journal of Speech and Hearing Research, 29(4), 434–446.

[127] Pickering, S. J., & Gathercole, S. E. (2004). Distinctive working memory profiles in children with special educational needs. Educational Psychology, 24, 393–408.

[128] Poulin, V., Korner-Bitensky, N., Dawson, D. R., & Bherer, L. (2012). Efficacy of executive function interventions after stroke: A systematic review. Topics in Stroke Rehabilitation, 19, 158–171.

[129] Purdy, S. C., Smart, J. L., Baily, M., & Sharma, M. (2009). Do children with reading delay benefit from the use of personal FM systems in the classroom? International Journal of Audiology, 48(12), 843–852.

[130] Racette, A., Bard, C., & Peretz, I. (2006). Making non-fluent aphasics speak: Sing along! Brain, 129(Pt. 10), 2571–2584.

[131] Rawool, V. W. (2012). Conservation and management of hearing loss in musicians. In V. W. Rawool (Ed.), Hearing conservation: In occupational, recreational, educational, and home settings (pp. 201–223). New York: Thieme.

[132] Recanzone, G. H., Schreiner, C. E., & Merzenich, M. M. (1993). Plasticity in the frequency representation of primary auditory cortex following discrimination training in adult owl monkeys. Journal of Neuroscience, 13(1), 87–103.

[133] Riley, K. G., & McGregor, K. K. (2012). Noise hampers children's expressive word learning. Language, Speech, and Hearing Services in Schools, 43(3), 325–337.

[134] Ronsse, L. M., & Wang, L. M. (2010). Effects of noise from building mechanical systems on elementary student achievement. ASHRAE Transactions, 116, 347–354.

[135] Ronsse, L. M., & Wang, L. M. (2013). Relationships between unoccupied classroom acoustical conditions and elementary student achievement measured in eastern Nebraska. Journal of the Acoustical Society of America, 133(3), 1480–1495.

[136] Rudner, M., Lunner, T., Behrens, T., Thorén, E. S., & Rönnberg, J. (2012). Working memory capacity may influence perceived effort during aided speech recognition in noise. Journal of the American Academy of Audiology, 23(8), 577–589.

[137] Rueda, M. R., Rothbart, M. K., McCandliss, B. D., Saccomanno, L., & Posner, M. I. (2005). Training, maturation, and genetic influences on the development of executive attention. Proceedings of the National Academy of Sciences USA, 102(41), 14931–14936.

[138] Schäffler, T., Sonntag, J., Hartnegg, K., & Fischer, B. (2004). The effect of practice on low-level auditory discrimination, phonological skills, and spelling in dyslexia. Dyslexia, 10(2), 119–130.

[139] Schum, D. J. (1997). Beyond hearing aids: Clear speech training as an intervention strategy. Hearing Journal, 50, 36–39.

[140] Searl, J., & Evitts, P. M. (2013). Tongue-palate contact pressure, oral air pressure, and acoustics of clear speech. Journal of Speech, Language, and Hearing Research, 56(3), 826–839.

[141] Shahin, A. J. (2011). Neurophysiological influence of musical training on speech perception. Frontiers in Psychology, 2, 126.

[142] Shalev, L., Tsal, Y., & Mevorach, C. (2007). Computerized progressive attentional training (CPAT) program: Effective direct intervention for children with ADHD. Child Neuropsychology, 13(4), 382–388.

[143] Shield, B., & Dockrell, J. (2008a). The effects of classroom and environmental noise on children's academic performance. Paper presented at the Ninth International Congress on Noise as a Public Health Problem (ICBEN), Foxwoods, CT.

[144] Shield, B. M., & Dockrell, J. E. (2008b). The effects of environmental and classroom noise on the academic attainments of primary school children. Journal of the Acoustical Society of America, 123(1), 133–144.

[145] Shinn-Cunningham, B. G., Kopco, N., & Martin, T. J. (2005). Localizing nearby sound sources in a classroom: Binaural room impulse responses. Journal of the Acoustical Society of America, 117(5), 3100-3115.

[146] Smiljanić, R., & Bradlow, A. R. (2011). Bidirectional clear speech perception benefit for native and high-proficiency non-native talkers and listeners: Intelligibility and accentedness. Journal of the Acoustical Society of America, 130(6), 4020–4031.

[147] Smith, E. E., & Jonides, J. (1997). Working memory: A view from neuroimaging. Cognitive Psychology, 33(1), 5–42.

[148] Smith, E. E., & Jonides, J. (1998). Neuroimaging analyses of human working memory. Proceeding of the National Academy of Sciences of the United States of America. 95(20). 12061–12068.

[149] Smith, E. E., Jonides, J., & Koeppe, R. A. (1996). Dissociating verbal and spatial working memory using PET. Cerebral Cortex, 6(1), 11–20.

[150] Smoski, W. J., Brunt, M. A., & Tannahill, J. C. (1992). Listening characteristics of children with central auditory processing disorders. Language, Speech, and Hearing Services in Schools, 23, 145–152.

[151] Solan, H. A., Shelley-Tremblay, J., Ficarra, A., Silverman, M., & Larson, S. (2003). Effect of attention therapy on reading comprehension. Journal of Learning Disabilities, 36(6), 556–563.

[152] Song, J. H., Skoe, E., Banai, K., & Kraus, N. (2012). Training to improve hearing speech in noise: Biological mechanisms. Cerebral Cortex, 22(5), 1180–1190.

[153] Spiers, H. J., & Bendor, D. (2014). Enhance, delete, incept: Manipulating hippocampus-dependent memories. Brain Research Bulletin, 105, 2-7.

[154] Sternberg, S. (1969). Memory-scanning: Mental processes revealed by reaction-time experiments. American Scientist, 57(4), 421–457.

[155] Stevens, C., Fanning, J., Coch, D., Sanders, L., & Neville, H. (2008). Neural mechanisms of selective auditory attention are enhanced by computerized training: Electrophysiological evidence from language-impaired and typically developing children. Brain Research, 1205, 55–69.

[156] Strenziok, M., Parasuraman, R., Clarke, E., Cisler, D. S., Thompson, J. C., & Greenwood, P. M. (2014). Neurocognitive enhancement in older adults: Comparison of three cognitive training tasks to test a hypothesis of training transfer in brain connectivity. Neuroimage, 85(Pt. 3), 1027–1039.

[157] Stroop, J. R. (1935). Studies of interference in serial verbal reactions. Journal of Experimental Psycholgy, 18, 643–662.

[158] Sweetow, R. W., & Sabes, J. H. (2010). Auditory training and challenges associated with participation and compliance. Journal of the American Academy of Audiology, 21(9), 586–593.

[159] Tallal, P., Miller, S. L., Bedi, G., et al. (1996). Language comprehension in language-learning impaired children improved with acoustically modified speech. Science, 271 (5245), 81–84.

[160] Tervaniemi, M., Kruck, S., De Baene, W., Schröger, E., Alter, K., & Friederici, A. D. (2009). Top-down modulation of auditory processing: Effects of sound context, musical expertise and attentional focus. European Journal of Neuroscience, 30 (8), 1636–1642.

[161] Thompson, W. F., Marin, M. M., & Stewart, L. (2012). Reduced sensitivity to emotional prosody in congenital amusia rekindles the musical protolanguage hypothesis. Proceedings of the National Academy of Sciences of the United States of America, 109(46), 19027–19032.

[162] Tye-Murray, N., & Witt, S. (1997). Communication strategies training. Seminars in Hearing, 18, 153–165.

[163] Vemuri, S., Schmandt, C., Bender, W., Tellex, S., & Lassey, B. (2004). An audio-based personal memory aid. Proceedings of UbiComp, 2004, 400-417.

[164] Wechsler, D. (2004). The Wechsler intelligence scale for children (5th ed.). London: Pearson Assessment.

[165] Weiskopf, N. (2012). Real-time fMRI and its application to neurofeedback. Neuroimage, 62(2), 682–692.

[166] Wilson, W. J., Jackson, A., Pender, A., et al. (2011). The CHAPS, SIFTER, and TAPS-R as predictors of (C)AP skills and (C)APD. Journal of Speech, Language, and Hearing Research, 54(1), 278–291.

[167] Wilson, R. H., & McArdle, R. (2012). Speech-in-noise measures: Variable versus fixed speech and noise levels. International Journal of Audiology, 51(9), 708–712.

[168] Woodford, C. M., Tomkowski, A. C., & Lawrence, L. D. (1998). Improving listening conditions in agriculture and forestry higher education classrooms. NACTA Journal, 42(1), 42–45.

[169] Wright, B. A., Buonomano, D. V., Mahncke, H. W., & Merzenich, M. M. (1997). Learning and generalization of auditory temporal-interval discrimination in humans. Journal of Neurosciences, 17(10), 3956–3963.

[170] Wright, B. A., & Sabin, A. T. (2007). Perceptual learning: How much daily training is enough? Experimental Brain Research, 180(4), 727–736.

[171] Yathiraj, A., & Maggu, A. R. (2013). Screening Test for Auditory Processing (STAP): A preliminary report. Journal of the American Academy of Audiology, 24(9), 867–878.

[172] Zekveld, A. A., George, E. L., Kramer, S. E., Goverts, S. T., & Houtgast, T. (2007). The development of the text reception threshold test: A visual analogue of the speech reception threshold test. Journal of Speech, Language, and Hearing Research, 50(3), 576–584.

[173] Zekveld, A. A., Kramer, S. E., Vlaming, M. S., & Houtgast, T. (2008). Audiovisual perception of speech in noise and masked written text. Ear and Hearing, 29(1), 99–111.

[174] Zhang, G., Yao, L., Zhang, H., Long, Z., & Zhao, X. (2013). Improved working memory performance through self-regulation of dorsal lateral prefrontal cortex activation using real-time fMRI. PLoS ONE, 8(8), e73735.

[175] Zhang, Y. X., Barry, J. G., Moore, D. R., & Amitay, S. (2012). A new test of attention in listening (TAIL) predicts auditory performance. PLoS ONE, 7(12), e53502.

[176] Zinke, K., Zeintl, M., Rose, N. S., Putzmann, J., Pydde, A., & Kliegel, M. (2014). Working memory training and transfer in older adults: Effects of age, baseline performance, and training gains. Developmental Psychology, 50(1), 304 –315.

Chapter 9

Training to Improve Auditory Temporal Processing

9 Training to Improve Auditory Temporal Processing

Individuals with temporal processing deficits should be provided with training to address their specific needs. Several studies have reported improvement with training in various aspects of auditory temporal processing. Many of the studies have used computerized training programs. However, some of the training tasks can be implemented using real-life activities and presented in motivating game-like formats. This chapter discusses the effectiveness of some of the training procedures used for improving auditory temporal processing.

9.1 Frequency Discrimination

Frequency information is partially coded in the auditory system through tonotopic organization and by the phase-locked activity of neurons. Thus, accurate temporal processing or phase-locking plays an important role in frequency discrimination. In a study by Jäncke, Gaab, Wüstenberg, Scheich, and Heinze (2001), listeners were asked to press a button to indicate when they heard a rare (14%) stimulus (952 Hz) that was presented among stimuli of another frequency (e.g., 950 Hz), which were presented more frequently (e.g., 86%).

The performance of some listeners improved within five sessions (1 week), whereas other participants did not show improvement with similar short-term training. The hemodynamic responses in the auditory cortex decrease significantly for the listeners who showed improvement with training, suggesting a reduction in internal noise. Such improvements were not apparent for listeners who did not show improvements or for listeners in the control group who did not receive any training. Note that, in this task, the listeners were expected to respond only to rare stimuli; no response was required for frequent stimuli (Jäncke et al., 2001).

If the oddball task is modified so that the listener is expected to identify the oddball, or rare, frequency stimulus as deviant and the frequent frequency stimulus as standard, frequency discrimination can improve rapidly in the first week with smaller but constant improvements over the next 2 weeks. During such training, listeners are provided with feedback about the accuracy of each response (▶ Fig. 9.1). Patient responses can be classified as shown in ▶ Fig. 9.2 for further analyses. Improvements following such training are accompanied by an increase in the amplitudes of the

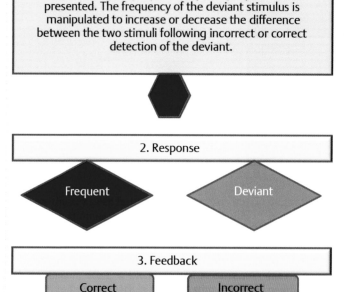

Fig. 9.1 Example of a training paradigm to improve frequency discrimination when the listener is required to listen to one stimulus on each trial and judge the stimulus as being either frequent or deviant.

1. Either a deviant (0.3) or a frequent (0.7) stimulus is presented. The frequency of the deviant stimulus is manipulated to increase or decrease the difference between the two stimuli following incorrect or correct detection of the deviant.

2. Response

Frequent | Deviant

3. Feedback

Correct | Incorrect

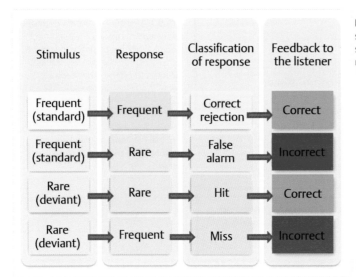

Stimulus	Response	Classification of response	Feedback to the listener
Frequent (standard)	Frequent	Correct rejection	Correct
Frequent (standard)	Rare	False alarm	Incorrect
Rare (deviant)	Rare	Hit	Correct
Rare (deviant)	Frequent	Miss	Incorrect

Fig. 9.2 Classification of patient responses with the use of the procedure shown in ▶ Fig. 9.1 (based on Menning, Roberts, & Pantev, 2000).

magnetoencephalographic mismatch negativity field to the deviant stimuli (Menning, Roberts, & Pantev, 2000).

Frequency discrimination can improve with training relatively quickly within 500 trials in normal-hearing listeners using a two-interval, two-alternative forced choice (2I-2AFC) task, as shown in ▶ Fig. 9.3. Approximately 76 to 98% of the improvement appears to be perceptual rather than procedural. Task-specific improvement accounts for only about 2 to 24% of such learning (Hawkey, Amitay, & Moore, 2004). Improvement in frequency discrimination can occur using a similar 2I-2AFC procedure and feedback of happy and sad faces (▶ Fig. 9.3) for accurate and inaccurate responses. Such improvement appears to be related to a decrease in internal noise (e.g., spontaneous firing of neurons) following training (Jones, Moore, Amitay, & Shub, 2013).

An example of the sequence of events used in training with feedback is shown in ▶ Fig. 9.4. If feedback about the accuracy of the responses is provided during behavioral training, as shown in ▶ Fig. 9.4, and the participant dedicates sufficient time, the degree of improvement in frequency discrimination can be relatively large. Using the training paradigm shown in ▶ Fig. 9.4, one of the listeners in a study by Cansino and Williamson (1997) managed to improve frequency discrimination thresholds from 50 to 10 Hz after approximately 74,000 trials. The listener needed more trials, as the difference between the standard and the probe tones became smaller than when the differences were larger. Reaction time decreases

and confidence levels increase with such training. Improved frequency discrimination in this study was accompanied by a decrease in the relative auditory magnetic field amplitude of the 100 ms component recorded from the primary and association auditory cortices (Cansino & Williamson, 1997).

A 3I-3AFC procedure (▶ Fig. 9.5) has also been used successfully to lead individuals to improve their frequency discrimination at 5 or 8 kHz. Although the improvement generalizes to tones of untrained frequencies, better improvement is apparent for the trained frequency (Irvine, Martin, Klimkeit, & Smith, 2000). After providing 12 hours of training to improve frequency discrimination at a trained frequency, minimal training (e.g., 2 hours) at untrained frequencies is sufficient to obtain finer frequency discrimination at untrained frequencies. In addition, the learning effect generalizes to the untrained ear. Which ear is used for training has no significant effect on the generalization of learning across ears (Delhommeau, Micheyl, & Jouvent, 2005). Frequency discrimination learning generalizes across some stimulus durations using a 3I-2AFC procedure. In this case, the listeners are presented with three tones, and the first tone is always of a fixed frequency (e.g., 1000 Hz). One of the remaining tones has the same frequency, and the other has a slightly higher frequency. The listeners' task is to indicate whether the second or the third tone has a pitch that is different from the pitch of the other two tones. In this case, if training is provided using stimuli lasting for 200 ms, the learning can generalize to stimuli

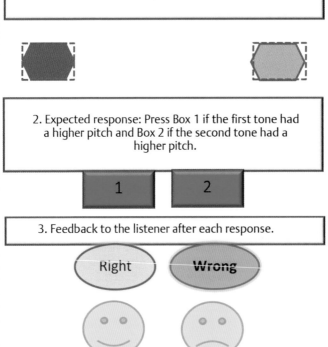

1. Presentation of two stimuli: A standard tone of 1000 Hz and another tone of higher frequency. The frequency of the higher tone is changed adaptively based on the response of the listener.

2. Expected response: Press Box 1 if the first tone had a higher pitch and Box 2 if the second tone had a higher pitch.

1   2

3. Feedback to the listener after each response.

Right   Wrong

Fig. 9.3 Sequence of events in the two-interval, two-alternative forced choice (2I-2AFC) testing and training procedure used by Hawkey, Amitay, and Moore (2004). The feedback provided by Jones, Moore, Amitay, and Shub (2013) consisted of happy or sad faces, as shown in the last row. This feedback was designed to encourage optimal response behavior and to minimize the use of non-stimulus-driven strategies.

with durations of 100 ms but not to stimuli with durations of 40 ms (Delhommeau, Micheyl, Jouvent, & Collet, 2002).

The ability to discriminate small changes in the carrier frequency of 40 Hz modulated tones can improve following 15 adaptive training sessions of 30 minutes each in nonmusicians. The improvement can generalize to a lesser degree to untrained frequencies and is accompanied by enhancement of the P2 and N1c (defined as the most negative peak occurring between 120 ms and 180 ms at electrodes T7 and T8 based on the radial orientation of this trough in each hemisphere) auditory evoked cortical potentials (Bosnyak, Eaton, & Roberts, 2004), suggesting improved phase-locked activity or finer neural tuning.

The effect of training on frequency discrimination and generalization to other frequencies in children may be dependent on the characteristics of the children, the attentional or memory demands of the specific training tasks, the duration of training, and the availability or lack of a learning

consolidation period. In one study, 100 normally hearing 6- to 11-year-old children received approximately 1 hour of training to improve frequency discrimination using a 3AFC procedure similar to that shown in ▶ Fig. 9.5, with the exception that the children received computerized game-like training and trial-by-trial visual feedback after each correct response. In addition, they could see tokens accumulating at the bottom of the touch screen as a reflection of their ongoing success. Following training, frequency discrimination thresholds improved across all age groups, including the 6- to 7-, 8- to 9-, and 10- to 11-year age groups, demonstrating that auditory learning can be induced within a short period in children. There was a marked variation in frequency discrimination ability before and after termination of the 1-hour training session. Approximately 20% of the children had frequency discrimination thresholds similar to those apparent in naive adults before the training began. Another 30% achieved thresholds similar to adults during training. The

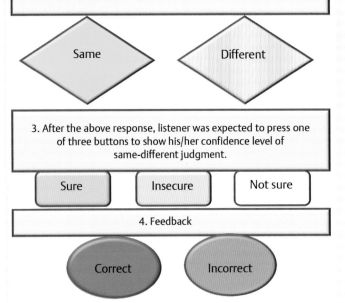

1. Stimulus presentation: Test stimulus (40 ms tone burst) is presented followed by presentation of the probe stimulus with an inter-stimulus interval of approximately 500 ms. The difference in the probe and the stimulus frequency varied from 5 and 50 Hz.

2. Response: The listener pressed one of the two buttons to indicate whether the two stimuli were same or different. The training is provided in 300 trial blocks. The test and probe stimuli are the same in half of the trials and different in the rest of the trials. The intertrial intervals were 1500, 2000, and 2500 ms presented in random order.

Same

Different

3. After the above response, listener was expected to press one of three buttons to show his/her confidence level of same-different judgment.

Sure

Insecure

Not sure

4. Feedback

Correct

Incorrect

Fig. 9.4 Auditory training procedures used by Cansino and Williamson (1997) to improve frequency discrimination.

remaining children did not achieve adultlike performance at any point during the 1-hour training. Learning did not generalize to a different standard frequency (Halliday, Taylor, Edmondson-Jones, & Moore, 2008). For children, greater variability in stimuli may be necessary for successful generalization to other stimuli and tasks.

Ten- to 15-minute daily sessions over 10 to 20 days of adaptive practice with feedback can lead to improvement of frequency discrimination thresholds in many (80%) children with dyslexia, and the effect of training along with training of other auditory tasks transfers to language-related phonological and spelling skills (Schäffler, Sonntag, Hartnegg, & Fischer, 2004).

Optimal learning regimens for frequency discrimination training using the 3AFC procedure

(▶ Fig. 9.5) presented in game-like formats with trial-by-trial feedback on task performance consist of short sessions that are spaced over several days during early learning stages. The group with the shortest training sessions lasting for approximately 8 minutes (100 trials daily) showed significantly faster learning in the early stages of training compared to groups receiving longer training sessions. In later training stages, the group with the longest training sessions lasting for more than 1 hour (800 trials daily) showed slower learning than other groups. The time between the training sessions allowed for maximum latent improvements or more opportunities for consolidation of perceptual learning (Molloy, Moore, Sohoglu, & Amitay, 2012). Compliance may be better with less intense regimens, and learning may be more efficient.

1. Listener initiates a trial by pushing first of three buttons on a handheld three key pad.

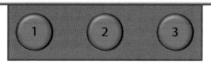

Fig. 9.5 Steps in a three-alternative forced choice (3AFC) procedure for improving frequency discrimination (Based on Irvine, Martin, Klimkeit, & Smith, 2000).

2. Stimuli presented in three intervals indicated by light. The frequency in two of the intervals is the same. In the third randomly selected interval, it is higher. The frequency difference is increased in the presence of each incorrect response and decreased following two consecutive correct responses.

3. The listener's task is to press one of the buttons to indicate which interval had the higher frequency.

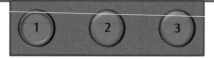

4. The difference limen for frequency (DLF) is determined after 11 reversals including 6 downward reversals. The geometric mean of the frequency difference in the last 8 reversals is determined to be the DLF.

5. After each DLF estimate, the listener is informed of his/her threshold.
(Note: No feedback is provided after each response.)

9.2 Gap Detection Thresholds

Gap detection thresholds using adaptive tasks in which the duration of the gap is varied based on the listener's performance (▶ Fig. 9.6) can improve with practice without any feedback over 4 days with practice sessions of approximately 1 hour each day. During such tasks, if the markers at the beginning or the end of the gap are fixed in duration, stimuli with gaps have longer duration than stimuli without gaps. Thus, listeners can use overall duration of the tonal pair to determine which pair has a gap. Because the longer duration pair can be judged as the one with a gap, the duration of the markers of each pair that have no gaps can be increased to match the overall duration of stimuli with gaps. Such manipulation can cause an increase in spectral power in the stimulus pair without the gap. To control for these confounds, gap and no-gap stimuli can be created by using markers consisting of a single pure tone which are temporally enveloped by a series of overlapping Gaussian windows (Schneider, Pichora-Fuller, Kowalchuk, & Lamb, 1994). Each Gaussian window can have a standard deviation of 1 ms, and the temporal offset between peaks of successive windows can be set to 1 ms. The duration of each marker in this case is defined as the number of Gaussian windows in the series

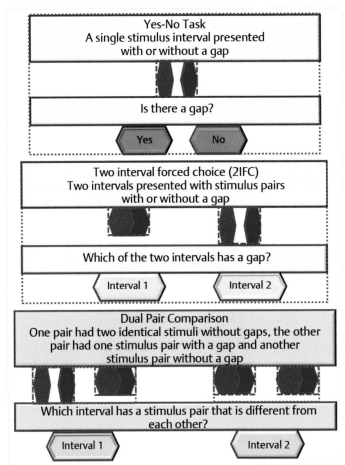

Fig. 9.6 Various procedures used for gap detection testing and training by Smith, Trainor, Gray, Plantinga, and Shore (2008). The duration of the gap is changed adaptively based on the response of the listener.

and gap size is defined as the number of 1-ms Gaussian windows between the last window of the first marker and the first window of the second marker. Spectral density functions for such stimuli with or without gaps show similar ranges and profiles. After practice on gap detection tasks (▶ Fig. 9.6), the greatest improvement is apparent under stimulus conditions where the initial performance is not near ceiling. The thresholds are initially better for gap markers closer in frequency than those further apart in frequency. Thus, more improvement is apparent in detecting gaps between tones of 1000 and 4000 Hz than when the gap markers are closer in frequency (e.g., gaps between 1000 and 1150 Hz). Gap detection thresholds are higher for the yes-no task (▶ Fig. 9.6) than the dual-pair comparison task. Thus, more improvement is apparent after training in the yes-no task (Smith, Trainor, Gray, Plantinga, & Shore, 2008).

In general, older adults exhibit significantly poorer gap detection thresholds than younger adults. However, in one study, following 10 training sessions spaced 1 or 2 days apart and using a 3I-3AFC procedure with visual feedback showing the correct answer, the mean gap detection thresholds of older adults appeared similar to those of younger adults (Kishon-Rabin, Avivi-Reich, & Roth, 2013). Younger adults also showed improved gap detection after training. No such improvement was apparent in the control group of younger and older adults. Both the trained younger and older adults in the study retained their improvement in performance 1 month after training.

Ten- to 15-minute daily sessions over 10 to 20 days of adaptive practice with feedback can lead to improvement of gap detection thresholds in many (77%) children with dyslexia; furthermore,

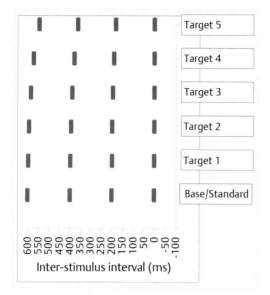

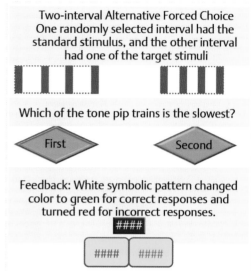

Fig. 9.7 Schematic of stimuli used in the temporal rate (modulation) discrimination training procedure used by van Wassenhove and Nagarajan (2007). The stimuli were 1 kHz tone pip trains with four tone pips in each train. The standard or base stimulus was modulated at the rate of 5 Hz with an interstimulus interval of 200 ms. The targets were modulated at higher rates: 5.03125 (target 1), 5.0625 (target 2), 5.125 (target 3), 5.25 (target 4), and 5.5 (target 5) Hz.

Fig. 9.8 The training task used by van Wassenhove and Nagarajan (2007) to improve temporal rate (modulation) discrimination.

the effect of training, along with training of other auditory tasks, transfers to language-related phonological and spelling skills (Schäffler et al., 2004).

9.3 Temporal Modulation Detection

The ability to detect sinusoidal amplitude modulations (SAMs; 80 Hz rate, 3–4 kHz band pass carrier frequency) in the temporal waveform can improve with adaptive training with feedback after each trial. During training, either the modulation depth or the rate is varied. There is a considerable amount of variability in the amount of training required. Some listeners can reach asymptomatic performance within one session, whereas others can continue to improve over a period of four to six sessions. The training effects can generalize to untrained modulation rates of 30 and 150 Hz. In addition, brief exposure to the tasks during a pre-training test session alone appears to lead to improved performance after 1 week in individuals in

an untrained control group (Fitzgerald & Wright, 2011).

9.4 Temporal Rate (Modulation) Discrimination

With a relatively short amount of training lasting for 3 days with 1 hour practice daily, listeners can improve their ability to distinguish between stimuli that differ in temporal modulation rates, as shown in ▶ Fig. 9.7. The training procedure in this investigation was 2I-2AFC, and feedback about accuracy of response was provided to the participants, as shown in ▶ Fig. 9.8. The improvement after training was reflected in lower discrimination thresholds and improved ability to detect modulation. The learning partially generalized to a gap duration discrimination task where, instead of four components, as shown in ▶ Fig. 9.7, only two components were presented in each stimulus interval. The improvement in temporal rate discrimination was accompanied by an increase in the amplitudes of the early magnetoencephalographic responses evoked by the trained stimuli, which indicated plastic changes in the auditory nervous system. In addition, there was an increase in the power of evoked activity in the high gamma (γ) band (62–98 Hz) located in the left inferior frontal cortex (van Wassenhove & Nagarajan,

2007). It should be noted that the stimuli (tone-pip trains) in this study differed not only in the stimulus rate but also in the overall durations of the tone-pip trains. At higher modulation rates, the stimuli had shorter overall duration, as shown in ▶ Fig. 9.7. Thus, either duration, rate, or both cues may have been used by listeners to improve their discrimination performance.

9.5 Temporal, Spectral, and Spectrotemporal Modulation Depth Discrimination

Sabin, Eddins, and Wright (2012) provided auditory training to normal-hearing listeners to improve their ability to discriminate the depth of spectral, temporal, or upward spectrotemporal modulation. The standard stimulus was a modulated noise with a 50 dB depth. The target stimuli had shallower depths. The standard stimuli were presented randomly in two of three stimulus intervals in each trial. The target stimulus was presented in the remaining third interval. Listeners had to identify the interval that contained the stimulus with the shallower depth by clicking the mouse on the appropriate visual display of one of the three intervals. After each trial they received feedback about the accuracy of their response. The noise modulation depth (peak-to-valley difference in dB) was adjusted adaptively. Listeners were able to improve their ability to discriminate the depth of spectral, temporal, or spectrotemporal modulation with 1 hour of training daily over a period of 7 days. A matched control group did not show such improvement (Sabin et al., 2012).

9.6 Discrimination of Spectral Profile

Profile analysis is a term used to describe a listener's ability to detect changes in the spectral shape or profile of a complex sound (Green, 1988). A spectral profile in this context consists of several pure tone components presented simultaneously. The spectral shape or profile can be changed by increasing the intensity of one of the components, thereby creating a spectral "bump." For example, a spectral profile can be composed of 11 pure tones of the same sound pressure level. The level of the middle component can be varied in small steps to see how much minimal change is necessary for the listener to detect a change in the spectral profile

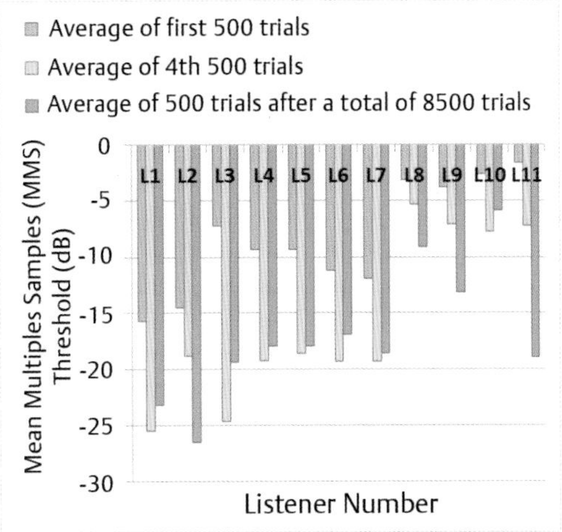

Fig. 9.9 Mean of multiple samples (MMS) thresholds (signal level relative to the context level) for detecting intensity change in the middle component of a stimulus with 11 pure tone components. The performance is shown for 11 listeners. The performance is averaged over a block of 500 trials. For some listeners, peak performance is apparent after 1500 trials (average of 4th 500 trials); for others, peak performance is apparent after 8500 trials (based on Drennan & Watson, 2001).

from the standard or reference profile. The listener's task is to select the profile that is different from the standard profile by listening to the standard and two other profiles, one of which is different from the standard. There is considerable variability in thresholds with a range of −1 to −25 dB (signal level relative to context level). The thresholds can improve with training. Good listeners can improve within 2000 trials, whereas some poor listeners may continue to improve with 9000 trials (▶ Fig. 9.9). Up to 6 hours of training is necessary to reach a plateau in performance following profile analyses training. In comparison, pure tone intensity discrimination training requires less training to reach asymptotic performance (Drennan & Watson, 2001).

9.7 Duration Discrimination Judgment

The ability to discriminate between a reference duration tone of 800 ms and another tone either shorter or longer in duration can improve following training with speech (consonant-vowel [CV] syllables) that is altered in such a way that the

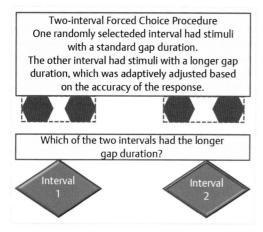

Two-interval Forced Choice Procedure
One randomly selecteded interval had stimuli with a standard gap duration.
The other interval had stimuli with a longer gap duration, which was adaptively adjusted based on the accuracy of the response.

Which of the two intervals had the longer gap duration?

Interval 1

Interval 2

Fig. 9.10 Schematic illustration of the procedure for improving gap duration discrimination used by Wright, Buonomano, Mahncke, and Merzenich (1997).

most rapidly changing components are extended to allow more processing time and are amplified by up to 20% to make them more salient (Nagarajan et al., 1998; Tallal et al., 1996). As the child gains proficiency in recognizing the components accurately, the rate and volume of the speech segments are adaptively and gradually returned to the levels found in average conversational speech. The modified speech is presented in computer game format to maintain attention and motivation. Children trained with the modified speech show improved accuracy on a task involving auditory duration discrimination of 1000 Hz tones (Agnew, Dorn, & Eden, 2004).

9.8 Gap Duration Discrimination

Gap duration discrimination thresholds can improve with adaptive practice and immediate feedback on accuracy of performance in many participants when they are expected to discriminate between a standard gap of 100 ms marked by short 1 kHz tone pips and a comparison gap (▶ Fig. 9.10). There is some individual variability in the amount of improvement, and the improvement can generalize to a similar 100 ms gap that is marked by tones of different frequencies, such as 4 or 3.75 kHz. However, the learning does not transfer to different standard gap durations of 50, 200, or 500 ms (Karmarkar & Buonomano, 2003; Wright, Buonomano, Mahncke, & Merzenich, 1997). Improvement in gap duration discrimination thresholds can generalize

to duration discrimination tasks if the standard gap and tone durations are similar (e.g., 100 ms gap or 100 ms tone; Karmarkar & Buonomano, 2003).

Bratzke, Schröter, and Ulrich (2014) used a gap duration training procedure with a single stimulus protocol. At the beginning of each block of trials, listeners were presented with 10 trials of the standard stimulus. After this presentation, they were presented with one of eight possible target stimuli with gap durations centered on the standard gap duration of 100 ms. This included durations shorter than the standard (79, 85, 91, or 97 ms) and gap durations longer than the standard (103, 109, 115, or 121 ms). The listeners were instructed to respond with their left index finger when the target was shorter than the standard gap duration and with their right index finger when the target was longer than the standard gap duration. In the presence of an incorrect response, participants received tactile stimulation on their right lower leg for 500 ms. With such a procedure, gap duration discrimination can improve following training offered only over 4 days with 30-minute sessions on each day (Bratzke, Seifried, & Ulrich, 2012). Most of the improvement appears to occur during the early period of training. The effect of training generalizes to visual modality, showing cross-modal transfer. The transfer effects are larger after a 24-hour consolidation period compared to a 5-minute consolidation period (Bratzke et al., 2014).

9.9 Temporal Asynchrony Detection

A 2I-2AFC procedure (▶ Fig. 9.11) can be used to improve the detection of temporal onset asynchrony within a two-tone stimulus complex consisting of 0.25 and 4 kHz frequencies. Within a training period of about 6 to 8 hours, the smallest onset difference that is detectable within the tonal complex can improve from the initial 80 ms difference in time (Δt) to approximately 20 ms Δt. The training effect does not generalize to untrained frequency pairs or the detection of temporal offsets. The perceptual learning is maintained over a period of at least 1 to 2 months. A brief 1-hour exposure to temporal asynchrony threshold tasks without any specific additional training can lead to some improvement in individuals in control or nonexperimental groups (Mossbridge, Fitzgerald, O'Connor, & Wright, 2006).

The detection of temporal asynchrony at stimulus offset (▶ Fig. 9.12) can also improve with 1-hour adaptive training on a daily basis for 6 to 9

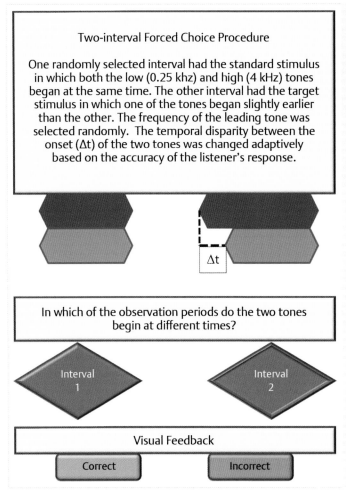

Two-interval Forced Choice Procedure

One randomly selected interval had the standard stimulus in which both the low (0.25 khz) and high (4 kHz) tones began at the same time. The other interval had the target stimulus in which one of the tones began slightly earlier than the other. The frequency of the leading tone was selected randomly. The temporal disparity between the onset (Δt) of the two tones was changed adaptively based on the accuracy of the listener's response.

Δt

In which of the observation periods do the two tones begin at different times?

Interval 1

Interval 2

Visual Feedback

Correct

Incorrect

Fig. 9.11 Schematic illustration of the procedure for improving temporal onset asynchrony detection used by Mossbridge, Fitzgerald, O'Connor, and Wright (2006).

days and can generalize to the detection of stimulus onset asynchrony. In addition, training on this task can improve temporal order judgment thresholds for detecting the order of tones within the two-tone complex, indicating generalization to an untrained temporal auditory task (Mossbridge, Scissors, & Wright, 2008). It appears that an efficient approach to improving temporal asynchrony detection may be to provide training for improving offset asynchrony.

9.10 Temporal Order Judgment Thresholds for Tones within a Two-Tone Complex

The smallest difference (Δt) in the onset of two tones needed to correctly judge the order of the two tones within a two-tone asynchronous complex can improve with adaptive training (▶ Fig. 9.13). In this task, listeners are provided with a standard asynchronous complex in which the low-frequency tone begins slightly earlier (Δt) than the high-frequency tone. In the target signal, the onset of the low-frequency tone lags behind the onset of the high-frequency tone. The smallest onset difference necessary to determine the observation interval in which the high-frequency tone begins sooner than the low-frequency tone is initially about 35 ms. Following approximately 6 to 8 hours of training, normal-hearing listeners can judge the temporal order of the tones correctly with onset asynchrony of about 15 ms. The learning effect does not generalize to untrained frequencies (Mossbridge et al., 2006). Similar improvements are possible after training for correctly judging the offset order of tones within a two-tone complex, and the training leads to improvement in

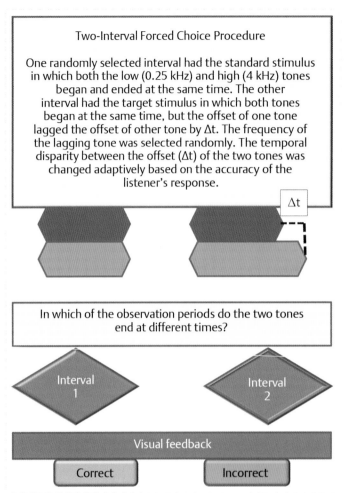

Two-Interval Forced Choice Procedure

One randomly selected interval had the standard stimulus in which both the low (0.25 kHz) and high (4 kHz) tones began and ended at the same time. The other interval had the target stimulus in which both tones began at the same time, but the offset of one tone lagged the offset of other tone by Δt. The frequency of the lagging tone was selected randomly. The temporal disparity between the offset (Δt) of the two tones was changed adaptively based on the accuracy of the listener's response.

Δt

In which of the observation periods do the two tones end at different times?

Interval 1   Interval 2

Visual feedback

Correct   Incorrect

Fig. 9.12 Schematic illustration of the procedure for improving temporal offset asynchrony detection used by Mossbridge, Fitzgerald, O'Connor, and Wright (2008).

correctly judging the onset order of the two tones (Mossbridge et al., 2008).

9.11 Interaural Temporal Order Judgment Thresholds

In the training task for improving interaural temporal order judgment thresholds, a stimulus is presented to each ear with a specific temporal interval between the two stimuli. The listeners are asked to indicate the ear that received the first of the two stimuli. The temporal interval between the stimuli presented to the right and the left ears is adjusted adaptively depending on the accuracy of the response. In a study by Mates, von Steinbüchel, Wittmann, and Treutwein (2001), patients with aphasia who needed 100 ms intervals to correctly judge the interaural temporal order could

judge the order correctly with 37 ms interstimulus intervals following adaptive training with feedback on the accuracy of their responses. This improvement generalized to the discrimination of /da/ versus /ta/ syllables. More specifically, their ability to discriminate /da/ and /ta/ syllables was significantly improved when compared to control groups with aphasia who received a no-temporal visual or auditory control training (Mates et al., 2001). Note that one of the cues important for the discrimination of the voiced /d/ and the voiceless /t/ is the voice onset time, which is shorter for /d/ when compared to that for /t/.

In one study, approximately 30 minutes of adaptive training with visual feedback on accuracy of response significantly improved the accuracy of interaural temporal order judgment performance, from 65 to 70%, for brief 10 ms noise bursts presented to the right and left ears in normal-hearing

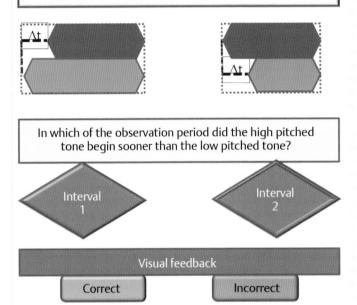

Two-Interval Forced Choice Procedure

One randomly selected interval had the standard stimulus in which the low (0.25 kHz) frequency tone began sooner (Δt) than the high (4 kHz) frequency tone. The remaining interval had the target stimulus in which the 0.25 kHz tone began later than the 4 kHz tone. The temporal disparity between the onset (Δt) of the two tones was the same in both intervals and was changed adaptively based on the accuracy of the listener's response.

In which of the observation period did the high pitched tone begin sooner than the low pitched tone?

Interval 1

Interval 2

Visual feedback

Correct

Incorrect

Fig. 9.13 Schematic illustration of the procedure for improving temporal onset order discrimination within an asynchronous two-tone complex used by Mossbridge, Fitzgerald, O'Connor, and Wright (2006).

individuals (Bernasconi, Grivel, Murray, & Spierer, 2010). At the beginning of the training, there was bilateral posterior sylvian region (PSR) activation, but at the end of the training, the activation pattern showed left hemisphere dominance. In addition, at the beginning of the training, there was a correlation between the left and right PSR activation, but at the end of the training, the left and right responses were uncorrelated (Bernasconi et al., 2010).

9.12 Stimulus Duration Thresholds for Accurate Temporal Order Judgment

For accurate judgment of temporal order of stimuli, the stimuli need to have a critical duration. The smallest duration necessary to judge the temporal order of four stimuli correctly presented one after another can be improved with training (▶ Fig. 9.14). There is individual variability in learning patterns (▶ Fig. 9.15), which may interact with such factors as the closeness of the spectral content of the stimuli included in the stimulus sequence (Neisser & Hirst, 1974).

Training can improve the ability of listeners to identify the correct order of unrelated sounds, such as hisses, tones, and buzzes lasting for 10 ms or less. Two mechanisms have been suggested to correctly judge the order of sounds. The first is fine resolution, which allows correct judgment of temporal order for sounds that are very brief (10 ms or less) in duration; training is often necessary to achieve such fine resolution. The second is a

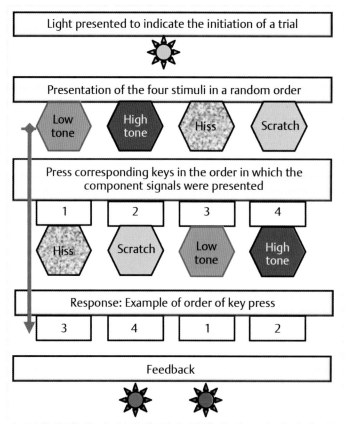

Light presented to indicate the initiation of a trial

Presentation of the four stimuli in a random order

| Low tone | High tone | Hiss | Scratch |

Press corresponding keys in the order in which the component signals were presented

| 1 | 2 | 3 | 4 |

| Hiss | Scratch | Low tone | High tone |

Response: Example of order of key press

| 3 | 4 | 1 | 2 |

Feedback

Fig. 9.14 The procedure used by Neisser and Hirst (1974) to improve the smallest duration of stimuli necessary to correctly judge the order of four sequential stimuli. The four stimuli were a low-frequency tone (500 Hz), a high-frequency tone (3,400 Hz), a hiss (broadband noise), and a scratch (made by passing white noise through a Schmitt trigger to maintain only the peaks, which were amplified). The durations of the stimuli were adjusted adaptively depending on the response of the listener.

course resolution mechanism that allows correct judgment of order for sounds that are usually longer than 200 ms in duration; this can be achieved without training in normal-hearing listeners (Warren, 1974).

9.13 Temporal Order Judgment with Sound-Emitting Toys

Simpler versions of temporal order judgment tasks can be implemented by using sound-emitting toys. Various sounds can be produced behind a child, and the child can then be asked to either create a similar sequence or name the toys/animals that produced the sounds in correct order or point to the toys in the correct order. Task difficulty can be varied by increasing or decreasing the duration of each sound, increasing or decreasing the interstimulus intervals, and varying the number of toys used in each trial. There are toys available that will sequentially play certain sounds, then allow the listener to play those back in the same sequence. An example of such a toy is the Mini Simon with

Carabiner, an electronic game of memory from Basic Fun (Boca Raton, FL). With each correct response, more sounds are added, and the speed of sound presentation is increased.

9.14 Improving Temporal Order Judgment with Applications

There are applications, or apps, that allow presentation of various sounds generated by animals, environmental sounds, or speech sounds. For example, free apps are available that have the potential to improve pitch-sequencing skills. One app, Blob Chorus: Pitch game (http://www.lumpty.com/music/training/blobPitch/blobPitch.html from Lumpty Learning, Penarth, United Kingdom), presents listeners with a series of vocals with different pitches. Listeners can then arrange the vocals from lower to higher using associated visual patterns (e.g., bars increasing in length). Another example is an Android app, Scenemon (http://www.joy-inn.com/scenemon/scenemon.html from Joy-inn, Paris, France), which is a version of the

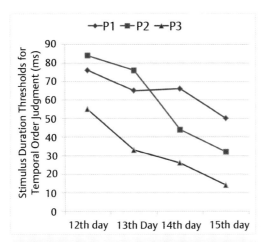

Fig. 9.15 Improvement in the smallest stimulus duration necessary for accurate judgment of the temporal order of a sequence of four stimuli for three normal participants (P). The durations of the four stimuli were changed adaptively based on the listener's response. The four stimuli were irregularly spaced by introducing a silent interval into each cycle of stimuli at a randomly determine point (based on Neisser & Hirst, 1975). Note the variability in the amount of improvement across listeners.

Simon game. Listeners are presented with a sequence of different tones along with corresponding visual cues. They then try to replicate the pattern by sequentially clicking on the related visual squares. The difficulty of the task is varied by increasing the number of sounds and the speed of presentation. In such applications, good working memory and visual skills are important for accurate response in the presence of several visual distractions on the screen. The benefits from such applications or generalization from training are unknown.

9.15 Frequency Order (Pitch Pattern Sequence) Judgment

Temporal order judgment for tonal sequences can improve after training. About 20 hours of experience spread over several weeks of daily practice may be necessary for long patterns consisting of 12 tones. Identification tends to be more accurate for initial (primacy effect) and final (recency effect) portions of each pattern compared to the middle portions. There is considerable individual variability in the learning patterns and the time required to reach near 90% accuracy in judging the

patterns (Leek & Watson, 1988). Approximately 64% of children with dyslexia showed performance below the 16th percentile rank on a temporal order judgment task involving two tones (1.00 and 1.12 kHz) of 200 ms duration. After training, the percentage of children showing performance below the 16th percentile dropped to 36% (Schäffler et al., 2004).

A related ability to judge temporal pitch/frequency patterns correctly is to detect individual tones in a complex pattern. This is similar to detecting a phoneme accurately in a complex sentence. Leek and Watson (1984) studied listeners' ability to hear all the details of an initially unfamiliar sequence of 10 tones of 45 ms duration by tracking detection thresholds for each tonal component. After a prolonged period of training, listeners were able to detect the presence or absence of individual tones even after attenuating the tones by 40 to 50 dB relative to the remaining tones in the pattern. Two different learning patterns were detected, with some listeners showing gradual improvement in detection thresholds over many trials, and others demonstrating abrupt reductions in thresholds following listening trials at high-intensity levels. Special training strategies such as improving the duration of the tones and reducing stimulus uncertainty improved the rate of training (Leek & Watson, 1984). Similar strategies have been incorporated in some of the current computerized training programs for improving speech perception. An application called Blob Chorus: Ear Training (http://www.lumpty.com/music/training/blobChorus/blobChorus.html) from Lumpty Learning, Penarth, United Kingdom, provides similar practice in detecting one sound among several sounds in a fun format.

9.16 Temporal Pattern Discrimination

Temporal pattern discrimination can improve with practice in which the listeners are expected to judge if the two presented patterns are the same or different. If tones within the pattern are presented at slower presentation rates (e.g., 5 components/s), the discrimination appears to be mainly based on discrimination of order of tones. However, at higher presentation rates of 62 or more components per second, listeners may rely primarily on the detection of spectral differences between the two patterns. For rates in between, either temporal order or spectral cues or a combination of the two cues may be used to discriminate between patterns (Nickerson & Freeman, 1974). Training in temporal pattern discrimination may be most effective if a wide range of frequencies are included during training, and the standard pattern is fixed during training (Barsz, 1996).

9.17 Backward Masking

Detection of a tone in the presence of a backward masker can improve with training in adults and some adolescents. The improvement occurs more slowly in adolescents than adults. The improvement can generalize to tones of untrained frequencies (Huyck & Wright, 2013). Adults can improve their performance after training incorporating feedback on performance by about 11 dB when the signal is a 1000 Hz tone, and the masker is composed of a narrow band (600–1400 Hz) centered around 1000 Hz. The effect of such training does not generalize to simultaneous masking tasks (Roth, Kishon-Rabin, & Hildesheimer, 2001).

9.18 Future Trends

Software tools are currently available that can assist in generating deficit-specific training to meet the needs of individuals with temporal processing deficits. For example, the System for Testing Auditory Responses (STAR, http://star.ihr.mrc.ac.uk/IHR_Software/STAR.aspx#auditorystar) tool from MRC Institute of Hearing Research (Nottingham, United Kingdom) allows presentation of N-alternative (2, 3, 4, etc.) forced choice sound discrimination tests with visual displays that appear on the screen along with the auditory stimuli and are used by the child to respond to the stimuli. More specifically, the Auditory STAR tool includes tasks such as frequency discrimination, backward masking, and simultaneous masking with flexibility for changing different parameters. Practice with these tasks has the potential for improving temporal processing skills. In the future, more such tools may be available to allow flexibility in designing deficit-specific training to meet the needs and interests of individual patients.

9.19 Review Questions

1. Compare and contrast the various training procedures used for improving frequency discrimination. Can frequency discrimination improve with training in children with dyslexia? What is the effect of duration of training on the efficiency of training designed to improve frequency discrimination? Discuss the physiological changes that can accompany improvement in frequency discrimination after training.

2. Discuss procedures used for improving gap detection thresholds. For which types of tasks and stimuli is maximum improvement in gap detection apparent? Is it possible to improve the gap detection thresholds of older individuals?

3. Review improvement of temporal modulation detection skills following training. Discuss the generalization effects apparent after such training.

4. Discuss the effect of auditory training on temporal rate discrimination. What types of changes are apparent in the auditory evoked responses after such training? Review the effects of training on modulation depth discrimination. What is profile analysis? What is the effect of training on the discrimination of spectral profile?

5. What is the effect of adaptive training with consonant-vowel (CV) syllables on tonal duration discrimination? What types of procedures can be used to improve gap duration discrimination? Review the effects of auditory training on gap duration discrimination and any associated transfer effects.

6. What types of procedures are used to improve temporal asynchrony detection? What is the most efficient approach for improving temporal synchrony detection? Review auditory training for improving the judgment of temporal order within an asynchronous two-tone complex.

7. Review auditory training for improving interaural temporal order judgment thresholds. Discuss training for improving the smallest stimulus duration necessary for accurate judgment of temporal order. How does the temporal order judgment differ for brief stimuli with durations within 10 ms and those with durations longer than 200 ms?

8. Outline a live training procedure for improving temporal order judgment in young children using sound-emitting toys. Locate and discuss some applications (apps) that can be used to improve temporal order judgment. Discuss the effect of auditory training on temporal order judgment in individuals with normal hearing and in children with dyslexia.

9. Discuss the effects of auditory training on temporal pattern discrimination and backward masking.

10. Briefly discuss potential future trends in training for addressing temporal processing deficits.

References

[1] Agnew, J. A., Dorn, C., & Eden, G. F. (2004). Effect of intensive training on auditory processing and reading skills. Brain and Language, 88(1), 21–25.

[2] Barsz, K. (1996). Accuracy of same/different judgments of sequences of complex tones differing in tonal order under various levels of fundamental frequency range, listener training, and type of standard sequence. Journal of the Acoustical Society of America, 99, 1660–1669.

[3] Bernasconi, F., Grivel, J., Murray, M. M., & Spierer, L. (2010). Plastic brain mechanisms for attaining auditory temporal order judgment proficiency. Neuroimage, 50(3), 1271–1279.

[4] Bosnyak, D. J., Eaton, R. A., & Roberts, L. E. (2004). Distributed auditory cortical representations are modified when non-musicians are trained at pitch discrimination with 40 Hz amplitude modulated tones. Cerebral Cortex, 14(10), 1088–1099.

[5] Bratzke, D., Schröter, H., & Ulrich, R. (2014). The role of consolidation for perceptual learning in temporal discrimination within and across modalities. Acta Psychologica (Amsterdam), 147, 75–79.

[6] Bratzke, D., Seifried, T., & Ulrich, R. (2012). Perceptual learning in temporal discrimination: Asymmetric cross-modal transfer from audition to vision. Experimental Brain Research, 221(2), 205–210.

[7] Cansino, S., & Williamson, S. J. (1997). Neuromagnetic fields reveal cortical plasticity when learning an auditory discrimination task. Brain Research, 764(1–2), 53–66.

[8] Delhommeau, K., Micheyl, C., & Jouvent, R. (2005). Generalization of frequency discrimination learning across frequencies and ears: Implications for underlying neural mechanisms in humans. Journal of the Association for Research in Otolaryngology, 6(2), 171–179.

[9] Delhommeau, K., Micheyl, C., Jouvent, R., & Collet, L. (2002). Transfer of learning across durations and ears in auditory frequency discrimination. Perception and Psychophysics, 64(3), 426–436.

[10] Drennan, W. R., & Watson, C. S. (2001). Sources of variation in profile analysis: 1. Individual differences and extended training. Journal of the Acoustical Society of America, 110(5, Pt. 1), 2491–2497.

[11] Fitzgerald, M. B., & Wright, B. A. (2011). Perceptual learning and generalization resulting from training on an auditory amplitude-modulation detection task. Journal of the Acoustical Society of America, 129(2), 898–906.

[12] Green, D. M. (1988). Profile analysis: Auditory intensity discrimination. New York, NY: Oxford University Press.

[13] Halliday, L. F., Taylor, J. L., Edmondson-Jones, A. M., & Moore, D. R. (2008). Frequency discrimination learning in children. Journal of the Acoustical Society of America, 123(6), 4393–4402.

[14] Hawkey, D. J. C., Amitay, S., & Moore, D. R. (2004). Early and rapid perceptual learning. Nature Neuroscience, 7(10), 1055–1056.

[15] Huyck, J. J., & Wright, B. A. (2013). Learning, worsening, and generalization in response to auditory perceptual training during adolescence. Journal of the Acoustical Society of America, 134(2), 1172–1182.

[16] Irvine, D. R. F., Martin, R. L., Klimkeit, E., & Smith, R. (2000). Specificity of perceptual learning in a frequency discrimination task. Journal of the Acoustical Society of America, 108(6), 2964–2968.

[17] Jäncke, L., Gaab, N., Wüstenberg, T., Scheich, H., & Heinze, H. J. (2001). Short-term functional plasticity in the human auditory cortex: An fMRI study. Brain Research. Cognitive Brain Research, 12(3), 479–485.

[18] Jones, P. R., Moore, D. R., Amitay, S., & Shub, D. E. (2013). Reduction of internal noise in auditory perceptual learning. Journal of the Acoustical Society of America, 133(2), 970–981.

[19] Karmarkar, U. R., & Buonomano, D. V. (2003). Temporal specificity of perceptual learning in an auditory discrimination task. Learning and Memory, 10(2), 141–147.

[20] Kishon-Rabin, L., Avivi-Reich, M., & Roth, D. A. (2013). Improved gap detection thresholds following auditory training: Evidence of auditory plasticity in older adults. American Journal of Audiology, 22, 343–346.

[21] Leek, M. R., & Watson, C. S. (1984). Learning to detect auditory pattern components. Journal of the Acoustical Society of America, 76(4), 1037–1044.

[22] Leek, M. R., & Watson, C. S. (1988). Auditory perceptual learning of tonal patterns. Perception and Psychophysics, 43(4), 389–394.

[23] Mates, J., von Steinbüchel, N., Wittmann, M., & Treutwein, B. (2001). A system for the assessment and training of temporal-order discrimination. Computer Methods and Programs in Biomedicine, 64(2), 125–131.

[24] Menning, H., Roberts, L. E., & Pantev, C. (2000). Plastic changes in the auditory cortex induced by intensive frequency discrimination training. NeuroReport, 11(4), 817–822.

[25] Molloy, K., Moore, D. R., Sohoglu, E., & Amitay, S. (2012). Less is more: Latent learning is maximized by shorter training sessions in auditory perceptual learning. PLoS ONE, 7(5), e36929.

[26] Mossbridge, J. A., Fitzgerald, M. B., O'Connor, E. S., & Wright, B. A. (2006). Perceptual-learning evidence for separate processing of asynchrony and order tasks. Journal of Neuroscience, 26(49), 12708–12716.

[27] Mossbridge, J. A., Scissors, B. N., & Wright, B. A. (2008). Learning and generalization on asynchrony and order tasks at sound offset: Implications for underlying neural circuitry. Learning and Memory, 15(1), 13–20.

[28] Nagarajan, S. S., Wang, X., Merzenich, M. M., et al. (1998). Speech modifications algorithms used for training language learning-impaired children. IEEE Transactions on Rehabilitation Engeering, 6(3), 257–268.

[29] Neisser, U., & Hirst, W. (1974). Effect of practice on the identification of auditory sequences. Perception and Psychophysics, 15(2), 391–398.

[30] Nickerson, R. S., & Freeman, B. (1974). Discrimination of the order of the components of repeating tone sequences: Effects of frequency separation and extensive practice. Perception and Psychophysics, 16(3), 471–477.

[31] Roth, D. A., Kishon-Rabin, L., & Hildesheimer, M. (2001). Auditory backward masking and the effect of training in normal hearing adults. Journal of Basic and Clinical Physiology and Pharmacology, 12(2, Suppl.), 145–159.

[32] Sabin, A. T., Eddins, D. A., & Wright, B. A. (2012). Perceptual learning evidence for tuning to spectrotemporal modulation in the human auditory system. Journal of Neuroscience, 32(19), 6542–6549.

[33] Schäffler, T., Sonntag, J., Hartnegg, K., & Fischer, B. (2004). The effect of practice on low-level auditory discrimination, phonological skills, and spelling in dyslexia. Dyslexia, 10(2), 119–130.

[34] Schneider, B. A., Pichora-Fuller,M. K., Kowalchuk, D., & Lamb, M. (1994). Gap detection and the precedence effect in young and old adults. Journal of the Acoustical Society of America, 95, 980–991.

[35] Smith, N. A., Trainor, L. J., Gray, K., Plantinga, J. A., & Shore, D. I. (2008). Stimulus, task, and learning effects on measures of temporal resolution: Implications for predictors of language outcome. Journal of Speech, Language, and Hearing Research, 51(6), 1630–1642.

[36] Tallal, P., Miller, S. L., Bedi, G., et al. (1996). Language comprehension in language-learning impaired children im-proved with acoustically modified speech. Science, 271 (5245), 81–84.

[37] van Wassenhove, V., & Nagarajan, S. S. (2007). Auditory cortical plasticity in learning to discriminate modulation rate. Journal of Neuroscience, 27(10), 2663–2672.

[38] Warren, R. M. (1974). Temporal discrimination by trained listeners. Cognitive Psychology, 6(2), 237–256.

[39] Wright, B. A., Buonomano, D. V., Mahncke, H. W., & Merzenich, M. M. (1997). Learning and generalization of auditory temporal-interval discrimination in humans. Journal of Neuroscience, 17(10), 3956–3963.

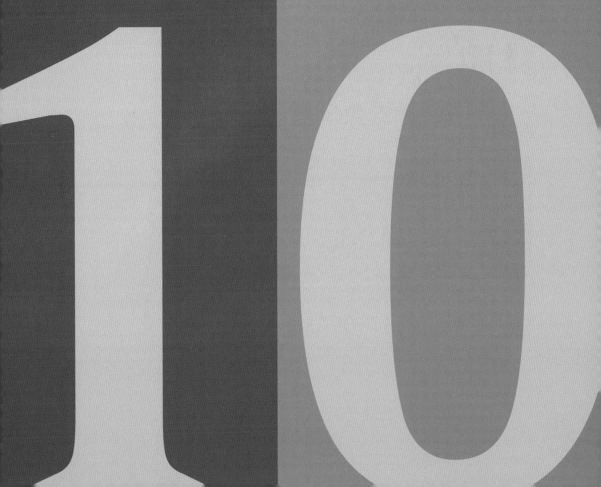

Chapter 10

Training to Improve Binaural Processing

10 Training to Improve Binaural Processing

Deficit-specific auditory training allows treatment of underlying deficits. If these are not addressed, listeners can continue to struggle in difficult environments and may have to use cognitive resources such as closure to cope with the difficulties. Such use of cognitive resources may leave limited resources for other operations, such as memorizing the presented information for later use. Thus, in the presence of binaural processing deficits, it is important to offer training to address the specific deficits. A review of various strategies that can be used to improve binaural processing is discussed in this chapter.

Performance on many auditory tasks can improve with neural maturity, experience, and task-specific training. For binaural processing, changes also occur with developmental changes in head size. Such improvements can co-occur with changes in the auditory nervous system. The stimuli used in training can be real, synthetic, or modified versions of speech or nonspeech stimuli. Training can occur in real-life environments, such as classrooms, or simulated real-life environments that are created in sound-attenuated booths or in therapy rooms. Binaural processing training also can be conducted in virtual listening environments using earphones. Computers allow the creation of training systems with a wide range of stimuli and competing messages. During training, fatigue should be controlled through short sessions, appropriate breaks, and reinforcements. Breaks between training sessions can consolidate the effects of training, leading to more efficient perceptual learning.

10.1 Masking-Level Difference

For masking-level differences (MLDs), training should focus on improving tonal or speech thresholds in out-of-phase configurations, in which either the noise or the signal is out of phase at both ears. The noise should be maintained at comfortable listening levels, and the speech or tonal signals should be presented initially below just above the threshold levels established during testing. Ongoing feedback should be provided to the listener about the accuracy of his or her performance while lowering the signal levels until the MLD is within normal limits for the listener's age. Hafter and Carrier (1970) used a two-interval forced choice procedure, as shown in ▶ Fig. 10.1. Detection of signals that are given out of phase in the presence of noise presented in phase at both ears improves over time using this procedure. The MLDs are largest at 500 Hz when compared to those at 250 or 1000 Hz (Hafter & Carrier, 1970).

10.2 Dichotic Listening

The types of deficits apparent on dichotic tasks can be classified using various categories based on those discussed in Chapter 6. Depending on the deficits apparent during testing, training sessions can be devised to address each type of deficit. For example, a patient may need training in ignoring information presented to one ear and focusing on information presented to the other ear (binaural separation), processing dichotic information presented to both ears, or resynthesizing dichotic information presented to both ears (binaural resynthesis or fusion). The three types of training can complement each other in improving performance on all three tasks.

10.2.1 Binaural Separation

Deficits on binaural separation tasks can be apparent in just one ear (e.g., left ear deficit) or appear in both ears. For example, when the target stimuli are presented to the right ear, and the listener is expected to ignore the stimuli presented to the left ear, the right ear performance may be within normal limits. However, when the listener is expected to repeat sentences presented to the left ear and ignore those presented to the right ear, the performance may be abnormally poor. In this case, training should be focused on improving the performance of the left ear during binaural separation tasks. Initially, the competing stimuli presented to the right ear can be softer than those presented to the left ear. When the stimuli presented to the right ear are sufficiently soft, the left ear performance is expected to improve. The interaural level asymmetry at first can be adjusted in 5 dB steps; during later training phases, the adjustment can occur in 2 or 1 dB steps. Over time the presentation level in the right ear can be slowly raised until the individual begins to show left ear performance similar to age-matched peers. A variety of competing stimuli can be used. The task can also be made easier initially by using competing stimuli that are dissimilar to the target stimuli. For example, if the

Each trial consisted of two bursts.
The first burst always contained the masker in phase at two ears. The second burst was set randomly to either be similar to the first burst or contained both the signal (out of phase at two ears) and masker. The level of the signal is changed adaptively.

Instructions: You will hear two bursts. The first will sound as though it is in the center of the head. The second might sound either the same as the first burst or may sound different with a slightly lateral (away from the center) perception of the sound image. Feel free to use any cues in addition to a lateral image perception to determine if the second burst is the same as the first burst or different than the first burst.

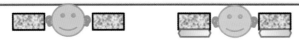

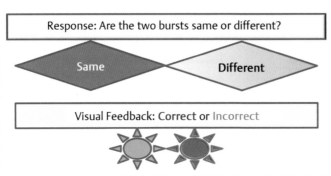

Response: Are the two bursts same or different?

Same   Different

Visual Feedback: **Correct** or Incorrect

Fig. 10.1 Procedure used by Hafter and Carrier (1970) to improve masking level difference (MLD). The MLDs improve over time with this procedure.

target stimuli are sentences, speech-shaped noise would be an easier competing stimulus compared to sentences. Binaural separation deficits in each ear should be addressed first before proceeding to more difficult dichotic tasks.

10.2.2 Binaural Recall of Dichotic Stimuli

This task is more advanced than the binaural separation task described above. In this case, stimuli presented to both ears have to be processed simultaneously and then recalled. Deficits can be apparent in stimuli presented to just one ear or stimuli presented to both ears. Strategies used for binaural separation training can be incorporated in binaural recall of dichotic stimuli. If one ear is weaker than the other, stimuli presented to the stronger ear can

initially be softer than those presented to the weaker ear that is being trained. Slowly over time the level in the stronger ear should be raised so that at the end of the training the level is the same in both ears, and the individual begins to show performance that is similar to his or her age-matched peers. Initially, the interaural level asymmetry can be adjusted in 5 dB steps (▶ Fig. 10.2); during later training phases, the adjustment can occur in 2 or 1 dB steps. This type of training has been referred to as *dichotic interaural intensity difference* (DIID) training (Musiek, Baran, & Shinn, 2004). Commercially available dichotic materials can be used for this type of training, including a dichotic training program titled Constrain Induced Auditory Therapy (CIAT) from Auditec, Inc. (St. Louis, MO). The materials in CIAT include numbers, syllables, words, sentences of various lengths, short stories, fables, and a longer story. The

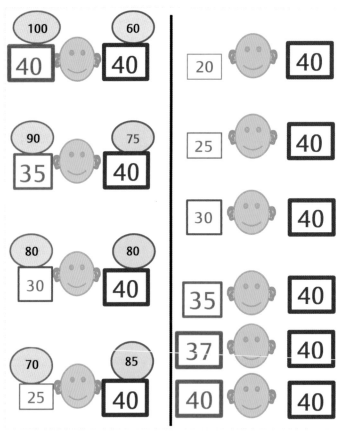

Fig. 10.2 Schematic illustration of dichotic interaural intensity difference (DIID) training. In this example, it is assumed that the patient shows poor left ear performance in dichotic listening tasks. The left panel illustrates the determination of the crossover point at which the performance in the left ear exceeds the performance in the right ear. The right panel illustrates binaural presentation levels through the training period. All presentation levels are given in dB sensation level (SL) (*squares*). The speech recognition performance is given in percentage (*circles*). During the training period, the presentation levels are maintained until the left ear performance is about 90 to 100%.

competition for the dichotic exercises is either the same material (e.g., different syllables in each ear) or a four talker babble (e.g., words in one ear and the four talker babble in the other ear (Hurley & Davis, 2011). DIID training in some children can improve performance in the weaker ear with a simultaneous improvement in language comprehension and word recognition (Hurley, 2011; Moncrieff & Wertz, 2008). Significant improvements following DIID training have been reported on dichotic tasks incorporating digits or words (Schochat, Musiek, Alonso, & Ogata, 2010). Easier competing stimuli can be used initially, proceeding to difficult competing stimuli during later phases of training. In some cases, for home-based training, an earplug with minimal attenuation can be fitted to the stronger ear while listening to TV for about 5 minutes. When the deficit is in only one ear, caution is necessary to ensure that the normal ear does not begin to show a deficit due to strengthening training provided to the weaker ear.

If the deficit is apparent in both ears, training should be devised to address weaknesses in each ear and systematically adjusted to improve performance. Initially, training can begin with presentation of just one word and/or digit to each ear, then proceed to two or more digits or words during later phases of the training.

10.2.3 Binaural Resynthesis

Deficits on this task indicate difficulty of the central auditory system in combining the information presented to the left and right ears. Improvements in dichotic fusion can be achieved by making use of stimuli that present one part of the information to each ear either in the spectral domain (e.g., low pass filtered to the right ear and high pass filtered to the left ear) or in the temporal domain (e.g., consonants to one ear and vowels to the other ear). Ideally, the information presented to just one ear should be insufficient to decode the message so that the central auditory system is pressed to combine the information presented to the two ears to decode the message.

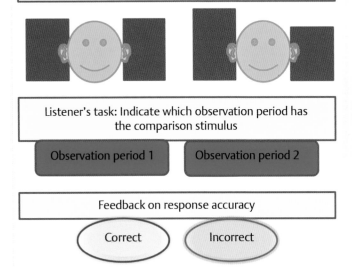

Two visually marked observation periods.
In one randomy selected period, a fixed ILD (standard stimulus) was presented. In the other observation period, the fixed ILD and ΔILD (comparison stimulus) were presented. The ΔILD was adaptively changed to find the smallest change in the two observation periods that was detectable to the listener. The ΔILD was increased after each incorrect response and decreased after three successive correct responses.

Listener's task: Indicate which observation period has the comparison stimulus

Observation period 1   Observation period 2

Feedback on response accuracy

Correct   Incorrect

Fig. 10.3 Procedure for improving interaural level difference discrimination used by Wright and Fitzgerald (2001).

10.3 Simulated Environments for Binaural Listening

Various systems can be used to create binaural listening environments for training in the clinical or home setting. These can include 2 to 16 speakers surrounding the listener or in the frontal listening field. Systems recommended for home-based training can consist of up to eight loudspeakers. Loudspeakers can be placed in such a way that the sound is presented at the ear level of the listener for horizontal localization training. For vertical localization training, the loudspeakers can be placed above, at, and below the ear level. Besides ear angle differences, the distance of the listener from the speakers can be varied for enhancing the use of level cues in predicting the distance of the sound source.

10.4 Localization Training

Good localization allows better recognition of acoustic targets in degraded listening environments.

For example, if a listener knows where a speaker is, he or she can understand the speech better in a crowded room. As noted in Chapter 6, two of the many cues that are important for localization are interaural time and interaural intensity differences. The learning patterns for these two cues are somewhat different.

10.4.1 Interaural Level Difference (ILD)

The procedure for improving interaural level difference (ILD) discrimination is shown in ▶ Fig. 10.3. In a study by Wright and Fitzgerald (2001), discrimination for ILD improved after approximately 9 hours of training for tonal stimuli presented at 4 kHz. There was a rapid stage of improvement from pre- to posttraining tests apparent in control group listeners without any specific training. A slower stage of improvement was apparent in trained listeners, adding to the improvement beyond that apparent in listeners in the

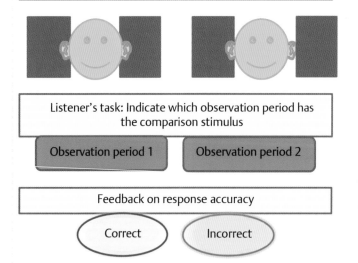

Two visually marked observation periods. In one randomly selected period, a fixed ITD (standard stimulus) was presented. In the other observation period, the fixed ITD and ΔITD (comparison stimulus) were presented. The ΔITD was adaptively changed to find the smallest change in the two observation periods that was detectable to the listener. The ΔITD was increased after each incorrect response and decreased after three successive correct responses.

Listener's task: Indicate which observation period has the comparison stimulus

Observation period 1   Observation period 2

Feedback on response accuracy

Correct   Incorrect

Fig. 10.4 Procedure for improving interaural time difference discrimination used by Wright and Fitzgerald (2001).

untrained control group. The learning was maintained over a period of at least 1 month. When tonal stimuli such as 4 kHz are used, the training may not generalize to other lower frequencies, such as 0.5 kHz (Wright & Fitzgerald, 2001).

Instead of using pure tones, if sinusoidally modulated tones with a carrier frequency of 4 kHz are used to improve ILD discrimination over a training period of 9 to 10 hours, learning effects can generalize to an untrained lower carrier frequency. In this case, the listener's task is to indicate which of the two stimuli appear to be furthest from the midline or the center. If, during training, the stimuli are adjusted in such a way that the sound image is always lateralized to the left hemifield (louder stimuli in the left ear), the perceptual learning may not generalize to the opposite, or right, hemifield (Kumpik, Ting, Campbell, Schnupp, & King, 2009). Thus, for complex stimuli such as sinusoidally modulated tones, training in each hemifield may be necessary to improve ILD discrimination in each hemifield.

10.4.2 Interaural Time Difference

Wright and Fitzgerald (2001) used the procedure shown in ▶ Fig. 10.4 in an attempt to improve interaural time difference (ITD) thresholds for tonal stimuli at 0.5 kHz. Mean thresholds for ITD discrimination improved during initial 2-hour testing sessions. An additional 9 hours of training did not lead to further improvements.

Zhang and Wright (2007) used a procedure similar to that shown in ▶ Fig. 10.4 for improving ITD thresholds for sinusoidally modulated tones. In their study, a total of 9 training sessions lasting for approximately 1 hour were provided to trained listeners. Before starting, listeners were provided practice in indicating the position of the perceived sound image on a schematic diagram of a human head. Both trained and untrained (control) listeners showed improvement on the posttraining tests probably due to practice during the pretest period. ITD thresholds for high-frequency amplitude-modulated stimuli may improve with more extensive training. The degree of improvement in ITD

Four binaural clicks presented on each trial. In the referent event, the clicks were presented dioticially with no interaural difference between clicks. In the comparison event, either the first or the second pair of clicks was presented with an interaural time difference. The IDT was varied adaptively in 10 μs steps based on the accuracy of the listener's response. For the referent event, the sound was perceived either at the right or left of the midline.

Fig. 10.5 Procedure for improving interaural time difference thresholds for clicks used by Saberi and Perrott (1990).

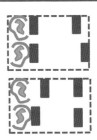

Listener's task: Indicate whether the second event was to the right or the left of the first event

| Left | Right |

Feedback on response accuracy

| Correct | Incorrect |

thresholds can be substantial in some listeners following multiple training sessions, including hundreds to thousands of training trials, and the effect may generalize to untrained stimuli (Rowan & Lutman, 2006).

Approximately 20 to 30 hours of training may be necessary to improve the perception of ITD cues for pairs of clicks (▶ Fig. 10.5) under headphones. However, once learned, the improvement can last well beyond the learning period (Saberi & Perrott, 1990).

10.4.3 Localization Accuracy

Systematic training provided using the procedure illustrated in ▶ Fig. 10.6 can improve localization accuracy. Terhune (1985) demonstrated the effects of practice on localization accuracy in a single

listener (▶ Fig. 10.7). The localization accuracy improved at all of the various azimuths used in the study. A similar task may improve the accuracy further if the listener is expected to indicate the degree of azimuth on a circular pad.

Localization training can be provided to children in a natural setting using simple game-like instructions, such as "Point to the talking [or singing] bear." The child can be asked to sit on a stool with his or her eyes closed or can be blindfolded. The bear is then placed at various locations around the child, and the child is asked to point at the bear. For variety and to maintain interest, any of the child's favorite toys can be used. Some toys allow remote activation of the sound generated by the toy. Such toys can be placed around the child, and the child can be asked to point to the direction from which the sound is coming. If the child makes

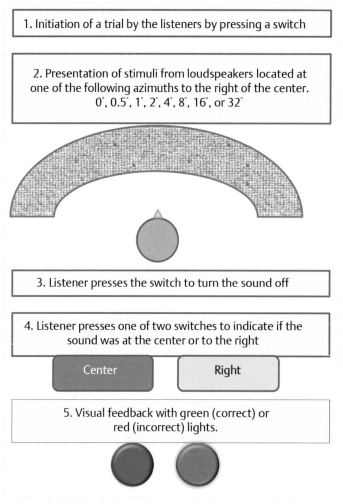

1. Initiation of a trial by the listeners by pressing a switch

2. Presentation of stimuli from loudspeakers located at one of the following azimuths to the right of the center. 0°, 0.5°, 1°, 2°, 4°, 8°, 16°, or 32°

3. Listener presses the switch to turn the sound off

4. Listener presses one of two switches to indicate if the sound was at the center or to the right

Center | Right

5. Visual feedback with green (correct) or red (incorrect) lights.

Fig. 10.6 Procedure used by Terhune (1985) for measuring and improving localization accuracy.

an error, he or she can initially be asked to perform the same activity with eyes open. Small rewards can be provided for correct responses. Another popular game that can enhance sound localization is hide and seek. In this case, instead of the child, the sound source is held steady, and the child is instructed to find the sound. Active feedback should be provided, such as by saying, "Warmer" or "You are heading in the wrong direction; I am here." Once the child masters the steady sound source, he or she can be blindfolded and requested to track a moving sound source.

10.4.4 Multisensory Cues for Localization

If the spectral cues offered by pinnae are altered by fitting custom-made molds in both ears within the concha that continue to provide consistent spectral information about stimulus elevation, the localization accuracy for the detection of sound elevation is initially reduced. However, after wearing the molds for up to 6 weeks, localization improves over time without any specific auditory training, suggesting marked ability of humans to adapt to the new spectral cues. In addition, after removal of the molds, the localization ability is as accurate as apparent before fitting the ear molds. Cognitive effort does not appear to be necessary for this adaptation given that the localization response latencies are below 300 ms. While wearing molds, participants are usually not aware of their localization deficits, which suggests that visual spatial information can dominate the perception of auditory location and may contribute to the adaptation to altered spectral cues. When visual cues are not

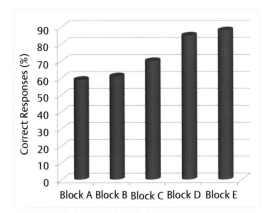

Fig. 10.7 Effect of practice on localization accuracy. In this case, a single subject was presented with a tone of 8 kHz over 2500 trials. In half of the trials, the tone was presented at 0 degree azimuth. In the remaining trials, the signal was presented at five locations: 1, 2, 4, 8, and 16 degree azimuths. The listener had to indicate if the signal was at the center or straight ahead (0 degree azimuth) or to the right of the center. After each response, visual feedback (a green or red light) was provided about the accuracy (based on Terhune, 1985).

available due to the occurrence of a sound source out of the retinal periphery or absent due to darkness, active eye and/or head movements may assist in adaptation (Hofman, Van Riswick, & Van Opstal, 1998). Similar results are obtained when the spectral cues are altered by fitting molds to just one ear, provided that the cues are sufficiently different from the subject's unoccluded ears (Van Wanrooij & Van Opstal, 2005). The importance of vision is apparent in ventriloquism experiments, in which repeated exposures to consistent disparity between auditory and visual location of a sound source can alter the perception of location of the auditory source (Recanzone, 1998). Such experiments suggest that visual feedback regarding the correct location of the sound source can enhance auditory training designed to improve sound localization.

ITD and ILD cues do not exist when the sound source is directly in front of the listener versus when it is behind the listener. In this case, sound localization of short-duration sounds is based on spectral cues. The sound levels in the frequency regions of approximately 3 and 7 kHz are higher when the sound is in front compared to when the sound source is behind the listener. Thus, analysis of sound levels in these frequency regions provides a cue about the sound location. There is individual variability in terms of the strategies used for front-back localization, and some listeners compare multiple

frequency bands to differentiate between front and back sound sources (Zhang & Hartmann, 2010). Such spectral cues are distorted when nonindividualized head-related transfer functions are incorporated in virtual auditory displays leading to errors in front-back localization (Wenzel, Arruda, Kistler, & Wightman, 1993). The errors appear in the form of reversals in which sound sources in the front are identified as being in the back, while sounds in the back hemifield are identified as being in the front hemifield. In real-life situations, most listeners have access to multisensory cues to determine the location of the sound source. Thus, a computerized perceptual training technique that provides listeners with auditory, visual, and proprioceptive/vestibular feedback about the true location of the sound source can be used to improve front-back sound localization (▶ Fig. 10.8). With training and feedback, some listeners appear to make better use of spectral cues in the frequency regions ranging from 3 to 7 kHz, leading to more accurate front-back localization. Listeners in the control group who practice without any feedback do not show such improvements (▶ Fig. 10.9; Zahorik, Bangayan, Sundaraswaran, Wang, & Tam, 2006).

The importance of visual cues in virtual listening environments was confirmed by Majdak, Goupell, and Laback (2010). In this study, 500 ms gaussian white noises filtered using subject-specific head-related transfer functions served as stimuli. The investigators compared sound localization without visual cues (darkness) and with visual cues using a virtual visual environment (VE) via a head-mounted display. A computer was used to create and present the acoustic stimuli, record the tracker data, and control the experimental procedure, while another computer was used to manipulate the 3D graphic based upon clients' responses. Localization in the horizontal plane was significantly better in the virtual VE condition. Virtual VE also reduced the number of front-back confusions. The investigators also compared head versus manual pointing tasks and noted no difference in localization accuracy across these two tasks. The training included feedback on localization accuracy. During training, listeners played a simple game while being immersed in a virtual VE in which they were positioned inside a yellow sphere with a diameter of 5 meters. Horizontal (every 5 degrees) and vertical (every 11.25 degrees) gridlines were used to improve listeners' orientation in the VE sphere. Visual feedback consisted of a red rotating cube at the position of the acoustic stimulus. When the acoustic target was outside the field of vision, an

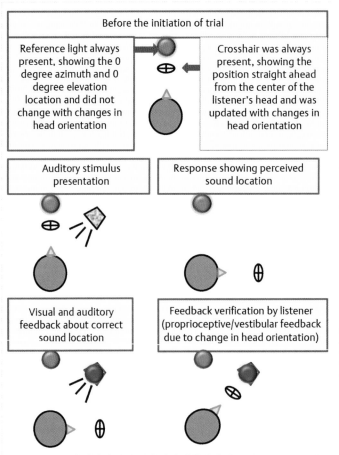

Fig. 10.8 Computerized training technique for improving front back localization in the presence of distorted spectral cues. Stimuli are presented through a personal computer (PC) –based three-dimensional computer graphics system coupled to a head-mounted display. An ultrasonic sensor tracked the orientation of the listener's head with 0.1 degree accuracy. The spatial locations of visual and auditory sound source were updated in real time with reference to changes in the head position (adapted from Zahorik, Bangayan, Sundareswaran, Wang, & Tam, 2006).

arrow appeared pointing toward the position of the acoustic target. Listeners were expected to find and point to the visual target and click the button on a handheld device. The click initiated a repetition of the acoustic stimulus, which allowed listeners to hear and see the location of the sound source. Listeners were then expected to return to the reference position and listen to the same acoustic target again. This procedure provided practice in associating the visual and auditory spatial positions of targets. A significant improvement was apparent during the first 400 training trials. The localization accuracy continued to improve up to 1600 trials, but the improvement was smaller (Majdak, Goupell, & Laback, 2010).

Important spatial cues for sound localization in the sagittal plane are encoded in the frequency range between 4 and 16 kHz. Some individuals have high-frequency hearing loss leading to reduction of high-frequency cues. These cues may be either band limited or spectrally warped following

hearing aid fittings. Band limiting can occur due to limited bandwidth in some hearing aids. Other hearing aids allow the option of frequency compression, which leads to a spectrally warped output. In a double-blind study involving audiovisual training covering the full three-dimensional space, normal-hearing listeners were trained 2 hours daily for 3 weeks to localize sounds that were either band limited up to 8.5 kHz or spectrally warped from the range of 2.8 to 16 kHz to the range of 2.8 to 8.5 kHz (Majdak, Walder, & Laback, 2013). The improvement in localization performance due to training in the warped condition exceeded the improvement that can be expected from procedural task learning. Performance in the band-limited stimulus conditions was even better than that in the warped stimulus conditions after training. These results suggest that adequate training can improve sound localization even after reduction or modification of high-frequency spectral cues (Majdak et al., 2013). Similar training for individuals

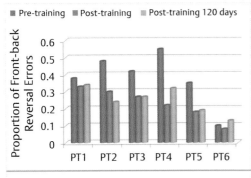

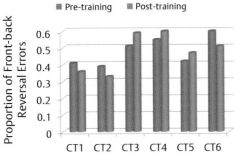

Fig. 10.9 Front-back reversal errors before and after practice. The top panel shows the errors before and after training with visual, auditory, and proprioceptive feedback in six participants (PT). The first and the last participant did not show improvement with training. Note that the last participant made few errors even prior to training. The second panel shows the performance of participants in the control group (CT) who practiced without any feedback (based on Zahorik, Bangayan, Sundareswaran, Wang, & Tam, 2006).

with hearing loss may be beneficial for improving their localization accuracy.

10.4.5 Commercial Computerized Training Systems

Computerized training programs are commercially available for localization training. An example of such training is the Localization Training Module of the Spatial Hearing Training System (Tyler, Witt, Dunn, & Wang, 2010). Some patients show improvement in localization with this training module. Different stimuli, including door knock, bell ringing, warning siren, and drums, are embedded in the localization training module. The home- and laboratory-based training modules use either two or eight loudspeakers. For two-speaker home-based training, listeners are encouraged to begin by placing the speakers toward the left and right

ears for easier localization, then to increase the task difficulty by slowly moving the speakers closer together in front of them. Two types of options are available for training: active exploring and guided listening.

Active Exploring

During active exploring, the listener chooses the specific configuration for the training session. An example of the selection choices are shown in ▶ Fig. 10.10. For example, a listener may decide that he or she wants to hear the door knock coming from the left speaker five times and the bell ringing from the right speaker twice. In the active exploring stage, the listener can listen to various sounds coming from various locations until he or she feels comfortable in locating and detecting the sound source.

Guided Listening

During guided listening, the ability of the listener to localize the sound can be assessed. A sound is randomly presented, and the listener is expected to indicate its location. The listener receives feedback about the accuracy of his or her response, and the same sound is presented again, along with visual indicators on the computer screen that indicate the correct location of the sound by illuminating the corresponding loudspeaker icons.

10.5 Speech Recognition Training for Spatially Separated Targets and Competition

As noted in Chapter 6, some individuals have spatial auditory processing disorders, meaning they are unable to take advantage of the spatial separation of the target message and a competing signal. Thus, they need a significantly better signal-to-noise ratio to achieve the same speech recognition threshold (SRT) as their age-matched peers (Cameron & Dillon, 2008). Among children who are referred for assessment of auditory processing deficits, 17% may be diagnosed with spatial processing deficits (Dillon, Cameron, Glyde, Wilson, & Tomlin, 2012). Some of these individuals may benefit from training designed to recognize speech from spatially separated competition. Localization cues, more specifically, ILD cues (Glyde, Buchholz, Dillon, Cameron, & Hickson, 2013), are important for taking advantage of spatial separation of target messages and competing backgrounds. Before

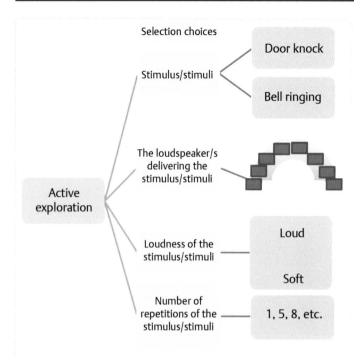

Fig. 10.10 Examples of selection choices during the active exploring training format in the Spatial Hearing Training System. Active exploration allows the experience of listening to various sounds arriving from different locations at various loudness levels.

initiating this training, some individuals may benefit from localization training. Computerized training programs are available for speech recognition training where the target speech stimuli are spatially separated from competing stimuli. Some of these training programs are discussed below.

10.5.1 Speech in Noise Training Module of the Spatial Hearing Training System

The Speech in Noise training module of the Spatial Hearing Training System (Tyler, Witt, Dunn, & Wang, 2010) is very similar to the localization module described above with the exception that the stimuli consist of a closed set of 12 spondee words that are presented in a background of male and female two-talker babble. During the active exploring stage, listeners can select the word they wish to hear and the loudspeakers presenting the words and the babble. This allows practice in listening to various words with various spatial separations between the words and the babble. During guided listening, the level of the speech is held constant, and the babble level is adjusted using an adaptive procedure to achieve 50% recognition. In this way, listeners are trained with a task that is neither too easy nor too hard. Feedback is

provided for correct responses. If a response is incorrect, the incorrect response is contrasted with the correct response. For the eight-speaker system, when listeners give a correct response, they receive positive feedback, and the spatial separation between the word and the babble is decreased during the next training trial. For the two-speaker home-based training system, listeners are encouraged to begin by placing the speakers toward the left and the right ears, then to decrease the spatial separation by slowly moving the speakers closer together in front of them. Some patients show improvement in recognizing speech in noise with this training module.

10.5.2 LiSN and Learn Auditory Training Software

The LiSN and Learn auditory training program (Cameron & Dillon, 2010) is specifically developed to remediate spatial processing deficits. The software simulates a three-dimensional auditory environment under headphones. Listeners hear words embedded in sentences that are presented in competing speech. The target sentences appear to come from directly in front of the listener, whereas the competing continuous stories appear to come from either the left or the right side. The same female voice is used for delivering target words and competing stories. Listeners are expected to rely on spatial separation of the target and competing speech stimuli. In the program, listeners identify the target words (nouns, verbs, or adjective) by selecting corresponding images on the computer screen. Initially, the target is presented at 62 dB sound pressure level (SPL), and the competing stories are presented at 55 dB SPL. Following the initial presentation, an adaptive procedure is used to adjust the level of the target. With a correct response, the target level is reduced by 1.5 dB to make the listening task more difficult; with an incorrect response, it is increased by 2.5 dB to make listening easier. If an unsure response is made, the level is increased by 1.5 dB. The software is capable of generating 131,220 unique sentences. Each game takes 5 to 10 minutes to complete.

In one study, after playing two games on a daily basis for 5 days/week over 12 weeks (120 games), listeners' ability to recognize speech in spatially separated competing stimuli appeared to improve (Cameron & Dillon, 2011). Participants also reported improved ability to listen to speech in noise; for most participants, the improvement was maintained for at least 3 months following training. In addition, the specific training offered by the software appears to be more effective in addressing spatial processing deficits when compared to other auditory training software, such as Earobics from Cognitive Concepts (2008). In addition to the improvement in spatial processing of speech stimuli, trained children showed improvement on Fisher's auditory problems checklist (Cameron, Glyde, & Dillon, 2012; Fisher, 2008). The repetitive nature of the tasks and the visual stimuli in this software may lead to boredom for some children. To improve the motivational aspects of training, the software has been upgraded with a supplementary training game, additional rewards, and an avatar, or buddy, who presents information to the child throughout the training (Cameron et al., 2012).

10.6 Future Trends

10.6.1 Virtual Auditory-Visual Displays

Virtual auditory-visual displays may provide more opportunities in the future to improve binaural listening and auditory visual integration. Although some studies have shown the effectiveness of training to improve sound localization using head-mounted displays, there is a need for studies that show how well these improvements are transferred in real-life situations. It is possible that some additional but minimal training may be necessary for accurate localization in real-life settings after training in virtual listening environments.

10.6.2 "Voices in the Head" Technologies

Generally, when sounds are presented via loudspeakers, they seem to be located somewhere outside the head. However, when the sounds are presented through headphones, they seem to be located inside the head. New technologies are allowing sound beams to be projected in the head without the use of headphones. One such technology is audio spotlight. Another technology has been referred to as "voice to skull" (V2K), voice of God, synthetic telepathy, or psychotronics.

Audio Spotlight

For a demonstration of the audio spotlight, readers can Google "Audio spotlight featured on the Smithsonian Channel's SciQ" or watch the video using the following link: http://www.youtube.com/watch?v=0tY_EOYqoVs.

With this technology, modulated ultrasounds are used to project sound beams. Ultrasounds are higher in frequency than what is generally considered within the audible range for human hearing. These sounds have extremely short wavelengths lasting only a few millimeters and thus naturally travel in an extremely narrow beam. As a modulated ultrasonic beam travels through the air, the inherent properties of the air change the shape of the ultrasound which allows the air within the beam to extract the modulation signal (e.g. music or speech) from the ultrasound. By generating the correct modulated ultrasonic signal, essentially any desired sound can be projected through the air. The sound can be projected over a very small, specific area similar to the projection of a spotlight and creates a spatialized sound distant from the transducer (Pompei, 1999). Only listeners within the path of the sound beam can hear the extracted signal; the signal remains inaudible to listeners outside the beam.

Voice to Skull (V2K)

The Center for Army Lessons Learned (CALL) defines voice to skull (V2K) devices as one of the following: (1) a neuro-electromagnetic device that transmits sounds in the skull of a person or animal using pulse-modulated microwave radiation; (2) a silent sound device that can transmit sound into the skull of a person or animal (http://www.fas.org/sgp/othergov/dod/vts.html as cited in FAS Project on Government Secrecy, 2004). The sound modulation can be sent as either voices or audio subliminal messages. With audio subliminal messages, the message is sent to the listener without the person being aware of it.

A patent titled "Hearing System" describes a device that is capable of inducing sounds in the head of a listener by radiating the head with microwaves in the range of 100 to 10,000 MHz that are modulated with a particular waveform (Brunkan, 1989). This type of hearing has been referred to as radio-frequency, or microwave auditory effect. More specifically, high-frequency electromagnetic energy is projected through the head of a listener. The modulation of the electromagnetic energy allows creation of signals that are intelligible to listeners regardless of their peripheral auditory sensitivity.

This microwave auditory effect was previously described by Frey (1962). He noted that his participants localized the sound source as being within or behind the head. He suggested that the electromagnetic field could interact with the fields generated by neurons and that the microwave or radiofrequency auditory effect can be nullified by placing a 22-inch-wide fly screen around the temporal area (Frey, 1962).

A similar approach is described in "A Method for Encoding and Transmitting Speech by Means of the Radio Frequency Hearing Phenomenon" (U.S. Air Force, 1994). A unique feature of this method is that it is unnecessary for the listener to use any specific devices such as hearing aids or earphones. Instead, it employs encoded speech using a combination of filtering, biasing, and nonlinear processing of the speech signal and suppressed carrier amplitude modulation. Such a speech (or music) signal is intelligible to humans by means of the radiofrequency hearing effect. The researchers describe possible uses of this method for communication in environments such as space missions and hostage situations. This is most likely possible because microwaves or radio-frequency signals can be sent from a remote location using a suitable apparatus, and the speech signal becomes perceptible only to the listener whose head is being radiated and remains inaudible to people surrounding the listener. Such psychotronic technologies have been discussed elsewhere (Thomas, 1998).

Applications of Beaming Sounds in the Head

Audio spotlight systems can be mounted 8 stories up on a building rooftop and can beam clearly audible sound to listeners at street level. Such a system was used to advertise the A&E channel show *Paranormal State,* which featured real-life mysteries that included poltergeists, ghosts, and hauntings. (The demonstration can be watched using this link: http://www.holosonics.com/v_ae.html.) The technology has several other practical uses beyond beaming of advertisements directly to customers' heads. For example, museums and libraries can keep large spaces quiet while using audio spotlight systems in specific areas. In automobiles, passengers can listen to music separately. At home, people can watch different TV sets with clearly audible sound without bothering others. In clubs, those who wish to dance can enjoy music spotlighted on them, which allows others to converse without being bombarded by music. If applied correctly, the technology may also minimize the possibility of music-induced hearing loss. In waiting areas or at art galleries, audio spotlight systems can deliver sound to those who are interested in listening while allowing quiet time for other visitors.

V2K technology allows subliminal messages to be sent to listeners. For example, subliminal messages could be used in substance abuse treatment centers to encourage clients with positive messages to enhance self-concepts and self-control (e.g., I can stay without drugs or alcohol) or in stores to discourage shoplifting ("I will pay for what I need") (US Patent No. 4395600 A, 1983). Subliminal messages that are delivered to the participants repeatedly without the participant being aware of the message can have more powerful effects on self-concepts and physical function than explicit messages (Levy, Pilver, Chung, & Slade, 2014). As cited in FAS Project on Government Secrecy (2004), CALL noted that V2K can be used as an electronic "scarecrow" to scare birds away from airports. For other potential uses of V2K technology in audiology, refer to the future trends section in Chapter 15.

Potential Misuse of "Voices in the Head" Technologies

As an example of the misuse of such technologies, consider the case of James Walbert, who went to court in 2008 to prevent his former business associate from blasting him using electronic technologies such as those described in the previous section. His associate had threatened him with "jolts of radiation" after a disagreement over a business deal. Later Walbert began hearing electronically generated tones, including popping and ringing sounds. On December 30, 2009, the court issued an order of protection banning Walbert's associate from electronically harassing him (Hambling, 2009).

At the very least, audiologists should be aware of psychotronic technology and the possibility of its abuse. Bullying, for instance, can take on an entirely new form, with "voices in the head" technologies such as audio spotlight, which are relatively cheap and easily available.

Given the growing use of psychotronic technology, audiologists should not assume that a patient who reports hearing voices or music in his or her head is mentally ill. Some psychoanalysts have expressed the need for new criteria for diagnosing mental illnesses with consideration for mind-invasive psychotronic technologies (Smith, 2003). Audiologists should be aware that the diagnostic criteria of schizophrenia have changed. According to the latest version of the *Diagnostic and Statistical Manual* (American Psychiatric Association, 2013), the diagnosis of schizophrenia requires at least two of the following symptoms: delusions, hallucinations, disorganized speech, grossly organized catatonic behavior, and negative symptoms such as diminished emotional expression or avolition. In the fourth edition of the *DSM* (American Psychiatric Association, 1994), only one of these five symptoms were needed if the patient reported hearing a voice providing a running commentary on the person's behavior or thoughts or two or more voices conversing with each other. Children are especially apt to be misdiagnosed and given unnecessary mind-altering medications that could lead to further complications. The possibility of a misdiagnosis of schizophrenia is greater in the presence of hearing loss or a family history of mental illness. Audiologists should also be aware that verbal and music hallucinations have been reported in healthy individuals. According to a recent review, auditory hallucinations can appear as an entity by themselves and are not necessarily indicative of transition along the psychosis continuum (de Leede-Smith & Barkus, 2013). In the future, individuals may need to be educated about differentiating between voices projected through the use of psychotronic technologies and their own inner voices.

10.7 Review Questions

1. Describe the dichotic interaural intensity difference training procedure to improve the recognition of dichotic stimuli presented to each ear. A child is experiencing difficulty with a binaural resynthesis task. What can you do to improve his performance?

2. Describe a procedure for improving the thresholds for interaural level difference. What sorts of generalization effects are possible after such training? What are some limits to such generalization?

3. Describe a procedure for improving the thresholds for interaural time difference. What types of generalizations are possible after such training?

4. How can you improve sound localization in children without the use of computers?

5. Discuss the importance of visual cues for sound localization.

6. Discuss a procedure for reducing front-back reversal errors in virtual auditory displays.

7. Is it possible to improve sound localization in the sagittal plane after modifying high-frequency spectral cues?

8. Describe the localization training module of the Spatial Hearing Training System.

9. Describe a computerized training program that could address a spatial processing deficit.

10. Discuss "voices in the head" technologies. What are the potential uses of such technologies? Why should audiologists be aware of such technologies?

References

[1] American Psychiatric Association (APA). (1994). Diagnostic and statistical manual of mental disorders (4th ed.). Washington, DC: Author.

[2] American Psychiatric Association (APA). (2013). Diagnostic and statistical manual of mental disorders (5th ed.). Arlington, VA: Author.

[3] Brunkan, W. B. (1989). Hearing system (U.S. Patent No. 4,877,027). Washington, DC: U.S. Patent and Trademark Office.

[4] Cameron, S., & Dillon, H. (2008). The Listening in Spatialized Noise-Sentences Test (LISN-S): Comparison to the prototype LISN and results from children with either a suspected (central) auditory processing disorder or a confirmed language disorder. Journal of the American Academy of Audiology, 19 (5), 377–391.

[5] Cameron, S., & Dillon, H. (2010). LISN & Learn auditory training software (Version 1.1.0) [Computer software]. Sydney, Australia: National Acoustic Laboratories.

[6] Cameron, S., & Dillon, H. (2011). Development and evaluation of the LiSN & Learn auditory training software for deficit-specific remediation of binaural processing deficits in children: Preliminary findings. Journal of the American Academy of Audiology, 22(10), 678–696.

[7] Cameron, S., Glyde, H., & Dillon, H. (2012). Efficacy of the LiSN & Learn auditory training software: Randomized blinded controlled study. Audiology Research, 2, e15.

[8] Cognitive Concepts. (2008). Earobics [CD-ROM]. Boston: Houghton Mifflin Harcourt.

[9] de Leede-Smith, S., & Barkus, E. (2013). A comprehensive review of auditory verbal hallucinations: Lifetime prevalence, correlates and mechanisms in healthy and clinical individuals. Frontiers in Human Neuroscience, 7, ID 367, 1-25. Retrieved from http://www.ncbi.nlm.nih.gov/pmc/articles/PMC3712258/pdf/fnhum-07-00367.pdf.

[10] Dillon, H., Cameron, S., Glyde, H., Wilson, W., & Tomlin, D. (2012). An opinion on the assessment of people who may have an auditory processing disorder. Journal of the American Academy of Audiology, 23(2), 97–105.

[11] FAS Project on Government Secrecy. (2004). Secrecy News, 64. Retrieved from http://fas.org/sgp/news/secrecy/2004/07/071204.html.

[12] Fisher, L. I. (2008). Fisher's auditory problems checklist. Tampa, FL: Educational Audiology Association.

[13] Frey, A. H. (1962). Human auditory system response to modulated electromagnetic energy. Journal of Applied Physiology, 17, 689-692.

[14] Glyde, H., Buchholz, J. M., Dillon, H., Cameron, S., & Hickson, L. (2013). The importance of interaural time differences and level differences in spatial release from masking. Journal of the Acoustical Society of America, 134(2), EL147–EL152.

[15] Hafter, E. R., & Carrier, S. C. (1970). Masking level differences obtained with a pulsed tonal masker. Journal of the Acoustical Society of America, 47, 1041-1047.

[16] Hambling, D. (2009). Court to defendant: Stop blasting that man's mind! Wired. Retrieved from http://www.wired.com/2009/07/court-to-defendant-stop-blasting-that-mans-mind/.

[17] Hofman, P. M., Van Riswick, J. G., & Van Opstal, A. J. (1998). Relearning sound localization with new ears. Nature Neuroscience, 1(5), 417–421.

[18] Hurley, A. (2011). Auditory remediation for patients with Landau-Kleffner syndrome. Retrieved from http://www.asha.org/Publications/leader/2011/110405/Auditory-Remediation-for-Patients-With-Landau-Kleffner-Syndrome.htm.

[19] Hurley, A., & Davis, D. (2011). Constrain induced auditory therapy (CIAT): A dichotic listening auditory therapy. St. Louis, MO: AudiTec.

[20] Kumpik, D., Ting, J., Campbell, R. A. A., Schnupp, J. W. H., & King, A. J. (2009). Specificity of binaural perceptual learning for amplitude modulated tones: A comparison of two training methods. Journal of the Acoustical Society of America, 125(4), 2221–2232.

[21] Levy, B. R., Pilver, C., Chung, P. H., & Slade, M. D. (2014). Subliminal strengthening: Improving older individuals' physical function over time with an implicit-age-stereotype intervention. Psychological science, DOI: 10.1177/0956797614551970.

[22] Lundy, R. R., & Tyler, D. L. (1983). U.S. Patent No. 4,395,600. Washington, DC: U.S. Patent and Trademark Office.

[23] Majdak, P., Goupell, M. J., & Laback, B. (2010). 3-D localization of virtual sound sources: Effects of visual environment, pointing method, and training. Attention, Perception, and Psychophysics, 72(2), 454–469.

[24] Majdak, P., Walder, T., & Laback, B. (2013). Effect of long-term training on sound localization performance with spectrally warped and band-limited head-related transfer functions. Journal of the Acoustical Society of America, 134(3), 2148–2159.

[25] Moncrieff, D. W., & Wertz, D. (2008). Auditory rehabilitation for interaural asymmetry: Preliminary evidence of improved dichotic listening performance following intensive training. International Journal of Audiology, 47(2), 84–97.

[26] Musiek, F. E., Baran, J. A., & Shinn, J. (2004). Assessment and remediation of an auditory processing disorder associated with head trauma. Journal of the American Academy of Audiology, 15(2), 117–132.

[27] Pompei, J. F. (1999). The use of airborne ultrasonics for generating audible sound. Journal of the Audio Engineering Society, 47(9), 726–731.

[28] Recanzone, G. H. (1998). Rapidly induced auditory plasticity: The ventriloquism aftereffect. Proceedings of the National Academy of Sciences of the United States of America, 95(3), 869–875.

[29] Rowan, D., & Lutman, M. E. (2006). Learning to discriminate interaural time differences: An exploratory study with amplitude-modulated stimuli. International Journal of Audiology, 45(9), 513–520.

[30] Saberi, K., & Perrott, D. R. (1990). Lateralization thresholds obtained under conditions in which the precedence effect is assumed to operate. Journal of the Acoustical Society of America, 87(4), 1732–1737.

[31] Schochat, E., Musiek, F. E., Alonso, R., & Ogata, J. (2010). Effect of auditory training on the middle latency response in children with (central) auditory processing disorder. Brazilian Journal of Medical and Biological Research, 43(8), 777–785.

[32] Smith, C. (2003). On the need for new criteria of diagnosis of psychosis in the light of mind invasive technology. Journal of Psycho-Social Studies, 2 (3). Retrieved from http://www.biblesabbath.org.uk/invasivetechnology.pdf.

[33] Terhune, J. M. (1985). Localization of pure tones and click trains by untrained humans. Scandinavian Audiology, 14(3), 125–131.

[34] Thomas, T. L. (1998). The mind has no firewall. Parameters, 84–92.

[35] Tyler, R. S., Witt, S. A., Dunn, C. C., & Wang, W. (2010). Initial development of a spatially separated speech-in-noise and localization training program. Journal of the American Academy of Audiology, 21(6), 390–403.

[36] U. S. Air Force. (1994). A method for encoding & transmitting speech by means of the radio frequency hearing phenomenon. Disclosure and record of invention, AF form 1279 to document inventions for consideration of patenting by the Air Force. Retrieved from http://cryptome.org/rf-speech/rf-speech-02.pdf.

[37] Van Wanrooij, M. M., & Van Opstal, A. J. (2005). Relearning sound localization with a new ear. Journal of Neuroscience, 25(22), 5413–5424.

[38] Wenzel, E. M., Arruda, M., Kistler, D. J., & Wightman, F. L. (1993). Localization using nonindividualized head-related transfer functions. Journal of the Acoustical Society of America, 94(1), 111–123.

[39] Wright, B. A., & Fitzgerald, M. B. (2001). Different patterns of human discrimination learning for two interaural cues to sound-source location. Proceedings of the National Academy of Sciences of the United States of America, 98(21), 12307–12312.

[40] Zahorik, P., Bangayan, P., Sundareswaran, V., Wang, K., & Tam, C. (2006). Perceptual recalibration in human sound localization: Learning to remediate front-back reversals. Journal of the Acoustical Society of America, 120(1), 343–359.

[41] Zhang, P. X., & Hartmann, W. M. (2010). On the ability of human listeners to distinguish between front and back. Hearing Research, 260(1-2), 30–46.

[42] Zhang, Y., & Wright, B. A. (2007). Similar patterns of learning and performance variability for human discrimination of interaural time differences at high and low frequencies. Journal of the Acoustical Society of America, 121(4), 2207–2216.

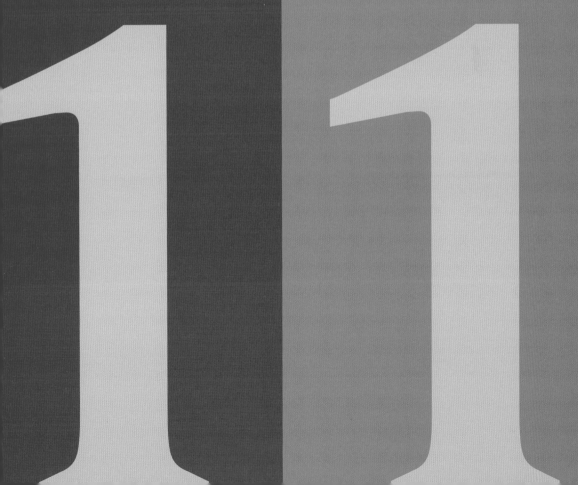

Chapter 11

Training to Improve Speech Recognition

11 Training to Improve Speech Recognition

Individuals who have difficulty recognizing speech, including low-redundancy speech stimuli, can benefit from training designed to improve speech recognition in quiet, noisy, or reverberant listening conditions. The stimuli can include phonemes, syllables, words, sentences, and paragraphs. This chapter reviews several studies that show the efficacy of auditory training in improving perception of normal and degraded speech.

11.1 Phoneme Discrimination

Phoneme discrimination training can successfully be employed with nonnative speakers to recognize phoneme features that are not part of their native languages. For example, English speakers have difficulty differentiating one of the phoneme contrasts in Hindi, /t(h)a/ versus /d(h)a/. However, through auditory training, they can learn to differentiate between the two phonemes (Werker & Tees, 1984). Similarly, the differentiation of /r/ versus /l/ is difficult for people from Japan, China, and Korea. Well-designed auditory training can improve the perception of the contrasts provided the

token contrasts used during training are articulated by multiple speakers (Lively, Logan, & Pisoni, 1993). The effects of training are long lasting (Lively, Pisoni, Yamada, Tohkura, & Yamada, 1994). The amount of time required for learning nonnative contrasts varies depending on the similarities and differences in native and nonnative languages (Iverson & Evans, 2009; Pruitt, Jenkins, & Strange, 2006).

The components of successful training protocols to improve phoneme perception are shown in ▶ Fig. 11.1 (Logan, Lively, & Pisoni, 1991). Training involving fewer repetitions of a more variable set of words recorded by multiple speakers leads to better generalization of learning to untrained stimuli compared to training that includes many repetitions of a limited set of words recorded by a single speaker (Sadakata & McQueen, 2013). Improved phoneme perception also improves the accuracy of phoneme production, which is maintained for a long duration following training (Bradlow, Akahane-Yamada, Pisoni, & Tohkura, 1999). Improvement in phoneme production may lead to further improvement in speech perception.

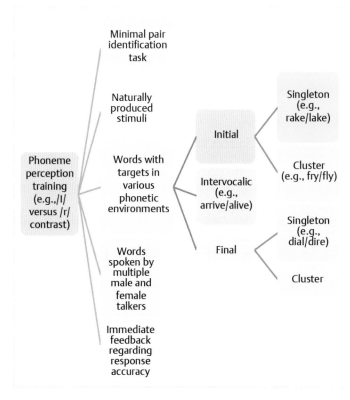

Fig. 11.1 Characteristics of effective training procedures for improving phoneme perception.

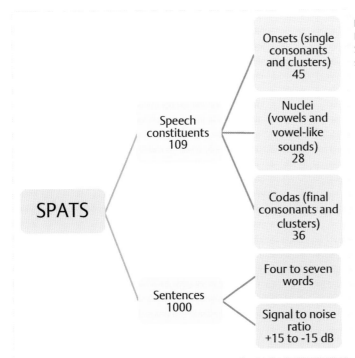

Fig. 11.2 Components of the Speech Perception Assessment and Training System (SPATS) (based on Miller, Watson, Kistler, Preminger, & Wark, 2008).

In a study by Lengeris and Hazan (2010), native speakers of Greek improved their ability to process vowels in English through auditory training for vowel processing in both languages; the improvement was related to frequency discrimination acuity. Individuals with acute frequency discrimination skills were more accurate in processing and producing English vowels following training. Although minimal pair words have been used for training, perception of vowel contrast can also be improved with exposure to words embedded in sentences containing the contrasts (Hirata, Whitehurst, & Cullings, 2007).

11.1.1 Speech Perception Assessment and Training System (SPATS)

The Speech Perception Assessment and Training System (SPATS) software consists of two modules: one designed to improve syllable or constituent perception and other to improve sentence recognition. The purpose of the constituent program is to sharpen the perception of spectral-temporal properties that specify the elements of syllables, as shown in ▶ Fig. 11.2. There are at least 212 different syllable constituents in spoken English, of which 109 were included in the software based

on those that are considered most important for perception of English. The importance was determined by the frequency with which the item occurred in running text and the number of different English words in which it occurred. To provide listening practice in various phonetic contexts, onsets (single consonants and clusters at the beginning of the syllable) are presented with four different vowels; nuclei (vowels and vowel-like sounds) are placed in an h(nucleus)d context (e.g., heed, had, head), and codas (consonants at the end of the syllable) are presented with five different stems. The resulting 388 syllables are recorded by eight different speakers with a middle-American accent. On each practice trial, the listener is presented with one of the constituents and is requested to first imitate the sound, then identify it by clicking on one of the related buttons on the computer display. Feedback on correct and incorrect responses is provided. The listener is encouraged to click on the highlighted button to rehear the target and to also hear the incorrect response. The greatest amount of training is directed toward those constituents that are identified as being moderately difficult for the client. Preliminary evaluation of the SPATS software suggests that it is effective in leading to improvement in the identification of syllable constituents (Miller, Watson, Kistler, Preminger, & Wark, 2008).

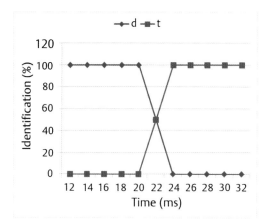

Fig. 11.3 Idealized results for a listener for the perception of voiced (/d/) versus voiceless stops (/t/) based on variation in voice onset time. In this example of categorical perception, categorization of voiced versus voiceless stops is based on voice onset time cues.

11.1.2 Categorical Speech Perception

Categorical speech perception refers to an ability to place consonants in different categories based on some distinct cues. One example of such a cue is the voice onset time. Voice onset time is the time interval between the onset of the bursts associated with stops and the vocal cord vibration. For initial consonant positions, the voice onset time is short (less than 20 ms) for voiced stops and longer for voiceless stops (Lisker & Abramson, 1964). An illustration of how the voice onset time cue changes the perception of consonants from voiced (d) to its voiceless counterpart (t) is shown in ▶ Fig. 11.3. In this figure, the listener perceives the sound as being /d/ for voice onset times less than 20 ms and as being /t/ for voice onset times greater than 24 ms.

Another example of a distinct cue that allows categorical perception is the transition of the second formant from its onset to its steady-state frequency. This transition is illustrated in ▶ Fig. 11.4. The frequency of the steady-state portion of the second formant in this example is 2160 Hz. The frequency of the steady-state portion of the first formant is 360 Hz. This combination of the first and second formant frequency is maintained through all the stimuli in ▶ Fig. 11.4, which allows the perception of the same vowel. The onset frequency of the second formant is changed from 1320 Hz in the first panel to 2880 Hz in the last, or the 14th, panel. The transition from the onset

frequency to the steady-state frequency of 2160 Hz is brief and lasts about 40 ms. The change in perception of the consonants from /b/ to /d/ to /g/ is illustrated in ▶ Fig. 11.5 for a hypothesized listener based on the data provided by Liberman, Harris, Hoffman, and Griffith (1957). In this illustration, the change in the onset frequency of the second formant is associated with various places of articulation categories moving from the front of the mouth for /b/ to the back of the mouth for /g/.

In the above examples of categorical perception, the perception is considered to vary across a continuum such as voice onset time. Musicians show superior discrimination across synthetic speech syllable continua compared to nonmusicians when the discrimination requires resolution of temporal cues (e.g., voice onset time). Their performance on discrimination tasks across the temporal syllable continua is positively correlated with the length and intensity of musical training. These results suggest that intensive auditory practice such as that provided by music training may improve temporal acuity (Zuk et al., 2013) required for discrimination of phonemes.

11.1.3 Phoneme Perception Training Based on Categorical Speech Perception

Phonomena

The game Phonomena, designed for children, has a training section called "Sound Game" and a reward arcade-style section called "3's Company" (Robinson, 2004). The 11 British English phoneme contrasts included in "Sound Game" are as follows:

- ± Labial (stop): /biː/ versus /diː/
- ± Labial (nasal): /maː/ versus /naː/
- ± Coronal: /daː/ versus /gaː/
- ± Low: /ɛ/ versus /a/
- ± Round: /əː/ versus /ɔː/
- ± High: /ɪ/ versus /ɛ/
- ± Lateral: /liː/ versus /ɹiː/
- ± Anterior: /saː/ versus /ʃaː/
- ± Distributed: /saː/ versus /θaː/
- ± Sonorant: /vaː/ versus /waː/
- ± Back: /a/ versus /ʌ/

The sound files in the sound game include either a single vowel or a consonant-vowel (CV) combination. Most of the syllables are meaningless. The end points of each continuum (e.g., /da/ versus /ga/) are derived by analysis and resynthesis of

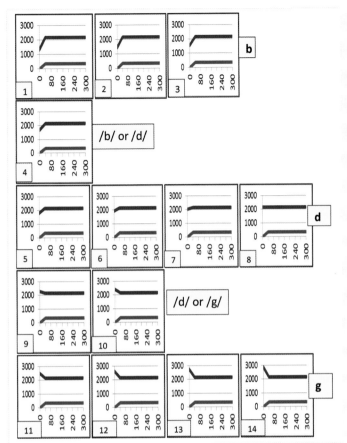

Fig. 11.4 The varying second formant transitions that elicit the perception of consonant stops (/d/, /b/, /g/). Frequency (Hz) is shown on the vertical Y-axis and time (ms) is shown on the horizontal X-axis. The onset frequency of the second formant is changed from 1320 to 2880 Hz in 120 Hz steps from panel 1 to panel 14 (based on Liberman, Harris, Hoffman, & Griffith, 1957). The perceived consonants associated with these transitions are shown in ▶ Fig. 11.5.

naturally spoken recordings of the syllables. These can be conceptualized as panels 5 and 14 in ▶ Fig. 11.4. The sound files between the end points are created by interpolating between the acoustic parameters of the end point files and presented adaptively during the sound game depending on the accuracy of the listener's response.

Each sound game consists of a total of 60 trials, and a brief animation is presented following each completed sound game. The training is embedded in a computer game. The embedded graphics are designed by a commercial game developer. On each trial in the sound game, a dinosaur character called Rex-T serves as a tutor and presents a syllable drawn from a library of sound sets. Following this presentation, two cavemen characters referred to as Mic and Mac each present a syllable, one of which is the same as that presented by the tutor. The response task is to identify the caveman who produced the same syllable that was presented by Rex-T. The presentation of the syllable is

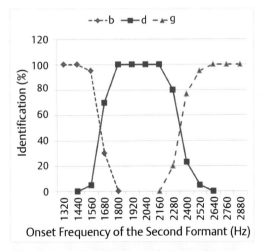

Fig. 11.5 Schematic illustration of categorical perception for /b/, /d/, and /g/ (based on Liberman, Harris, Hoffman, & Griffith, 1957). Note that there is individual variability in perception; some listeners cannot consistently identify such boundaries.

accompanied by a simple change from closed to open mouth position. Thus, there are no obvious visible cues for recognizing the syllable. The difficulty of the syllable-matching task is varied adaptively depending on the listener's response. Correct responses lead to the syllables sounding more similar, and incorrect responses lead to the syllables sounding more apart from each other. Feedback for correct and incorrect responses is provided in the form of a bell or a hooter sound after each response. Additional feedback is provided in the form of a cumulative correct trial score in the top right corner of the computer screen.

Moore, Rosenberg, and Coleman (2005) used the above game to train typically developing children ages 8 to 10 years. The training was offered over a period of 4 weeks and included 12 sessions, with each session lasting for 30 minutes. Enhancement on the trained phoneme discrimination contrasts were weak and variable following training probably due to the relatively large number of phonetic contrasts and several contrasting steps within each contrast. Because the end points across each pair are based on natural speech, the task can be expected to be harder when the pair has fewer differences than the end points. However, the age-equivalent scores of the trained children improved by approximately 2 years on the Word Discrimination Test and the Phonological Assessment Battery (PhAB). No improvement was apparent on the PhAB in the children in the age-matched untrained control group. The improvement apparent in the trained children was maintained for at least 5 to 6 weeks following training. Children enrolled in speech and language therapy can also benefit from this type of training (Rosenberg & Moore, 2003). The benefit may be greater for children who have auditory processing deficits (APDs) and/or accompanying reading deficits.

11.1.4 Earobics

The Earobics software (Cognitive Concepts, Inc., Evanston, IL; http://www.earobics.com/), designed for children, has some interactive games that can improve phoneme perception. For example, in one of the games, titled Paw Park Sassy Seals, a cartoon character presents a target word, then several other words are presented in association with different fish. The listener's task is to click on the fish that is associated with a word with the same phoneme in the target word. For example, the target word could be *win*. The listener can select a word from the following choices: *pen, wait, date, who,*

and *new*. If the response is correct (e.g., wait), the associated fish is put in a jar at the top left of the screen. This lets the player see his or her progress in terms of an increase in the number of fish in the corner jar.

The tasks referred to as auditory processing in the Woodcock-Johnson Psycho-education Battery Revised (WJ-R; Woodcock & Johnson, 1989) are sound blending and incomplete words. Sound blending involves analysis of acoustic waveforms to identify phonological elements and blending of the identified phonological elements to match the previously stored lexical entries. Incomplete Words requires closure skills (see Chapter 8) and involves extraction of phonological features from the acoustic signal and completion of the incomplete signal with stored representation of similar complete words to fill in missing elements.

Children with learning problems show improvement in sound blending and auditory processing scores on the WJ-R test battery after 35 to 40 1-hour training sessions with the Earobics software over an 8-week period. These improvements are accompanied by accelerated maturational pattern of the cortical responses to speech stimuli (/ga/ and /da/) in quiet and higher resistance of speech evoked cortical responses to degradation when speech stimuli (/da/) are presented in noise. Similar improvements are not apparent in a control group of children with learning problems (Hayes, Warrier, Nicol, Zecker, & Kraus, 2003).

11.1.5 Neuroplastic Changes Associated with Improvement in Phoneme Discrimination

In one study, listeners were provided with training on 5 days to differentiate between two synthesized versions of the syllable /ba/ (Ross, Jamali, & Tremblay, 2013). One version had a voice onset time of 20 ms, and the other had a voice onset time of 10 ms. Before training, most English-speaking listeners could not differentiate between these stimuli. After training, they could learn to identify the stimulus with 20 ms voice onset time as *mba* and the 10 ms voice onset time stimulus as *ba*. The improvement in differentiation between the two versions of the syllable was accompanied by an enhancement of the amplitude of the P2 m magneto-encephalographic wave that occurs 200 ms after the onset of the stimuli. The increase in amplitude persisted over time, suggesting that the change is neuroplastic in nature (Ross et al., 2013).

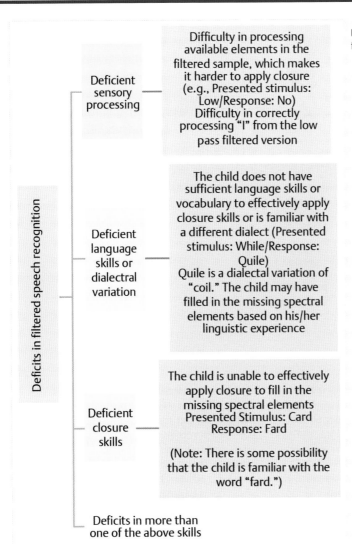

Fig. 11.6 Reasons for deficits in filtered speech recognition.

Deficits in filtered speech recognition

- Deficient sensory processing — Difficulty in processing available elements in the filtered sample, which makes it harder to apply closure (e.g., Presented stimulus: Low/Response: No) Difficulty in correctly processing "I" from the low pass filtered version

- Deficient language skills or dialectral variation — The child does not have sufficient language skills or vocabulary to effectively apply closure skills or is familiar with a different dialect (Presented stimulus: While/Response: Quile) Quile is a dialectral variation of "coil." The child may have filled in the missing spectral elements based on his/her linguistic experience

- Deficient closure skills — The child is unable to effectively apply closure to fill in the missing spectral elements Presented Stimulus: Card Response: Fard

  (Note: There is some possibility that the child is familiar with the word "fard.")

- Deficits in more than one of the above skills

11.2 Degraded Speech

Failure to recognize degraded speech can occur for various reasons. The results of an auditory processing test battery along with the responses of the listener on degraded speech tasks can provide an insight into the reasons which are applicable for each patient. Depending on the applicable reason, the appropriate strategy or multiple strategies can be used to improve recognition of degraded speech. For children who do not have age-appropriate linguistic skills, language therapy can enhance performance on degraded speech tasks. Training in improving closure skills can enhance performance of those listeners who have difficulty

implementing closure or are hesitant in applying closure (see Chapter 8). The specific stimuli used in assessing the deficits should not be used during training to minimize the possibility of learning effects that can confound the assessment of benefits derived from training.

11.2.1 Filtered Speech

▶ Fig. 11.6 shows the possible reasons for failure in recognizing filtered speech, including deficient sensory processing, limited linguistic skills, and deficits in adequate use of closure skills. Depending on the deficit or deficits, several strategies can be used to improve the perception of filtered

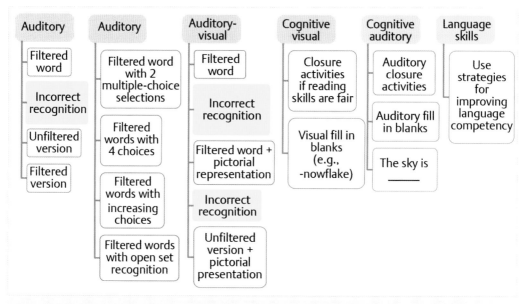

Fig. 11.7 Stimulus presentation sequences (first three columns) or strategies (last three columns) for improving recognition of filtered speech. The blocks titled "Incorrect recognition" indicate patient responses.

speech (▶ Fig. 11.7). For example, training can occur for addressing sensory processing deficits by presenting filtered words. Whenever the listener gives an incorrect response, the correct unfiltered version of the target is provided. Verbal feedback is also provided for correctly recognized stimuli. Several repetitions of the same target stimuli can occur until the listener begins to recognize the word correctly. Another way to improve sensory auditory processing is to supplement it by visual stimuli. This can be accomplished by presenting written or pictorial versions of the target stimuli whenever an incorrect response is given. If the listener is having great difficulty in recognizing filtered speech, a multiple choice response task can be used. Initially, only two response foils can be used; with increasing success, more response foils can be added until the listener can provide age-appropriate response accuracy in an open set task.

11.2.2 Spectrally Smeared or Shifted Speech

The auditory, auditory-visual-pictorial, or auditory-visual-print presentations of the targets can be presented to the listener repeatedly to improve the performance of spectrally smeared speech. Improvement in performance on spectrally smeared

speech may improve performance on listening to reverberant speech.

Improvement of phoneme perception may be more important for implanted children with limited speech recognition abilities or language skills. Such children must develop a central speech template based on the stimulation they receive through cochlear implants. Training that targets vowel contrasts using monosyllable words may result in the best overall phoneme recognition for spectrally shifted speech stimuli (Fu, Nogaki, & Galvin, 2005).

11.2.3 Noise-Vocoded Speech

A brief training session including exposure to 30 noise-vocoded sentences can significantly improve the recognition of words within sentences (Davis, Johnsrude, Hervais-Adelman, Taylor, & McGettigan, 2005). An example of a procedure to improve the perception of noise-vocoded speech is given in ▶ Fig. 11.8. Learning to recognize noise-vocoded stimuli is more efficient when the feedback consists first of a nondistorted or clear version of the stimulus, followed by the noise-vocoded version, compared to when the noise-vocoded version is presented first, followed by the clear version of the stimulus. This suggests that a process that critically evaluates clear and noise-vocoded stimuli is involved in learning, which allows mapping of

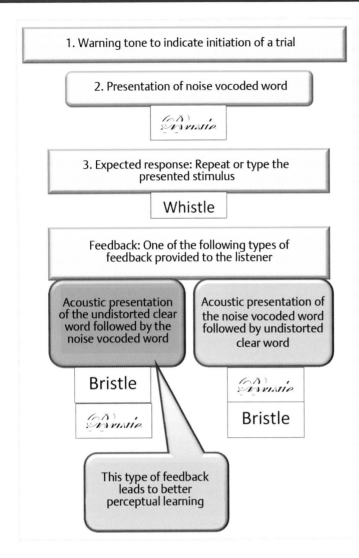

Fig. 11.8 Example of procedures for improving recognition of noise-vocoded speech (based on Heravis-Adleman, Davis, Johnsrude, & Carlyon, 2008).

future distorted input onto the correct internal representation. The learning can occur for words and nonwords and can generalize to untrained stimuli, suggesting the involvement of a sublexical level of processing, in which the representations that encode nondistorted phonemes or phonetic features are changed to improve the perception of noise-vocoded speech (Hervais-Adelman, Davis, Johnsrude, & Carlyon, 2008). Effective learning of noise-vocoded speech can also occur when a written form of the stimulus is presented concurrently with the noise-vocoded version (Davis et al., 2005).

Word- (▶ Fig. 11.9) or sentence-based (▶ Fig. 11.10) auditory training with feedback on correct and incorrect responses can improve the ability of listeners with normal hearing to perceive noise-vocoded speech that is spectrally shifted to simulate tonotopic misalignment. Training during a single session lasting for about 1 to 2 hours can improve speech recognition by 7 to 12%. An additional three sessions can lead to improvements in the range of 13 to 18% (Stacey & Summerfield, 2007). Word-based training can improve discrimination of noise-vocoded vowels and consonants, but no such improvement is apparent with sentence- or phoneme-based training. Significantly larger improvements in identification of words in noise-vocoded sentences are apparent with word- or sentence-based training compared to phoneme-based training (Stacey & Summerfield, 2008).

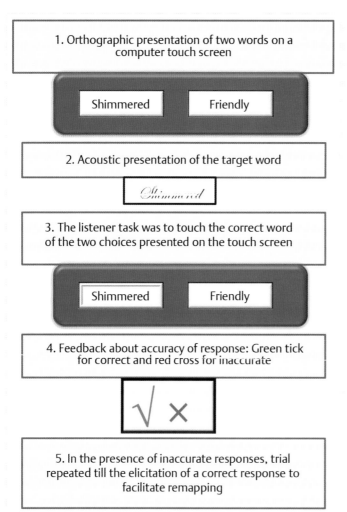

Fig. 11.9 Training procedure used by Stacey and Summerfield (2008) for improving recognition of noise-vocoded words.

1. Orthographic presentation of two words on a computer touch screen

Shimmered   Friendly

2. Acoustic presentation of the target word

Shimmered

3. The listener task was to touch the correct word of the two choices presented on the touch screen

Shimmered   Friendly

4. Feedback about accuracy of response: Green tick for correct and red cross for inaccurate

√ ×

5. In the presence of inaccurate responses, trial repeated till the elicitation of a correct response to facilitate remapping

These series of studies suggest that in improving perception of degraded speech, it may be better to initially use words as stimuli compared to sentences, which can place higher demand on preserving memory traces of the clear stimulus patterns. For some individuals with APDs, clear speech feedback followed by the distorted version may be useful in improving speech recognition in degraded listening environments. In addition, if literacy skills are good, a written version of the stimulus may improve the efficiency in learning to recognize speech under degraded listening environments.

11.2.4 Frequency Transposed Speech

For patients who have no usable hearing in the higher frequencies, lowering the higher frequencies

and adding the processed signal to the original unprocessed signal can improve audibility of sounds. The patient's ability to make use of these processed signals can be improved through auditory training. A computer-based training program has been developed to improve the recognition of frequency transposed speech (Kuk, Keenan, Peeters, Lau, & Crose, 2007). This 10-day program with 20- to 30-minute daily sessions targets voiceless consonants (/p, t, k, s, f, ʃ, tʃ/) that are most amenable to frequency transposition. The patient's attention is directed to different sounds every day. Training for each sound is provided at syllable, word, and sentence levels. The ease of the interactive training games is maintained at the sixth-grade reading level. The exercises are divided into different interactive games. In the discrimination exercise, the target word pair (e.g., *cat, cats*) is presented in a

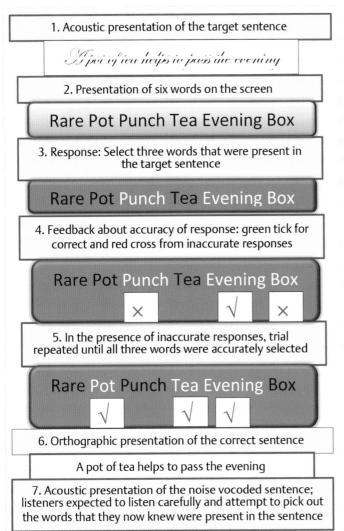

Fig. 11.10 Training procedure used by Stacey and Summerfield (2008) for improving recognition of noise-vocoded sentences.

1. Acoustic presentation of the target sentence

A pot of tea helps to pass the evening

2. Presentation of six words on the screen

Rare Pot Punch Tea Evening Box

3. Response: Select three words that were present in the target sentence

Rare Pot Punch Tea Evening Box

4. Feedback about accuracy of response: green tick for correct and red cross from inaccurate responses

Rare Pot Punch Tea Evening Box
× √ ×

5. In the presence of inaccurate responses, trial repeated until all three words were accurately selected

Rare Pot Punch Tea Evening Box
√ √ √

6. Orthographic presentation of the correct sentence

A pot of tea helps to pass the evening

7. Acoustic presentation of the noise vocoded sentence; listeners expected to listen carefully and attempt to pick out the words that they now knew were present in the sentence

sentence. In the attention exercise, the patient is expected to count the number of times a target phoneme is uttered in a sentence. A crossword puzzle is included in the identification exercise, and the patient can get cues to solving the puzzle by listening to sentences. A memory exercise requires the patient to hear the target sound, then select the target from a list of options. All of the exercises are designed to increase awareness of the target voiceless consonant sounds while promoting various auditory skills. The training materials are spoken by two female speakers and one male speaker to improve generalizability (Kuk et al., 2007). Training can improve the perception of many of the targeted frequency transposed consonants in normal-hearing listeners with simulated high-frequency hearing loss (Korhonen & Kuk, 2008) and in children (Auriemmo et al., 2009) and adults (Kuk, Keenan, Korhonen, & Lau, 2009) with hearing loss.

11.2.5 Interrupted Speech

A deficit in the recognition of interrupted speech is most likely related to deficits in filling the missing information in the temporal domain. There is a significant correlation between receptive vocabulary and verbal intelligence and perception of interrupted speech (Benard, Mensink, & Başkent, 2014). Thus, improving vocabulary is an important strategy for improving perception of interrupted speech. Training in improving closure skills (see

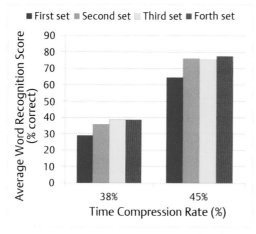

Fig. 11.11 Average word recognition scores with exposure to four sets of time-compressed sentences with five sentences in each set (based on Dupoux & Green, 1997).

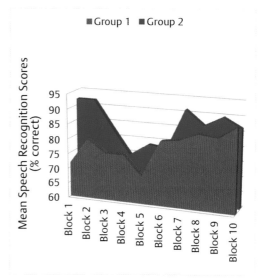

Fig. 11.12 Mean speech recognition scores (percentage correct) across 10 blocks for rapid speech. Each block contained six sentences spoken at a fast rate. Group 2 received prior practice in listening to 60 time-compressed sentences. Scores of group 2 are initially higher, suggesting some transfer of perceptual learning from time-compressed speech. Note that the performance of group 1 improves over time, which indicates adaptation to listening to fast speech (based on Adank & Janse, 2009).

Chapter 8) using auditory stimuli and visual cues can assist in improving the recognition of interrupted speech. Training incorporating visual sentence text and auditory playback of interrupted and uninterrupted speech can also improve performance due to more active and effective use of top-down closure skills. The training is generalizable to interrupted speech in which the silent gaps are filled with noise and leads to a reduction in the amount of perceived mental effort in recognizing the sentences. The training effects are maintained over a period of several weeks (Benard & Başkent, 2013).

11.2.6 Time-Compressed Speech

Recognition of time-compressed speech requires the ability to apply closure in the temporal domain to fill in the missing elements of speech as is required in the recognition of interrupted speech. It also requires faster processing speed. During the processing of a regular version of a word or sentence, more time is available for processing the message than what is available during the processing of a time-compressed version of the same signal. For example, with 50% compression, half of the time is available for processing the sentence when compared to an uncompressed version of the same sentence. Thus, any activities that can improve processing speed are expected to improve the recognition of time-compressed speech provided that the

listener has good closure skills in the temporal domain.

Some improvement in the recognition of words within time-compressed sentences is apparent with relatively limited exposure to time-compressed sentences. ▶ Fig. 11.11 shows improvement in the word recognition scores following exposure to four sets of time-compressed sentences with five sentences in each set (Dupoux & Green, 1997). Note that the most improvement is apparent between the first and second sets. Reliable improvements in the perception of time-compressed sentences have been reported using various exposure paradigms, including continuous exposure to time-compressed sentences and exposure to time-compressed sentences interspersed with exposure to natural uncompressed sentences. The improvement is apparent in both younger and older adults (Golomb, Peelle, & Wingfield, 2007). Exposure to time-compressed nonsense sentences (Altmann & Young, 1993) or time-compressed materials in a nonnative language that is similar to the native language can also lead to improvement in the perception of

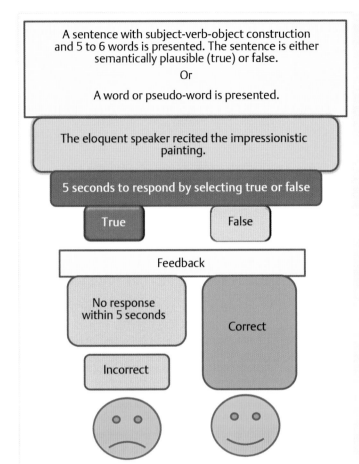

A sentence with subject-verb-object construction and 5 to 6 words is presented. The sentence is either semantically plausible (true) or false.

Or

A word or pseudo-word is presented.

The eloquent speaker recited the impressionistic painting.

5 seconds to respond by selecting true or false

True   False

Feedback

No response within 5 seconds

Correct

Incorrect

Fig. 11.13 Procedure for improving recognition of time-compressed speech used by Banai and Lavner (2012). The time compression rate was changed adaptively depending on the patient's response.

time-compressed speech, which suggests that adaptation to phonological information is important in improving the perception of time-compressed speech (Sebastián-Gallés, Dupoux, Costa, & Mehler, 2000).

Adult listeners who receive practice in listening to time-compressed speech are better at recognizing naturally fast sentences than those who have not received such practice (▶ Fig. 11.12). However, listeners who do not receive prior practice with time-compressed speech can improve their recognition of rapid speech with practice (Adank & Janse, 2009).

Children also adapt to time-compressed and rapid speech after listening practice (Guiraud, Ferragne, Bedoin, & Boulenger, 2013), which suggests that children's perception of rapid speech may improve with well-designed training in which the rate of speech is changed in an adaptive fashion, and feedback is provided for correct and incorrect responses. Banai and Lavner (2012) changed the

rate of speech adaptively to train normal young adults to improve their recognition of time-compressed speech. Training sessions were administered over the course of 10 days in 5 adaptive blocks of 60 trials. Listeners were presented with sentences that were either semantically plausible (true) or false and words that were real or pseudo-words. After presentation of stimuli, listeners had 5 seconds to respond by selecting either true or false on the computer screen. Feedback was provided about accuracy of responses by showing smiley faces for correct responses and sad faces for incorrect responses (▶ Fig. 11.13). Failure to respond within 5 seconds was counted as an incorrect response. Training led to improvement in the accuracy of responses that was more than what was apparent in the control group. The results in the trained group were generalized to untrained conditions when different talkers presented the trained speech materials (Banai & Lavner, 2012).

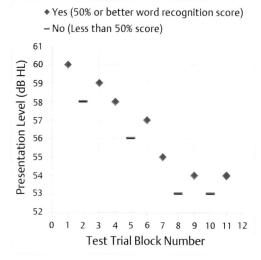

◆ Yes (50% or better word recognition score)
– No (Less than 50% score)

Fig. 11.14 Hypothetical example of adaptive training for improving speech recognition in competing background. The competing speech-shaped noise is presented at a constant level of 50 dB effective masking (EM). The listener initially needed the speech to be presented at 60 dB hearing level (HL) to correctly recognize 50% of the words. Through adaptive changes in presentation level and listening practice at each presentation level, the patient is able to achieve 50% recognition at 54 dB HL at the end of the training period. In this case, the speech recognition threshold in the competition of 50 dB EM speech-shaped noise improved by 6 dB.

11.2.7 Speech in Competing Backgrounds

For training in understanding speech in competing backgrounds, noise can be presented at a fixed level that will not cause discomfort during a relatively long presentation period of up to 30 minutes. For example, for listeners with normal peripheral hearing, the level of the speech-shaped noise can be 40 or 45 dB effective masking (EM), which is equivalent to a level of 60 to 65 dB sound pressure level (SPL). Keeping the noise constant, the presentation levels for target stimuli can be adjusted in an adaptive manner. An example of this is given in ▶ Fig. 11.14. At each presentation level, four spondees are presented, and the percent of words correctly repeated by the listener are noted. If the listener repeats 50% or more words correctly, the speech presentation level is decreased. If the listener recognizes less than 50% of words, then the level is increased. In some investigation, the speech presentation level is held constant, and the

competition level is varied. Systematic training can improve speech discrimination in the background of both speech-shaped noise and multitalker babble with slightly greater improvement when the competition is the latter (Cainer & Rajan, 2008).

Children trained to listen to sentences in the presence of an interrupted noise masker show improvement in the recognition of speech in the background of both interrupted and continuous noise, which indicates generalization of listening skills to continuous noise (Sullivan, Thibodeau, & Assmann, 2013). Thus, it may be more beneficial to begin training in the presence of an interrupted instead of a continuous noise masker. For training children, a response task similar to that shown in ▶ Fig. 11.15 can be used with certain modifications. The words can be shown on a background of a picture representing the words, and feedback can be provided after each trial (Sullivan et al., 2013).

Training on a monosyllabic word recognition task in noise can lead to better improvement on a sentence recognition in noise task in children ages 8 to 10 years compared to untrained children in a control group (Millward, Hall, Ferguson, & Moore, 2011). The background noise in this case consisted of a modulated speech-shaped noise. During training, the masker noise was maintained at a level of 60 dB(A), and the speech level was changed adaptively depending on the responses provided by the child. The training task involved a three-interval, three-alternative forced choice (3I-3AFC) procedure. Each interval was marked by a cartoon character. One of the intervals had a standard stimulus, and the remaining intervals had either the same or a different stimulus. The response task involved selecting the interval that had the different stimulus. The training was presented in the form of computer games, and children received stickers depending on the number of tasks they completed during each session. Additional reinforcements were provided in the form of prizes. Children had the option of choosing two smaller prizes (bouncing balls, magic playing cards, or glitter putty) that were awarded at the middle and at the end of the training period or a larger prize (kites, crayons, and Doctor Who activity packs) to be collected at the end of the training period (Millward et al., 2011).

Practice in the discrimination of CV syllables (/da/ vs. /ga/) embedded in increasing levels of noise can reflect the significant, robust, latent effects of training. The improvement is apparent 6 hours and not earlier than 4 hours following the

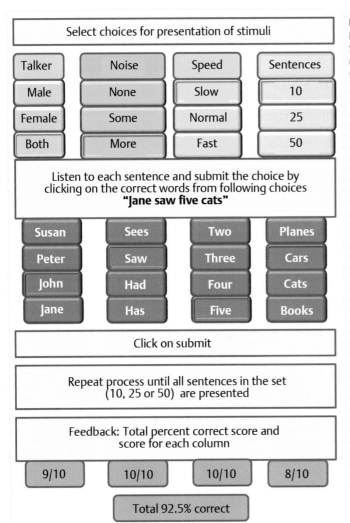

Fig. 11.15 The sequence of activities in the sentence Matrix 1 module of the Soundscapes program by MedEl (http://www.medel.com/us/sound-scape/).

SPATS

As mentioned previously, the SPATS software has a sentence recognition module with 1000 sentences varying in length from four to seven words, which are presented at signal-to-noise ratios varying from +15 to −15 dB (▶ Fig. 11.2). The listener can select responses from the target and three foils for each word. If a foil is selected for a word, the color

training sessions. The improvement is maintained over a period of at least 6 months after training (Roth, Kishon-Rabin, Hildesheimer, & Karni, 2005). Such results show the importance of rest periods between training sessions to consolidate the effects of training and to improve efficiency.

of the foil changes to red, and the sentence is replayed. The process is repeated until all of the words in the sentence are correctly identified. The sentences are structured in such a way that if the first word or first two words in the sentence are identified correctly, the identification of the remaining words is easier with the use of contextual cues. Listeners are encouraged to use the contextual cues and to identify all of the words as rapidly as possible to promote the use of cognitive resources. Preliminary data suggest that the software can lead to improvement equivalent to about a 5 dB reduction in the signal-to-noise ratio required to achieve targeted performance, and the improvement is generalized to better performance on other speech recognition tests (Miller et al., 2008).

Listening and Communication Enhancement (LACE)

The Listening and Communication Enhancement (LACE) software from Neurotone Inc. (Redwood City, CA) provides adaptive training with immediate feedback for improving speech recognition in the presence of single- or multitalker babble and can improve speech perception in many individuals (Sweetow & Sabes, 2006). New hearing aid users derive greater benefit from the LACE training exercises when compared to experienced hearing aid users (Olson, Preminger, & Shinn, 2013). There is a considerable amount of variability in the amount of improvement following training. Listeners with poorer scores on measures of degraded and competing speech show more improvement with the use of LACE software compared to those with better scores (Henderson Sabes, & Sweetow, 2007).

I Hear What You Mean

The software program I Hear What You Mean emphasizes meaning-based training (Barcroft et al., 2011). It includes 12 lessons; each with five activities that gradually increase in listening demands. Activity 1 is focused on sound identification, activity 2 includes a picture-based four-choice discrimination task, activity 3 requires completion of sentences, contextualized sentence identification is required in activity 4, and listening comprehension is expected in activity 5. Training can be provided in the background of four-talker babble. The speech-to-babble ratio is changed adaptively to allow 80% correct recognition during training. Many patients show improvement in their speech discrimination skills following 6 weeks of training (Barcroft et al., 2011).

MED-EL Soundscape

SoundScape speech training software from MED-EL Corp. (Durham, NC; http://www.medel.com/us/soundscape/) offers tasks in the form of games for improving speech recognition in quiet and noisy surroundings. For adults, Matrix sentences are available for practice at easier (level 1) and more difficult listening levels (level 2). At the easier level, the sentences are shorter and consist of four words (e.g., Susan has five cats). The listener chooses the correct words from a list of 16 words, which are presented in four columns and four rows, as shown in ▶ Fig. 11.15. Because there are no contextual cues, the listener cannot guess. Thus, the listener is required to pay close attention to each word. The sentences in level 2 are made up of 10 words, and the listener is required to recognize 7 of the words (e.g., the underlined words in the following sentence: He will cancel the appointment on Monday at 6:10). The words the, on, and at appear in all sentences. The listener can choose noisy or quiet backgrounds, as shown in ▶ Fig. 11.15. In addition, the listener can change the background noise from restaurant to music at the more difficult listening level 2.

For children younger than age 2 years, SoundScape includes reading materials and video clips to demonstrate activities for improving listening skills. For children between the ages of 2 and 6 years, listening activities become more difficult as children progress through the games. For example, in "Ms. MacDonald's Shed," listeners are presented with pictures of a number of vehicles in a farm setting and are expected to follow directions by clicking or dragging the mouse. Feedback is provided for correct and incorrect responses. Examples of responses from activities 2 to 6 are shown below:

- Level 2: Find the scooter.
- Level 3: Drag the fire truck into the shade.
- Level 4: Where are the hot air balloon and the scooter?
- Level 5: Put the scooter beside the cat.
- Level 6: Click on the one you hear. This vehicle is red, it has four wheels and two doors.

Similar games are available for children older than 6 years. In "Let's Go Shopping," children put different items in a cart or a shopping bag. In "Telling Tales," children answer questions for 13 different stories of various difficulty levels.

11.2.8 Combined Speech Degradations

Speech that is degraded through multiple modifications can improve with practice. The results of two listeners on the time-compressed plus reverberation task are shown in ▶ Fig. 11.16. The data was collected by presenting 50 words to each listener. Improvement is apparent in performance over the first set of 10 words, with peak performance during the third set of 10 words suggesting adaptation to degraded speech. The results reveal that listeners can adapt to this type of speech without any feedback. The results further suggest that perception on such tasks may improve with

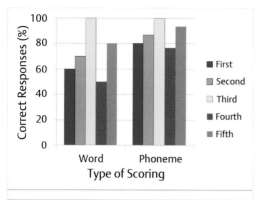

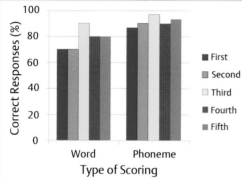

Fig. 11.16 Left ear performance of two 21-year-old female listeners on the Northwestern University Auditory Test No. 6 (NU-6) words time compressed at 45% mixed with reverberation of 0.3 second. The 50 words were presented at 45 dB HL. Performance is shown for each set of 10 words. Peak performance is apparent on the third set.

systematic training with reinforcement and feedback and that the improvements are expected to be greater for listeners who show poor perception during baseline tests. The required training duration may be longer for more difficult stimuli (e.g., 65% vs. 45% time compression).

11.3 Effect of Speech Discrimination Training on Related Skills

11.3.1 Phonological Awareness

Students in one study who received three 1-hour daily intervention sessions showed significant improvement in phonological awareness after 6 weeks of intervention (Pokorni, Worthington, & Jamison, 2004). In this study, the successful training programs were Earobics Step 2 (Cognitive

Concepts Inc., 1998) and the Lindamood Phonemic Sequencing Program (LiPS; Lindamood & Lindamood, 1998). The Earobics software provided auditory training in a fun, interactive game format. The various discrimination tasks involved discrimination of vowels and consonants; recognition of diphthongs and tense, and lax vowels in a word; and identification of consonant sound positions in a word. Examples of other skills targeted during training were blending of two to four syllables into a word, blending of three or four phonemes into a word, and word closure. The LiPS program was implemented without the use of computers by an intervention leader and presented to children in a group format, with each group comprising four children. The LiPS program divides auditory training into five categories: sensory input, perception, conceptualization, storage, and retrieval. For example, one of the concepts in the LiPS program involves identification and classification of speech sounds by place and manner of articulation. Learners in the study were guided through the oral-motor features of sounds and their relationships using labels such as "brother," "cousin," and "borrower" sounds. Participants were required to practice and track both vowels and consonants (Pokorni et al., 2004).

Another study focused on auditory training designed to teach discrimination of phoneme representatives of the major phonological categories of British English (Moore et al., 2005). The training was active and adaptive. Auditory training was embedded in a computer game and provided in 30-minute sessions interleaved with intrinsic arcade-style reward games. In addition, coaches provided verbal reinforcements and redirected attention as necessary. After each 5-minute game, children were rewarded with stickers that could be redeemed for prizes. Because the training for each stimulus set was brief, no improvement was apparent in phoneme discrimination. However, trained children showed dramatic improvement in phonological awareness, whereas untrained children showed no such improvement (Moore et al., 2005). Improvements in phonological awareness have also been reported by other investigators following training with acoustically modified speech (Habib et al., 1999).

11.3.2 Auditory Temporal Discrimination

Intensive training with acoustically modified speech can lead to improvement in auditory duration discrimination without any improvement in visual duration discrimination. Thus, the effect of intensive training with modified speech generalizes to temporal discrimination and is restricted to the auditory modality (Agnew, Dorn, & Eden, 2004).

11.4 Future Trends

11.4.1 Immersive Virtual Environments

Immersive virtual environments can allow listeners the experience of being immersed in a realistic environment. Total sensory interfaces use either head-mounted displays or immersive virtual reality rooms for visual immersion, stereoscopic sounds for acoustic immersion, and haptic technologies (simulation of forces, vibrations, and motions) for tactile immersion. For example, Cai and colleagues (2013) developed a virtual dolphin interaction program called Virtual Dolphinarium that allows children with autism the sense of being fully immersed in a simulated dolphin lagoon. The goal of this program is to teach children hand-based communication in an entertaining format by enabling them to play the role of a dolphin trainer. Children with autism are varied in their interest in interacting with the virtual pink dolphins. The researchers found that some children with autism had no problem wearing three-dimensional (3-D) glasses and expressed much interest in interacting with the virtual dolphins. Other children, however, refused to wear the glasses or showed limited interest (Cai et al., 2013). This study demonstrates that some children can benefit from immersive virtual reality environments.

Wade and Holt (2005) evaluated the effect of an interactive multimodal training format on the perceptual learning of spectrally complex nonspeech auditory categories. Listeners played a computer game that required them to navigate through a 3-D virtual space while encountering animated characters. The players' job was either to shoot enemy characters or to capture friendly characters. Each time a character was encountered, the listeners heard a distinctive sound category always associated with that character. Their goal was to maintain a high score, which was determined by the number of characters successfully shot. More points were awarded for faster shooting and at higher levels of game play. At higher levels, the characters became harder to identify visually, and players benefited by paying attention to the associated sound patterns to identify them. Although

participants were neither informed about the auditory patterns associations with each character nor asked to pay close attention to the sound patterns, they demonstrated reliable learning of the acoustic patterns during posttraining tests. These types of activities may lead to efficient learning of phoneme contrasts but should be modified to remove the violence related to the games.

Immersive virtual environments for improving speech recognition will be developed in the future that will help listeners understand speech spoken by various talkers under normal or degraded listening conditions. Users of these virtual systems should be able to control the type of degradation, including background noises, the types of noises (restaurant vs. sports arena), the type of speech (fast vs. slow), reverberation conditions (no reverberation vs. reverberation), and the number and spatial locations of talkers, including the distance and azimuth from the listener. The transfer of any improvements in speech recognition in the immersive virtual environments to real-life environments will need to be evaluated.

11.4.2 Socially Assistive Robotic Systems

Socially assistive robots can help people with special needs in social interactions. For example, such robots have been used to evoke attention and prosocial behavior in children with autism (Scassellati, Admoni, & Matarić, 2012). A robotic ball called Roball has the capability of performing intentional self-propelled movements and can generate a variety of interplay situations using motion, messages, sounds, illuminated parts, and other sensors (Michaud et al., 2005). Another robotic toy, IROMEC (Interactive RObotic social MEdiators as Companions), can play a therapeutic role for children with autism by encouraging the development of social interactions and communication in an interactive manner. The toy is programmable and allows various play scenarios to target various objectives. For example, the play scenario called "Make It Move" fosters nonverbal vocal communication (Ferrari, Robins, & Dautenhahn, 2009).

A baby harp seal robot, Paro (PARO Robots U.S., Inc. Schaumburg, IL), has been used in treating patients with dementia (Marti, Bacigalupo, Giusti, Mennecozzi, & Shibata, 2006). The robot is equipped with four senses: sight, tactile, balance, and hearing. Hearing includes sound source localization and speech recognition. Paro can perform vertical and horizontal neck movements, front and rear paddle movements, and independent movements of each eyelid to allow facial expressions. These features allow the robot to react to various stimuli. For example, after a sudden loud sound, Paro pays attention and looks in the direction of the sound (Marti et al., 2006).

A talking robot consisting of motor-controlled organs, including vocal chords, a vocal tract, and a nasal cavity, has been developed to generate a natural voice that allows simulation of human vocalization (Sawada, Kitani, & Hayashi, 2008). By allowing auditory feedback learning with an adaptive control algorithm of pitch and phoneme, the robot can vocalize stable vocal sounds imitating human speech. Preliminary data suggest that the talking robot can help hearing-impaired individuals improve their articulation and voice.

All of the above studies suggest the potential benefit of socially assistive robots for young clinical populations. In the future, socially assistive robots may be used to motivate young children to differentiate between phonemes. The robots can be programmed to provide a variety of auditory stimuli and reinforcements for correct responses (e.g., Good listening!) and may be specially useful for children with auditory processing and other co-morbid deficits such as language or attention deficits. Such robots may also be used to improve the speech recognition skills of older adults who are living alone or are in nursing homes and have difficulty using computers.

11.5 Review Questions

1. Review the characteristics of training protocols that can improve phoneme perception. Discuss the module designed to improve syllable or constituent perception in the Speech Perception Assessment and Training System (SPATS).

2. What is categorical speech perception? Discuss phoneme perception training based on categorical speech perception. Discuss how Earobics games can improve phoneme perception. What types of neuroplastic changes are apparent following improvements in phoneme discrimination?

3. What types of strategies can be used to improve the perception of filtered speech? What strategies can maximize the efficiency of training designed to improve noise-vocoded speech?

4. Describe a training program designed to improve the perception of frequency transposed consonants.

5. How can the perception of interrupted speech be improved?

6. What types of strategies can be used to improve the perception of time-compressed speech? What is the effect of training on time-compressed speech on the recognition of rapid speech?

7. Review studies that have shown the efficacy of training for improving speech perception in noise. Review the components of the computerized training programs SPATS, SoundScape, and LACE that can be used to improve speech recognition in noise.

8. Review the potential impact of speech recognition training on phonological awareness and auditory temporal discrimination.

9. What are immersive virtual environments? How can these environments be designed to improve speech recognition?

10. Describe socially assistive robotic systems. What are the potential applications of such systems for improving phoneme perception in children?

References

[1] Adank, P., & Janse, E. (2009). Perceptual learning of time-compressed and natural fast speech. Journal of the Acoustical Society of America, 126(5), 2649–2659.

[2] Agnew, J. A., Dorn, C., & Eden, G. F. (2004). Effect of intensive training on auditory processing and reading skills. Brain and Language, 88(1), 21–25.

[3] Altmann, G. T. M., & Young, D. H. (1993). Factors affecting adaptation to time-compressed speech. Proceedings of Eurospeech, Berlin, 9(1), 333–336.

[4] Auriemmo, J., Kuk, F., Lau, C., et al. (2009). Effect of linear frequency transposition on speech recognition and production of school-age children. Journal of the American Academy of Audiology, 20(5), 289–305.

[5] Banai, K., & Lavner, Y. (2012). Perceptual learning of time-compressed speech: More than rapid adaptation. PLoS ONE, 7(10), e47099.

[6] Barcroft, J., Sommers, M. S., Tye-Murray, N., Mauze, E., Schroy, C., & Spehar, B. (2011). Tailoring auditory training to patient needs with single and multiple talkers: Transfer appropriate gaines on a four-choice discrimination text. International Journal of Audiology, 50, 802–880.

[7] Benard, M. R., & Başkent, D. (2013). Perceptual learning of interrupted speech. PLoS ONE, 8(3), e58149.

[8] Benard, M. R., Mensink, J. S., & Başkent, D. (2014). Individual differences in top-down restoration of interrupted speech: Links to linguistic and cognitive abilities. Journal of the Acoustical Society of America, 135(2), EL88.

[9] Bradlow, A. R., Akahane-Yamada, R., Pisoni, D. B., & Tohkura, Y. (1999). Training Japanese listeners to identify English /r/ and /l/: Long-term retention of learning in perception and production. Perception and Psychophysics, 61(5), 977–985.

[10] Cai, Y., Chia, N. K., Thalmann, D., Kee, N. K., Zheng, J., & Thalmann, N. M. (2013). Design and development of a Virtual Dolphinarium for children with autism. IEEE Transactions

on Neural Systems and Rehabilitation Engineering, 21(2), 208–217.

[11] Cainer, K. E., James, C., & Rajan, R. (2008). Learning speech-in-noise discrimination in adult humans. Hearing Research, 238(1-2), 155–164.

[12] Cognitive Concepts, Inc. (1998). Earobics auditory development and phonics program step 2. Evanston, IL: Author.

[13] Davis, M. H., Johnsrude, I. S., Hervais-Adelman, A., Taylor, K., & McGettigan, C. (2005). Lexical information drives perceptual learning of distorted speech: Evidence from the comprehension of noise-vocoded sentences. Journal of Experimental Psychology: General, 134(2), 222–241.

[14] Dupoux, E., & Green, K. (1997). Perceptual adjustment to highly compressed speech: Effects of talker and rate changes. Journal of Experimental Psychology: Human Perception and Performance, 23(3), 914–927.

[15] Ferrari, E., Robins, B., & Dautenhahn, K. (2009). Therapeutic and educational objectives in robot assisted play for children with autism. In Proceedings of the 18th IEEE International Symposium on Robot and Human Interactive Communication (RO-MAN 2009), Sept. 27–Oct. 2, Toyama, Jpn. (pp. 108–114). Piscataway, NJ: IEEE.

[16] Fu, Q. J., Nogaki, G., & Galvin, J. J. III. (2005). Auditory training with spectrally shifted speech: Implications for cochlear implant patient auditory rehabilitation. Journal of the Association for Research in Otolaryngology, 6(2), 180–189.

[17] Golomb, J. D., Peelle, J. E., & Wingfield, A. (2007). Effects of stimulus variability and adult aging on adaptation to time-compressed speech. Journal of the Acoustical Society of America, 121(3), 1701–1708.

[18] Guiraud, H., Ferragne, E., Bedoin, N., & Boulenger, V. (2013). Adaptation to natural fast speech and time-compressed speech in children. In F. Bimbot, C. Cerisara, C. Fougeron, G. Gravier, L. Lamel, F. Pellegrino, & P. Perrier (eds.), Interspeech (pp. 1370–1374). Baixas, France: International Speech Communication Association.

[19] Habib, M., Espesser, R., Rey, V., Giraud, K., Bruas, P., & Gres, C. (1999). Training dyslexics with acoustically modified speech: Evidence of improved phonological performance. Brain and Cognition, 40(1), 143–146.

[20] Hayes, E. A., Warrier, C. M., Nicol, T. G., Zecker, S. G., & Kraus, N. (2003). Neural plasticity following auditory training in children with learning problems. Clinical Neurophysiology, 114(4), 673–684.

[21] Henderson Sabes, J., & Sweetow, R. W. (2007). Variables predicting outcomes on listening and communication enhancement (LACE) training. International Journal of Audiology, 46(7), 374–383.

[22] Hervais-Adelman, A., Davis, M. H., Johnsrude, I. S., & Carlyon, R. P. (2008). Perceptual learning of noise vocoded words: Effects of feedback and lexicality. Journal of Experimental Psychology: Human Perception and Performance, 34(2), 460–474.

[23] Hirata, Y., Whitehurst, E., & Cullings, E. (2007). Training native English speakers to identify Japanese vowel length contrast with sentences at varied speaking rates. Journal of the Acoustical Society of America, 121(6), 3837–3845.

[24] Iverson, P., & Evans, B. G. (2009). Learning English vowels with different first-language vowel systems: 2. Auditory training for native Spanish and German speakers. Journal of the Acoustical Society of America, 126(2), 866–877.

[25] Korhonen, P., & Kuk, F. (2008). Use of linear frequency transposition in simulated hearing loss. Journal of the American Academy of Audiology, 19(8), 639–650.

[26] Kuk, F., Keenan, D., Korhonen, P., & Lau, C. C. (2009). Efficacy of linear frequency transposition on consonant identifica-

tion in quiet and in noise. Journal of the American Academy of Audiology, 20(8), 465–479.

[27] Kuk, F., Keenan, D., Peeters, H., Lau, C., & Crose, B. (2007). Critical factors in ensuring efficacy of frequency transposition: 2. Facilitating initial adjustment. Hearing Review, 14(4), 90–96.

[28] Lengeris, A., & Hazan, V. (2010). The effect of native vowel processing ability and frequency discrimination acuity on the phonetic training of English vowels for native speakers of Greek. Journal of the Acoustical Society of America, 128(6), 3757–3768.

[29] Liberman, A. M., Harris, K. S., Hoffman, H. S., & Griffith, B. C. (1957). The discrimination of speech sounds within and across phoneme boundaries. Journal of Experimental Psychology, 54(5), 358–368.

[30] Lindamood, C. H., & Lindamood, P. C. (1998). Lindamood Phoneme Sequencing Program (LiPS). Austin, TX: PRO-ED.

[31] Lisker, L., & Abramson, A. S. (1964). A cross-language study of voicing in initial stops: Acoustical measurements. Word, 20, 384–422.

[32] Lively, S. E., Logan, J. S., & Pisoni, D. B. (1993). Training Japanese listeners to identify English /r/ and /l/: 2. The role of phonetic environment and talker variability in learning new perceptual categories. Journal of the Acoustical Society of America, 94(3, Pt. 1), 1242–1255.

[33] Lively, S. E., Pisoni, D. B., Yamada, R. A., Tohkura, Y., & Yamada, T. (1994). Training Japanese listeners to identify English /r/ and /l/: 3. Long-term retention of new phonetic categories. Journal of the Acoustical Society of America, 96(4), 2076–2087.

[34] Logan, J. S., Lively, S. E., & Pisoni, D. B. (1991). Training Japanese listeners to identify English /r/ and /l/: A first report. Journal of the Acoustical Society of America, 89(2), 874–886.

[35] Marti, P., Bacigalupo, M., Giusti, L., Mennecozzi, C., & Shibata, T. (2006). Socially assistive robotics in the treatment of behavioural and psychological symptoms of dementia. Paper presented at the First IEEE/RAS-EMBS International Conference on Biomedical Robotics and Biomechatronics (BioRob 2006), Pisa, Italy. Retrieved from http://ieeexplore.ieee.org.

[36] Michaud, F., Laplante, J. F., Larouche, H., et al. (2005). Autonomous spherical mobile robot for child-development studies. IEEE Transactions on Systems, Man, and Cybernetics, Part A: Systems and Humans, 35(4), 471–480.

[37] Miller, J. D., Watson, C. S., Kistler, D. J., Preminger, J. E., & Wark, D. J. (2008). Training listeners to identify the sounds of speech: 2. Using SPATS software. Hearing Journal, 61(10), 29–33.

[38] Millward, K. E., Hall, R. L., Ferguson, M. A., & Moore, D. R. (2011). Training speech-in-noise perception in mainstream school children. International Journal of Pediatric Otorhinolaryngology, 75(11), 1408–1417.

[39] Moore, D. R., Rosenberg, J. F., & Coleman, J. S. (2005). Discrimination training of phonemic contrasts enhances phonological processing in mainstream school children. Brain and Language, 94(1), 72–85.

[40] Olson, A. D., Preminger, J. E., & Shinn, J. B. (2013). The effect of LACE DVD training in new and experienced hearing aid users. Journal of the American Academy of Audiology, 24(3), 214–230.

[41] Pokorni, J. L., Worthington, C. K., & Jamison, P. J. (2004). Phonological awareness intervention: Comparison of Fast ForWord, Earobics, and LiPS. Journal of Educational Research, 97(3), 147–157.

[42] Pruitt, J. S., Jenkins, J. J., & Strange, W. (2006). Training the perception of Hindi dental and retroflex stops by native

speakers of American English and Japanese. Journal of the Acoustical Society of America, 119(3), 1684–1696.

[43] Robinson, B. (2004). Phonomena: Sound game & 3's company game. [CD-ROM]. United Kingdom: Mindweavers (http://www.mindweavers.co.uk).

[44] Rosenberg, J. F., & Moore, D. R. (2003). Winning game (Auditory training in speech and language therapy: A field trial). Bulletin of the Royal College Speech Language Therapy, June Edition, 5–6.

[45] Ross, B., Jamali, S., & Tremblay, K. L. (2013). Plasticity in neuromagnetic cortical responses suggests enhanced auditory object representation. BMC Neuroscience, 14, ID 151.

[46] Roth, D. A., Kishon-Rabin, L., Hildesheimer, M., & Karni, A. (2005). A latent consolidation phase in auditory identification learning: Time in the awake state is sufficient. Learning and Memory, 12(2), 159–164.

[47] Sadakata, M., & McQueen, J. M. (2013). High stimulus variability in nonnative speech learning supports formation of abstract categories: Evidence from Japanese geminates. Journal of the Acoustical Society of America, 134(2), 1324–1335.

[48] Sawada, H., Kitani, M., & Hayashi, Y. (2008). A robotic voice simulator and the interactive training for hearing-impaired people. Journal of Biomedicine and Biotechnology, 2008, ID 768232.

[49] Scassellati, B., Admoni, H., & Matarić, M. (2012). Robots for use in autism research. Annual Review of Biomedical Engineering, 14, 275–294.

[50] Sebastián-Gallés, N., Dupoux, E., Costa, A., & Mehler, J. (2000). Adaptation to time-compressed speech: Phonological determinants. Perception and Psychophysics, 62(4), 834–842.

[51] Stacey, P. C., & Summerfield, A. Q. (2007). Effectiveness of computer-based auditory training in improving the perception of noise-vocoded speech. Journal of the Acoustical Society of America, 121(5, Pt. 1), 2923–2935.

[52] Stacey, P. C., & Summerfield, A. Q. (2008). Comparison of word-, sentence-, and phoneme-based training strategies in improving the perception of spectrally distorted speech. Journal of Speech, Language, and Hearing Research, 51(2), 526–538.

[53] Sullivan, J. R., Thibodeau, L. M., & Assmann, P. F. (2013). Auditory training of speech recognition with interrupted and continuous noise maskers by children with hearing impairment. Journal of the Acoustical Society of America, 133 (1), 495–501.

[54] Sweetow, R. W., & Sabes, J. H. (2006). The need for and development of an adaptive Listening and Communication Enhancement (LACE) Program. Journal of the American Academy of Audiology, 17(8), 538–558.

[55] Wade, T., & Holt, L. L. (2005). Incidental categorization of spectrally complex non-invariant auditory stimuli in a computer game task. Journal of the Acoustical Society of America, 118(4), 2618–2633.

[56] Werker, J. F., & Tees, R. C. (1984). Phonemic and phonetic factors in adult cross-language speech perception. Journal of the Acoustical Society of America, 75(6), 1866–1878.

[57] Woodcock, R., & Johnson, M. (1989). Woodcock Johnson psycho-educational battery–revised: Tests of cognitive ability. Allen, TX: DLM Teaching Resources.

[58] Zuk, J., Ozernov-Palchik, O., Kim, H., et al. (2013). Enhanced syllable discrimination thresholds in musicians. PLoS ONE, 8 (12), e80546.

Chapter 12

Evidence-based Practice and Effectiveness of Intervention

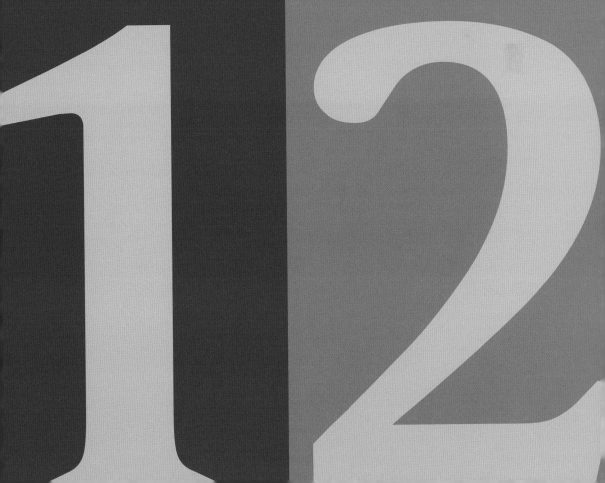

12 Evidence-based Practice and Effectiveness of Intervention

When intervention is provided to address auditory processing deficits (APDs), the measurement of outcomes is important for several reasons. For example, if the intervention is not effective, it is important to make changes to the intervention approach to improve outcomes. Outcome measurements are also important in terms of documenting the effectiveness of the intervention approach for third-party reimbursements. This chapter addresses three concepts related to measuring outcomes—efficacy, effectiveness, and efficiency (Haynes, 1999; Marley, 2000). In addition, evidence based-practice and single case research are also reviewed.

12.1 Efficacy

Efficacy can be defined as the degree to which an intervention approach has the ability to improve the intended auditory processing skills under ideal research conditions, such as in a randomized clinical trial. Randomized controlled trials (RCTs) are assumed to be very good at assessing efficacy or answering the question, Can a treatment work? However, RCTs have their own limitations. For example, one bias is that individuals participating in trials may be highly screened. They may have perfectly normal hearing, for example, and may not have any other comorbid conditions. Also, in the case of RCTs devised for adults, young adults are often included, possibly skewing the outcomes. Because of this selection bias, the results of RCTs may not apply to a typical patient with APD. For example, adults with APD may have hearing loss, they may be older (see Chapter 17), they may have been exposed to ototoxins (see Chapter 16), or they may have other health conditions, such as diabetes. Young children may have other comorbid conditions, such as attention deficit hyperactivity disorder (ADHD).

12.2 Effectiveness

Effectiveness can be defined as the extent to which an intervention approach can lead to improved auditory processing in usual or typical clinical settings. In typical clinical settings, several variables, including the knowledge, skills, and experience of the treatment provider, the motivation and resources of caregivers, and the motivation and preferences of the patient, can cause variation in treatment delivery and effectiveness. For example, practitioner bias (▶ Fig. 12.1) and patient preference (▶ Fig. 12.2) may lead to different outcomes. Effectiveness can be evaluated qualitatively and quantitatively through observational studies in clinical settings.

12.3 Efficiency

Efficiency is related to the cost-effectiveness of the intervention to individuals and society. For example, a treatment may appear to have high efficacy using RCTs but may not be the most cost-effective option for individual patients. When considering cost, monetary, time, and psychological costs to the patient, caregivers, and society should be considered. With reference to psychological cost, a treatment with high efficacy may not be an acceptable option to a patient or caregivers. For example,

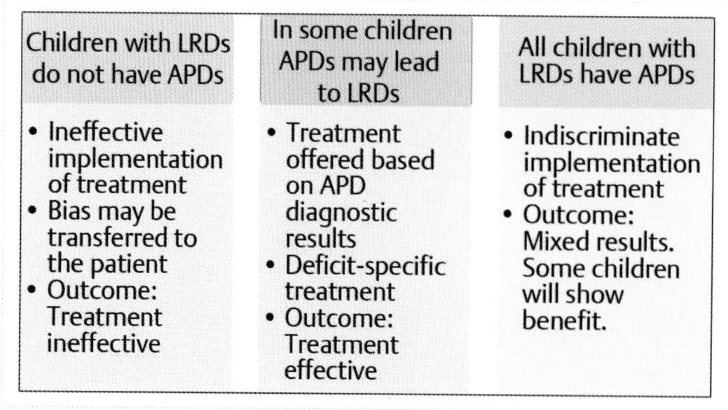

Children with LRDs do not have APDs	In some children APDs may lead to LRDs	All children with LRDs have APDs
• Ineffective implementation of treatment • Bias may be transferred to the patient • Outcome: Treatment ineffective	• Treatment offered based on APD diagnostic results • Deficit-specific treatment • Outcome: Treatment effective	• Indiscriminate implementation of treatment • Outcome: Mixed results. Some children will show benefit.

Fig. 12.1 An example of potential effects of practitioner belief on treatment effectiveness. The first row shows three different beliefs related to LRDs and APDs. APD, auditory processing deficit; LRD, language-related disorders.

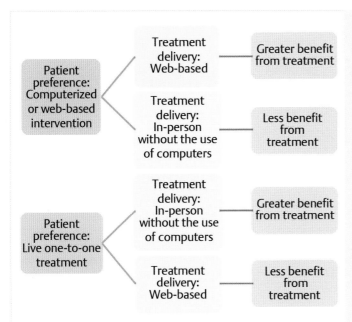

Fig. 12.2 Example of potential effects of patient preference on the effectiveness of treatment.

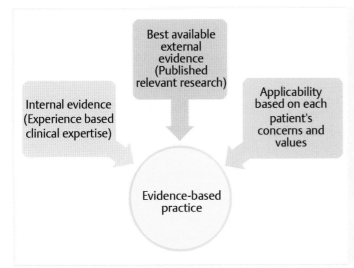

Fig. 12.3 Major components of evidence-based practice.

an 88-year-old may not wish to undergo computerized auditory training because he or she may be unfamiliar or uncomfortable with computers and related technology.

12.4 Evidence-based Practice

Evidence-based practice involves the judicious use of current evidence in providing services to individual patients (Sackett, Rosenberg, Gray, Haynes, & Richardson, 1996). In medical and paramedical fields, evidence-based practice (▶ Fig. 12.3) is recommended. There are two types of evidence: internal and external. Internal evidence refers to the clinical experience or expertise of the audiologist in providing effective and efficient services. External evidence refers to evidence published in scientific or clinical journals by other investigators. Without consideration of clinical experience and expertise, quality of services can be compromised by external evidence. This is because even so-called top-level external evidence may be ineffective for

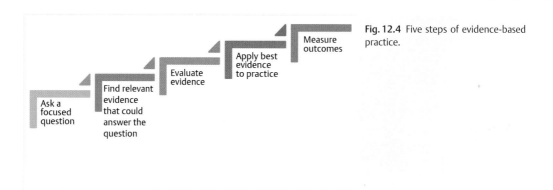

Fig. 12.4 Five steps of evidence-based practice.

an individual patient. However, external evidence has the potential to replace older diagnostic and treatment procedures with newer, more accurate, more powerful, and more effective approaches. Without current best external evidence, service delivery can become outdated. External evidence is not restricted to randomized trials and meta-analyses. It is the best evidence that will support the best outcomes for a patient based on his or her specific deficit, cultural values, and linguistic background.

Some clinical questions do not necessarily require RCTs (e.g., "How can we help this child to hear better in noisy classrooms"?), and in some children with APDs, waiting for RCTs may lead to the loss of critical periods of care or to the implementation of ineffective approaches with no apparent improvement. If RCTs have not been conducted, the next best available evidence (e.g., published reports based on cohort studies) should be used. It should be noted that even if the diagnostic test results of two patients appear to be similar, each patient has unique preferences, concerns, and expectations that should be taken into account in providing services.

12.4.1 Steps for Conducting Evidence-based Practice

Generally, there are five steps in conducting evidence-based practice: asking focused questions, searching for the evidence, appraising the evidence, applying the evidence to practice, and evaluating outcomes (▶ Fig. 12.4).

Asking Focused Questions

Focused questions should facilitate the search for a precise answer. There are several considerations relevant in phrasing a question, as shown in

▶ Fig. 12.5. First, the question should include the deficit or concerns of the specific patient. For example, the question may include "in patients who are performing poorly on dichotic listening tasks and report difficulty understanding speech in noisy conditions." Second, the question should consider the outcomes that the patient would like to have. For example, the patient may want to improve his or her ability to understand conversations at the dinner table. Third, the question should include the kind of intervention or interventions being considered based on patient acceptability. If markedly different interventions are under consideration, the question should include these interventions.

Searching for the Evidence

Based on the question, a variety of searches can be performed to find the external evidence to answer it. Sometimes clinicians are already familiar with the best evidence because of continuing education requirements. Regular attendance at professional conferences can keep clinicians aware of new treatment avenues. Such familiarity will allow clinicians to more quickly focus their search further or apply the available evidence immediately. Resources such as the Cochrane Library (http://www.thecochranelibrary.com/view/0/index.html) can provide quick access to current evidence in various areas of study.

Some investigators have identified several levels of evidence, as shown in ▶ Fig. 12.6, which are described below.

Level 1: Meta-Analyses of Randomized Controlled Trials

In this case, data from several RCTs are analyzed to determine the effectiveness of a treatment

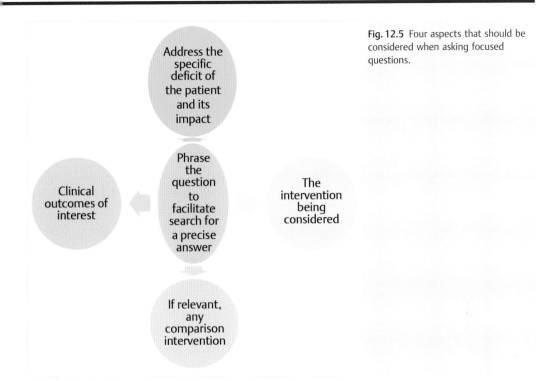

Fig. 12.5 Four aspects that should be considered when asking focused questions.

approach for a specific population. For example, in one meta-analysis, the effectiveness of auditory integration therapy or other methods of sound therapy was evaluated for individuals with autism spectrum disorders (Sinha, Silove, Hayen, & Williams, 2011). The intended goal of auditory integration therapy (Berard, 1993) is to reduce the abnormal response to auditory stimuli in the form of hypersensitivity (ear covering or screaming) or hyposensitivity (the appearance of being deaf) by some children with autism spectrum disorders. The results of the meta-analysis suggested that there was no evidence that auditory integration or other sound therapies are effective as treatment for autism spectrum disorders. There was also insufficient evidence to prove that this treatment was not effective. The authors of the meta-analysis noted that of the seven studies including 182 participants that had been reported, only two (with an author in common), involving a total of 35 participants, reported statistically significant improvements in the group receiving auditory integration therapy and for only two outcome measures, including the Aberrant Behavior Checklist and Fisher's Auditory Problems Checklist (Sinha et al., 2011).

Level 2: Systematic Reviews

In this case, investigators identify a specific question of clinical relevance and conduct an extensive literature search to identify studies with valid findings and good methodology. The studies are then reviewed and evaluated for quality. The results are summarized using predetermined criteria to answer the specific question. Brouns, El Refaie, and Pryce (2011) conducted a systematic review to answer the following question: Does auditory training improve speech discrimination in hearing-impaired adults? The answer to the question can inform clinicians about whether or not they should implement auditory training in addition to hearing aids during the provision of audiology services. The authors identified six studies that provided preliminary evidence suggesting an improvement due to various auditory training paradigms. However, the treatment effect size was modest.

Level 3: Randomized Controlled Trials

RCTs involve the use of two groups of participants: one that receives treatment and a control group that does not. The participants are randomly assigned to either group. In one study on the need

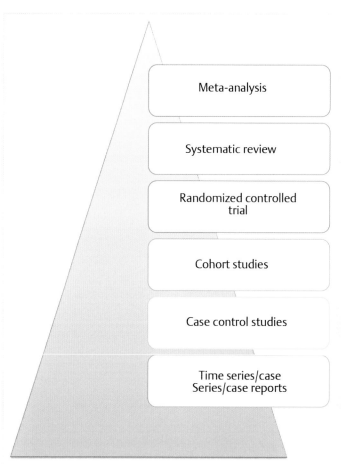

Fig. 12.6 Different types of external evidence to support a treatment approach.

for and development of an adaptive Listening and Communication Enhancement (LACE) program, 65 participants were randomly placed in one of two groups (Sweetow & Henderson Sabes, 2006). One group received auditory training immediately following baseline tests; the other served as a control for 1 month and then received training. The training was offered over a period of 4 weeks with 1-hour sessions for 5 days weekly. Outcome measures included speech perception in noise and subjective questionnaires. A significant improvement was noted in the training tasks and several of the subjective and objective measures. However, there was individual variability in outcomes, with some listeners showing substantial improvement and others showing no or minimal improvement (Sweetow & Henderson Sabes, 2006).

Level 4: Cohort Studies

In a cohort study, a group of patients who are undergoing a particular treatment are followed over time and compared to another group who is not receiving the treatment.

Level 5: Case Control Studies

In a case control study, patients with a specific condition are compared to those who do not have the condition. For example, Dlouha, Novak, and Vokral (2007) compared a group of children with specific language impairment (SLI) to a group of age-matched normal peers. They administered a dichotic listening task involving two bisyllabic words to all of the children. The performance of children with SLI was significantly poorer than that of normal children, as shown in ▶ Fig. 12.7.

Level 6: Time Series Studies

In a time series study, each participant serves as his or her own control. The person is evaluated before and after treatment on the same outcome measures to detect any improvement.

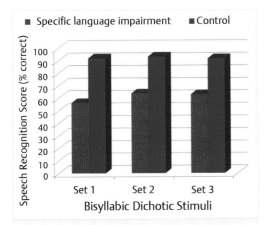

Fig. 12.7 Example of data from a case control study. In this case, the performance of children with specific language impairment is compared to the performance of those without any impairment. The dichotic listening task involved presentation of bisyllabic words simultaneously to both ears. The performance is measured using three different sets of dichotic words (based on Dlouha, Novak, & Vokral, 2007). The figure shows average word recognition scores.

The design allows elimination of confounding variables such as gender and genetic factors. In one time series study, adolescents (11–17 years, $n = 20$) and adults (≥ 18 years, $n = 11$) received computerized auditory training to improve detection of a backward-masked tone for about 1 hour daily for 10 days (Huyck & Wright, 2013). Nearly every adult and half of the adolescents improved across sessions, and the adolescents who learned did so more slowly than adults. Clinicians can implement such a design in their audiology practice more easily than other types of research design. Multiple baseline and outcome measures and incorporation of objective measures can enhance confidence in the effectiveness of a particular treatment in a time series research design.

Case Series versus Case Reports

Case series include reports on the treatment of several individual patients. Case reports usually include a report of the effect of intervention on one patient. For example, in one study, two school-aged children with auditory processing disorders received the Fast ForWord training program (Krishnamurti, Forrester, Rutledge, & Holmes, 2013). Significant changes were noted in the speech-evoked auditory brainstem responses (ABRs) following intervention compared to the responses

before intervention. In some case reports, the patient may have a unique or rare deficit. In other cases, the intervention may be unique or different in some way.

Appraising the Evidence

The evidence should be evaluated to determine its validity, clinical relevance, and applicability (▶ Fig. 12.8). Based on the appraisal, the best evidence should be selected. In evaluating research, clinicians should ask if the research question is pertinent to the patient, if the study was properly designed to answer the question and generated data of high quality, and if appropriate statistical procedures were used (Concato et al., 2010).

Although a hierarchy of levels of evidence has been suggested, the evidence should not be judged based only on the hierarchy shown in ▶ Fig. 12.6. Although randomized controlled studies are considered by some as the gold standard for research designs, the quality of a study should not be evaluated using only the research design criterion (Concato, 2013). Cross-sectional, cohort, and case control studies, often referred to as observational studies, can offer important information and insights for evidence-based practice. The hierarchical notion of research designs as shown in ▶ Fig. 12.6 can lead to automatic and unscientific discounting of valid results generated through individual observational studies (Concato et al., 2010) that could be applicable to a specific patient. Clinicians should note the following limitations of RCTs.

Limitations of Randomized Controlled Trials

Concato (2013) summarized the limitations of RCTs:
- Results of several RCTs can often disagree. In a previously mentioned meta-analysis, it was noted that out of the seven RCTs, two studies revealed a significant effect on some of the measures, and five studies showed no effect (Sinha et al., 2011). Such differences can occur because of the eligibility criteria used in selecting participants, the baseline differences in populations across case studies, and the experience of service providers.
- Results of meta-analyses and large RCTs often disagree. In theory, the results of meta-analyses that analyzed data from several RCTS and results of RCTs using a large number of participants should agree. In one investigation, the results of

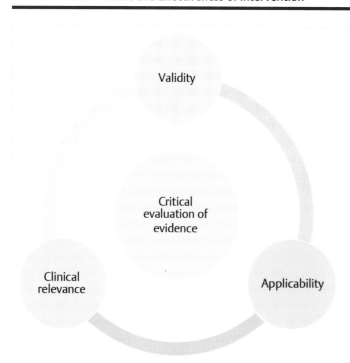

Fig. 12.8 Three considerations for critical evaluation of external evidence or published research. The research needs to be valid, relevant, and applicable to the clinical population being considered.

12 large RCTs and 19 meta-analyses were compared. Although results from previous meta-analyses should allow accurate prediction of outcomes of future large RCTs, about 35% of the time the prediction was not accurate (LeLorier, Grégoire, Benhaddad, Lapierre, & Derderian, 1997). This disagreement in the results between meta-analyses and RCTs shows that the top-level evidence status given to these two research designs may mislead clinicians. Clinicians may assume that the evidence will apply to their patients if the results are significant and that it will not apply if a theoretically sound treatment is found to have no efficacy in an RCT. Clinicians should note that, in the past, the U.S. Food and Drug Administration approved some treatments without RCTs, and these continue to be effective in clinical practice. For example, the drug Cisplatin was initially approved to treat testicular cancer in 1978 without a randomized controlled trial. The use of this drug was later expanded to treat ovarian and bladder cancer (Tsimberidou, Braiteh, Stewart, & Kurzrock, 2009). In some cases, blind application of results of RCT can lead to negative unpredictable outcomes (Juurlink et al., 2004).

- RCTs have limited generalizability. Following large RCTs, a treatment may show efficacy but may deliver an uneven mix of benefits to individual patients. This problem is referred to as *heterogeneity of treatment effects* (Greenfield, Kravitz, Duan, & Kaplan, 2007). Large RCTs may include populations that are highly selective or are more likely to respond to an intervention. For example, in selecting an APD population, children with comorbid reading deficits may be excluded. The results of such a trial may not apply to all children with APDs given that some children with APDs are likely to have dyslexia. Because the APD population is highly heterogeneous, the heterogeneity of treatment effects may make the treatment effects less predictable. Stated differently, the "one size fits all' approach based on the results of RCTs is less likely to apply to the APD population (Gabler, Duan, Vohra, & Kravitz, 2011).

Asking Questions for Appraising Evidence

In appraising any external evidence, clinicians should ask several questions. For example, if a randomized controlled study is being appraised, the following questions should be asked:
- How was randomization achieved (computerized randomization is best), or how were patients assigned to the treatment or control groups?

- Were the treatment and control groups similar at the beginning of the trial on the outcome measures and other relevant criteria, such as intelligence and age?
- Were at least some outcome measures objective (e.g., speech-evoked ABR), or were individuals recording the measures blind to who received the treatment and who did not?
- Were appropriate statistical procedures used?
- How large was the treatment effect?
- Do these results apply to your patient? Are patients included in the RCT similar to your patient? If they are not, the treatment may not be effective for your patient. Is the treatment feasible in your clinical setting? Will the treatment be acceptable to the patient in terms of compliance? Will it be cost-effective?

Applying the Evidence to Practice

The best evidence should be applied to the particular patient. In clinical practice, clinical expertise and patient values may require slight modifications to the intervention protocol.

Evaluating Outcomes

Although the evidence was selected with the expectation of good outcomes for the patient, the outcomes may not always be as expected. Thus, it is important to evaluate the outcomes. If the outcomes are not achieved, a change in the intervention is necessary.

12.5 Conducting Single-Case Research

Clinicians can use a single-subject design in applying the evidence they gathered, in measuring outcomes, and in sharing the results with other clinicians and patients. In sharing results with other clinicians and researchers, the focus is sometimes on whether or not a particular treatment approach worked or not. In sharing the results with patients, clinicians should note that the focus of patients or, in the case of children, the patients' parents is on whether or not the patients improved and concerns were addressed.

The most easily applicable single-subject design in clinical settings is a time series. In this type of study, clinicians gather data on multiple measures to record patient concerns and deficits. When the baseline measures are obtained more than once, the design is referred to as a *multiple baseline*. The data

obtained during the baseline phase are used along with external evidence and clinical experience to implement interventions (see Chapter 8). Outcomes are then measured again to determine if the intervention approaches worked. These are sometimes referred to as *treatment phase data*. An example of outcome measurements is shown in ▶ Fig. 12.9. If intervention did not work, the treatment should be modified to address any failures. Various approaches have been recommended for analyzing data obtained from single subjects. Because populations with APDs tend to be heterogeneous, single-subject designs can generate valuable information. It should be noted that when the same measures are used before and after training, some improvement may appear due to the ease in performing the task. Also, some measures have inherent test–retest variability that may seem like improvement.

To yield high-quality single-case research, it has been suggested that at least three attempts should be made to demonstrate an intervention effect at three different points. To assess the effects of treatment in single-case studies, the following six data features can be examined within and across the preintervention (baseline) and postintervention (treatment) phases of outcome measures (Kratochwill et al., 2010):

1. Level: This is the mean score for the data within a phase.
2. Trend: This is the slope of the best-fitting trend line for the data within a phase.
3. Variability: This is the range or standard deviation of data around the best-fitting straight line.
4. Immediacy of the effect: This refers to the change in the outcome measures close in time after the beginning of the intervention. Visual examination of the level, trend (slope), and variability can be used to examine the immediacy effect.
5. Overlap: This refers to the number of data points within the baseline and posttreatment measures that overlap.
6. Consistency of data patterns within the same or similar phases: This is related to less variability in the outcome measures.

12.5.1 Examples of Outcomes Presented in Single-Subject Studies

Percentage Change in Baseline Measures

Weihing and Musiek (2013) presented a case study of a 58-year-old man who experienced a stroke

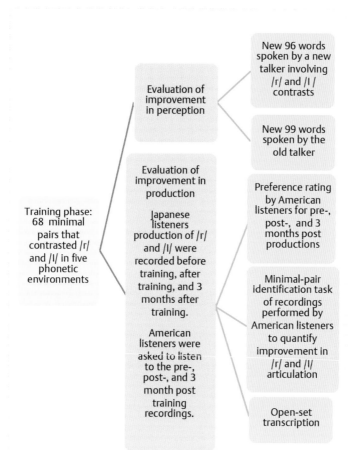

Fig. 12.9 Example of outcome measures used for auditory training designed to improve perception and production of English /r/–/l/ minimal pairs by Japanese listeners (based on Bradlow, Akahane-Yamada, Pisoni, & Tohkura, 1999).

with a large subcortical bleed in the left parieto-temporal region in June 2002 with resultant global aphasia. By October 2004, he had improved, with a mild-to-moderate anomia for both nouns and verbs and mild apraxia. He could understand short sentences with simple syntax but continued to experience difficulty with longer, more complex materials. Because of his auditory complaints, peripheral and central audiological evaluations were completed. The results showed more hearing loss in the left ear but more central difficulties in the right. The patient showed normal performance on duration and frequency pattern tests. His performance on the dichotic rhyme, double dichotic digits, and auditory closure tests was outside the normal limits in both ears. With single dichotic digits, performance was poor only in the left ear. The patient was provided with dichotic interaural intensity difference (DIID) training. His posttraining minus pretraining test performance in the left ear was presented as a percentage change, which showed

22 to 25% improvement on both the dichotic rhyme and single dichotic digits tasks. This case illustrates the effectiveness of DIID training even in the presence of mild to moderate receptive aphasia and mild apraxia.

Pre- and Postquantitative and Qualitative Measures

A boy was diagnosed with ADHD at the age of 6 years and APDs at the age of 9 years. His reading and spelling skills were 2 years below grade level. He received two 50-minute auditory therapy sessions weekly for 9 weeks. All sessions included two phonemic synthesis training lessons, visual-rhyming therapy, speech reading (use of available visual cues including lip reading and any other contextual cues to understand speech), and instruction in improving listening in noisy environments. The various outcome measures performed for this case are shown in ▶ Fig. 12.10. In this case,

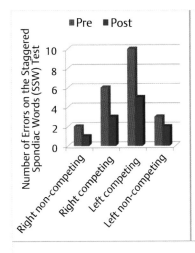

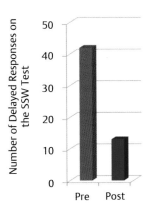

Fig. 12.10 Example of qualitative and quantitative outcome measures. Outcomes of auditory therapy are shown for a boy with attention deficit hyperactivity disorder and auditory processing deficits (based on Tillery, 1998).

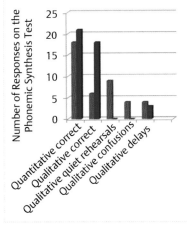

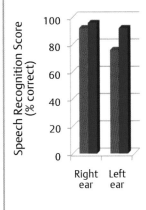

both quantitative and qualitative measures showed improvement following auditory training. For example, qualitatively, there was a decrease in the number of delayed responses on the Staggered Spondaic Word (SSW) test and the number of quiet reversals on the phonemic synthesis test (Tillery, 1998). This case study suggests the potential benefit of auditory training for children with comorbid APDs and ADHD.

Age-Appropriate Norms

▶ Fig. 12.11 shows an example of a case study where pre- and posttreatment scores are shown in comparison to age-matched norms. As apparent from the figure, some scores were below age-matched normative criteria and improved beyond the age-matched norms. The patient in this case was a 7-year-old boy. He also showed improvement on the Test of Nonverbal Intelligence (TONI).

The age-matched norms for the test range from 85 to 115. His pretraining score was 64, and the post training score was 84. The effectiveness of treatment was further supported in this case through electrophysiological measures. Speech-evoked ABR showed an increase in the amplitude of peak V, suggesting neuroplastic changes following training (Krishnamurti et al., 2013).

Improvement of at Least 1 Standard Deviation

▶ Fig. 12.12 shows an example where the outcome is measured as improvement of at least 1 standard deviation (SD) between pre- and posttraining and pretraining and long-term follow-up measures. In this figure, children APD04 and APD08 received training with Fast ForWord software (see Chapter 8), child APD09 received training with the Earobics software (see Chapter 11), and child APD03

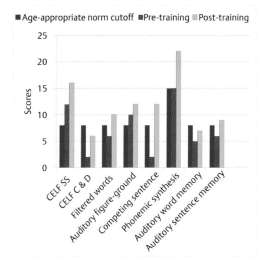

Fig. 12.11 Example of treatment outcomes presented with age-appropriate norms. As can be seen in some of the tasks, the performance was below the normative cutoff before training and exceeded the normative cutoff criteria after training (based on Krishnamurti, Forrester, Rutledge, & Holmes, 2013).

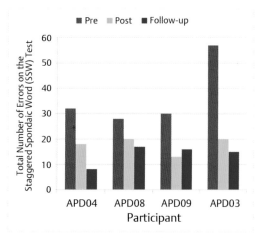

Fig. 12.12 Example of outcomes measured as at least 1 standard deviation (SD) improvement from pre- to posttraining and pretraining to follow-up tests. Follow-up testing occurred 3 to 6 months after the completion of intervention (based on Miller et al., 2005).

received live, in-person training designed to improve the following skills: auditory memory, auditory discrimination, auditory closure, auditory synthesis, multisensory integration, and auditory figure-ground (Miller et al., 2005).

Visual Examination of Graphed Data

▶ Fig. 12.13 shows the pre- and posttraining performance of a female subject for speech recognition in noise. The speech stimuli consisted of Northwestern University Auditory Test No. 6 (NU-6) words presented at 45 dB hearing level (HL) in the left ear in the presence of ipsilateral speech-shaped noise of 45 dB effective masking (EM). Performance is shown in terms of word recognition and phoneme recognition scores for four different NU-6 word lists. These probe stimuli were not used during training. The training was conducted once a week for a period of 10 weeks. Each auditory training session lasted for approximately 10 minutes. During training, various procedures were used to improve performance. During some segments of the sessions, a list of words was presented, and the presentation level of the words was adjusted adaptively depending on the spoken response of the listener. When the listener seemed hesitant or less confident in her response, immediate feedback about the accuracy of the response

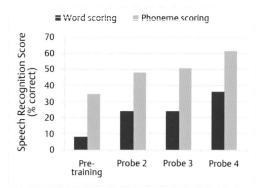

Fig. 12.13 Effects of auditory training on speech recognition in noise for a 21-year-old listener.

was provided. In other segments of training, a list of printed words was provided to the listener. She was asked to say the word, and then the same word was presented at a level where performance was about 50%. After presentation of the word, she was asked to repeat the word again to strengthen the kinesthetic feedback loop. ▶ Fig. 12.13 suggests improvement in word and phoneme recognition scores over time and indicates that performance may have improved further with additional training. Visual examination of graphed data is considered an essential initial step before performing statistical analyses in single-case research (Manolov, Solanas, Sierra, & Evans, 2011).

12.6 Statistical Analyses for Single-Case Research

Statistical analyses yielding statistical significance and effect size can complement visual analysis and summary statistics generated in single-subject research. Quantification of intervention outcomes is important when more precise reports are necessary about the amount of improvement. Such precision is helpful in the following circumstances:

1. Documenting the effectiveness of clinical services for legal, government, or insurance agencies
2. Comparing the effectiveness of two or more potentially useful interventions
3. Contributing to and enhancing the knowledge base necessary for evidence-based practice
4. Contributing to the meta-analyses that could pool results based on single-case research

12.6.1 Using the Available Baseline Data

In some cases, baseline measures are available from various sources. Some of these measures can be used in determining the outcomes of treatment. For example, a child diagnosed with a specific language impairment may have been enrolled in speech therapy. The child may have received various probe measures (e.g., phonological processing, working memory) during the therapy sessions that showed no or minimal improvement. After the child is diagnosed as having an APD, he or she may receive training to address the specific APD and may show marked improvement on the previously obtained probe measures. Another example is when the impact of a deficit is apparent before the specific APD is diagnosed. Thus, before the deficit is diagnosed and addressed, the child may show poor academic achievements for a relatively long period. After the APD is addressed, immediate and marked improvement in academics is noted. An example of using available data for determining the effectiveness of treatment is shown in ▶ Table 12.1.

12.6.2 McNemar's Test of Correlated Proportions

When outcome data are obtained on several different measures, as shown in ▶ Table 12.1, the data can be analyzed using McNemar's test of correlated proportions (McNemar, 1947). A table can be

Table 12.1 Hypothetical Examples of Outcomes Showing Improvement*

Baseline Measures	Intervention (4 Months)	Outcome Measures
Left ear deficit on dichotic listening tasks	Training to improve speech recognition in the left ear during dichotic listening tasks using speech stimuli within the linguistic abilities of the child. Test items included in the baseline dichotic task are not used during training.	Age-appropriate performance during dichotic listening in both ears
Receptive language skills similar to children 1 year younger	Usual language therapy offered before the diagnosis of APD continued with the addition of FM device use in noisy therapeutic conditions	Age-appropriate performance on receptive language skills
Academic: behind grade level in all subject areas	Use of FM device in classroom until reduction of dichotic listening deficit	Grade-level performance on standardized tests
Teacher concerns: appears to have difficulty processing information		Good ability to process information presented in the classroom
Parents' perception: poor understanding of speech in noisy conditions	Training to improve speech in noisy backgrounds under monaural, binaural, and spatial separation listening conditions	Some improvement in detecting speech in noise; however, in some situations, struggle is still apparent.

* In this case, improvement is apparent on several measures. There may be some scope for improvement in more noisy conditions. Thus, speech training in noise may continue by simulating the specific noisy environments reported by the parents of the patient.
Abbreviations: APD, auditory processing deficit; FM, frequency modulation.

Table 12.2 Creating a Table for Applying McNemar's Test of Correlated Proportions to Outcomes of a Single-Case Study

		After the Intervention		Total
		Score within age-appropriate norms	Scores below age-appropriate norms	
Prior to the intervention	Scores within age-appropriate norms	4	0	4
	Scores below age-appropriate norms	5	1	6
Total		9	1	10

created, similar to ▶ Table 12.2, and subjected to statistical analyses. Such analyses can allow clinicians to examine the significance of the treatment effect. The example in ▶ Table 12.2 assumes that a total of 10 measures (deficit and impact) were used before and after the training. Thus, data are available on 10 measures showing whether or not the patient's performance was within the normative range for his or her age. Scores were within age-appropriate norms for four of the measures prior to intervention and for nine of the 10 measures after the intervention. For this example, the probability of significance for a one-tailed test is .03, and that for a two-tailed test is .06. These results suggest that the training was effective in reducing the deficit and/or related impact. Criteria for the normative range can vary from standard scores, performance within 1 or 2 SDs of normative data, performance in the 10th or 25th percentile rank, and grade-equivalent scores, depending on the measures used.

12.6.3 Statistical Analyses for Multiple Measures of Single Outcomes

Other types of analyses have been suggested when repeated measurements are available for a single variable (e.g., Parker, Vannest, & Davis, 2011). Nonoverlap of all pairs (NAP) and improvement rate difference (IRD) are two examples.

Nonoverlap of All Pairs (NAP)

One accepted indicator of treatment effectiveness is the extent to which baseline and postintervention measures do not overlap. For example, the percentage of nonoverlapping data (PND) is defined as the percentage of postintervention data points that exceed the single highest data point during the baseline measures. PND has been suggested as an index of treatment effectiveness (Scruggs & Casto, 1987). NAP is an improved index based on this concept of nonoverlapping data.

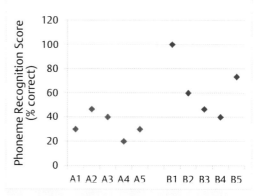

Fig. 12.14 Phoneme recognition scores in speech-shaped noise obtained prior to auditory training (A) and after training (B). These scores are based on the baseline data obtained before initiation and after termination of auditory training (last probe in ▶ Fig. 12.13). Within each phase, each data point is based on the scores obtained after presenting 5 words (15 phonemes) from one of the Northwestern University Auditory Test No. 6 (NU-6) word lists. Each list has a total of 25 words, yielding a total of 5 data points in each phase. The calculation of the nonoverlap of all pairs (NAP) index based on this data is shown in ▶ Table 12.3.

NAP is the percentage of nonoverlapping data points between the baseline and treatment phases. It attempts to determine the probability (0.5–1.0) of a score drawn at random from a treatment phase exceeding a score drawn at random from a baseline phase. In this case, the term *nonoverlap* means the score after treatment exceeds the score obtained during the baseline phase or that there was no overlap between the scores during the baseline and treatment phases.

Five sets of phoneme recognition scores across pre-and post- auditory training sessions are displayed in ▶ Fig. 12.14 and are shown in ▶ Table 12.3 as preliminary preparation for the calculation of the NAP index. The NAP index is calculated as the number of comparison pairs showing no overlap divided by the total number of

Table 12.3 Matrix for Determining Nonoverlap of All Pair Based on Phoneme Recognition Score Data

		B1	B2	B3	B4	B5	Number of overlapping Pairs
	Score (% correct)	100	60	46.67	40	73.33	
A1	30	+	+	+	+	+	0
A2	46.67	+	+	Tie	-	+	1.5
A3	40	+	+	+	Tie	+	0.5
A4	20	+	+	+	+	+	0
A5	30	+	+	+	+	+	0
Total overlapping pairs							2

A=Baseline scores; B=post-intervention scores.

pairs compared. Based on expert visual judgments of 200 datasets from single-case studies, the treatment effects with the NAP index can be tentatively interpreted as follows. If the NAP index is within 0.50 to 0.65, the treatment effect is considered weak. If the index is within 0.66 to 0.92, the effect is considered moderate. If the index is within 0.93 to 1.00, the effect is considered strong (Parker & Vannest, 2009). To determine the significance of the findings, the data in ▶ Table 12.3 were subjected to Kendall Rank Correlation analyses (http://www.wessa.net/rwasp_kendall.wasp/; Wessa, 2012), as suggested by Parker, Vannest, and Davis (2011). The data were entered as X (A=baseline phase) and Y (B=treatment phase) variables after rank ordering the values. The analyses yielded a significance value of $p = .043$, which suggests a significant treatment effect.

When a data point in the treatment phase (B) in ▶ Table 12.3 exceeds that in the baseline phase (A), the comparison is marked as + and is considered a nonoverlap. In this case, the data following treatment (phase B) exceed the data obtained during the baseline (phase A) for all paired comparisons except A2 versus B3 (tie), A2 versus B4 (decrease in score marked as −), and A3 versus B4 (tie). A2 versus B4 is considered one overlapping pair, while each tie is considered a half overlapping pair.

Total pairs compared in this example = 25 (5 baseline phase data points multiplied by 5 post-treatment phase data points)

Number of overlapping pairs = 2

Number of nonoverlapping pairs = total pairs − overlapping pairs = 25 − 2 = 23

NAP index = number of nonoverlapping pairs/total pairs = 23/25 = 0.92, or 92%

As mentioned previously, NAP indices of 0.66 to 0.92 suggest medium treatment effects (Parker &

Vannest, 2009). Thus, the current data suggest a medium effect of auditory training on phoneme recognition scores in noise. Note that the training was terminated before the listener showed a plateau in performance. With further training, a larger treatment effect may have occurred.

Improvement Rate Difference

Assume that a clinician obtained five ABR waveforms by averaging 1000 clicks presented at the rate of 30/s and determined the I to V interpeak latency for each of the waveforms. She then provided treatment to improve processing speed, including the use of frequency modulation (FM) devices and auditory training using both nonspeech and speech stimuli. At the end of the treatment, she again obtained five ABRs waveforms. The hypothetical data are shown in ▶ Fig. 12.15.

Improvement Rate

The improvement rate for each phase (baseline and treatment) is the improved data points divided by the total data points in that phase.

Improved Data Point in the Baseline Phase

An improved data point in the baseline phase is any data point that equals or shows better response than any data point in the treatment phase. In this case, the second data point in the baseline phase shows shorter latency (4.2 ms) than the third data point (4.25 ms) obtained following treatment. Thus, the improvement rate in the baseline phase is 1/5, or 0.20, as there are a total of five data points in the baseline phase.

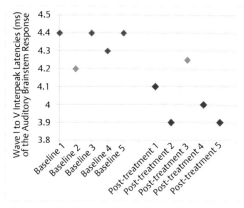

Fig. 12.15 Illustration of the procedure to determine the effect of treatment for improving processing speed using hypothetical data for waves I to V interpeak latencies of the auditory brainstem response (ABR) obtained using clicks presented at the rate of 30/s. It is assumed that ABRs were recorded five times prior to and five times after the treatment on a single subject.

Improved Data Point in the Treatment Phase

An improved data point in the treatment phase is any point that exceeds all data points in the baseline phase. In this case. Four data points in the treatment phase show shorter inter-peak latencies than all of the data points in the baseline phase. Thus, the improvement rate in the treatment phase is 4/5, or 0.80, as there are a total of five data points in the treatment phase.

Calculating the Improvement Rate Difference

IRD is the difference between the two improvement rates. In this case, the difference is 0.80 − 0.20 = 0.60, or 60%. Thus, the improvement that occurred following treatment is above the chance level of 50%. Confidence intervals around the IRD can also be determined (Parker et al., 2009). The chance level performance for the IRD statistics is very likely to be less than 50% and is expected to decrease with an increase in the number of data points recorded before and after intervention.

12.7 Sharing Single-Case Research

Many journals publish single-case research, and many conferences allow presentations of single-case

research in podium or poster formats. Clinicians are encouraged to share the outcomes of their intervention with other professionals. Single-case research can be pooled together for meta-analyses, and statistical procedures are available for pooling the data (Manolov & Solanas, 2013).

12.8 Future Trends

Single-patient trials are likely to be widely accepted by both patients and clinicians. Personalized clinical application of single-patient trials may improve in the future as a result of improvements in methodologies for the precise assessment of outcomes in such trials. With such improvements, single-patient trials have the potential to make strong contributions to comparative effectiveness research and patient-centered outcomes research. By allowing direct estimation of individual treatment effects, single-case trials can facilitate finely individualized intervention, enhance therapeutic efficiency, improve patient outcomes, and reduce costs that are involved in conducting RCTs (Duan, Kravitz, & Schmid, 2013).

12.9 Review Questions

1. Compare the terms *efficacy, effectiveness,* and *efficiency* with reference to intervention.
2. Discuss the key aspects of evidence-based practice.
3. Describe five steps involved in evidence-based practice.
4. Describe and compare different types and levels of external evidence for clinical practice.
5. What should you consider in appraising the available external evidence? Appraise the evidence provided in the following study: Hornickel, J., Zecker, S. G., Bradlow, A. R., & Kraus, N. (2012). Assistive listening devices drive neuroplasticity in children with dyslexia. *Proceedings of the National Academy of Sciences of the United States of America, 109*(41), 16731–16736.
6. Discuss the potential limitations of evidence generated in randomized controlled trials.
7. Minimally, how many data points should be collected during the pre- and post-training phases to generate high-quality, single-case research?
8. Which data features can be used in evaluating the effects of treatment in single-case research? Provide examples of outcomes that have been presented in single-case research related to auditory processing deficits.

9. Discuss the relevance of statistical significance for single-case research. Discuss McNemar's test of correlated proportions. What types of statistical analyses are possible when multiple measures are available for a single outcome?

10. Discuss future trends related to treatment effectiveness research.

References

[1] Berard, G. (1993). Hearing equals behavior. New Canaan, CT: Keats Publishing.

[2] Bradlow, A. R., Akahane-Yamada, R., Pisoni, D. B., & Tohkura, Y. (1999). Training Japanese listeners to identify English /r/ and /l/: Long-term retention of learning in perception and production. Perception and Psychophysics, 61(5), 977–985.

[3] Brouns, K., El Refaie, A., & Pryce, H. (2011). Auditory training and adult rehabilitation: A critical review of the evidence. Global Journal of Health Science, 3(1), 49–63.

[4] Concato, J. (2013). Study design and "evidence" in patient-oriented research. American Journal of Respiratory and Critical Care Medicine, 187(11), 1167–1172.

[5] Concato, J., Lawler, E. V., Lew, R. A., Gaziano, J. M., Aslan, M., & Huang, G. D. (2010). Observational methods in comparative effectiveness research. American Journal of Medicine, 123(12, Suppl. 1), e16–e23.

[6] Dlouha, O., Novak, A., & Vokral, J. (2007). Central auditory processing disorder (CAPD) in children with specific language impairment (SLI): Central auditory tests. International Journal of Pediatric Otorhinolaryngology, 71(6), 903-907.

[7] Duan, N., Kravitz, R. L., & Schmid, C. H. (2013). Single-patient (N-of-1) trials: A pragmatic clinical decision methodology for patient-centered comparative effectiveness research. Journal of Clinical Epidemiology, 66(8, Suppl.), S21–S28.

[8] Gabler, N. B., Duan, N., Vohra, S., & Kravitz, R. L. (2011). N-of-1 trials in the medical literature: A systematic review. Medical Care, 49(8), 761–768.

[9] Greenfield, S., Kravitz, R., Duan, N., & Kaplan, S. H. (2007). Heterogeneity of treatment effects: Implications for guidelines, payment, and quality assessment. American Journal of Medicine, 120(4, Suppl. 1), S3–S9.

[10] Haynes, B. (1999). Can it work? Does it work? Is it worth it? The testing of healthcare interventions is evolving. BMJ, 319 (7211), 652–653.

[11] Huyck, J. J., & Wright, B. A. (2013). Learning, worsening, and generalization in response to auditory perceptual training during adolescence. Journal of the Acoustical Society of America, 134(2), 1172–1182.

[12] Juurlink, D. N., Mamdani, M. M., Lee, D. S., et al. (2004). Rates of hyperkalemia after publication of the Randomized Aldactone Evaluation Study. New England Journal of Medicine, 351(6), 543–551.

[13] Kratochwill, T. R., Hitchcock, J., Horner, R. H., et al. (2010). Single-case designs technical documentation. Retrieved from http://ies.ed.gov/ncee/wwc/pdf/wwc_scd.pdf.

[14] Krishnamurti, S., Forrester, J., Rutledge, C., & Holmes, G. W. (2013). A case study of the changes in the speech-evoked auditory brainstem response associated with auditory training in children with auditory processing disorders. International Journal of Pediatric Otorhinolaryngology, 77(4), 594–604.

[15] LeLorier J., Grégoire, G., Benhaddad, A., Lapierre, J., & Derderian, F. (1997). Discrepancies between meta-analyses and subsequent large randomized, controlled trials. New England Journal of Medicine, 337(8), 536–542.

[16] Manolov, R., & Solanas, A. (2013). Assigning and combining probabilities in single-case studies: A second study. Behavior Research Methods, 45(4), 1024–1035.

[17] Manolov, R., Solanas, A., Sierra, V., & Evans, J. J. (2011). Choosing among techniques for quantifying single-case intervention effectiveness. Behavior Therapy, 42(3), 533–545.

[18] Marley, J. (2000). Efficacy, effectiveness, efficiency. Australian Prescriber, 23(6), 114–115.

[19] McNemar, Q. (1947). Note on the sampling error of the difference between correlated proportions or percentages. Psychometrika, 12(2), 153–157.

[20] Miller, C. A., Uhring, E. A., Brown, J. J. C., Kowalski, E. M., Roberts, B., & Schaefer, B. A. (2005). Case studies of auditory training for children with auditory processing difficulties: A preliminary analysis. Contemporary Issues in Communication Science and Disorders, 32, 93–107.

[21] Parker, R. I., & Vannest, K. (2009). An improved effect size for single-case research: Nonoverlap of all pairs. Behavior Therapy, 40(4), 357–367.

[22] Parker, R. I., Vannest, K. J., & Davis, J. L. (2011). Effect size in single-case research: A review of nine nonoverlap techniques. Behavior Modification, 35(4), 303–322.

[23] Parker, R. I., Vannest, K. J., & Brown, L. (2009). The improvement rate difference for single-case research. Exceptional Children, 75(2), 135–150.

[24] Sackett, D. L., Rosenberg, W. M., Gray, J. A., Haynes, R. B., & Richardson, W. S. (1996). Evidence based medicine: What it is and what it isn't. BMJ, 312(7023), 71–72.

[25] Scruggs, M., & Casto, B. (1987). The quantitative synthesis of single-subject research. Remedial and Special Education, 8, 24–33.

[26] Sinha, Y., Silove, N., Hayen, A., & Williams, K. (2011). Auditory integration training and other sound therapies for autism spectrum disorders (ASD). Cochrane Database of Systematic Reviews, 12, CD003681.

[27] Sweetow, R. W., & Sabes, J. H. (2006). The need for and development of an adaptive Listening and Communication Enhancement (LACE) program. Journal of theAmerican Academy of Audiology, 17(8), 538–558.

[28] Tillery, K. L. (1998). Central auditory processing assessment and therapeutic strategies for children with attention deficit hyperactivity disorder. In M. G. Masters, N. A. Stecker, & J. Katz (Eds.), Central auditory processing disorders: Mostly management (pp. 175–194). Boston: Allyn & Bacon.

[29] Tsimberidou, A.-M., Braiteh, F., Stewart, D. J., & Kurzrock, R. (2009). Ultimate fate of oncology drugs approved by the US Food and Drug Administration without a randomized trial. Journal of Clinical Oncology, 27(36), 6243–6250.

[30] Weihing, J., & Musiek, F. E. (2013). Dichotic Interaural Intensity Difference (DIID) training. In D. Geffner & D. Ross-Swain (Eds.), Auditory processing disorders: Assessment, management, and treatment (pp. 447–468). San Diego, CA: Plural Publishing.

[31] Wessa, P. (2012). Kendall tau rank correlation (v1.0.11). In Free Statistics Software (v1.1.23-r7), Office for Research Development and Education. Retrieved from http://www.wessa.net/rwasp_kendall.wasp.

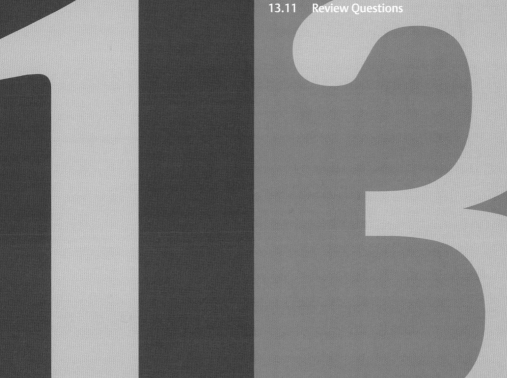

Chapter 13

Attention Deficit Hyperactivity Disorder and Auditory Processing Deficits

13 Attention Deficit Hyperactivity Disorder and Auditory Processing Deficits

Auditory processing disorders (APDs) and attention deficit hyperactivity disorder (ADHD) can co-occur in some children. In some cases, children with APD can appear to have ADHD due to overlapping symptoms such as difficulty following oral instructions. This chapter includes a description of ADHD, possible reasons for co-occurrence of ADHD and APD, auditory processing test results in individuals with ADHD, and strategies for diagnosing and treating children with comorbid ADHD and APD.

ADHD is characterized by inattention and/or hyperactivity and impulsive behaviors that cannot be better explained by any other mental disorders. The symptoms associated with the disorder are listed in ▶ Tables 13.1, ▶ 13.2, ▶ 13.3, and ▶ 13.4. The disorder is considered mostly of the inattention type if, in addition to the presence of at least six of the symptoms for inattention in ▶ Table 13.1, no more than five of the symptoms for hyperactivity or impulsivity in Table 13.3 are apparent. It is considered to be of the predominantly hyperactive/impulsive type if six or more symptoms for hyperactivity/impulsivity are apparent, and less than six of the symptoms for inattention are apparent. If the criteria for both inattention and hyperactivity/impulsivity are met with six or more symptoms in each category, the disorder is considered to be of the combined type. The various presentations of the disorder are shown in ▶ Table 13.5. When full criteria were previously met, but fewer than six symptoms in Table 1 or 2 are apparent for the previous six months with continuing negative impact on social, academic or occupational performance the disorder can be specified as being "in partial remission". (▶ Fig. 13.1) (American Psychiatric Association, 2013).

When there is demonstrable abnormality of attention, activity, and impulsivity at home and another setting, such as school, the term *hyperkinetic disorder* is used to discribe the condition (World Health Organization, WHO, 1992). According to the WHO, at least three of the inattention problems, three of the hyperactivity symptoms, and one of the impulsivity symptoms should be apparent at home to diagnose the disorder. In addition, at least two of the inattention symptoms and three of the hyperactivity symptoms should be apparent in the school or preschool setting.

Furthermore, these findings should be confirmed by evidence of abnormal inattention or hyperactivity by direct observation in the clinic or laboratory or by documentation of impaired performance on psychometric measures of attention (World Health Organization, WHO, 1992).

13.1 Prevalence

Parent reports suggest that ADHD was diagnosed in 8.2% of schoolchildren in the United States in 2007, corresponding to slightly more than 4 million cases (Larson, Russ, Kahn, & Halfon, 2011). Interestingly, higher rates of ADHD were noted among multiracial children (14.2%) compared to white (9.9%) and African American (10.1%) children in 2007. In the same year, high rates of ADHD were reported for children covered by Medicaid (13.6%) compared to those who had non-Medicaid health coverage (8.1%) (Centers for Disease Control and Prevention, CDC, 2010).

An older review of four U.S. studies and nine non-U.S. studies using the criteria from the fourth edition of the *Diagnostic and Statistical Manual of Mental Disorders* (*DSM-IV*) for diagnosing ADHD estimated the prevalence between 2.4 and 19.8%. The prevalence tended to vary depending on the assessment criteria and the study sample (Faraone, Sergeant, Gillberg, & Biederman, 2003). A more recent meta-analysis suggests that the prevalence using *DSM-IV* criteria is 5.9 to 7.1% in adolescents and adults when determined by either a best estimate diagnostic procedure or by parent or teacher ratings. Self-report measures by young adults suggest the prevalence to be slightly lower, at 5% (Willcutt, 2012).

13.2 Risk Factors

ADHD is most likely caused by an interaction of various genetic and environmental factors (▶ Fig. 13.2). In addition, increased exposure to environmental factors may modify gene function, as suggested by the increase in the incidence of disorders such as ADHD and autism (Latham, Sapienza, & Engel, 2012). However, because the predictive value of associated genes is small, clinical testing for susceptibility genes is not recommended

Table 13.1 Inattention Checklist Based on the *DSM-5* (American Psychiatric Association, 2013).

Inattention characterized by frequent occurrence of at least six or more of the following symptoms for at least 6 months	Circle the number that corresponds to the best description of the individual's behavior over the previous 6 months considering his/her developmental level.						
	Setting/Observer	Never	Rarely	Sometimes	Often	Always	Score
Fails to give close attention to details OR makes careless errors in schoolwork, at work, or during other activities	Home/parent or guardian	−2	−1	0	1	2	
	Outside home/teacher or parenting class instructor	−2	−1	0	1	2	
	Home, school, and/or work/self	−2	−1	0	1	2	
	Average score for this question						
Cannot sustain attention during tasks or play activities	Home/parent or guardian	−2	−1	0	1	2	
	Outside home/teacher or parenting class instructor	−2	−1	0	1	2	
	Home, school, and/or work/self	−2	−1	0	1	2	
	Average score for this question						
Avoids or appears reluctant to involve in activities that require sustained mental effort or dislikes such activities (e.g., homework)	Home/parent or guardian	−2	1	0	1	2	
	Outside home/teacher or parenting class instructor	−2	−1	0	1	2	
	Home, school, and/or work/self	−2	−1	0	1	2	
	Average score for this question						
Does not seem to listen when spoken to even without any obvious distractions	Home/parent or guardian	−2	−1	0	1	2	
	Outside home/teacher or parenting class instructor	−2	−1	0	1	2	
	Home, school, and/or work/self	−2	1	0	1	2	
	Average score for this question						
Easily distracted by extraneous stimuli and unrelated thoughts	Home/parent or guardian	−2	−1	0	1	2	
	Outside home/teacher or parenting class instructor	−2	−1	0	1	2	
	Home, school, and/or work/self	−2	−1	0	1	2	
	Average score for this question						
Does not follow through on instructions; failure to complete chores, schoolwork, or duties in the workplace	Home/parent or guardian	−2	−1	0	1	2	
	Outside home/teacher or parenting class instructor	−2	−1	0	1	2	
	Home, school, and/or work/self	−2	−1	0	1	2	
	Average score for this question						

Table 13.1 continued

Inattention characterized by frequent occurrence of at least six or more of the following symptoms for at least 6 months	Circle the number that corresponds to the best description of the individual's behavior over the previous 6 months considering his/her developmental level.						
	Setting/Observer	Never	Rarely	Sometimes	Often	Always	Score
Has organization difficulties	Home/parent or guardian	-2	-1	0	1	2	
	Outside home/teacher or parenting class instructor	-2	-1	0	1	2	
	Home, school, and/or work/self	-2	-1	0	1	2	
	Average score for this question						
Loses things required for tasks or activities (e.g., school supplies)	Home/parent or guardian	-2	-1	0	1	2	
	Outside home/teacher or parenting class instructor	-2	-1	0	1	2	
	Home, school, and/or work/self	-2	-1	0	1	2	
	Average score for this question						
Forgetful in daily activities (e.g., errands)	Home/parent or guardian	-2	-1	0	1	2	
	Outside home/teacher or parenting class instructor	-2	-1	0	1	2	
	Home, school, and/or work/self	-2	-1	0	1	2	
	Average score for this question						
Total score out of 18							
Do the assigned scores appear reliable?						Y	N
Is there an underreporting bias as indicated by more than 3 "never" responses? Even normal individuals are expected to sometimes show the above symptoms.						Y	N
Is there an overreporting bias as indicated by more than 3 "always" responses? Even ADHD individuals can occasionally perform well on many of the indicators.						Y	N
Is there too much discrepancy in the scores assigned by different observers? For example, one observer selects "sometimes" or "rarely," and another observer selects "often." Further questioning of the observers on the questions may allow the service providers to determine if one or the other observers is biased and is under- or overreporting on the indicator.						Y	N
What is the adjusted average score after correcting for underreporting or overreporting bias or discrepancies in observer ratings?							

From American Psychiatric Association (2013). Abbreviations: ADHD, attention deficit hyperactivity disorder; DSM-5, Diagnostic and Statistical Manual of Mental Disorders (5th ed.).

(National Collaborating Center for Mental Health, NCCMH, 2009).

Several biological factors that have a negative impact on pre- and postnatal brain development increase the risk of ADHD. A significant prenatal risk factor is smoking during pregnancy (Sciberras, Ukoumunne, &Efron, 2011). Prenatal tobacco exposure may account for approximately 270,000 excess cases of ADHD in the United States (Braun, Kahn, Froehlich, Auinger, & Lanphear, 2006). ADHD symptoms are associated with both maternal and paternal smoking during pregnancy. Paternal smoking in the absence of maternal smoking is also associated with ADHD in the offspring

Table 13.2 Evaluating the Presence of Inattention

Carefully consider the following questions to evaluate inattention presentation.	Yes	No
1. Does the individual have a score of 1 or 2 from each of the observers on at least 6 of the questions listed in Table 13.1?		
2. Is there clear evidence that the symptoms have a negative impact on social or academic/occupational function?		
3. Were several of the symptoms present before the age of 12 years?		
4. Are any of the symptoms apparent exclusively during the course of schizophrenia or another psychotic disorder or are accounted better by another mental disorder (e.g., mood disorder, anxiety disorder, dissociative disorder, or a personality disorder)?		
If the answers to questions 1 to 3 are yes, and the answer to question 4 is no, the deficit is confirmed.		

(Langley, Heron, Smith, & Thapar, 2012), which may be related to the effect of passive smoking by the mother. In addition, maternal smoking appears to be associated with a severe form of ADHD with severe symptoms and poorer neuropsychological performance (Thakur et al., 2013).

Perinatal factors such as prematurity (birth before 37 weeks of gestation) are associated with ADHD (Chu et al., 2012), especially when coupled with medically induced delivery due to placental complications, including obstruction and decreased maternal spiral artery conversion (Talge et al., 2012). Extreme prematurity with birth prior to 28 weeks of gestation is associated with a 5-fold increased risk of ADHD (Halmøy, Klungsøyr, Skjærven, & Haavik, 2012). In addition, birth weight under 2500 g (5.5 lb) is associated with attention deficits (Chu et al., 2012; Halmøy et al., 2012). Five-minute Apgar scores lower than 4 and 7 are associated with 2.8- and 1.5-fold increased risks of ADHD, respectively (Halmøy et al., 2012).

An important postnatal risk factor for ADHD is exposure to lead (Braun et al., 2006). Lead is sometimes present in older plumbing fixtures and paint in older buildings. Exposure is possible through lead-contaminated soil, folk remedies, cooking in imported pottery painted with lead-containing paint or glaze, toys, and dust (Arizona Department of Health Services, 2003; U.S. Environmental Protection Agency, 2006). For example, Greta and Azarcon (also known as alarcon, coral, luiga, maria luisa, or rueda) are Hispanic remedies given for an upset stomach (empacho), constipation, diarrhea, and vomiting and to teething babies. The lead content of Greta and Azarcon can be as high as 90%. Ghasard, an Indian folk medicine, is used as a tonic and contains lead. Ba-baw-san, a Chinese herbal remedy used to treat colic pain or to pacify young children contains lead. Daw Tway, used as a

digestive aid in Thailand and Myanmar (Burma) contains as much as 970 parts per million (ppm) of lead. The paints used to paint some of the toys can contain lead. Another source of lead exposure is lead pellets used in game hunting (Lévesque et al., 2003). The association between ADHD and lead is apparent at relatively low blood lead levels between 1.6 and 2.7 µg/dL (Boucher et al., 2012). Children exposed to lead are also at higher risk for delinquency probably due to the direct negative impact on brain development and neuronal function but also due to impaired cognitive abilities and the failure to achieve academic goals (Needleman, McFarland, Ness, Fienberg, & Tobin, 2002).

Other risk factors are traumatic brain injury (Gerring et al., 1998); epilepsy and some genetic conditions, such as neurofibromatosis type 1 (Mautner et al., 2002); and syndromes such as fragile X (Hagerman, Murphy, & Wittenberger, 1988), Angelman, Prader-Willi, Smith-Magenis, and velocardiofacial syndromes. Among epileptic children with well-controlled seizures and no intellectual disability, ADHD occurrence is similar to that seen in the general population (Kim et al., 2012). Early psychosocial adversity also increases the risk of ADHD. For example, early deprivation of 6 or more months due to institutional raring is associated with ADHD, possibly because of adverse neurodevelopmental programming during critical developmental periods (Stevens, Sonuga-Barke, et al., 2008). Another possible reason is a failure to acquire cognitive and emotional control (NCCMH, 2009).

13.3 Knowledge Competencies for Professionals

A child suspected of ADHD may be seen initially by general practitioners or by other primary care,

Table 13.3 Hyperactivity/Impulsivity ADHD Checklist Based on *DSM-5*

Hyperactivity/impulsivity characterized by frequent occurrence of at least six or more of the following symptoms for at least 6 months	Circle the number that corresponds to the best description of the individual's behavior over the previous 6 months considering his/her developmental level.						
	Setting/Observer	Never	Rarely	Sometimes	Often	Always	Score
Squirms in seat or fidgets with or taps hands or feet	Home/parent or guardian	−2	−1	0	1	2	
	Outside home/teacher or parenting class instructor	−2	−1	0	1	2	
	Home, school, and/or work/self	−2	−1	0	1	2	
	Average score for this question						
Cannot remain seated when expected	Home/parent or guardian	−2	−1	0	1	2	
	Outside home/teacher or parenting class instructor	−2	−1	0	1	2	
	Home, school, and/or work/self	−2	−1	0	1	2	
	Average score for this question						
Runs about or climbs inappropriately	Home/parent or guardian	−2	−1	0	1	2	
	Outside home/teacher or parenting class instructor	−2	−1	0	1	2	
	Home, school, and/or work/self	−2	−1	0	1	2	
	Average score for this question						
Unable to play or engage in leisure activities quietly	Home/parent or guardian	−2	−1	0	1	2	
	Outside home/teacher or parenting class instructor	−2	−1	0	1	2	
	Home, school, and/or work/self	−2	−1	0	1	2	
	Average score for this question						
Moves or acts as if driven by a motor	Home/parent or guardian	−2	−1	0	1	2	
	Outside home/teacher or parenting class instructor	−2	−1	0	1	2	
	Home, school, and/or work/self	−2	−1	0	1	2	
	Average score for this question						
Talks excessively	Home/parent or guardian	−2	−1	0	1	2	
	Outside home/teacher or parenting class instructor	−2	−1	0	1	2	
	Home, school, and/or work/self	−2	−1	0	1	2	
	Average score for this question						

Table 13.3 continued

Hyperactivity/impulsivity characterized by frequent occurrence of at least six or more of the following symptoms for at least 6 months	Circle the number that corresponds to the best description of the individual's behavior over the previous 6 months considering his/her developmental level.						
	Setting/Observer	Never	Rarely	Sometimes	Often	Always	Score
Blurts out a response before the completion of a question	Home/parent or guardian	−2	−1	0	1	2	
	Outside home/teacher or parenting class instructor	−2	−1	0	1	2	
	Home, school, and/or work/self	−2	−1	0	1	2	
	Average score for this question						
Has difficulty waiting his or her turn (e.g., while waiting in line)	Home/parent or guardian	−2	−1	0	1	2	
	Outside home/teacher or parenting class instructor	−2	−1	0	1	2	
	Home, school, and/or work/self	−2	−1	0	1	2	
	Average score for this question						
Interrupts or intrudes on others	Home/parent or guardian	−2	−1	0	1	2	
	Outside home/teacher or parenting class instructor	−2	−1	0	1	2	
	Home, school, and/or work/self						
	Average score for this question						

Total inattention score out of 18	
Do the assigned scores appear reliable?	
Is there an underreporting bias as indicated by more than 3 "never" responses? Even normal individuals are expected to sometimes show the above symptoms.	
Is there an overreporting bias as indicated by more than 3 "always" responses? Even ADHD individuals can occasionally perform well on many of the indicators.	
Is there too much discrepancy in the scores assigned by different observers? For example, one observer selects "sometimes" or "rarely" and another observer selects "often". Further questioning of the observers on the questions may allow the service provider to determine if one or the other observers is biased and is under- or over-reporting on the indicator.	
What is the adjusted score after correcting for underreporting or overreporting bias or discrepancies in observer ratings?	

Abbreviations: ADHD, attention deficit hyperactivity disorder; DSM-5, Diagnostic and Statistical Manual of Mental Disorders (5th ed.).

education, or social work professionals, including teachers, speech-language pathologists, and audiologists. The goals of screening at this tier 1 stage are to answer the following questions (Scottish Intercollegiate Guidelines Network, SIGN, 2009):

1. Are the symptoms consistent with the diagnostic criteria for any of the types of ADHD?
2. If the answer to question 1 is yes, then how severe is the problem, considering the negative impact on family, social, and/or educational domains?

Table 13.4 Evaluation of the Presence of Hyperactivity/Impulsivity

Carefully consider following questions to evaluate "hyperactivity-impulsivity" presentation.	Yes	No
1. Does the individual have a score of 1 or 2 from each of the observers on at least 6 of the questions listed in Table 13.3?		
2. Is there clear evidence that the symptoms have a negative impact on social or academic/occupational function?		
3. Were several of the symptoms present before the age of 12 years?		
4. Are any of the symptoms apparent exclusively during the course of schizophrenia or another psychotic disorder or are accounted better by another mental disorder (e.g., mood disorder, anxiety disorder, dissociative disorder, or a personality disorder)?		
If the answers to questions 1 to 3 are yes, and the answer to question 4 is no, the deficit is confirmed.		

Table 13.5 Different Presentations of ADHD

Adjusted Hyperactivity/Impulsivity Score from Table 13.4, Last Row	Adjusted Inattention Score from Table 13.2, Last Row	Presentation
6 or more	6 or more	Combined ADHD
5 or less	6 or more	Predominantly inattentive presentation
6 or more	5 or less	Predominantly hyperactive/impulsive

Abbreviation: ADHD, attention deficit hyperactivity disorder.

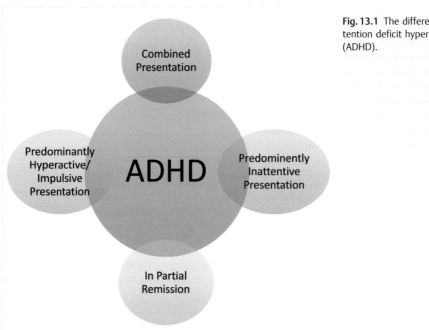

Fig. 13.1 The different types of attention deficit hyperactivity disorder (ADHD).

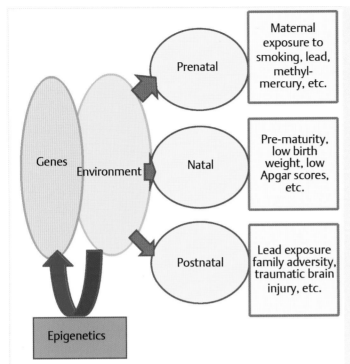

Fig. 13.2 Risk factors for attention deficit hyperactivity disorder (ADHD).

Prenatal — Maternal exposure to smoking, lead, methyl-mercury, etc.

Natal — Pre-maturity, low birth weight, low Apgar scores, etc.

Postnatal — Lead exposure family adversity, traumatic brain injury, etc.

Genes — Environment

Epigenetics

If preliminary screening suggests the possibility of ADHD with significant impairment, the individual should be referred for a more comprehensive assessment (SIGN, 2009). The knowledge competencies required for tier 1 professionals are as follows (NCCMH, 2009):

1. Knowledge of the three core symptoms of ADHD, including inattention, hyperactivity, and impulsivity
2. Knowledge that the core symptoms need to have been present before the age of 12 years
3. Recognition that direct observation of a child/ young adult for a short time in a clinical setting may not always reveal obvious features of ADHD
4. Knowledge that symptoms should occur in all environments even though related impairment may not be apparent in all settings
5. Knowledge of symptom checklists for parents, children, or teachers that can be helpful in determining the need for further referral when used in association with clinical assessment
6. Awareness of comorbid conditions
7. Ability to consider family circumstances because recent changes in behavior can occur as a result of family issues, such as loss of employment and divorce

8. Awareness of the individual's developmental and medical history, including hearing or sleep problems

With respect to the last knowledge competency in the above list, the SIGN (2009) guidelines note that hearing should be assessed and formally tested if indicated as part of the clinical examination for ADHD. Some psychologists have suggested that a diagnosis of ADHD should not be made without ruling out the possibility that the individual may be inattentive due to the presence of an auditory processing deficit (APD; Keller, 1992). Others have suggested that individuals with ADHD who do not respond adequately to medications may actually have APDs (Bailey, 2010).

Audiologists who are attempting to perform evaluations for individuals suspected of APDs may come across some who either have been diagnosed with ADHD or are suspected of having the disorder. There are three reasons for this:

- Comorbidity: Patients may have ADHD in addition to APDs. This may be especially true for children with ADHD who are suspected of having language or learning disorders.
- Individuals with APDs may have difficulty attending to stimuli over a longer period and thus may seem inattentive.

- Individuals with ADHD may often say "Huh?" or "What did you say?," thus giving the impression of difficulty in processing auditory stimuli.

A sufficient knowledge base will allow audiologists to differentiate between ADHD and APD and minimize the adverse effects of any comorbid ADHD on APD test and treatment outcomes. With such a knowledge base, audiologists will be able to fully participate in team efforts in providing high-quality services to children affected by both APD and ADHD.

The SIGN (2009) guidelines note that the history and examination of an individual with ADHD may suggest the need for further ancillary assessments to rule out other disorders or to identify comorbid disorders. Detailed speech and language assessment may be recommended as part of the ancillary assessment. The American Speech-Language-Hearing Association has noted that, in addition to providing assessment and intervention services for children with ADHD and comorbid language disorders, a speech-language pathologist can assist multidisciplinary teams in observing pre- and postmedication behaviors, changing the classroom environment, improving communication in social situations, and enhancing study skills.

13.4 Diagnoses

The diagnostic evaluation of ADHD includes collecting information from parents and schools and, for adolescents and adults, from self-reports. Two components are necessary for making the diagnosis. The first is the documentation of age-inappropriate levels of inattentive, hyperactive, and/or impulsive behaviors. The second is the presence of significant clinical and psychosocial impairments in two or more settings. The level of impairment can be estimated by using a global adjustment scale, such as the Children's Global Assessment Scale (CGAS; Shaffer et al., 1983), and using a predetermined score, such as less than 60, on the scale (NCCMH, 2009).

Several pieces of information should be collected from parents or guardians. A case history can be useful for this purpose. A sample case history form is included in the appendix of Chapter 4.

13.4.1 Information from the Family

It is important to note the age of onset and any changes in symptoms over time, in addition to chief concerns. Family history is important because the siblings and/or parents of a child with ADHD can also have ADHD, which requires special management strategies. The past medical history can reveal any need for evaluation of comorbid disorders. Parents can be requested to release the medical history from relevant medical settings.

Prenatal history can reveal smoking by the mother during pregnancy. In addition, hypertensive disorders during pregnancy should be noted given that these can lead to premature delivery and associated attention deficits (Talge et al., 2012). History related to other potential risk factors, including alcohol or drug (e.g., opium) consumption during pregnancy and maternal depression, should be noted.

Postnatal history should include questions related to exposure to lead. Other significant elements are a history of delayed milestones, including language delays in isolation or with other delays, such as acquisition of fine motor and adaptive social skills (Venkatesh, Ravikumar, Andal, & Virudhagirinathan, 2012).

The psychosocial history can allow the assessment of impact of ADHD on psychosocial functioning. Parents should be asked to complete a validated ADHD instrument to document the presentation of related symptoms in the home setting. They also should be asked to report the child's strengths and weaknesses. Family dynamics should be assessed to note any issues such as divorce or poverty due to loss of employment that can negatively impact a child's behavior. Clinicians should note whether parental reports of a child's poor behavior are possibly associated with maternal depression resulting in the mother's reduced ability to interact positively with the child (Kiernan & Huerta, 2008). Excessively anxious and stress-reactive parents, including fathers, appear to be vulnerable to significant distress and impairment in the face of daily exposure to behavior problems shown by their children (Kashdan et al., 2004). Parents should be requested to report on school performance and to release relevant information from school and other settings (sports programs, music/dance classes, etc.).

13.4.2 Information from Schools and Important Community Informants

Following parent and/or patient consent/assent, teachers should be asked about any concerns they may have about a child who is being evaluated and should be requested to complete a validated ADHD instrument. Teachers and community informants can report on how well the child functions in academic or work settings and the extent and quality of his or her social interactions. Academic records covering performance on psychoeducational evaluations, standardized tests, and oral evaluations can provide valuable information about the function of the child in basic areas such as reading, spelling, and mathematics. Teachers can provide qualitative information about underachievement, learning style, attention span, work efficiency, impulsivity, and self-confidence. For example, a child just barely making passing grades may have done so as a result of grade inflation due to curving or addition of bonus points for mere attendance. Any administrative records related to disciplinary actions should also be carefully evaluated.

13.4.3 Information from the Patient

Clinicians can obtain valuable information from the patient while at the same time observing his or her behavior directly. A child may behave very well during a short session and not reveal any symptoms related to ADHD. Thus, direct observations in a clinical setting cannot be used to rule out ADHD. However, in some severe cases, direct observations can reveal hyperactivity and impulsivity, allowing direct confirmation of the deficit. Depending on their age, patients can be asked about any concerns they have about their behaviors, family relationships, peers (bullying), and schools. Their own perception of their educational performance and psychosocial function should be evaluated. They should be requested to specify both strengths and weaknesses in each area. Physicians usually are expected to perform physical and neurologic examinations to evaluate or rule out any comorbid disorders.

Adolescents and adults can be requested to complete a validated self-report instrument of ADHD.

13.4.4 Documenting Symptoms through Rating Scales

For all individuals, criteria listed in ▸ Table 13.1, ▸ Table 13.2, Table 13.3 and ▸ Table 13.4 can be used in deciding the presence of ADHD-related deficits. Several scales are available for evaluation.

Standardized rating scales can be used that appear to have fair reliability and validity, but the normative samples may not be representative of the United States or other countries. Thus, generalization of the standardization data to lower socioeconomic groups and individuals of different ethnicities, including Asians and Hispanics, should be made with caution (McGoey, DuPaul, Haley, & Shelton, 2007).

An example of a scale for preschoolers is the ADHD Rating Scale IV, Preschool Version. On this 18-item questionnaire, respondents rate each item on a Likert scale of 0 (not at all) to 3 (very often). The items are based on ADHD symptoms listed in the text revision of the *DSM-IV* (American Psychiatric Association, 2000). During the development of the scale, examples appropriate for the developmental level of preschool children were included. The scale was then reviewed by a panel of experts in early childhood development and assessment, preschool teachers, and parents of preschool children. Based on the panel's recommendations, the scale was modified and pilot tested to ensure clarity and readability in a clinic experienced in assessing behavior problems in preschool children. The scale yields scores for inattentive, hyperactive/impulsive, and total subscales. Two examples of items from this rating scale are "Does not seem to listen when spoken to directly (tunes you out)" and "Does not follow through on instructions and fails to finish tasks (i.e., 'Go upstairs, get your shoes, and socks')." Future research on the scale is recommended to explore the effect of ethnicity, disability, and gender on teacher and parent ratings and to determine its discriminant validity and clinical utility (McGoey et al., 2007).

A review (Taylor, Deb, & Unwin, 2011) of 14 scales used for identifying adults with ADHD noted that the Conners' Adult ADHD Rating Scale (CAARS; Conners, Erhardt, & Sparrow, 1999) and the short version of the Wender Utah Rating Scale (WURS; Ward, Wender, & Reimherr, 1993) have the best psychometric properties (e.g., internal consistency, test–retest reliability, sensitivity, and specificity) and have been widely studied. However, several of the studies were considered to be of poor quality.

The short version of the CAARS has 26 items and takes about 10 minutes to complete. The generated report provides information about the patient's score, how the results compare with other adults, and the specific subscales that show elevated scores. The subscales include inattention/memory problems, hyperactivity/restlessness, impulsivity/emotional lability, and problems with self-concept. An overall ADHD index and inconsistency index scores are also computed to rule out or to indicate the presence of ADHD.

The WURS short version includes 25 items that were found to be associated with ADHD. The patient rates a sentence that begins with "As a child, I had…" and ends with one of the symptom choices, such as "concentration problems." The rating scale ranges from not at all or very slightly (0) to very much (4). Thus, the score for each item varies from 0 to 4, and the total score for the scale varies from 0 to 100. A score higher than 46 is associated with the presence of ADHD in the absence of depression; a score higher than 36 is associated with ADHD and comorbid depression.

Further research on the CAARS and WURS scales is necessary (Taylor et al., 2011). A study completed on the Finnish translation of the WURS concluded that three of out of the five domains of WURS—Conduct Problems, Impulsivity Problems, Mood Difficulties, Inattention/Anxiety, Academic Concerns—are reliable indicators of ADHD. In one study, individuals with ADHD and dyslexia did not show differences on the mood difficulties and academic concerns domains (Kivisaari, Laasonen, Leppämäki, Tani, & Hokkanen, 2012).

An online version of the WHO Adult ADHD self-report scale (ASRS v1.1) is available (http://psychology-tools.com/adult-adhd-self-report-scale/). The ASRS v1.1 may also be useful for adolescents (ages 13 to 17 years) with high internal consistency (Adler et al., 2012), but further studies are necessary to confirm these findings.

Although rating scales can be useful in assisting with the diagnosis, ADHD should not be diagnosed based on rating scales alone. The findings of the entire test battery should be considered (NCCMH, 2009). Studies show that self-report rating scales do not allow the detection of feigned ADHD (Tucha, Sontag, Walitza, & Lange, 2009). There is substantial need for developing measures specifically for detecting malingered ADHD (Musso & Gouvier, 2012).

13.4.5 Careful Consideration of Developmental Level

In making observations, each child's developmental level should be considered, and the child's behavior should be assessed with careful consideration of the behaviors of normal age-matched peers. For example, a young normal child may seem inattentive due to limited ability to attend to a task, but this ability improves over time.

Similarly, a preschool child may appear hyperactive as a result of a constant need to move around and increased demands on caregivers.

If the child's developmental level is not carefully considered, there is a risk of overdiagnosing the youngest children in each classroom as having attention deficits due to the behavioral differences between the youngest and oldest children (Evans, Morill, & Parente, 2010). In a cohort study involving 937,943 children in British Columbia, Canada, who were 6 to 12 years of age at any time between December 1, 1997, and November 30, 2008, the youngest children in classrooms were found to be at a greater risk for being diagnosed as having ADHD compared to the oldest children. More specifically, the youngest boys were 41% more likely and the youngest girls were 77% more likely to be given a prescription for ADHD medication compared to their oldest counterparts (Morrow et al., 2012). In another study, the youngest children in fifth and eighth grades were found to be nearly twice as likely as their older classmates to use stimulants regularly prescribed to treat ADHD. The study findings also suggested that teachers may perceive the youngest children as having the poorest behaviors (Elder, 2010). According to one estimate based on health surveys conducted during the 1996 to 2006 period, approximately 1.1 million children in the United States were inappropriately diagnosed with ADHD, resulting in over 800,000 receiving stimulant medications due only to relative age immaturity compared to their peers (Evans et al., 2010). Thus, as shown in ▶ Table 13.1, ▶ Table 13.2, Table 13.3 and ▶ Table 13.4, any discrepancies in the rating of two observers (e.g., a parent and a teacher) should be carefully questioned and resolved.

During early school years, a child with ADHD may be able to control excessive movements in some situations but will still show excessive movements compared to his or her peers in situations where calm is expected. During adolescence, he or she may be able to control whole body movements but will appear excessively fidgety compared to his or her peers. As an adult, he or she frequently will feel restless (NCCMH, 2009).

13.4.6 Documentation of Initiation of Symptoms before the Age of 12 Years

Several of the ADHD symptoms should be present before the age of 12 years (American Psychiatric Association, 2013; NCCMH, 2009). The rationale for requirement for the onset of symptoms in childhood is based on the assumption that ADHD is a developmental disorder. Some studies have indicated that most children (83%) with late-onset ADHD tend to be younger than 12 years of age (Faraone et al., 2006). In addition, the use of a younger age of onset criterion such as 7 years can exclude several (43%) children with predominantly inattentive-type and some (18%) children with the combined-type ADHD (Applegate et al., 1997). Clinicians should note that the recall of age of onset of symptoms by parents and other observers may not always be accurate. For example, one study reported a significant increase in the retrospectively reported age of onset of symptoms for ADHD for both parental and self-reports after a period of 5 years (Todd, Huang, & Henderson, 2008).

13.4.7 Existence of the Symptoms Continuously for at Least 6 Months

Symptoms that appear to be similar to ADHD can occur in life crisis situations, such as the death of a family member and divorce. In these types of circumstances, the child or adult may appear inattentive or restless at home, in school, or in work situations. However, in most cases, these symptoms are not long lasting. Therefore, to confirm a diagnosis of ADHD, it is necessary to ensure that the symptoms have existed for a period of at least 6 months and that the initiation of the symptoms are not related to any critical life situations.

13.4.8 Minimal Age for Diagnosis

Children must be at least 4 years old before a diagnosis can be made. Before this age, there is considerable variability in children's behaviors to make reliable judgments about abnormality.

13.4.9 Documentation from at Least Two Observers in Two Different Settings

The presence of symptoms in at least two settings is required to confirm the diagnosis (▶ Table 13.1, ▶ Table 13.2, Table 13.3 and ▶ Table 13.4). If a child is not yet attending school, a primary care provider can encourage the child's parents to enroll him or her in preschool to obtain observations or ratings of the symptoms from a preschool teacher. The physician may also recommend that the parents take parenting classes to teach them about

age-appropriate expectations and managing problem behaviors. Following parent consent, the parenting class instructors can inform the clinician about the ability of the parents to manage the child and, if they can observe the child directly, provide information about the child to allow confirmation of ADHD-related behaviors.

Adolescents may underreport symptoms because of personal bias or expected stigma. In such cases, it is important to obtain ratings from other observers in addition to teachers, such as coaches, school guidance counselors, and community leaders who may be involved in extracurricular activities with the adolescents. Parent and patient consent should be obtained before seeking such information.

The prevalence of diversion and misuse of pharmaceutical stimulants is relatively high among adults with ADHD (Kaye & Darke, 2012). Some adolescents may overreport symptoms if they are dependent on drugs or to gain medication prescriptions to distribute among peers. Drug dependency should be carefully considered or ruled out. In cases of suspected drug dependency, it is particularly important to ensure that behaviors and symptoms are not apparent in only one environmental setting, such as home, and are not restricted to only one type of impairment, such as academic underachievement. Such occurrence in only one setting and restricted to only one type of impairment is insufficient to make the diagnosis.

13.4.10 Comprehensive Assessment of ADHD

Following referral for suspected ADHD, a diagnosis is based on various assessment procedures with consideration of the needs of the individual. A physical evaluation is performed to detect any underlying medical problems and to identify potential contraindications to pharmacological therapy, such as cardiovascular deficits. Comprehensive vision and hearing evaluations may be recommended if indicated by the case history or clinical examination.

More in-depth physical investigations should be carried out as needed based on the case history and initial physical examination. Such assessment can include blood analyses for lead, chromosome testing for fragile X syndrome, electroencephalography, and magnetic resonance imaging for suspected neurologic disorders or space-occupying lesions. Referrals to specialists may be necessary to exclude other diagnoses or to identify comorbid disorders. These may include detailed audiological, psychiatric, neurologic, psychological, psychoeducational, speech and language, and occupational therapy assessments.

The comprehensive assessment can be completed by experienced specialists from various backgrounds, including pediatricians. However, if there are concerns about the existence of comorbid psychiatric disorders or if a differential diagnosis is difficult, a child and adolescent mental health professional should be involved in the assessment.

Although psychological tests can provide information about how a child functions in a structured environment, they are not considered a routine part of the ADHD diagnostic procedure. Although executive functions such as the management and integration of complex information and behaviors may be poor in children with ADHD, tests of executive function may not reliably differentiate children with ADHD. The correlations between ratings of executive function and results of psychometric tests of executive function are minimal. It is possible that the two measures capture different aspects of executive function. The performance measures may reflect the processing efficiency of the individual in a structured environment, whereas the rating measures may provide an indication of individual goal pursuit (Toplak, West, & Stanovich, 2012) or how the individual functions in real life, in the presence of or in spite of deficits in executive function.

13.4.11 Continuous Performance Tests

Continuous performance tests (CPTs) are designed to measure sustained attention and usually require a response (e.g., a button press) to a "target"

stimulus and inhibition of responses for all other stimuli. CPTs have good sensitivity, but they do not consistently and reliably differentiate children with ADHD (Mahone, 2005; SIGN, 2009). Also, boys may do significantly worse than girls on measures of impulsivity (Hasson & Fine, 2012). However, CPTs may be useful in detecting feigned ADHD in adults (Quinn, 2003) and differentiating comorbid APDs in individuals with ADHD (Tillery, Katz, & Keller, 2000). Performance on some APD tasks, such as the frequency pattern test, appears to show a modest correlation with performance on CPT tasks (Sharma, Purdy, & Kelly, 2009). In addition, if a child performs well on a CPT, this may suggest that the child's performance can be improved by using highly structured test situations or environments (Toplak et al., 2012). Therefore, a brief discussion of CPTs is included here.

In the original CPT test, X and AX type visual letters (illustrated in the first two columns of ▶ Fig. 13.3) were used and shown to be sensitive in differentiating the performance of patients with and without brain damage (Rosvold, Mirsky, Sarason, Bransome, & Beck, 1956. Since then, several different variations have been added to CPT tasks. Examples of some of these variations are shown in ▶ Fig. 13.3. Instead of letters, digits, words, playing cards, geometrical figures, math equations, and pictures of objects and persons can be used. Auditory stimuli can be used (Keith, 1994), and some tests use both auditory and visual stimuli (Sandford & Turner, 1995). CPT tests can vary in other ways, including how frequently the target stimulus appears, stimulus duration, stimulus quality, interstimulus interval, distracting stimuli, and feedback on performance as shown in ▶ Fig. 13.4.

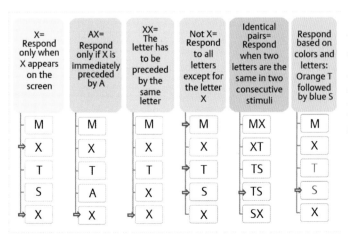

Fig. 13.3 Example of task variations in Visual Continuous Performance tests. Arrows indicate correct responses. Letters can be replaced by digits, words, playing cards, pictures of objects, or pictures of persons. In auditory continuous performance tests, instead of visual stimuli, auditory stimuli are used.

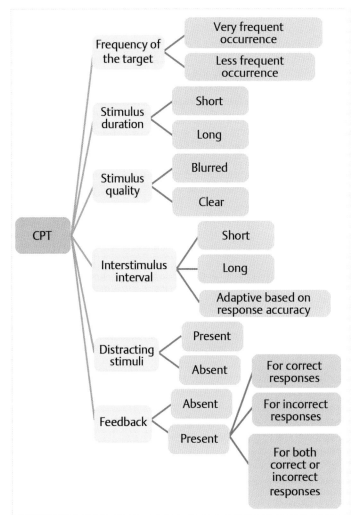

Fig. 13.4 Variables that can change performance on continuous performance test (CPTs).

The most frequently measured CPT responses are the following:

- Errors of omission: No response in the presence of a target; this is used as an index of inattention.
- Errors of commission: Response to a nontarget stimulus; frequently, this is used as an index of impulsivity.
- Response latency: The time taken to make a response after the appearance of the target; this can be indexed as part of the processing speed measure.
- Response variability or stamina: Accuracy of responses or reaction times of correct responses at the beginning (e.g., the first 50 trials) compared to the same at the end (e.g., the last 50 trials); this is used as an index of sustainability of attention.

Some investigators have categorized the above measures into subtypes. For example, if errors of commission are committed with fast response latency, they are associated with hyperactivity/impulsivity. If such errors are committed with slow reaction times, they are considered to be more indicative of inattention (Halperin, Wolf, Greenblatt, & Young, 1991). Other measures are consistency, which takes into account the reliability and variability of response times and is used to index the ability to stay on task, and focus, which is derived by considering the total variability of response latencies for all correct responses (Sandford & Turner, 1995).

13.5 ADHD Treatments

Compared to normal peers, children with ADHD are more likely to show problems in other areas, such as school difficulties (repeating a grade or dropping out of school), teen pregnancy, development of sexually transmitted diseases, substance abuse, accident-prone behavior (e.g., repeated car accidents), arrests, incarceration, and employment difficulties (e.g., being fired from jobs). It is important to treat ADHD to minimize such problems. Various treatment approaches are used for managing children and adults with ADHD, including nonpharmacological and pharmacological interventions.

13.5.1 Behavioral Interventions

Behavioral interventions can be offered to parents of children diagnosed with ADHD and/or to the individual suffering from ADHD.

Behavioral Parent Training

Behavioral interventions by trained facilitators with parents of preschool children are recommended (SIGN, 2009). Interactions between children identified with ADHD and their parents tend to show conflicts and an increase in parenting stress (Deault, 2010). Behavioral parent training (BPT) is designed to improve parenting skills and to teach parents the application of successful child management strategies with an emphasis on positive reinforcement for socially appropriate behaviors and timeout or negative reinforcement for inappropriate behaviors. Improving delay tolerance may be another important goal (Dalen, Sonuga-Barke, Hall, & Remington, 2004). Most BPT programs cover the following aspects (SIGN, 2009):

- Teaching parents procedures for targeting and changing specific behaviors and monitoring relevant changes
- Teaching parents strategies for the management of misbehavior:
  - Setting clear rules with consequences for not following rules
  - Using boundaries, routine, countdowns, reminders, and limit setting
  - Being firm without being coercive
  - Using quiet time, planned ignoring, and timeouts
  - Being consistent
  - Maintaining a calm emotional environment (e.g., communicating without shouting)
- Teaching parents strategies for encouraging appropriate behaviors:
  - Praising

- Showing physical affection
- Providing rewards and incentives
- Teaching parents strategies for promoting positive parenting experience through engagement in play and child-centered activities
- Providing constructive feedback to parents using direct observation of interactions between the child and parents.

Evidence of the effectiveness of BPT is more encouraging for parents and caregivers for reducing parental stress and building confidence in parenting skills than for successfully modifying child behaviors (Zwi, Jones, Thorgaard, York, & Dennis, 2011). BPT appears to improve child behavior, parent behavior, and parental perceptions of parenting immediately following treatment. However, the effect of BPT on child behavior can dissipate rapidly with termination of behavioral contingencies. Thus, at follow-up, the effect of BPT on child behavior can decrease from moderate to zero, and the effect on parental perception of parenting can decrease from high to moderate (Lee, Niew, Yang, Chen, & Lin, 2012). Because ADHD is a chronic condition, any behavioral contingencies need to be well integrated in daily routines for young children to allow maintenance of the BPT effect on child behavior.

Both fathers and mothers should be involved in BPT. One study investigated the effectiveness of a BPT specifically designed for fathers. Results suggested that the BPT was effective in reducing the rate of negative talk and increasing the rate of praise when compared to those in the wait-listed group. In addition, the father rating of the intensity of problem behaviors was reduced after BPT (Fabiano et al., 2012).

Behavioral Teacher Training

The addition of a behavioral teacher training (BTT) component may improve the benefits of behavioral intervention. Interventions involving both parents and teachers can reduce the number of children meeting ADHD and/or oppositional defiant disorder (ODD) criteria. Teachers who have students with more problematic classroom behaviors appear to benefit most from such intervention (Ostberg & Rydell, 2012).

The school environment should be included in all treatment plans for ADHD (American Academy of Pediatrics, AAP, 2011). Depending on the existence of comorbid conditions, such as a learning disability, a child with ADHD may have an individualized education plan (IEP) or a 504 plan that provides a list of special accommodations. Some examples of accommodations are preferential seating, use of simple, concise instructions, teaching compensatory strategies, monitoring child fatigue and adjusting activities to allow time away from seating, modifying test procedures, and modifying the environment to minimize distractions. According to Section 504 of the Rehabilitation Act (173), all entities that receive federal funds, including public schools, colleges, and universities, must offer services that provide access to their programs. Section 504 is designed to protect qualified individuals from discrimination due to their disability. Some children with ADHD may perform at grade levels due to significant efforts by parents and children. Such children may not have an individualized educational plan (IEP) due to their grade level performance. A 504 plan can be used to provide services to these children so that they have access to educational and other services. Note that such accommodations can also help children with APDs.

Behavioral Training for Preadolescent Children

Behavioral therapy should be considered for children who have a mild form of ADHD as a first line of treatment. Along with pharmacological interventions, behavioral therapy has been recommended for school-aged children when the ADHD is accompanied by comorbid symptoms, such as generalized anxiety, aggressive behavior, and oppositional defiant disorder (SIGN, 2009).

13.5.2 Pharmacological Interventions

Primary care providers can prescribe medications approved by the U.S. Food and Drug Administration for ADHD. For children ages 4 to 5 years, methylphenidate should be considered if behavior interventions fail to provide significant improvement in the presence of moderate to severe dysfunction. If behavioral interventions are not available, the risks of starting medications are weighed against the harm of delaying treatment (AAP, 2011).

Pharmacological interventions are recommended for school-aged children who have no comorbid conditions and for those who show comorbid symptoms, including ODD, aggressive behaviors, and generalized anxiety. Such interventions are more effective when they are combined with behavioral programming (SIGN, 2009).

Psychostimulants such as amphetamines and methylphenidate are considered the first choice of medication when pharmacological interventions are considered to treat ADHD symptoms for individuals older than 6 years, except for individuals who have known cardiac abnormalities or who are at risk for cardiac abnormalities (e.g., a family history). If one psychostimulant is found to be ineffective, a trial with another is recommended. If psychostimulants are not appropriate, not tolerated, or are ineffective, atomoxetine is recommended for treating the symptoms (SIGN, 2009). The evidence of effectiveness is strong for stimulant medications and sufficient but less strong for atomoxetine, extended-release guanfacine, and extended-release clonidine (AAP, 2011). The course of ADHD in very young children with moderate to severe ADHD appears to be generally chronic, with high impairment, despite the use of medications. Thus, development of more effective interventions is necessary for this group of children (Riddle et al., 2013).

Where there is the possibility of drug abuse or addiction, consideration of modified-release formulations or atomoxetine is recommended (SIGN, 2009). In addition to abuse, drug diversion, which refers to the transfer of medication to other individuals who do not have a prescription for the drug, may occur. Psychostimulants have the potential to induce abuse and addiction because of their action on the neurotransmitter system and are among the most commonly abused drugs. The most commonly reported reasons for misuse or abuse are to improve attention, concentration, and alertness, to improve study habits and academic performance, and to get "high" (Kaye & Darke, 2012). Particularly when injected in the immediate-release form, the stimulants can produce subjective effects similar to illicit psychostimulants. Extended- or controlled-release formulations may have lower abuse potential than immediate-release formulations (Kollins, Rush, Pazzaglia, & Ali, 1998).

Adverse Effects

Parents and individuals should be informed about the potential adverse effects of medications. Potential adverse effects of stimulants include appetite loss, abdominal pain, headaches, and sleep disturbances. There is also a possibility of decrease in growth velocity with diminished growth in the range of 1 to 2 cm (0.4–0.8 in.; Swanson et al., 2007). There is some possibility of increased mood lability and dysphoria in preschool-aged children (Greenhill et al., 2006).

Potential adverse effects of the nonstimulant atomoxetine are somnolence, gastrointestinal tract symptoms (e.g., nausea, vomiting, and loss of appetite), irritability, and headaches (Vaughan & Kratochvil, 2012). There are warnings related to suicidal thoughts (Bangs, Tauscher-Wisniewski, et al., 2008) and hepatotoxicity. In the presence of jaundice or other evidence of liver injury, permanent discontinuation of atomoxetine is recommended (Bangs, Jin, et al., 2008).

Drug Monitoring

Any individual under pharmacological intervention should be carefully monitored for ongoing effectiveness and for any adverse effects, including on growth, pulse, and blood pressure. Additional vigilance is required for those at increased cardiovascular, hepatobiliary, and seizure risks and those with potential suicidal tendencies (SIGN, 2009).

13.6 Conditions that Can Co-occur with ADHD

Comorbid conditions are quite common in individuals with ADHD (Larson et al., 2011; SIGN, 2009). These include specific learning difficulties, ODD or conduct disorder, anxiety disorder (Venkatesh et al., 2012), mood disorders, specific developmental disorders, language-based difficulties, and motor coordination difficulties (SIGN, 2009).

In a study involving 61,779 children, including 5028 children with ADHD, 10 potential comorbid disorders were identified through parent reports (Larson et al., 2011). The prevalence of comorbid disorders identified in the study in children with and without ADHD is shown in ▶ Fig. 13.5. As shown in the figure, speech problems were reported in 2.5% of the non-ADHD population and 11.8% of the ADHD population. Hearing problems were reported in 1.2% of the non-ADHD population and 4.2% of the ADHD population. Children with ADHD were also found to have higher odds of school problems, grade repetition, and poor parent–child communication compared to their non-ADHD peers. Thirty-three percent of the ADHD children had at least one comorbid disorder, 16% had two, and 18% of the ADHD children had three

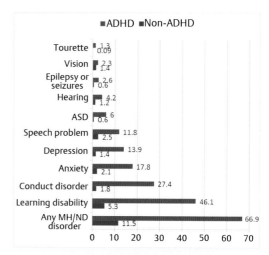

Fig. 13.5 Prevalence of comorbid disorders in children with and without ADHD (based on Larson, Russ, Kahn, & Halfon, 2011).

or more comorbid disorders. Odds of the ADHD child using special education services increased depending on the number of comorbid conditions. The odds were 16.04 (95% confidence interval [CI] 9.84–26.14) with three comorbid conditions (Larson et al., 2011).

Comorbidity with antisocial, mood, and anxiety disorders is one of the predictors of persistence of ADHD over a longer period. Children without these comorbid conditions may have better prognosis (Biederman, Petty, Clarke, Lomedico, & Faraone, 2011).

13.6.1 Comorbidity of ADHD with Auditory Processing Deficits

Overall, studies suggest that among children with ADHD, 50 to 80% may have comorbid APDs (Cook et al., 1993; Effat, Tawfik, Hussein, Azzam, & El Eraky, 2011; Gascon, Johnson, & Burd, 1986; Riccio, Hynd, Cohen, Hall, & Molt, 1994; Tillery et al., 2000). The incidence of comorbidity is likely to vary based on the complexity or simplicity of measures used to diagnose APDs with reference to attention or vigilance requirements and the precautions taken to control inattention. The specific criteria used to diagnose APDs and the presence of other comorbid conditions also may have an effect on the reported incidence of comorbidity. Without treatment, both ADHD and APDs can have a similar negative impact on academic performance and socialization skills.

13.6.2 Possible Reasons for Co-occurrence of ADHD and Auditory Processing Deficits

ADHD and APDs can co-occur for a variety of reasons (▶ Table 13.6)—common environmental risk factors, shared genetic influences, involvement of common brain regions—which are described below.

Common Environmental Risk Factors

Some of the common risk factors are lead exposure, smoking by parents, otitis media, and traumatic brain injury. Maternal smoking during pregnancy increases the risk of ADHD and is associated with a more severe form of ADHD (Thakur et al., 2013). Parental smoking increases the risk of chronic otitis media in children and is linked to increased risk of both APDs and ADHD. In one study, among children referred for evaluation due to school failure, 50% of nonhyperactive children had a history of 3 or more middle ear infections, and 20% had more than 10 infections. In comparison, 94% of the children medicated for hyperactivity had a history of 3 or more episodes of otitis media, and 69% had more than 10 episodes. In addition, a higher frequency of otitis media infections in early childhood was correlated with the presence and severity of hyperactive behaviors (Hagerman & Falkenstein, 1987).

Shared Genetic Influences

Many genes have broad effects on development and can lead to several developmental phenotypes (Chow, Ho, Wong, Waye, & Bishop, 2013). Preliminary results suggest possible genetic influences on certain auditory processing tasks. Analyses of test correlations among 106 monozygotic and 33 dizygotic twin pairs showed that dichotic listening ability is a highly heritable trait similar to height or insulin-dependent diabetes (Morell et al., 2007). Dichotic listening performance is poor in patients with mutations of the *PAX6* gene with associated reduction of the interhemispheric fibers (Bamiou et al., 2004). At least one gene appears to promote the genesis of absolute pitch (the rare ability to label tones with their musical note names without using a reference) in individuals of European ancestry (Theusch, Basu, & Gitschier, 2009). Twin studies show that the variation in musical pitch recognition as measured by a distorted tunes test, which requires subjects to judge whether simple popular melodies contain notes with incorrect pitch, is primarily related to highly heritable differences (Drayna, Manichikul, deLange, Snieder, & Spector, 2001). Congenital amusia, which is a deficit in processing musical pitch but not musical time, tends to be present in 39% of first-degree

Table 13.6 Examples of Commonalities in ADHD and APD

Common Elements	ADHD	APD
Potential genetic influences	Genes implicated in ADHD: • Serotonergic genes, including *5HTT* and *HTR1B* • Dopamine receptor gene polymorphisms, such as *DAT1*, *DRD4*, and *DRD5* • Synaptosomal associated protein SNAP-25, which plays an integral role in synaptic transmission	• In the primary auditory cortex, dopamine release is apparent during auditory training • D2 family of receptors activated by dopaminergic inputs to the auditory cortex may be required for sound sequence discrimination • At least one gene appears to promote the genesis of absolute pitch
Environmental risk factors	Lead exposure, smoking during pregnancy, otitis media	Lead exposure, otitis media (risk increases with increase in parental smoking)
Implicated brain regions	Temporal lobe, posterior regions of the corpus callosum	
Symptoms	Does not seem to listen when spoken to even without any obvious distractions, easily distracted by extraneous stimuli, does not follow through on instructions	
Impact	Poor academic performance, socialization problems	

Abbreviations: ADHD, attention deficit hyperactivity disorder; APD, auditory processing deficit.

relatives, which suggests genetic transmission of the deficit (Peretz, Cummings, & Dubé, 2007). There appears to be a close phenotypic and genetic relationship between absolute pitch and synesthesia with linkage on chromosomes 6q and 2 (Gregersen et al., 2013).

Although additional studies are necessary, serotonergic genes, including *5HTT* and *HTR1B*, dopamine receptor gene polymorphisms, such as *DAT1*, *DRD4*, and *DRD5* (Lasky-Su, Banaschewski, et al., 2007a; Lasky-Su, Biederman, et al, 2007), and the synaptosomal-associated protein SNAP-25, which plays an integral role in synaptic transmission, have been implicated in ADHD (Thapar, Cooper, Eyre, & Langley, 2013). Alteration of serotonin in the brain of depressed individuals can modulate auditory processing skills (Gopal, Briley, Goodale, & Hendea, 2005). In the primary auditory cortex, dopamine release is apparent during auditory training (Stark & Scheich, 1997). More specifically, the D2 family of receptors activated by dopaminergic inputs to the auditory cortex may be required for sound sequence discrimination (Kudoh & Shibuki, 2006). Stimulation of the ventral tegmental area, which contains dopamine neurons, together with a particular tone, expands the area representing the tonal frequency in the auditory cortex while simultaneously decreasing cortical representations of neighboring frequencies (Bao, Chan, & Merzenich, 2001). In addition, dopaminergic inputs regulate rapamycin (mTOR)–mediated, protein synthesis–dependent mechanisms in the auditory cortex, thus controlling for hours or days the consolidation of memory required for the discrimination of complex auditory stimuli (Schicknick et al., 2008). Thus, dopaminergic inputs, along with the auditory cortex, are involved in decoding sounds and in learning their behavioral significance (Scheich & Zuschratter, 1995).

Involvement of Common Brain Regions

Alterations across Brain Regions

Several alterations have been reported in the brains of children with ADHD, including significantly smaller volumes in the dorsolateral frontal cortex, caudate, pallidum, corpus callosum, and cerebellum (Seidman, Valera, & Makris, 2005). Many of these regions are involved in processing complex auditory stimuli. For example, during a task requiring repetition of the last word of a sentence in the presence of multitalker babble, the temporal cortex and several other regions, including the right anterior lobe of the cerebellum, the left posterior lobe of the cerebellum, and the right medial frontal gyrus, are involved (Salvi et al., 2002).

Temporal Lobe

Alterations in temporal lobe volume have been reported in individuals with ADHD (Castellanos et al., 2002; Sowell et al., 2003). One study has identified the temporal lobe as the main location of differences in boys with ADHD versus controls (Kobel et al., 2010). In addition, there are significant correlations between temporal gray matter volume and parent- and clinician-rated severity measures in the ADHD sample (Castellanos et al., 2003).

Corpus Callosum

The isthmus/splenium of the corpus callosum has fibers that link the auditory cortices in the left and right hemispheres (Fabri & Polonara, 2013) and appears to play an important role in interhemispheric communication involved in tasks such as verbal labeling of melodies. In one study, a 6-year-old diagnosed with ADHD showed complete agenesis of the corpus callosum (Roessner, Banaschewski, Uebel, Becker, & Rothenberger, 2004). Other studies suggest abnormalities, such as smaller size, in the posterior regions, including the isthmus/splenium of the corpus callosum, suggesting fewer interhemispheric connections (Hill et al., 2003; Luders et al., 2009; Lyoo et al., 1996). Abnormalities of the corpus callosum in children include macrostructural changes such as decreased thickness. In addition, diffused tensor imaging (DTI) has revealed significant reduction in the mean fractional anisotropy values assumed to reflect fiber density, axonal diameter, and myelination in white matter in children with ADHD (Cao et al., 2010). Although the macrostructure of the corpus callosum is normal in adults with ADHD, microstructural deficiencies continue, which suggests persistent impairment (Dramsdahl, Westerhausen, Haavik, Hugdahl, & Plessen, 2012).

13.7 Auditory Processing in Children with ADHD

Several studies have reported on auditory processing skills in children with ADHD. A brief review of some of these findings is presented below.

13.7.1 Acceptable Noise Level

During the measurement of acceptable noise level, listeners adjust the level of background noise (e.g., multitalker babble) to the maximum level of noise they are willing to accept without becoming tense or tired while listening to and following the words of a story or target signal. The adjusted level is referred to as the background noise level (BNL). The difference between the speech or signal presentation level and the BNL is referred to as the tolerated background noise level, or acceptable noise level (Nabelek, Tucker, & Letowski, 1991). Following stimulant medication, women with ADHD are able to accept higher BNL. As a result, with medication, the signal-to-noise ratio can be 2 to 3 dB lower without reduction in the willingness to listen to the signal. Thus, women with ADHD may be more tolerant of noise in noisy situations such as classrooms, work situations, and shopping venues following ADHD medications (Freyaldenhoven, Thelin, Plyler, Nabelek, & Burchfield, 2005).

13.7.2 Hypersensitivity to Sounds

Children with ADHD may be hypersensitive to sounds, as suggested by lower maximum comfortable loudness levels, than normal children (Lucker, Geffner, & Koch, 1996), but as adults they appear to outgrow the hypersensitivity, as suggested by normal maximum comfortable levels. In addition, stimulant medications do not change maximum comfortable levels in women with ADHD (Freyaldenhoven et al., 2005). Hypersensitivity to sounds in children with ADHD may depend on comorbid conditions, such as separation anxiety disorders. Children with comorbid separation anxiety disorders show more hypersensitivity than those without such disorders (Ghanizadeh, 2009).

13.7.3 Hyposensitivity to Sounds

Children with ADHD and ODD may exhibit more hyposensitivity to sounds than ADHD children without the disorder (Ghanizadeh, 2009). Such children may seek loud sounds, including loud music.

13.7.4 Central Masking

In the presence of contralateral masking, thresholds for a 500 Hz tone increase similarly for both ADHD and APD children. However, children with ADHD show a higher false alarm rate, suggesting difficulty with inhibiting response in the absence of a tonal stimulus, when compared to children with APD (Breier, Gray, Klaas, Fletcher, & Foorman, 2002).

13.7.5 Speech Recognition in Noise

Children with ADHD have significantly more difficulty recognizing speech in background noise when compared to children with dyslexia and normal children (Abdo, Murphy, & Schochat, 2010; Cook et al., 1993; Geffner, Lucker, & Koch, 1996; Pillsbury, Grose, Coleman, Conners, & Hall, 1995). Similarly, among children who are referred for the possibility of auditory or language processing deficits, children with ADHD perform significantly worse than those without ADHD on the figure-ground subtest of SCAN (Keith, Rudy, Donahue, & Katbamna, 1989). However, using the same subtest, Gomez and Condon (1999) reported no significant differences among children with attention deficit disorder and normal children.

13.7.6 Filtered Words

Children with ADHD show normal performance on tasks such as filtered words, showing normal closure skills (Cook et al., 1993; Gomez & Condon, 1999). However, among children who are referred for the possibility of auditory or language processing deficits, children with ADHD perform significantly worse than those without ADHD (Keith et al., 1989).

13.7.7 Binaural Interaction

ADHD children show binaural advantage similar to that apparent in normal children on masking-level difference (MLD) tasks for both tonal and speech stimuli (Pillsbury et al., 1995).

13.7.8 Dichotic Listening

Children with ADHD yield poorer performance for the dichotic digits task compared to normal children (Abdo et al., 2010). Other investigators have failed to show significant differences in children with ADHD and normal children in tasks such as the Staggered Spondaic Word (SSW) test (Cook et al., 1993) or SCAN competing words test (Gomez & Condon, 1999). Also, among children who are referred for the possibility of auditory or language processing deficits, there are no differences in children with or without ADHD on the SCAN competing words test (Keith et al., 1989). It appears that poor performance on a dichotic listening task is more likely to occur when ADHD is accompanied by comorbid conditions such as dyslexia (Gomez & Condon, 1999). A significant left ear deficit on the dichotic digits test has been noted in patients with APDs and ADHD compared to those with only ADHD (Effat et al., 2011).

13.7.9 Binaural Separation

Children with ADHD may show poorer performance in the left ear compared to normal children on the competing sentences Test (Cook et al., 1993). However, among children who are referred for the possibility of auditory or language processing deficits, there is no difference in children with or without ADHD on the test (Keith et al., 1989).

13.7.10 Binaural Fusion

Children with ADHD may show poorer performance on the Rapidly Alternating Speech Test compared to normal children, which suggests difficulty in fusing the information presented to the two ears (Cook et al., 1993).

13.7.11 Temporal Resolution (Gap Detection)

Some children with ADHD have difficulty in detecting gaps (Effat et al., 2011).

13.7.12 Temporal Pattern Recognition

Some children with ADHD may perform poorly when compared to children with dyslexia and normal children on the Pitch Pattern Sequence Test (Abdo et al., 2010; Effat et al., 2011).

13.7.13 Temporal Pitch Pattern Discrimination

Some children with ADHD show deficits in discriminating pitch patterns (Effat et al., 2011).

13.7.14 Duration Discrimination

ADHD children yield elevated visual and auditory duration discrimination thresholds when compared to normal controls, and the performance on

the auditory duration discrimination task is related to auditory memory for longer duration targets (400–1000 ms). The deficits in duration discrimination for shorter targets (200 ms) in both visual and auditory modes suggest the possibility of a basic internal timing deficit in ADHD children (Toplak, Rucklidge, Hetherington, John, & Tannock, 2003; Toplak & Tannock, 2005).

13.7.15 Summary of Auditory Processing Skills in Children with ADHD

As discussed above, at least some ADHD children perform poorly on many auditory processing skills. The performance of children varies across studies. Such variability is expected due to variation in auditory stimuli, response tasks, control of attention and fatigue during the task, the number of children in the ADHD group with comorbid conditions, including APDs, and the specific subtypes of ADHD included in the ADHD group. Because all children with ADHD do not have APDs, instead of reporting group differences, the percentage of children with ADHD showing poorer than normal performance should be reported in future studies, along with any comorbid conditions. Similarly, clinicians involved in the diagnosis and intervention of children with APDs should note that not all children with ADHD have APDs.

13.8 Auditory Processing Deficit Testing in the Presence of ADHD

The act of paying attention activates a network of localized brain regions and also enhances activation of specific sensory regions. Thus, in administering tests for assessing auditory processing skills, in addition to other factors, the influence of attention (▶ Fig. 13.6) should be considered both for differentiating ADHD and APDs and for evaluating the co-occurrence of the disorders. The following recommendations can improve the chances of obtaining reliable results from children with ADHD.

13.8.1 Ensure Good Sleep

In testing children, encourage parents to maximize the possibility of good sleep on the night prior to the day of testing. For example, the child should go to bed early if he or she is expected to wake up

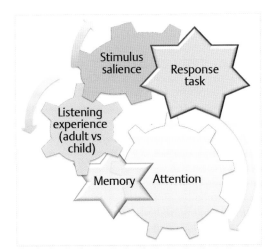

Fig. 13.6 Factors affecting responses on auditory processing tasks.

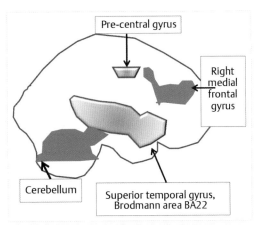

Fig. 13.7 Example of activation of additional regions (*green*) when speech is presented with reduced intelligibility in the presence of multitalker babble. Only blue regions are activated when speech is presented in quiet with 100% intelligibility (based on Salvi et al., 2002).

early to go to school. Staying away from drinks with caffeine might also help.

13.8.2 Consider Comorbid Conditions

When testing for ADHD, consider the presence of other comorbid conditions. When possible, adjust test environments, stimuli, and response modes to accommodate for the identified conditions. For example, in one study, children with ADHD performed as well as children in a control group in discriminating between pairs of monosyllabic words differing in one consonant and two- to five-syllable nonwords with contrasting vowels. Children with ADHD and movement coordination disorders performed well on monosyllabic words differing in one consonant but performed poorly on nonword tasks that involved a higher working memory load (Norrelgen, Lacerda, & Forssberg, 1999).

13.8.3 Check for Clear Audibility of Stimuli

When testing children with ADHD, check for clear audibility of stimuli. Stimuli that occur near thresholds involve more brain regions. Salvi and colleagues (2002) compared positron emission tomography (PET) scans elicited using clearly audible (100% intelligibility) speech in quiet with barely recognizable speech (50% intelligibility) presented in the background of multitalker babble. The

combination of both the background babble and 50% intelligibility led to the involvement of several brain regions in addition to those involved in listening to speech that had 100% intelligibility (▶ Fig. 13.7). This is most likely because when word intelligibility is lower, more cognitive effort is spent on guessing words occurring at the end of sentences. If the signal-to-babble ratio is adjusted so that the speech is highly intelligible, less cognitive effort is required.

13.8.4 Monitor and Regulate the Test Situation

External control provided by the examiner can yield performance similar to normal children in hyperactive children during auditory attention tasks. However, in the absence of such control, the performance of hyperactive children shows greater deterioration than that apparent in normal children (Draeger, Prior, & Sanson, 1986). Thus, it is important to observe the child carefully; if symptoms of inattention or hyperactivity appear, breaks should be provided at the end of each subtest. Breaks for water or a brief walk outside the booth may help to sustain attention and improve motivation. Providing a more vigorous activity such as jumping for a brief duration also may help improve attention on task without causing fatigue. If inattention is apparent, insertion of pauses and provision of verbal reinforcements can be helpful (see examples below under Test Interpretation). Highly unique reinforcers such as money should be avoided, as these can lead to a temporary and artificial improvement in performance that is unlikely to reflect the child's struggles in real-world environments.

13.8.5 Use Tasks that Require Interaction

When testing children with ADHD, use tasks that require interaction. For example, after presenting four stimuli, a response should be required. The presentation of lengthy stimuli without requiring a response can reduce vigilance and confound the scores on auditory processing tasks.

13.8.6 Use Tasks that Require Simple Responses

Use tasks that require simple responses, such as humming or linguistic labeling with minimal linguistic load (e.g., digits) or a linguistic load that is appropriate considering the child's language skills. For example, in assessing binaural interactions, use the 500 Hz tonal stimulus instead of speech.

13.8.7 Avoid Tasks Involving Other Sensory Modes

With patients with ADHD, it is important to avoid using auditory tasks that involve other sensory modes. In one study, when the response tasks involved complex visual displays and shifting of attention between auditory and visual modes, attention and cognition fluctuation had more impact on test results (Moore, Ferguson, Edmondson-Jones, Ratib, & Riley, 2010).

13.8.8 Consider ADHD Medications

When different sensory modes are involved in performing auditory tasks, such as frequency discrimination or frequency modulation (FM), children may perform better if they are on medications for ADHD compared to when they are off medications (Sutcliffe, Bishop, Houghton, & Taylor, 2006). Thus, if a child is taking medications, performing the test battery before the medication wears off may be helpful in controlling for any impact of inattention or hyperactivity on test results. It should be noted

that for auditory processing tests that involve a simple verbal response, the performance of children with ADHD is similar with or without medications (Tillery et al., 2000). If parents are unwilling to place the child on medications to control ADHD symptoms, such tests can be administered with appropriate controls (e.g., good sleep during the previous night, breaks during testing, pauses for re-instruction and reinforcement, etc.) for inattention and fatigue, as described above.

13.8.9 Use Tasks Involving Easier Understanding of Procedures

The use of complex tasks should be minimized. For example, determining the most comfortable level (MCL) does not require complex cortical function, whereas determining the acceptable noise level (ANL) does, perhaps because of the presence of a distracting background. This is suggested by the fact that the ANL improves with stimulant medication, whereas the medication has no effect on the MCL (Freyaldenhoven et al., 2005).

13.8.10 Avoid Tasks with Great Performance Variability

Avoid auditory processing tasks that show great performance variability in the normal population and require a considerable amount of training to stabilize performance (e.g., difference limen of frequency or intensity).

13.8.11 Minimize the Influence of Attention Deficits on Test Interpretation

Use a Team Approach

Use a team approach involving all related professionals (Keller & Tillery, 2002).

Use Intratest Comparisons

As discussed in Chapter 6, the SSW test yields scores under four different conditions: right competing, left competing, right noncompeting, and left noncompeting. If a patient yields poor scores in all four conditions, the influence of supramodal factors on the scores should be considered (Katz & Tillery, 2005).

Example 1

Consider the performance of a 7-year-old diagnosed with combined-type ADHD. In this example, the child's performance does not appear to be affected by ADHD based on the following behavioral observations and test result patterns.

Behavioral observations: The child appeared cooperative and alert through the test session. This is not unexpected, as children with ADHD often function well in structured environments (U.S. Department of Health Services, National Institute of Health, National Institutes of Mental Health, 2008).

Test result pattern examination:

- The number of errors on the first 20 items (31 errors) of the SSW test was similar to that on the second 20 (32 errors) items.
- Performance is within normal limits on various tests, including spondee MLD and filtered words, confirming no adverse effects of inattention or hyperactivity.
- On the competing words test, a significant right ear advantage was apparent in the right ear first condition (right ear 80%, left ear 13.33%). On the SSW test, a significant right ear advantage was apparent, with significantly more errors in the left ear, in the right ear first condition. On the competing sentences test, the child scored 80% in the right ear and 30% in the left ear. Using recommendations from Bellis (2003), the right ear performance is considered within normal limits, but the left ear performance is below the normal cutoff of 35% for 7-year-olds, suggesting a left ear deficit. ► Fig. 13.8 shows the percent correct scores on three different dichotic tasks for this child. As shown in the figure, a left ear deficit is apparent in three dichotic (competing) conditions: right ear first SSW, right ear first competing words, and competing sentences tests. Note that the deficit is apparent when the child is asked to repeat the stimuli presented to the right ear first and then those presented to the left ear as required in the competing words task. It is also apparent when the first part of the spondee begins in the right ear compared to when the first part of the spondee begins in the left ear as presented in the SSW test. As noted in Chapter 6, in the competing sentences test, in the right ear condition, the child is asked to repeat sentences presented only in the right ear and ignore those presented in the left ear. In the left ear condition, the child is asked to repeat sentences presented only in the left ear while ignoring those presented in the right ear. Recommendations for

this child included further testing to assess temporal resolution and temporal patterning skills, dichotic interaural intensity difference (DIID) training (see Chapter 10), and use of a personal FM device in the classroom to improve attention and to deliver the teacher's speech clearly without background competition to the child's ears.

Example 2

Consider the performance of an 8-year-old girl diagnosed with ADHD and a comorbid anxiety disorder on the random gap detection test, as shown in ► Fig. 13.9. Possible influence of both ADHD and anxiety is evident in the test pattern. Although the child has performed well on the screening/practice run, the overall results are somewhat questionable. Responses in the red circles show that the child is indicating the perception of two sounds when there is no gap between the sounds (2000 and 4000 Hz). The possible minimum gaps that are detected by this child are indicated by the green circles. In testing such children, close attention should be paid to the response behaviors, and appropriate feedback should be provided by pausing the test. For example, note the first blue arrow in the second row in ► Fig. 13.9. Just before the arrow, the patient indicated that she heard two sounds when the gap was only 2 ms; however, her previous performance indicates that she heard only

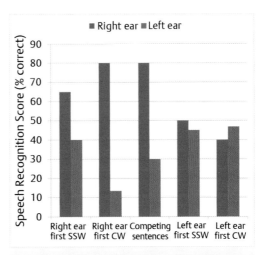

Fig. 13.8 Speech recognition scores of a child diagnosed with ADHD during three dichotic tasks. Left ear deficit is apparent in the first three conditions. CW, competing words; SSW, staggered spondaic words. For descriptions of these tests, see Chapter 6. For SSW, only the scores in the dichotic conditions are displayed.

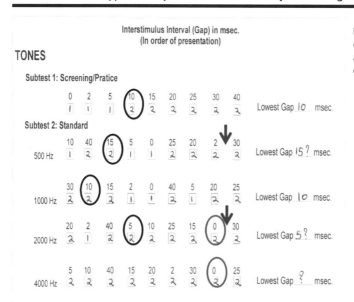

Fig. 13.9 Performance of an 8-year-old girl diagnosed with ADHD and anxiety disorders on the random gap detection test.

one sound with a larger gap of 5 ms, suggesting she could not detect the 5 ms gap. Similarly, note the response before the second arrow in the fourth row. She indicated that she heard two sounds when the gap was 0 ms. In this case, providing a brief pause where the arrows are placed and offering reinforcement and a reminder to the child to continue to pay close attention may have helped the child to stay attentive until the end of the test and could have allowed determination of a reliable gap detection threshold at 4000 Hz. Proper documentation of her gap detection skills is importance because the child did poorly on the pitch pattern sequencing test, suggesting a temporal processing deficit.

Use a Test Battery Approach

If the patient performs well within normal limits on various tests, then the presence of an APD can be ruled out, even if he or she has been diagnosed with ADHD. If a patient is exhibiting an APD, and the cognitive assessment shows normal nonverbal performance but a reduced verbal intelligence quotient (IQ), the potential impact of the APD on the verbal IQ should be considered.

13.9 Intervention for Auditory Processing Deficits in the Presence of ADHD

13.9.1 Assistive Listening Devices

Assistive listening devices can be recommended for children with APDs and/or ADHD. Such devices

deliver the teacher's speech to a child's ears with minimal contamination from noise or reverberation in the classroom. This allows the child to consistently hear better with the least amount of cognitive effort, which allows for better attention and easier learning. The most adequate type of assistive listening device for such children should be based on their specific learning environment and needs. Children with ADHD and APDs show significant improvement in teacher rating on questions related to social behavior, attentiveness, and hearing profiles following the use of bilateral ear-level FM devices (Friederichs & Friederichs, 2005). Attending behaviors of children with learning disabilities can improve following FM use. Such behaviors include motivation to participate, eye contact with teachers, response time, ability to follow directions, and body control. In addition, teachers have noted reduction in attention to extraneous classroom stimuli following FM use (Blake, Field, Foster, Platt, & Wertz, 1991). In one study, children with autism spectrum disorders and/or ADHD showed significantly better speech recognition in noise, improvement in on-task behaviors such as sitting quietly when expected or asked, and improvement in teacher ratings of listening behaviors following FM system use, suggesting that assistive listening devices can be useful for all ADHD children, including those with comorbid disorders (Schafer et al., 2013).

13.9.2 Other Interventions

Interventions described in Chapters 8 to 11 can be used to address APDs with accommodation for

ADHD. For example, during deficit-specific training activities, such as dichotic interaural intensity difference (DIID) training (see Chapter 10), before each stimulus item provide an alerting stimulus, such as "Are you ready?" and require a response from the child. After each response, provide feedback about the accuracy of the response. Vary stimuli in terms of difficulty and complexity to ensure that the child remains somewhat challenged and motivated to continue training. Use stimuli that are of specific interest to the child. Note that children with ADHD can often sustain their attention if the task is of interest to them. Some computerized training programs include attention control features such as a requirement to indicate readiness by clicking on an icon. A national field trial reported that children with diagnoses of attention deficit disorders can improve their language and processing skills using a computerized training program titled Fast ForWord Language (Scientific Learning Corporation, Oakland, CA) (Agocs, Burns, DeLey, Miller, & Calhoun, 2006). In addition, the neural mechanisms of selective auditory attention can improve through training (Stevens, Fanning, Coch, Sanders, & Neville, 2008). Additional studies could allow further documentation of the effectiveness of APD intervention in children with comorbid ADHD and APDs.

13.10 Future Trends

In the near future, most individuals—more specifically, children but also some young adults—who are considered to be at risk for ADHD will be referred for complete auditory processing evaluations. They will be evaluated by audiologists using a test battery that is minimally influenced by attention deficits. With appropriate breaks in testing as necessary, most of these individuals are expected to behave well in structured test settings that are used during audiological evaluations. Such evaluations may decrease the overdiagnosis of ADHD in some of this population, including those with primarily inattention deficits and those who do not respond well to stimulant medications (Bailey, 2010). Appropriate diagnoses of APDs in these individuals with or without accompanying ADHD is likely to result in better outcomes.

13.11 Review Questions

1. List the main subtypes of attention deficit hyperactivity disorder (ADHD) and describe the characteristics of each subtype.

2. What is the prevalence of ADHD? List the factors that increase the risk of ADHD.

3. How is ADHD diagnosed?

4. Describe continuous performance tests, their intended goals, and limitations.

5. What types of approaches are available for treating and/or managing ADHD? What are some potential side effects of pharmacological interventions?

6. List some conditions that co-occur more frequently in individuals with ADHD than in the general population.

7. What are the possible reasons for the comorbidity of auditory processing deficits (APDs) and ADHD?

8. What precautions should be taken in administering APD tests to children at risk for ADHD or diagnosed with ADHD?

9. How can APD test results be interpreted in the presence of ADHD?

10. What types of intervention techniques are available for children with comorbid APD and ADHD?

References

[1] Abdo, A. G., Murphy, C. F., & Schochat, E. (2010). Hearing abilities in children with dyslexia and attention deficit hyperactivity disorder. Pro Fono, 22(1), 25–30.

[2] Adler, L. A., Shaw, D. M., Spencer, T. J., et al. (2012). Preliminary examination of the reliability and concurrent validity of the attention-deficit/hyperactivity disorder self-report scale v1.1 symptom checklist to rate symptoms of attention-deficit/hyperactivity disorder in adolescents. Journal of Child and Adolescent Psychopharmacology, 22(3), 238–244.

[3] Agocs, M. M., Burns, M. S., DeLey, L. E., Miller, S. L., & Calhoun, B. M. (2006). Fast ForWord language. In R. J. McCauley and M. E. Fey (Eds.), Treatment of language disorders in children (pp. 471–508). Baltimore, MD: Brookes.

[4] American Academy of Pediatrics, Subcommittee on Attention-Deficit/Hyperactivity Disorder, Steering Committee on Quality Improvement and Management. (2011). ADHD: Clinical practice guideline for the diagnosis, evaluation, and treatment of Attention-Deficit/Hyperactivity Disorder in children and adolescents. Pediatrics, 128, 1007-1022. Retrieved from http://pediatrics.aappublications.org/content/128/5/1007.full.pdf+html.

[5] American Psychiatric Association. (2000). Diagnostic and statistical manual of mental disorders (4th ed.). Arlington, VA: Author.

[6] American Psychiatric Association. (2013). Diagnostic and statistical manual of mental disorders (5th ed.). Arlington, VA: Author.

[7] American Speech-Language-Hearing Association. (n. d.). Attention Deficit/Hyperactivity Disorder. Retrieved from http://www.asha.org/public/speech/disorders/ADHD/.

[8] Applegate, B., Lahey, B. B., Hart, E. L., et al. (1997). Validity of the age-of-onset criterion for ADHD: A report from the DSM-IV field trials. Journal of the American Academy of Child and Adolescent Psychiatry, 36(9), 1211–1221.

[9] Arizona Department of Health Services. (2003). Arizona's children and the environment: A summary of the primary environmental health factors affecting Arizona's children. Retrieved from http://www.azdhs.gov/phs/oeh/pdf/gov_chldrn_hlth_rpt.pdf.

[10] Bailey, T. (2010). Auditory pathways and processes: Implications for neuropsychological assessment and diagnosis of children and adolescents. Child Neuropsychology, 16(6), 521–548.

[11] Bamiou, D. E., Musiek, F. E., Sisodiya, S. M., et al. (2004). Deficient auditory interhemispheric transfer in patients with PAX6 mutations. Annals of Neurology, 56(4), 503–509.

[12] Bangs, M. E., Jin, L., Zhang, S., et al. (2008). Hepatic events associated with atomoxetine treatment for attention-deficit hyperactivity disorder. Drug Safety, 31(4), 345–354.

[13] Bangs, M. E., Tauscher-Wisniewski, S., Polzer, J., et al. (2008). Meta-analysis of suicide-related behavior events in patients treated with atomoxetine. Journal of the American Academy of Child and Adolescent Psychiatry, 47(2), 209–218.

[14] Bao, S., Chan, V. T., & Merzenich, M. M. (2001). Cortical remodelling induced by activity of ventral tegmental dopamine neurons. Nature, 412(6842), 79–83.

[15] Beck, L. H., Bransome, E. D., Jr, Mirsky, A. F., Rosvold, H. E., & Sarason, I. (1956). A continuous performance test of brain damage. Journal of Consulting Psychology, 20(5), 343–350.

[16] Bellis, T. J. (2003). Assessment and management of central auditory processing disorders in the educational setting: From science to practice (2nd ed.). Clifton Park, NY: Delmar Learning.

[17] Biederman, J., Petty, C. R., Clarke, A., Lomedico, A., & Faraone, S. V. (2011). Predictors of persistent ADHD: An 11-year follow-up study. Journal of Psychiatric Research, 45(2), 150–155.

[18] Blake, R., Field, B., Foster, C., Platt, F., & Wertz, P. (1991). Effect of FM auditory trainers on attending behaviors of learning-disabled children. Language, Speech, and Hearing Services in Schools, 22, 111–114.

[19] Boucher, O., Jacobson, S. W., Plusquellec, P., et al. (2012). Prenatal methylmercury, postnatal lead exposure, and evidence of attention deficit/hyperactivity disorder among Inuit children in Arctic Québec. Environmental Health Perspectives, 120(10), 1456–1461.

[20] Braun, J. M., Kahn, R. S., Froehlich, T., Auinger, P., & Lanphear, B. P. (2006). Exposures to environmental toxicants and attention deficit hyperactivity disorder in U.S. children. Environmental Health Perspectives, 114(12), 1904–1909.

[21] Breier, J. I., Gray, L. C., Klaas, P., Fletcher, J. M., & Foorman, B. (2002). Dissociation of sensitivity and response bias in children with attention deficit/hyperactivity disorder during central auditory masking. Neuropsychology, 16(1), 28–34.

[22] Cao, Q., Sun, L., Gong, G., et al. (2010). The macrostructural and microstructural abnormalities of corpus callosum in children with attention deficit/hyperactivity disorder: A combined morphometric and diffusion tensor MRI study. Brain Research, 1310, 172–180.

[23] Castellanos, F. X., Lee, P. P., Sharp, W., et al. (2002). Developmental trajectories of brain volume abnormalities in children and adolescents with attention-deficit/hyperactivity disorder. Journal of the American Medical Association, 288 (14), 1740–1748.

[24] Centers for Disease Control and Prevention (CDC). (2010). Increasing prevalence of parent-reported attention-deficit/hyperactivity disorder among children—United States, 2003 and 2007. Morbidity and Mortality Weekly Report, 59(44), 1439–1443.

[25] Chow, B W., Ho, C. S., Wong, S. W., Waye, M. M., & Bishop, D. V. (2013). Generalist genes and cognitive abilities in Chinese twins. Developmental Science, 16(2), 260–268.

[26] Chu, S. M., Tsai, M. H., Hwang, F. M., Hsu, J. F., Huang, H. R., & Huang, Y. S. (2012). The relationship between attention deficit hyperactivity disorder and premature infants in Taiwanese: A case control study. BMC Psychiatry, 12, 85–90.

[27] Conners, C. K., Erhardt, D., & Sparrow, E. (1999). Conners' adult ADHD rating scales. New York: Multi-Health Systems.

[28] Cook, J. R., Mausbach, T., Burd, L., et al. (1993). A preliminary study of the relationship between central auditory processing disorder and attention deficit disorder. Journal of Psychiatry and Neuroscience, 18(3), 130–137.

[29] Dalen, L., Sonuga-Barke, E. J., Hall, M., & Remington, B. (2004). Inhibitory deficits, delay aversion and preschool AD/HD: Implications for the dual pathway model. Neural Plasticity, 11(1-2), 1–11.

[30] Deault, L. C. (2010).A systematic review of parenting in relation to the development of comorbidities and functional impairments in children with attention-deficit/hyperactivity disorder (ADHD). Child Psychiatry and Human Development, 41(2), 168–192.

[31] Draeger, S., Prior, M., & Sanson, A. (1986). Visual and auditory attention performance in hyperactive children: Competence or compliance. Journal of Abnormal Child Psychology, 14(3), 411–424.

[32] Dramsdahl, M., Westerhausen, R., Haavik, J., Hugdahl, K., & Plessen, K. J. (2012). Adults with attention-deficit/hyperactivity disorder: A diffusion-tensor imaging study of the corpus callosum. Psychiatry Research, 201(2), 168–173.

[33] Drayna, D., Manichaikul, A., de Lange, M., Snieder, H., & Spector, T. (2001). Genetic correlates of musical pitch recognition in humans. Science, 291(5510), 1969–1972.

[34] Effat, S., Tawfik, S., Hussein, H., Azzam, H., & El Eraky, S. (2011). Central auditory processing in attention deficit hyperactivity disorder: An Egyptian study. Middle East Current Psychiatry, 18, 245–252.

[35] Elder, T. E. (2010). The importance of relative standards in ADHD diagnoses: Evidence based on exact birth dates. Journal of Health Economics, 29(5), 641–656.

[36] Evans, W. N., Morrill, M. S., & Parente, S. T. (2010). Measuring inappropriate medical diagnosis and treatment in survey data: The case of ADHD among school-age children. Journal of Health Economics, 29(5), 657–673.

[37] Fabiano, G. A., Pelham, W. E., Cunningham, C. E., et al. (2012). A waitlist-controlled trial of behavioral parent training for fathers of children with ADHD. Journal of Clinical Child and Adolescent Psychology, 41(3), 337–345.

[38] Fabri, M., & Polonara, G. (2013). Functional topography of human corpus callosum: An FMRI mapping study. Neural Plasticity, Volume 2013, Article ID 251308, 15 pages.

[39] Faraone, S. V., Sergeant, J., Gillberg, C., & Biederman, J. (2003). The worldwide prevalence of ADHD: Is it an American condition? World Psychiatry, 2, 104.

[40] Faraone, S. V., Biederman, J., Spencer, T., et al. (2006). Diagnosing adult attention deficit hyperactivity disorder: Are late onset and subthreshold diagnoses valid? American Journal of Psychiatry, 163(10), 1720–1729, quiz 1859.

[41] Friederichs, E., & Friederichs, P. (2005). Electrophysiologic and psycho-acoustic findings following one-year application of a personal ear-level FM device in children with attention deficit and suspected central auditory processing disorder. Journal of Educational Audiology, 12, 31–36.

[42] Freyaldenhoven, M. C., Thelin, J. W., Plyler, P. N., Nabelek, A. K., & Burchfield, S. B. (2005). Effect of stimulant medication on the acceptance of background noise in individuals with attention deficit/hyperactivity disorder. Journal of the American Academy of Audiology, 16(9), 677–686.

[43] Gascon, G. G., Johnson, R., & Burd, L. (1986). Central auditory processing and attention deficit disorders. Journal of Child Neurology, 1(1), 27–33.

[44] Geffner, D., Lucker, J. R., & Koch, W. (1996). Evaluation of auditory discrimination in children with ADD and without ADD. Child Psychiatry and Human Development, 26(3), 169–179.

[45] Gerring, J. P., Brady, K. D., Chen, A., et al. (1998). Premorbid prevalence of ADHD and development of secondary ADHD after closed head injury. Journal of the American Academy of Child and Adolescent Psychiatry, 37(6), 647–654.

[46] Ghanizadeh, A. (2009). Screening signs of auditory processing problem: Does it distinguish attention deficit hyperactivity disorder subtypes in a clinical sample of children? International Journal of Pediatric Otorhinolaryngology, 73(1), 81–87.

[47] Gomez, R., & Condon, M. (1999). Central auditory processing ability in children with ADHD with and without learning disabilities. Journal of Learning Disabilities, 32(2), 150–158.

[48] Gopal, K. V., Briley, K. A., Goodale, E. S., & Hendea, O. M. (2005). Selective serotonin reuptake inhibitors treatment effects on auditory measures in depressed female subjects. European Journal of Pharmacology, 520(1-3), 59–69.

[49] Greenhill, L., Kollins, S., Abikoff, H., et al. (2006). Efficacy and safety of immediate-release methylphenidate treatment for preschoolers with ADHD. Journal of the American Academy of Child and Adolescent Psychiatry, 45(11), 1284–1293.

[50] Gregersen, P. K., Kowalsky, E., Lee, A., et al. (2013). Absolute pitch exhibits phenotypic and genetic overlap with synesthesia. Human Molecular Genetics, 22(10), 2097–2104.

[51] Hagerman, R. J., & Falkenstein, A. R. (1987). An association between recurrent otitis media in infancy and later hyperactivity. Clinical Pediatrics, 26(5), 253–257.

[52] Hagerman, R. J., Murphy, M. A., & Wittenberger, M. D. (1988). A controlled trial of stimulant medication in children with the fragile X syndrome. American Journal of Medical Genetics, 30(1–2), 377–392.

[53] Halmøy, A., Klungsøyr, K., Skjærven, R., & Haavik, J. (2012). Pre- and perinatal risk factors in adults with attention-deficit/hyperactivity disorder. Biological Psychiatry, 71(5), 474–481.

[54] Halperin, J. M., Wolf, L. E., Greenblatt, E. R., & Young, G. (1991). Subtype analysis of commission errors on the continuous performance test in children. Developmental Neuropsychology, 7, 207–217.

[55] Hasson, R., & Fine, J. G. (2012). Gender differences among children with ADHD on continuous performance tests: A meta-analytic review. Journal of Attention Disorders, 16(3), 190–198.

[56] Hill, D. E., Yeo, R. A., Campbell, R. A., Hart, B., Vigil, J., & Brooks, W. (2003). Magnetic resonance imaging correlates of attention-deficit/hyperactivity disorder in children. Neuropsychology, 17(3), 496–506.

[57] Katz, J., & Tillery, K. L. (2005). Can central auditory processing tests resist supramodal influences? American Journal of Audiology, 14(2), 124–127, discussion 143–150.

[58] Kashdan, T. B., Jacob, R. G., Pelham, W. E., Lang, A. R., Hoza, B., Blumenthal, J. D., & Gnagy, E. M. (2004). Depression and anxiety in parents of children with ADHD and varying levels of oppositional defiant behaviors: Modeling relationships with family functioning. Journal of Clinical Child and Adolescent Psychology, 33(1), 169-181.

[59] Kaye, S., & Darke, S. (2012). The diversion and misuse of pharmaceutical stimulants: What do we know and why should we care? Addiction, 107(3), 467–477.

[60] Keith, R. W. (1994). Auditory continuous performance test. San Antonio, TX: Psychological Corp.

[61] Keith, R. W., Rudy, J., Donahue, P. A., & Katbamna, B. (1989). Comparison of SCAN results with other auditory and language measures in a clinical population. Ear and Hearing, 10(6), 382–386.

[62] Keller, W. (1992). Auditory processing disorder or attention deficit disorder? In J. Katz, N. Stecker, & D. Henderson (Eds.), Central auditory processing: A transdisciplinary view (pp. 107–114). St. Louis, MO: Mosby.

[63] Keller, W. D., & Tillery, K. L. (2002). Reliable differential diagnosis and effective management of auditory processing and attention deficit hyperactivity disorders. Seminars in Hearing, 23, 337–347.

[64] Kiernan, K. E., & Huerta, M. C. (2008). Economic deprivation, maternal depression, parenting and children's cognitive and emotional development in early childhood. British Journal of Sociology, 59(4), 783–806.

[65] Kim, G. H., Kim, J. Y., Byeon, J. H., et al. (2012). Attention deficit hyperactivity disorder in epileptic children. Journal of Korean Medical Science, 27(10), 1229–1232.

[66] Kivisaari, S., Laasonen, M., Leppämäki, S., Tani, P., & Hokkanen, L. (2012). Retrospective assessment of ADHD symptoms in childhood: Discriminatory validity of Finnish translation of the Wender Utah Rating Scale. Journal of Attention Disorders, 16(6), 449–459.

[67] Kobel, M., Bechtel, N., Specht, K., et al. (2010). Structural and functional imaging approaches in attention deficit/hyperactivity disorder: Does the temporal lobe play a key role? Psychiatry Research, 183(3), 230–236.

[68] Kollins, S. H., Rush, C. R., Pazzaglia, P. J., & Ali, J. A. (1998). Comparison of acute behavioral effects of sustained-release and immediate-release methylphenidate. Experimental and Clinical Psychopharmacology, 6(4), 367–374.

[69] Kudoh, M., & Shibuki, K. (2006). Sound sequence discrimination learning motivated by reward requires dopaminergic D2 receptor activation in the rat auditory cortex. Learning and Memory, 13(6), 690–698.

[70] Langley, K., Heron, J., Smith, G. D., & Thapar, A. (2012). Maternal and paternal smoking during pregnancy and risk of ADHD symptoms in offspring: Testing for intrauterine effects. American Journal of Epidemiology, 176(3), 261–268.

[71] Larson, K., Russ, S. A., Kahn, R. S., & Halfon, N. (2011). Patterns of comorbidity, functioning, and service use for US children with ADHD, 2007. Pediatrics, 127(3), 462–470.

[72] Lasky-Su, J., Banaschewski, T., Buitelaar, J., et al. (2007). Partial replication of a DRD4 association in ADHD individuals using a statistically derived quantitative trait for ADHD in a family-based association test. Biological Psychiatry, 62(9), 985–990.

[73] Lasky-Su, J., Biederman, J., Laird, N., et al. (2007). Evidence for an association of the dopamine D5 receptor gene on age at onset of attention deficit hyperactivity disorder. Annals of Human Genetics, 71(Pt. 5), 648–659.

[74] Latham, K. E., Sapienza, C., & Engel, N. (2012). The epigenetic lorax: Gene-environment interactions in human health. Epigenomics, 4(4), 383–402.

[75] Lee, P. C., Niew, W. I., Yang, H. J., Chen, V. C., & Lin, K. C. (2012). A meta-analysis of behavioral parent training for children with attention deficit hyperactivity disorder. Research in Developmental Disabilities, 33(6), 2040–2049.

[76] Lévesque, B., Duchesne, J. F., Gariépy, C., et al. (2003). Monitoring of umbilical cord blood lead levels and sources assessment among the Inuit. Occupational and Environmental Medicine, 60(9), 693–695.

[77] Lucker, J. R., Geffner, D., & Koch, W. (1996). Perception of loudness in children with ADD and without ADD. Child Psychiatry and Human Development, 26(3), 181–190.

[78] Luders, E., Narr, K. L., Hamilton, L. S., et al. (2009). Decreased callosal thickness in attention-deficit/hyperactivity disorder. Biological Psychiatry, 65(1), 84–88.

[79] Lyoo, I. K., Noam, G. G., Lee, C. K., Lee, H. K., Kennedy, B. P., & Renshaw, P. F. (1996). The corpus callosum and lateral ventricles in children with attention-deficit hyperactivity disorder: A brain magnetic resonance imaging study. Biological Psychiatry, 40(10), 1060–1063.

[80] Mahone, E. M. (2005). Measurement of attention and related functions in the preschool child. Mental Retardation and Developmental Disabilities Research Reviews, 11(3), 216–225.

[81] Mautner, V. F., Kluwe, L., Thakker, S. D., & Leark, R. A. (2002). Treatment of ADHD in neurofibromatosis type 1. Development Medicine and Child Neurology, 44(3), 164–170.

[82] McGoey, K. E., DuPaul, G. J., Haley, E., & Shelton, T. L. (2007). Parent and teacher ratings of attention deficit/hyperactivity disorder in preschool: The ADHD Rating Scale-IV Preschool Version. Journal of Psychopathology and Behavioral Assessment, 29, 269–276.

[83] Moore, D. R., Ferguson, M. A., Edmondson-Jones, A. M., Ratib, S., & Riley, A. (2010). Nature of auditory processing disorder in children. Pediatrics, 126(2), e382–e390.

[84] Morell, R. J., Brewer, C. C., Ge, D., et al. (2007). A twin study of auditory processing indicates that dichotic listening ability is a strongly heritable trait. Human Genetics, 122(1), 103–111.

[85] Morrow, R. L., Garland, E. J., Wright, J. M., Maclure, M., Taylor, S., & Dormuth, C. R. (2012). Influence of relative age on diagnosis and treatment of attention-deficit/hyperactivity disorder in children. Canadian Medicak Association Journal, 184(7), 755–762.

[86] Musso, M. W., & Gouvier, W. D. (2014). "Why is this so hard?": A review of detection of malingered ADHD in college students. Journal of Attention Disorders, 18, 186-201.

[87] Nabelek, A. K., Tucker, F. M., & Letowski, T. R. (1991). Toleration of background noises: Relationship with patterns of hearing aid use by elderly persons. Journal of Speech and Hearing Research, 34(3), 679–685.

[88] National Collaborating Center for Mental Health (NCCMH). (2009). Attention Deficit Hyperactivity Disorder: Diagnosis and management of ADHD in children, young people and adults. Leicester and London: The British Psychological Society and the Royal College of Psychiatrists.

[89] Needleman, H. L., McFarland, C., Ness, R. B., Fienberg, S. E., & Tobin, M. J. (2002). Bone lead levels in adjudicated delinquents: A case control study. Neurotoxicology and Teratology, 24(6), 711–717.

[90] Norrelgen, F., Lacerda, F., & Forssberg, H. (1999). Speech discrimination and phonological working memory in children with ADHD. Developmental Medicine and Child Neurology, 41(5), 335–339.

[91] Ostberg, M., & Rydell, A. M. (2012). An efficacy study of a combined parent and teacher management training programme for children with ADHD. Nordic Journal of Psychiatry, 66(2), 123–130.

[92] Peretz, I., Cummings, S., & Dubé, M.-P. (2007). The genetics of congenital amusia (tone deafness): A family-aggregation study. American Journal of Human Genetics, 81(3), 582–588.

[93] Pillsbury, H. C., Grose, J. H., Coleman, W. L., Conners, C. K., & Hall, J. W. (1995). Binaural function in children with attention-deficit hyperactivity disorder. Archives of Otolaryngology–Head and Neck Surgery, 121(12), 1345–1350.

[94] Quinn, C. A. (2003). Detection of malingering in assessment of adult ADHD. Archives of Clinical Neuropsychology, 18(4), 379–395.

[95] Riccio, C. A., Hynd, G. W., Cohen, M. J., Hall, J., & Molt, L. (1994). Comorbidity of central auditory processing disorder and attention-deficit hyperactivity disorder. Journal of the American Academy of Child and Adolescent Psychiatry, 33(6), 849–857.

[96] Riddle, M. A., Yershova, K., Lazzaretto, D., et al. (2013). The Preschool Attention-Deficit/Hyperactivity Disorder Treatment Study (PATS) 6-year follow-up. Journal of the American Academy of Child and Adolescent Psychiatry, 52(3), 264–278.

[97] Roessner, V., Banaschewski, T., Uebel, H., Becker, A., & Rothenberger, A. (2004). Neuronal network models of ADHD—lateralization with respect to interhemispheric connectivity reconsidered. European Child and Adolescent Psychiatry, 13 (Suppl. 1), I71–I79.

[98] Rosvold, H. E., Mirsky, Al. F., Sarason, I., Bransome Jr., E. D., & Beck, L. H. (1956). A continuous performance test of brain damage. Journal of Consulting Psychology, 20, 343-350.

[99] Salvi, R. J., Lockwood, A. H., Frisina, R. D., Coad, M. L., Wack, D. S., & Frisina, D. R. (2002). PET imaging of the normal human auditory system: Responses to speech in quiet and in background noise. Hearing Research, 170(1-2), 96–106.

[100] Sandford, J. A., & Turner, A. (1995). Manual for the Integrated Visual and Auditory Continuous Performance Test. Richmond, VA: Braintrain.

[101] Sciberras, E., Ukoumunne, O. C., & Efron, D. (2011). Predictors of parent-reported attention-deficit/hyperactivity disorder in children aged 6-7 years: A national longitudinal study. Journal of Abnormal Child Psychology, 39(7), 1025–1034.

[102] Schafer, E. C., Mathews, L., Mehta, S., et al. (2013). Personal FM systems for children with autism spectrum disorders (ASD) and/or attention-deficit hyperactivity disorder (ADHD): An initial investigation. Journal of Communication Disorders, 46(1), 30–52.

[103] Scheich, H., & Zuschratter, W. (1995). Mapping of stimulus features and meaning in gerbil auditory cortex with 2-deoxyglucose and c-Fos antibodies. Behavioural Brain Research, 66(1–2), 195–205.

[104] Schicknick, H., Schott, B. H., Budinger, E., et al. (2008). Dopaminergic modulation of auditory cortex-dependent memory consolidation through mTOR. Cerebral Cortex, 18(11), 2646–2658.

[105] Scottish Intercollegiate Guidelines Network (SIGN). (2009). Management of attention deficit and hyperkinetic disorders in children and young people: A national clinical guideline (SIGN Pub. No. 112). Retrieved from http://www.sign.ac.uk/pdf/sign112.pdf.

[106] Seidman, L. J., Valera, E. M., & Makris, N. (2005). Structural brain imaging of attention-deficit/hyperactivity disorder. Biological Psychiatry, 57(11), 1263–1272.

[107] Shaffer, D., Gould, M. S., Brasic, J., et al. (1983). A children's global assessment scale (CGAS). Archives of General Psychiatry, 40(11), 1228–1231.

[108] Sharma, M., Purdy, S. C., & Kelly, A. S. (2009). Comorbidity of auditory processing, language, and reading disorders. Journal of Speech, Language, and Hearing Research, 52(3), 706–722.

[109] Sowell, E. R., Thompson, P. M., Welcome, S. E., Henkenius, A. L., Toga, A. W.,& Peterson, B. S. (2003). Cortical abnormalities in children and adolescents with attention-deficit hyperactivity disorder. Lancet, 362(9397), 1699–1707.

[110] Stark, H., & Scheich, H. (1997). Dopaminergic and serotonergic neurotransmission systems are differentially involved in auditory cortex learning: A long-term microdialysis study of metabolites. Journal of Neurochemistry, 68(2), 691–697.

[111] Stevens, C., Fanning, J., Coch, D., Sanders, L., & Neville, H. (2008). Neural mechanisms of selective auditory attention are enhanced by computerized training: Electrophysiological evidence from language-impaired and typically developing children. Brain Research, 1205, 55–69.

[112] Stevens, S. E., Sonuga-Barke, E. J., Kreppner, J. M., et al. (2008). Inattention/overactivity following early severe institutional deprivation: Presentation and associations in early adolescence. Journal of Abnormal Child Psychology, 36(3), 385–398.

[113] Sutcliffe, P. A., Bishop, D. V. M., Houghton, S., & Taylor, M. (2006). Effect of attentional state on frequency discrimination: A comparison of children with ADHD on and off medication. Journal of Speech, Language, and Hearing Research, 49(5), 1072–1084.

[114] Swanson, J. M., Elliott, G. R., Greenhill, L. L., et al. (2007). Effects of stimulant medication on growth rates across 3 years in the MTA follow-up. Journal of the American Academy of Child and Adolescent Psychiatry, 46(8), 1015–1027.

[115] Talge, N. M., Holzman, C., Van Egeren, L. A., et al. (2012). Late-preterm birth by delivery circumstance and its association with parent-reported attention problems in childhood. Journal of Developmental and Behavioral Pediatrics, 33(5), 405–415.

[116] Taylor, A., Deb, S., & Unwin, G. (2011). Scales for the identification of adults with attention deficit hyperactivity disorder (ADHD): A systematic review. Research in Developmental Disabilities, 32(3), 924–938.

[117] Thakur, G. A., Sengupta, S. M., Grizenko, N., Schmitz, N., Pagé, V., & Joober, R. (2013). Maternal smoking during pregnancy and ADHD: A comprehensive clinical and neurocognitive characterization. Nicotine and Tobacco Research, 15(1), 149–157.

[118] Thapar, A., Cooper, M., Eyre, O., & Langley, K. (2013). What have we learnt about the causes of ADHD? Journal of Child Psychology and Psychiatry, 54(1), 3–16.

[119] Theusch, E., Basu, A., & Gitschier, J. (2009). Genome-wide study of families with absolute pitch reveals linkage to 8q24.21 and locus heterogeneity. American Journal of Human Genetics, 85(1), 112–119.

[120] Tillery, K. L., Katz, J., & Keller, W. D. (2000). Effects of methylphenidate (Ritalin) on auditory performance in children with attention and auditory processing disorders. Journal of Speech, Language, and Hearing Research, 43(4), 893–901.

[121] Todd, R. D., Huang, H., & Henderson, C. A. (2008). Poor utility of the age of onset criterion for DSM-IV attention deficit/hyperactivity disorder: Recommendations for DSM-V and ICD-11. Journal of Child Psychology and Psychiatry, 49(9), 942–949.

[122] Toplak, M. E., Rucklidge, J. J., Hetherington, R., John, S. C. F., & Tannock, R. (2003). Time perception deficits in attention-deficit/hyperactivity disorder and comorbid reading difficulties in child and adolescent samples. Journal of Child Psychology and Psychiatry, 44(6), 888–903.

[123] Toplak, M. E., & Tannock, R. (2005). Time perception: Modality and duration effects in attention-deficit/hyperactivity disorder (ADHD). Journal of Abnormal Child Psychology, 33(5), 639–654.

[124] Toplak, M. E., West, R. F., & Stanovich, K. E. (2013). Practitioner review: Do performance-based measures and ratings of executive function assess the same construct? Journal of Child Psychology and Psychiatry, 54(2), 131–143.

[125] Tucha, L., Sontag, T. A., Walitza, S., & Lange, K. W. (2009). Detection of malingered attention deficit hyperactivity disorder. Attention Deficit Hyperactivity Disorder, 1(1), 47–53.

[126] U. S. Department of Health Services, National Institute of Health, National Institutes of Mental Health. (2008). Attention Deficit Hyperactivity Disorder (NIH Publication No. 08-3572). Retrieved from http://www.nimh.nih.gov/health/publications/attention-deficit-hyperactivity-disorder/adhd_booklet_cl508.pdf.

[127] U.S. Environmental Protection Agency. (2006). Air quality criteria for lead (Vol. 1, Section 3.1.2). Research Triangle Park, NC: Author, Office of Research and Development, National Center for Environmental Assessment–RTP Division. Retrieved from http://cfpub.epa.gov/ncea/cfm/recordisplay.cfm?deid=158823.

[128] Vaughan, B., & Kratochvil, C. J. (2012). Pharmacotherapy of pediatric attention-deficit/hyperactivity disorder. Child and Adolescent Psychiatric Clinics of North Ericaca, 21(4), 941–955.

[129] Venkatesh, C., Ravikumar, T., Andal, A., & Virudhagirinathan, B. S. (2012). Attention-deficit/hyperactivity disorder in children: Clinical profile and co-morbidity. Indian Journal of Psychological Medicine, 34(1), 34–38.

[130] Ward, M.F., Wender, P. H., & Reimherr, F. W. (1993). The Wender Utah Rating Scale: An aid in the retrospective diagnosis of childhood attention deficit hyperactivity disorder. American Journal of Psychiatry, 150(6), 885–890.

[131] Willcutt, E. G. (2012). The prevalence of DSM-IV attention-deficit/hyperactivity disorder: A meta-analytic review. Neurotherapeutics, 9(3), 490–499.

[132] World Health Organization (WHO). (1992). International classification of diseases (10th ed.). Retrieved from http://www.who.int/classifications/icd/en/GRNBOOK.pdf.

[133] Zwi, M., Jones, H., Thorgaard, C., York, A., & Dennis, J. A. (2011). Parent training interventions for attention deficit hyperactivity disorder (ADHD) in children aged 5 to 18 years. Cochrane Database of Systematic Reviews, 7(12), CD003018.

Chapter 14

Language-related Impairments and Auditory Processing Deficits

14 Language-related Impairments and Auditory Processing Deficits

Difficulties in processing rapidly occurring acoustic elements in speech have the potential to slow down speech and language acquisition and/or make the ongoing processing of such stimuli difficult, especially in demanding listening environments, including background noise. As expected, some children with auditory processing deficits (APDs) have speech, language, and reading impairments. In a sample of children suspected of APDs, 67% had language and/or reading deficits (Sharma, Purdy, & Kelly, 2009). Thus, comprehensive language evaluations of children diagnosed with APDs are recommended (Fey et al., 2011).

Some children with language or related impairments show APDs, although considerable individual variability has been noted in children with specific language impairments (Bishop & McArthur, 2005), as well as phonological impairments (Lallier, Thierry, & Tainturier, 2013). APDs are more obvious in children who have both language and reading impairments (McArthur & Bishop, 2001). Performance in some auditory processing tasks, such as frequency discrimination, is highly correlated with formant discrimination (speech perception), reading abilities (Ahissar, Protopapas, Reid, & Merzenich, 2000), and detecting verb-agreement violations (Weber-Fox, Leonard, Wray, & Tomblin, 2010). In children with dyslexia, subtypes have been identified showing that some of these children have phonological deficits (O'Brien, Wolf, & Lovett, 2012), and some with severe phonological dyslexia can have relatively intact orthographic coding (Peterson, Pennington, & Olson, 2013). Individuals with dyslexia may have difficulty generating or exploiting neural discharges that are phase-locked to the fine structures in auditory stimuli, as apparent from reduced frequency discrimination, masking level differences (MLDs), and amplitudes of frequency following responses (McAnally & Stein, 1996).

Because of the co-occurrence of APD and language-related impairments (▶ Fig. 14.1), this chapter offers a brief review of speech and language-related impairments and APDs in such children. The review focuses on school-aged children, as the diagnoses of APD are confirmed at age 7 years. However, as discussed in other chapters in this book, children who are at risk for APD can be screened at an earlier age, and appropriate management can begin earlier. For more detailed information related to speech/language impairments, readers are encouraged to refer to several textbooks that are devoted to this topic (e.g., Kaderavek, 2014; Leonard, 2014).

14.1 Language

Language can be considered a code for representing ideas about the world through a conventional system of signals for communication (Bloom & Lahey, 1978) using specific rules. The things that the symbols such as apple represent are called referents. Referents can be objects, concepts, or ideas. Specific rules guide how symbols can be combined and in what sequence or how to use them in various situations. The various components of language are represented in ▶ Fig. 14.2. Humans are usually born with an innate ability to learn language, but language is learned using the code of the linguistic community in which an infant is reared.

14.2 Speech

Speech is the oral expression of language and is possible through the sensorimotor processes stored in the central nervous system. Each spoken language has specific sounds referred to as phonemes and specific sound combinations. Speech includes other dimensions, such as rate, voice quality, intonation, and fluency.

14.3 Risk Factors for Speech/ Language Impairments

Prenatal risk factors for language-related impairments include a family history of language disorders, premature birth, and alcohol consumption during pregnancy leading to fetal alcohol spectrum disorder. Natal risk factors include low birth weight. Postnatal risk factors include poor nutrition, failure to thrive, and poor speech/language environments. Other more obvious causes of speech/language impairment are hearing loss, intellectual disabilities, syndromes such as Down and fragile X, cerebral palsy, tumors, strokes, and brain injury. In many of these cases, language impairment is accompanied by other conditions, such as

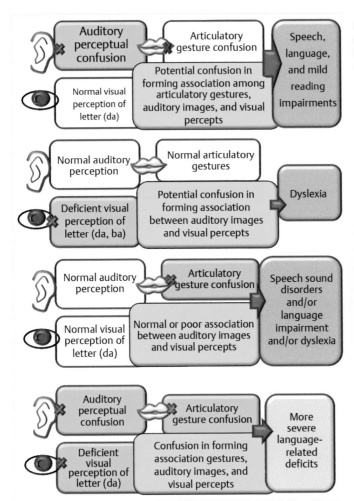

Fig. 14.1 A highly simplistic model showing the relationship of different language-related deficits using visual and/or auditory input /da/.

attention deficit hyperactivity disorder (ADHD) and learning disabilities. In some children, the causes of the impairments are not known. Physiological defects such as cleft palate or lip, if not repaired early, can lead to some speech sound disorders.

14.4 Communication Disorders

Three subtypes of communication disorders can be identified, as shown in ▶ Fig. 14.3. These are social communication, language, and speech disorders. The term *social communication disorders* refers to persistent difficulties in the social uses of verbal and nonverbal communication in the absence of restrictive repetitive behaviors, interests, and activities. In some cases, underlying language impairments can lead to a social communication disorder.

14.4.1 Language Impairment

Some children fail to learn language, and some or all components of language that are depicted in ▶ Fig. 14.2 can be affected. Language impairments can be further classified into two subtypes: late language emergence and specific language impairment. Language development can be delayed in some children due to various causes discussed above. Effective strategies used for managing developmental delays should address the underlying cause (e.g., poor nutrition) or deficit (e.g., hearing loss).

Specific Language Impairment

Children with specific language impairment do not learn language as rapidly and as effectively as their normal peers in the presence of normal hearing,

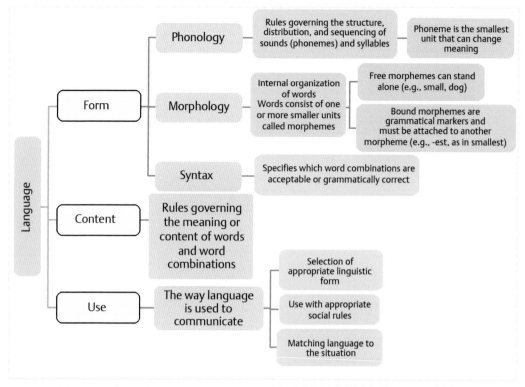

Fig. 14.2 The components of language.

normal nonverbal intelligence test scores, and no obvious neurologic damage (Leonard, 1998). Impairment can be apparent in several aspects of language shown in ▶ Fig. 14.2, including phonology (production of intelligible speech), morphology (e.g., difficulty with plurals, as in *boys* and *girls*), syntax (e.g., use of syntactically simpler sentences, shorter length of utterances), semantics (e.g., smaller vocabulary, word-finding difficulties), and pragmatics (e.g., fewer occurrences of communication initiations). In some children with specific language impairments, the difficulties in proper use of language or pragmatics may be related to underlying deficits in phonology, morphology, and syntax of language.

14.4.2 Speech Disorders

Speech disorders can be classified as voice, speech sound, motor speech, and child onset fluency disorders. Central auditory processing plays an important role in the development and use of normal speech (Tekieli Koay, 1992). An underlying APD may be the cause of some speech sound disorders.

Speech Sound Disorders

Different classification systems have been used to describe the subtypes of speech sound disorders. One such classification is depicted in ▶ Fig. 14.4.

Potential Impact of Speech Impairment in Childhood

A systematic review by Baker and McLeod (2011) suggested that speech impairment in childhood may be associated with the following activity limitations and/or participation restrictions:
- Communication
- Forming relationships with friends/peers, siblings, and parents
- Relating to persons in authority
- Learning to read, write, and calculate
- Educational achievements
- Focusing attention and thinking
- Mobility and self-care
- Acquiring, maintaining, and terminating a job

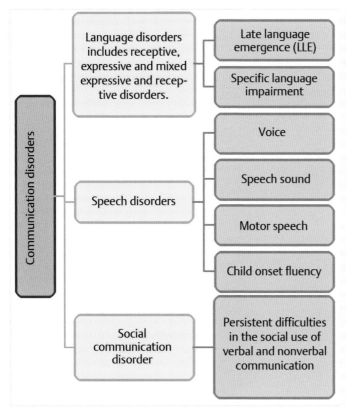

Fig. 14.3 Subtypes of communication disorders as given in the fifth edition of the *Diagnostic and Statistical Manual of Mental Disorders* (American Psychiatric Association, 2013).

14.5 Indicators for Speech and/or Language Assessment

Assessments are usually performed when a child is referred after screening of speech and/or language abilities. The screenings are performed at periodic intervals during regularly scheduled visits to pediatricians or at preschools or schools. Referrals for assessments can be made by related professionals, such as neurologists, audiologists, and special education teachers. Assessments can be performed on children who are considered at risk for speech and/or language impairments due to comorbid conditions such as ADHD (see Chapter 13). In addition, ongoing assessments are performed for individuals who have known speech and/or language impairments.

14.6 Purpose of Assessing Individuals with Speech/Language Impairments

The assessment can serve a variety of purposes, including the following:

- Deciding if a child has a speech and/or language problem or is at risk for related problems, such as reading or writing difficulties
- Detecting the cause of the problem or the factors that are related to the problem, such as malnutrition and chronic otitis media
- Specifying strengths and weaknesses (For example, the individuals may have strong phonemic awareness, but may have poor expressive language skills. In this case, the strength in phonemic awareness can be used to improve expressive language.)
- Determining the impact of speech, language, or communication impairment on activities and participation
- Determining any barriers or facilitators for normal speech and/or language acquisition and use
- Determining if a child is qualified for services
- Developing an intervention plan

14.7 Language Assessment

Ideally, a comprehensive language assessment includes the following components (American Speech-Language-Hearing Association [ASHA], 2004):

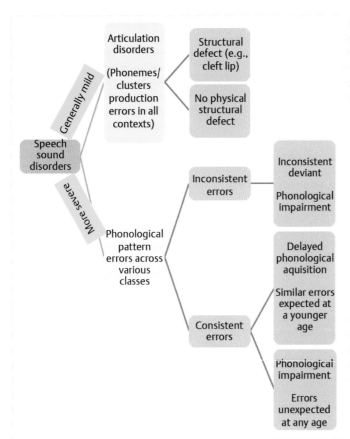

Fig. 14.4 Classification of speech sound disorders with a milder or more severe impact on speech intelligibility.

- Case history, including relevant prenatal, natal, and postnatal factors, current medical status, current performance in education settings, and socioeconomic, cultural, and linguistic backgrounds. Information obtained through written case history forms should be verified and augmented through patient/client and family interviews.
- Review and analysis of the current status of relevant modalities that can affect language acquisition or maintenance, including the auditory, visual, motor, and cognitive status
- Standardized measures of spoken and nonspoken language and cognitive communication with consideration for documented ecological validity. Effective communication encompassing listening, reading, speaking, writing, reading facial expressions, understanding tone of voice, etc., results from a complex interaction between cognition, language, and speech. Cognition includes attention, memory, abstract reasoning, awareness, and executive functions such as self-monitoring, flexibility, etc. Deficient cognition (e.g., from traumatic brain injuries) can lead to

inefficient communication or cognitive communication disorders. Cognitive communication disorders are communication impairments related to nonlinguistic cognitive functions such as attention, perception and memory and impairment of linguistic skills such as semantic, syntactic or pragmatic skills (Coelho, DeRuyter, & Stein, 1996). Ecological validity refers to the extent to which results from the standardized measures reflect communication problems experienced by the patient in real-life settings.

- Nonstandardized sampling or observation of spoken and nonspoken language and cognitive communication with consideration for ecological validity with reference to the individual's sociocultural experiences, educational curriculum, and vocational needs
- Assessment of knowledge and use of language for listening, speaking, reading, writing, and thinking across the following components:
  - Phonology and printed, orthographic symbols
  - Syntactic structures
  - Semantic relationships
  - Discourse structures

○ Pragmatic conventions (verbal and nonverbal)
○ Effective use of metacognitive and self-regulatory strategies to meet language and literacy demands. Metacognition involves awareness of, thinking about, and understanding one's own thought process. For example, someone with memory deficits may chunk large pieces of information into smaller units by grouping similar concepts and objects together to enhance memory and recall of information. An individual with an auditory processing deficit may use self-regulating coping strategies such as recognizing when they have difficulty in recognizing a message and finding a solution for improving communication. Thus, if there is TV in the background, they may turn the volume of the TV down before proceeding with communication.
• Assessment of the impact of speech/language impairments on the individual's participation in educational, social, and vocational activities
• Examination of strengths and contextual factors that influence the individual's relative success or difficulty in educational, social, and vocational activities (e.g., for adults with aphasia)
• Exploration of potential effective intervention and any compensatory strategies
• Identification of follow-up services, including monitoring of cognitive communication status for children and adolescents with identified spoken and written language disorders

14.8 Speech Assessment

In addition to the case history and the review of current auditory, visual, motor (including oral motor screen), and cognitive status, speech assessment can include the following measures (ASHA, 2004):
• Standardized measures of articulation accuracy and/or phonological assessment with documented ecological validity
• Spontaneous speech samples in different communication environments
• Assessment of speech intelligibility for connected speech:
○ One unfamiliar listener can listen to the sample of 100 or more words and can write down words that are intelligible and note the words that are unintelligible by placing a dash. Intelligibility percentage is calculated by dividing the number of intelligible words by the total number of words sampled. Approximate estimates

of age-appropriate intelligibility are 50% at age 2 years, 75% at age 3, and 100% at age 4. A child with poorer than expected speech intelligibility is considered to be at risk for language impairments (Coplan & Gleason, 1988).
• Perform error analyses to determine if the deficit is primarily related to difficulty in producing speech or is associated with phonological constraints. For example, a child might be deaffricating affricates (e.g., *chew* replaced by *shoe*).
• Perform relational analysis to compare the patient's performance with adult or age-expected target performance
• Independent analyses using a phonetic inventory
• Identification of follow-up intervention and support services as necessary

14.8.1 Speech Consistency

In addition to the above, consistency of speech sound productions can be assessed. A child may be asked to repeat 25 words three different times to determine how consistently the words are repeated. He or she may show inconsistent production of a particular phoneme in different word positions. For example, the child may correctly say /f/ in the initial position, as in *fig,* may replace it with /p/ in a final position (*cup* for *cuff*), and may replace it with /t/ in the middle position (*cate* for *cafe*). Another type of inconsistency occurs when a particular sound is replaced by various phonemes in the same position within a word. A third type of inconsistency is marked by inconsistent production of a particular phoneme in multiple repetitions of the same word and is considered to be a definitive characteristic of inconsistent speech disorder if the child has age-appropriate oral-motor skills and normal prosodic patterns and shows improved accuracy on imitation (Dodd, Holm, Crosbie, & McCormick, 2005). Typically developing children show generally consistent speech patterns with minor improvement in consistency with age. Inconsistency is not a prominent feature of speech development, even in 3-year-olds (Holm, Crosbie, & Dodd, 2007). Children between the ages of 3 and 3½ years yield a mean inconsistency score of 12.96%. Based on 2.5 standard deviations (SD) above the mean, 40% inconsistency scores are considered to be indicative of an inconsistent speech disorder (Dodd, 1995).

14.9 Interventions for Language Impairments

Various intervention approaches have been used for treating children with language impairments. Examples of some of the general approaches are shown in ▶ Table 14.1. Examples of approaches that attempt to address underlying causes or deficits are shown in ▶ Table 14.2. In addition to the above, factors leading to the maintenance of the impairment should be addressed (e.g., dysfunctional caregiver–child relationships, chronic otitis media, and malnutrition).

The authors of one systematic review found relatively little evidence supporting the language intervention practices used with school-aged children with language disorders and identified the following critical needs in the study of language intervention practices (Cirrin & Gillam, 2008).

1. High-quality language intervention studies with school-aged children with language disorders
2. Quality research examining the use of contingent language facilitation procedures (e.g., modeling, imitation, recasts, and focused stimulation) or other language facilitation strategies
3. Research on the long-term effectiveness of various language interventions
4. Research that examines the efficacy and effectiveness of language intervention on the receptive language abilities of school-aged students with language disorders
5. Efficacy and effectiveness studies of computer-based language intervention programs used in school settings
6. Efficacy and effectiveness studies of intervention methods designed to teach topic initiation, topic maintenance and relevance, and other conversational discourse skills, including the use of language to form and enhance peer social interactions within and outside the classroom
7. Narrative outcomes for prestory interventions (e.g., semantic word mapping and directed reading/thinking activities), during-story intervention methods (e.g., extensions, questioning, and episode/story mapping), poststory intervention methods (e.g., question–answer relationships, dramatic play, and story generation), and interventions for narrative and expository text comprehension questions
8. Studies on positive effects of language intervention on students' classroom language performance and related outcomes, such as progress in reading, writing, and math
9. Studies to show the amount and frequency of intervention required to make significant progress on language targets

14.10 Interventions for Speech Sound Disorders

Several approaches have been recommended for addressing speech sound disorders. Three of these are described below.

14.10.1 Phonological Awareness Program

The goal of phonological awareness intervention is to improve awareness of the sound structure and the links between the spoken forms of letters/words and their written forms. Examples of the different types of awareness taught during phonological intervention are given in ▶ Fig. 14.5 (Anthony & Lonigan, 2004). For linking speech to print, grapheme–phoneme correspondence activities are included in the training. An example of an activity related to this is identifying the named letter from a choice of letters (Gillon, 2002).

Direct instruction with explicit focus on phoneme segmentation is more effective than indirect instruction in phonological awareness. Direct instruction is most effective if it is offered after an initial treatment for building literacy consisting of exposure to various experiences with oral and written language. For increasing effectiveness, general language instruction should be offered before phonological awareness training (Ayres, 1995). Korkman and Peltomaa (1993) assigned 26 boys with language impairments to a program aimed at minimizing future reading/writing difficulties. The treatment included phonemic awareness exercises and grapheme-phoneme conversions on a two-letter syllable level. A control group of 20 boys with language impairments received mostly conventional speech/language therapy. At the end of the first school year, the experimental group performed significantly better than the control group on three of four reading and spelling tests, and also improved significantly on four tests of language and attention. The control group showed no significant improvement on any tests. In another study, children with specific language impairment improved their speech articulation, phonological awareness ability, and reading development following phonological awareness intervention (Gillon, 2000), and these improvements were maintained over time (Gillon, 2002).

Table 14.1 Examples of Techniques that Focus on Targeting Symptoms of Language Impairment

Treatment	Primary Target Population	Primary Goals	Key Features
Focused stimulation approach (Leonard, 1981; Weismer & Robertson, 2006)	Toddlers with language delays and children with developmental disabilities, or specific language impairments	Promoting form, content, and use of language	Exposure of the child to multiple examples of a specific linguistic target (e.g., a specific word or grammatical morpheme) within meaningful communications contexts Facilitation of spontaneous production of the target by taking advantage of natural contexts that enhance use of the target
Enhanced milieu teaching (Hancock, & Kaiser, 2006)	Children who are capable of imitating verbal models of adults but have specific language impairment, intellectual disabilities, autism spectrum disorders, or severe disabilities	Promotion of functional uses of productive language and communication skills in naturalistic interactions	A hybrid naturalistic conversation-based strategy with three components: 1. Environmental arrangement to support language learning and teaching (e.g., arranging for the occurrence of natural opportunities to promote language and natural positive consequences of using language) 2. Responsive interaction, which includes a set of behaviors that maintain the child's interest and provides linguistic models that are a little ahead of the child's current skills 3. Milieu teaching, which can include modeling an elaboration of a child-initiated utterance (e.g., *doll*: "I want the doll"), requesting a verbal utterance from the child (e.g., the child points at the ball and the clinician says, "What do you want?"), and encouraging a verbal utterance by pausing or using time delay
Conversational recast intervention (Camarata & Nelson, 2006; Nelson, 1977)	Children with specific language impairment, hearing impairment, intellectual disability, or autism spectrum disorders	Increasing use of all linguistic forms, including phonemes, words, grammatical morphemes, grammar, and complex sentences	Child's utterances are immediately recast to provide linguistic models that maintain the intended meaning of the child's utterance but are somewhat linguistically more advanced than the child's original utterance (e.g., grammatical forms are corrected or added or alternative grammatical forms are provided)

Table 14.2 Examples of Techniques that Attempt to Address Deficits Underlying Language-related Impairments

Treatment	Primary Target Population	Primary Goals	Key Features
HOPE Words based on auditory verbal therapy (http://hope.cochlearamericas.com/listen-ing-tools/HOPEWords)	Children with cochlear implants	Exposing children to all speech sounds through listening to establish strong auditory skills. Provide practice in auditory self-monitoring skills. Facilitate vocabulary development.	Interactive flash cards for the full alphabet are organized by the speech sounds in the English language. For each letter of the alphabet, there are 20 different flash cards illustrating words and images that contain the letter. For letters that have two different associated speech sounds (A as in *way* and *cat*), the flash cards are organized by the speech sound and are assigned 10 different flash cards. Children touch on a word or image on a mobile device, and the image enlarges, accompanied by a voice narration. The child can practice auditory self-monitoring by listening to a word and matching his or her speech production to what he or she heard. Vocabulary development is facilitated as the child begins to attach meaning to the spoken word paired with the pictured image. Parents are expected to encourage their children to listen and imitate the words and to interact with children and talk about the pictures.
Functional communication training (Carr & Durand, 1985; Lambert, Bloom, & Irvin, 2012)	Individuals with challenging or problematic behaviors, including severe and profound intellectual disabilities, autism spectrum disorders, and pervasive developmental disorders	Decreasing the frequency of problem behaviors and increasing functionally equivalent and socially acceptable communication behaviors with the assumption that problem behaviors may function as a means of communication	Assessment of the communication function of each problem behavior and replacing the behavior with a socially acceptable communication behavior that serves the same function using behavioral or operant teaching techniques

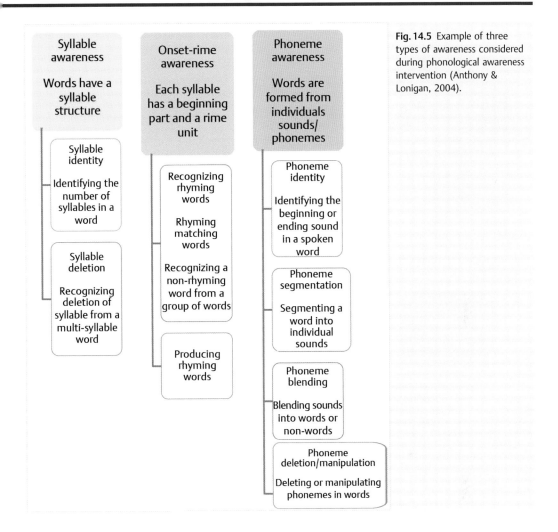

Fig. 14.5 Example of three types of awareness considered during phonological awareness intervention (Anthony & Lonigan, 2004).

14.10.2 Cycles of Phonological Patterns Approach

The cycles approach to improving speech intelligibility targets deficient phonological patterns apparent in a child's speech 40% or more of the time. The major steps incorporated in the cycles approach are shown in ▶ Fig. 14.6. In this approach, the child is cycled through several different targeted phonological patterns (▶ Fig. 14.7 and ▶ Fig. 14.8) regardless of the level of accuracy achieved on each pattern and with a rest period before recycling a previous pattern. The cycles approach exposes the child to various model phonological patterns without overemphasizing mastery of specific targets (Hodson, 2011; Hodson & Paden, 1991; Stoel-Gammon, Stone-Goldman, & Glaspey, 2002).

14.10.3 Ling's Approach to Improving Speech Intelligibility in Children with Hearing Loss

Ling's (1976) speech development program for children is based on the assumption of the requirement of five distinctive mechanisms for the development of spoken language, as shown in ▶ Fig. 14.9. The approach assumes that the child must meet the following conditions before being able to acquire speech: (1) differentiate between speech sounds, (2) derive meaning from the sounds made by other individuals in the environment, and (3) be aware of how well his or her speech sounds compare to those made by other individuals. In this approach, close attention is paid to breathing, voicing, and suprasegmental patterns, in addition to articulation

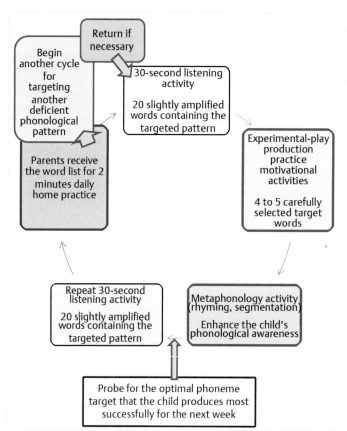

Fig. 14.6 Key steps for targeting each deficient phonological pattern in the cycles approach.

patterns to improve speech intelligibility. Most easily audible (voiced vs. unvoiced) and/or visible (front vs. back) speech sounds or characteristics (voiced vs. unvoiced or front vs. back) are targeted first before progressing to sounds that are difficult to hear or see. Examples of target behaviors for voice in increasing order of difficulty are shown in ▶ Fig. 14.10.

14.10.4 Need for Research in the Treatment of Speech Sound Disorders

In a narrative review of evidence-based practice for children with speech sound disorders, Baker and MacLeod (2011) identified a need for collaborative research with rigorous experimental designs. Other conclusions from this review are as follows.

Limited Generalizability to Clinical Practice

Most intervention studies had a small sample size. In addition, studies with a higher level of evidence used specific inclusion/exclusion criteria, limiting generalizability to the usual clinical settings.

Uncertainty about the Amount and Type of Sufficient Intervention

There is a need to understand the average amount and type of intervention that is sufficient to lead to intelligible speech.

Need for Effectiveness Studies

There is a need for studies designed to examine the outcomes of previously established efficacious interventions within the constraints of regular

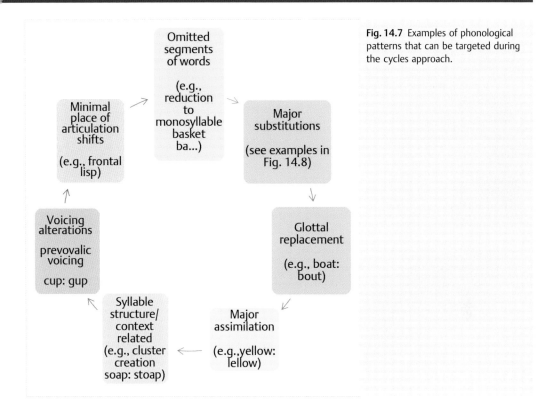

Fig. 14.7 Examples of phonological patterns that can be targeted during the cycles approach.

clinical practice settings that have to address complex circumstances, such as missed appointments and variations in cooperation from parents and caregivers (Fey & Finestack, 2009).

Lack of Consensus on the Sounds or Phonological Processes that Should Be Targeted First for Treatment

Some investigators recommend prioritization of stimulable early-developing phonemes to build on the child's preexisting strengths and to stabilize emerging forms (Rvachew & Bernhardt, 2010; Rvachew & Nowak, 2001), whereas others recommend priority for nonstimulable later-developing phonemes (Gierut et al., 1996).

Need for Studies Comparing the Effectiveness of Different Approaches

Twenty-three different approaches, as cited in Baker and MacLeod (2011), have been studied,

and the results suggest that intervention is better than no intervention. However, rigorous, well-designed studies designed to compare the efficacy and effectiveness of various approaches are necessary.

Need for Assessment of Long-Term Benefits of Intervention

Because children with speech sound disorders are at increased risk for literacy and math difficulties, an assessment of the long-term benefits of intervention is needed that focuses on attention, thinking, and other difficulties (McCormack, McLeod, McAllister, & Harrison, 2009). Long-term follow-up is necessary to ensure that children achieve their full potential. Children with comorbid speech sound disorders and language impairment may be especially at risk for deficits in preliteracy skills or dyslexia (Peterson, Pennington, Shriberg, & Boada, 2009; Sices, Taylor, Freebairn, Hansen, & Lewis, 2007).

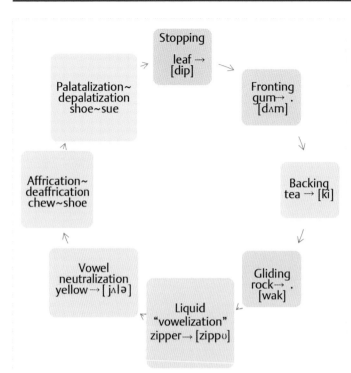

Fig. 14.8 Examples of major substitutions that can be targeted during the cycles approach for improving speech intelligibility.

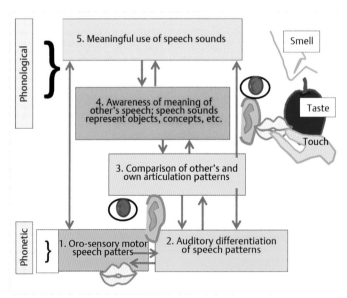

Fig. 14.9 Five mechanisms considered necessary for the development of spoken language (based on Ling, 1976).

14.11 Difficulty in Establishing Best Evidence

It is difficult to provide best evidence using the medical model of randomized controlled trials in children with speech, language, and auditory processing impairments because of the tremendous amount of heterogeneity among children presenting with these impairments and the variability of impact of these deficits on language, educational, and social development. Some children with language impairments may recover spontaneously, whereas others may be left with a significant language disability despite long-term therapy

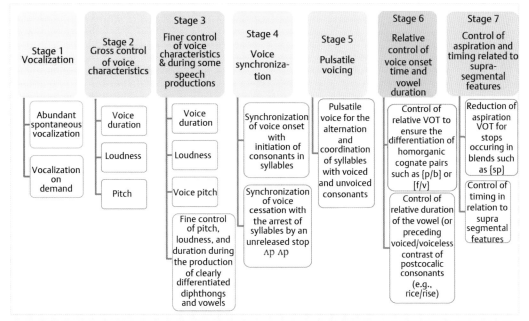

Fig. 14.10 Target behaviors for voice based on the Ling (1976) model for speech training for children with hearing loss. VOT, voice onset time.

(Leonard, 1998). For example, many adolescents with a specific language impairment appear to be less sensitive to tense-marking and non-tense-marking morpheme errors in sentences (Leonard, Miller, & Finneran, 2009; Miller, Leonard, & Finneran, 2008) even after therapy during childhood. Each child has unique needs that can only be met with unique interventions that consider family and cultural dynamics. It is well known that a single-treatment approach cannot be used with all children. Management of some children requires accurate selection and sequencing of different approaches (Dodd & Bradford, 2000).

In clinical settings, efficient clinicians are likely to follow a hybrid approach that includes a variety of speech and language interventions that target the impaired components of speech and/or language, consider any underlying deficits (including APDs) in planning sessions, accommodate for family and cultural dynamics, ensure the use of learned skills in all environments, and minimize future language-related impairments, such as reading and writing difficulties. The effectiveness of such interventions is difficult to document using large samples, which is possible in clinical drug trials with diseases using medical models of treatment effectiveness. Also, from an ethical standpoint, it is difficult to justify the inclusion of some

children who need treatment in the no treatment or control groups due to the relatively limited time window of critical periods of language development and the impact of language impairments on social and educational achievement. However, clinicians can employ single-subject designs (see Chapter 12) in ensuring that the treatment is effective for each child and make appropriate changes if it appears ineffective. In addition, clinicians need to be aware of current research literature and evaluate the possibility of revising their techniques.

14.12 Auditory, Speech, and Oral Language Processing

The auditory signal that conveys oral language is marked by brief or transient spectrotemporal events that follow each other very rapidly. For example, stop consonant syllables [ba] and [pa] are differentiated by the voice onset time (VOT), which is the brief gap between the release burst by the articulators and the onset of voicing. In American English, the VOT for [ba] is usually less than 25 ms, and that for [pa] is usually greater than 40 ms. Thus, oral language processing is partially based on exquisite temporal resolution over extended

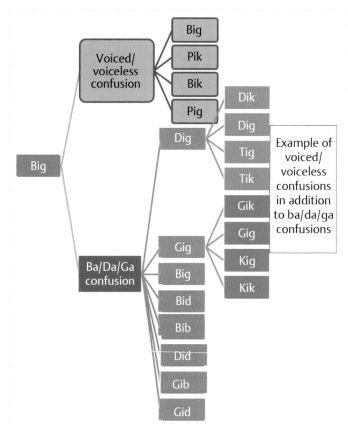

Fig. 14.11 Examples of perceptual confusion due to difficulty in discriminating gap durations (voice onset times) and/or capturing of rapid spectral transitions occurring within short time periods.

time periods (Hickok & Poeppel, 2007; Johnson, Nicol, Zecker, & Kraus, 2007; Telkemeyer et al., 2009).

Children with specific language impairments have temporal processing deficits that can lead to difficulties in developing phonological abilities necessary to map phonemes and to effectively and automatically code and decode words (▶ Fig. 14.11) and sentences. In one study, investigators hypothesized that, because syntactic processing is dependent on the correct ordering of different elements, it would be correlated with temporal pattern perception (Fortunato-Tavares et al., 2009). They found that children with specific language impairments performed poorly on the Test of Syntactic Complexity Comprehension compared to a control group, and their performance on the frequency or pitch pattern test (see Chapter 5) was poor. In addition, their performance on the pitch pattern test was correlated with syntactic complexity comprehension, and the correlation was stronger for sentences with higher syntactic complexity compared to those with

lower syntactic complexity (Fortunato-Tavares et al., 2009). Deficits involved in processing rapid stimuli may explain the particular difficulties children with specific language impairments have with short-duration grammatical inflections as shown by frequent omissions of such inflections (Leonard, 1998).

14.13 Auditory Processing Skills in Children with Language-related Impairments

14.13.1 Temporal Resolution

Studies that evaluate the ability to detect the minimal gap between two sounds by indicating whether one or two sounds are heard suggest that children with specific language impairments show significantly poorer temporal resolution compared to children in the control group at 4 kHz. These significant group differences occur due to a subgroup of children with poorer temporal resolution,

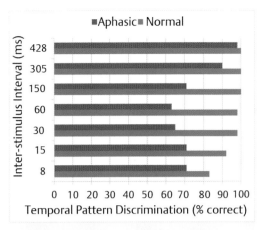

Fig. 14.12 Effect of the interstimulus interval on temporal pattern discrimination accuracy (average % correct scores) in children with aphasia and age-matched controls (based on Tallal & Piercy, 1973).

suggesting that only some children with specific language impairments demonstrate poorer temporal resolution at 4 kHz (Ahmed, Parker, Adams, & Newton, 2006). At lower frequencies, such as 1 kHz, the gap detection of children with language or literacy impairment appears to be normal (Boets, Wouters, van Wieringen, & Ghesquière, 2007; Lowe & Campbell, 1965).

14.13.2 Temporal Order Judgment Threshold

Children with specific language impairments need significantly longer interstimulus intervals (mean 400 ms) than a control group (mean 26 ms) for the accurate judgment of temporal order of auditory stimuli (Nickisch & Massinger, 2009). In one study, 1 out of 14 children with oral language delays and reading disorders could not perform the temporal order judgment threshold, and 5 of out 11 children in the oral language delay group showed abnormally high temporal order judgment thresholds (Heath, Hogben, & Clark, 1999). This led to significantly higher temporal order judgment thresholds in children with oral language delays and reading disorders (mean 237.7 ms) compared to normal age-matched children (mean 73 ms). In another study, the temporal order judgment thresholds of eight children with aphasia ranged from 55 to 700 ms (mean 357 ms), while those of eight children in the control group ranged from 15 to 80 ms (mean 36.1 ms). The difference in the two groups was statistically significant (Lowe & Campbell,

1965). In one early study, adults with expressive aphasia and lesions in the left temporal cortex needed a separation of approximately 575 ms to achieve 100% correct temporal order judgment and approximately 400 ms to achieve 75% correct judgments. Although phonemes occurred every 80 ms, these patients could understand speech probably due to redundancies inherent in spoken language (Efron, 1963).

14.13.3 Temporal Pattern Judgment

The performance of many children with dyslexia is poorer than normal children on the pitch pattern sequence task (Simões & Schochat, 2010) and the duration pattern sequence task (King, Lombardino, Crandell, & Leonard, 2003).

14.13.4 Temporal Pattern Discrimination

Children with reading impairments yield more errors than average readers in making "similar" or "different" judgments when presented with two rhythmic patterns, each with two tones (McGiven, Berka, Languis, & Chapman, 1991). Likewise, children with aphasia have difficulty in making "similar" or "different" judgments when presented with two 75 ms complex tone patterns containing two tones differing in their fundamental frequency (100 and 305 Hz). They need a separation of 305 ms to achieve 90% accuracy. The same accuracy can be achieved by age-matched normal children when the two tone patterns are separated by lower (15 ms) interstimulus intervals, as shown in ▶ Fig. 14.12 (Tallal & Piercy, 1973). Similar difficulties are apparent in adults with dysphasia with damage to the left hemisphere (Tallal & Newcombe, 1978).

14.13.5 Processing of Structural and Acoustic Attributes of Music

Individuals who have difficulty processing acoustic and structural attributes of music are characterized as having amusia. Individuals with congenital amusia have more difficulty decoding emotional expressions (e.g., happy, tender, irritated, or sad) in spoken phrases compared to matched controls. They also report difficulty understanding emotional prosody in their daily lives (Thompson, Marin, & Stewart, 2012). This may lead to difficulty in social

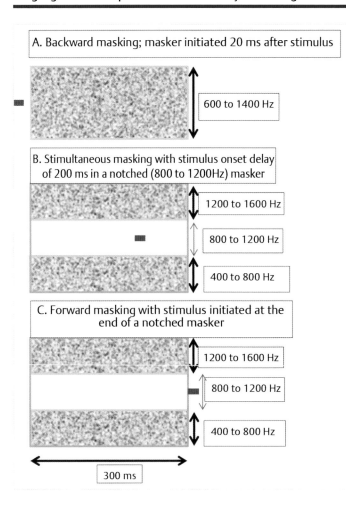

A. Backward masking; masker initiated 20 ms after stimulus

600 to 1400 Hz

B. Stimultaneous masking with stimulus onset delay of 200 ms in a notched (800 to 1200Hz) masker

1200 to 1600 Hz

800 to 1200 Hz

400 to 800 Hz

C. Forward masking with stimulus initiated at the end of a notched masker

1200 to 1600 Hz

800 to 1200 Hz

400 to 800 Hz

300 ms

Fig. 14.13 Approximate illustrations of backward, simultaneous, and forward masking configurations used by Wright et al. (1997). The stimulus was a 20 ms, 1000 Hz tone (*purple*).

communication situations where nonprosodic cues about emotions may not be available.

14.13.6 Stream Segregation Thresholds

Significantly higher auditory stream segregation thresholds (182 ms ± 32 ms) have been reported in patients with phonological disorders compared to a control group (125 ms ± 25 ms) with a significant correlation between these thresholds and phonological skills. More specifically, up to 78% (7/9) of individuals with comorbid phonological disorders and dyslexia yielded significantly higher auditory stream segregation thresholds (Lallier et al., 2013).

14.13.7 Backward Masking

Several studies have shown poorer performance on backward-masking tasks (▶ Fig. 14.13 a) by children with language impairments compared to children in control groups (Marler, Champlin, & Gillam, 2001; Wright et al., 1997). In addition, better backward-masking performance is related to better ability to repeat sentences (Marler, Champlin, & Gillam, 2002). A subset of children with both language and reading impairment yield poorer thresholds in backward-masking tasks compared to normal children (McArthur & Hogben, 2001)

14.13.8 Notched Masking

Simultaneous Masking with Stimulus Onset Delay

Children with language impairments have poorer thresholds compared to normal children when the 20 ms tone of 1000 Hz begins with a 200 ms delay after the initiation of a 300 ms noise (400

–1600 Hz) with a notch at the center around 1000 Hz (800–1200 Hz) (▶ Fig. 14.13 b) (Wright et al., 1997).

Forward Masking with a Notched Masker

Children with language impairment have poorer thresholds compared to normal children when a 20 ms tone of 1000 Hz is turned on immediately after a 300 ms noise (400–1600 Hz) with a notch at the center around 1000 Hz (800–1200 Hz) (▶ Fig. 14.13 c) (Wright et al., 1997).

14.13.9 Intensity Discrimination

A subset of children with specific language impairment or reading impairments yield poorer intensity discrimination thresholds than children in the control group (McArthur & Hogben, 2001).

14.13.10 Duration Discrimination

Some adults with reading disabilities show deficits in duration discrimination for a 1000 Hz tone (Watson, 1992). Several other studies have indicated duration discrimination deficits (see Chapter 5) in individuals with dyslexia.

Just Noticeable Differences in Voice Onset Time

As mentioned previously, the perception of contrasts between certain consonants, such as /d/ versus /t/, is dependent on the VOT, or the time between the release of the initial part of the consonant sound and the beginning of voicing. The minimum VOT difference necessary to differentiate between /d/ and /t/ can be defined as the just noticeable difference (JND) for /d/ or /t/. For example, when the VOT is within 20 ms, in most instances the sound is recognized as /d/; when the VOT increases to 35 ms, most often the sound is perceived as /t/ (Liberman, Delattre, & Cooper, 1958). Thus, the detection of the differences in duration between VOTs (e.g., 20 ms or less vs. 35 ms or more, or approximately 15 ms difference) provides an important cue for the differentiation between voiced and voiceless consonants. Children with language-based impairments need larger differences in VOTs to differentiate between voiced and voiceless consonants compared to children in a control group. These findings suggest that children with language impairments may confuse words such as *bet* versus *pet* that differ minimally or are spoken by someone in a nonstandard dialect (Elliott, Hammer, & Scholl, 1989). This is confirmed by a study that showed that children with specific language impairments have more difficulty in differentiating voicing contrasts (/apa/ vs. /aba/) in the presence of background noise when compared to children in a control group (Ziegler, Pech-Georgel, George, & Lorenzi, 2011).

14.13.11 Frequency Discrimination Deficits

Children with specific language impairments are less accurate than normal children in detecting a 2000 Hz target tone among other standard tones of 1000 Hz when the tones are presented with either 200 or 1000 ms interstimulus intervals (Weber-Fox et al., 2010). Individuals with reading difficulties have difficulty in discriminating brief tones of different frequencies (deWeirdt, 1988). Difficulties with frequency discrimination can continue in adulthood and appear to be related to retention of reading difficulties. In addition, frequency discrimination is highly correlated with both formant discrimination (speech perception) and reading abilities (Ahissar et al., 2000).

Just Noticeable Differences in Frequency

The JNDs for frequency are significantly poorer in children with specific language impairments (mean 126 Hz, range 85–155 Hz) than those in the control group (mean 24 Hz, range 7–79 Hz) (Nickisch & Massinger, 2009). Adults with dyslexia need larger differences in frequency to notice a change in frequency compared to individuals in a control group (France et al.; 2002; McAnally & Stein, 1996). JNDs in frequency are significantly correlated with phonological skills in children (Talcott et al., 2000, 2002).

Just Noticeable Differences in Second and Third Formant Frequencies

A continuum of consonant-vowel (CV) stimuli can be created representing the place-of-articulation feature embedded in syllables ([ba-da-ga]). The major acoustic differences along this continuum are the onset frequencies of the second and third formants. The smallest acoustic difference among the CV syllables that can be detected is the JND, which can be measured relative to /da/. Thus, the minimal difference necessary to detect the change from /da/ to /ba/ can be referred to as JNDB, or the minimum difference necessary to detect the change from /da/ to /ga/ can be referred to as JNDG. Children with language-based impairments need larger frequency differences to detect the changes compared to children in a control group (Elliott et al., 1989).

14.13.12 Frequency Modulation Detection

Patients with Wernicke aphasia (severely impaired single-word comprehension) show significant impairment in detecting frequency modulation (FM) at both fast (40 Hz) and slow (2 Hz) rates when the carrier frequency is 500 Hz compared to controls (Robson, Grube, Lambon Ralph, Griffiths, & Sage, 2012). Children with reading impairments need larger modulation depths to detect a 2 Hz frequency modulation of a 1 kHz carrier tone compared to children in a control group (Boets et al., 2007).

14.13.13 Dynamic Modulation Detection

Patients with Wernicke aphasia show significant impairment in detecting dynamic modulation at slow, intermediate, and high rates when compared to controls, which suggests a deficit in the spectro-temporal analysis of dynamic cues relevant to speech. In addition, their detection thresholds are significantly correlated with their speech comprehension and phonological scores (Robson et al., 2012).

14.13.14 Masking Level Difference

Adults with dyslexia have a smaller MLD for a 1000 Hz tone compared to a matched control group (McAnally & Stein, 1996).

14.13.15 Dichotic Speech Listening

Children with specific language impairments show poorer performance on dichotic tests (Dlouha, Novak, & Vokral, 2007), such as the Staggered Spondaic Word (SSW) test and dichotic digits, with deficient performance in the left ear when compared to children who do not have language impairments (Miller & Wagstaff, 2011). Some individuals with dyslexia show poorer performance in the left ear when listening to dichotic words (Moncrief & Musiek, 2002) and digits and poorer performance in the right ear when listening to dichotic CV syllables (Moncrieff & Black, 2008). Poor performance on the dichotic digits task by some individuals with dyslexia has been confirmed in other studies (Simões & Schochat, 2010).

14.13.16 Dynamic Localization

When children with specific language impairments are asked to track the apparent motion of a fused auditory image in front of them, moving from 45 degrees on the left side and 45 degrees on the right side with a 6-degree step size, using a laser pointer, their tracking accuracy is poorer than age-matched controls even though they show normal sensorimotor reaction times and normal tracking accuracy of a visual image (Visto, Cranford, & Scudder, 1996).

14.13.17 Dichotic Pitch

Some individuals with dyslexia have difficulty perceiving dichotic pitch when compared to average readers, which suggests a deficit in the use of binaural cues to extract sound streams from noisy backgrounds (Dougherty, Cynader, Bjornson, Edgell, & Giaschi, 1998). Individuals with dyslexia and poor dichotic pitch thresholds yield greater cortical activity for random noise and lower activity for a dichotic melody. Behavioral performance on phonological reading is correlated to cortical activity generated by dichotic pitch in the right Heschl gyrus and the right superior temporal sulcus (Partanen et al., 2012).

14.14 Electrophysiological Evidence of Auditory Processing Deficits in Language-related Impairment

14.14.1 Frequency Following Response

The frequency following responses of children with specific language impairments show degraded phase-locked activity (significantly reduced amplitudes), suggesting difficulty in faithfully tracking tonal sweeps, especially at higher stimulus rates, compared to age-matched children (Basu, Krishnan, & Weber-Fox, 2009). Children with language-related learning problems yield smaller amplitudes of the frequency following response over the 229 to 686 Hz range in response to /da/, which is the first formant of the /da/ stimulus, suggesting poor representation of crucial components of speech sounds that could cause perceptual confusions (Wible, Nicol, & Kraus, 2004). Similarly, the average amplitudes of the frequency following response are significantly smaller in adults with dyslexia when compared to those in a matched control group (McAnally & Stein, 1996)

14.14.2 Auditory Brainstem Response

Children with specific language impairments show significantly longer latencies of wave III of the click-evoked auditory brainstem response (ABR). In addition, a greater prolongation of wave III is apparent with an increase in stimulus rates when compared to children in a control group (Basu et al., 2009).

Binaural Interaction Component of the Click-Evoked Auditory Brainstem Response

The binaural interaction component of the ABR tends to be less prominent in children with specific language impairments. In addition, some children with specific language impairments yield smaller amplitudes of the binaural interaction component of the ABR evoked with clicks compared to age-matched children. Some aspects of the binaural interaction component are correlated with the measures of expressive and receptive morphosyntactic skills (Clarke & Adams, 2007). Children with severe to moderate language impairments similarly show reduced amplitude of the binaural interaction component in the domain of ABR wave V compared to children in a control group (Gopal & Pierel, 1999).

Speech-Evoked Auditory Brainstem Response

The ABR evoked with the five-formant syllable /da/ in children with language impairments shows longer latencies and smaller amplitudes of the harmonics in the frequency range of 721 to 1154 Hz when compared to typically developing children

(Rocha-Muniz, Befi-Lopes, & Schochat, 2012). Some children with language-based learning problems show significantly shallower slopes of wave V-V(n) and less sharpness in response to the onset of /da/ compared to normal children (Wible et al., 2004). These studies confirm deficient encoding of important acoustic features that could lead to perceptual confusions as are apparent in behavioral measures.

14.14.3 Steady-State Evoked Response

Children with receptive language impairments show absent or diminished steady-state auditory evoked responses for FM depths ranging from 20 to 100 Hz compared to normal children, showing deficient FM analyses (Stefanatos, Green, & Ratcliff, 1989).

14.14.4 Late Auditory Potentials

Bishop and McArthur (2005) reported immature or abnormal late auditory potentials (N1-P2-N2) evoked by using oddball (600 vs. 700 Hz tones of 25 ms duration) paradigm in a large proportion of individuals with specific language impairments. Most of the differences were related to waveform shapes rather than the traditionally reported measures of latencies or amplitudes.

14.14.5 Cortical Potentials in Response to Speech in Noise

Cortical responses to /da/ in the presence of noise are not as well correlated as normal children in some children with language-related impairments (Wible, Nicol, & Kraus, 2002).

14.14.6 P300

Adolescents with specific language impairments show significantly reduced amplitudes of the P300 in response to an oddball stimulus paradigm, including a target tone of 2000 Hz and a standard tone of 1000 Hz, when the interstimulus interval is 200 ms (Weber-Fox et al., 2010).

14.14.7 Evoked Auditory Gamma Activity

Children with language learning impairments show reduced amplitude and phase synchronization of

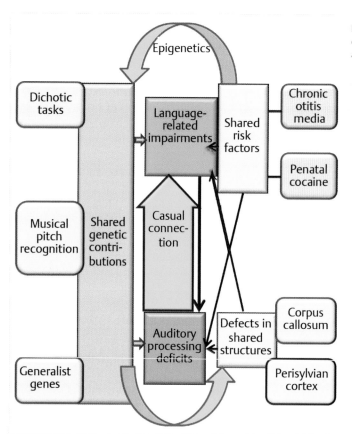

Fig. 14.14 Possible reasons for the comorbidity of auditory processing and language impairment.

early (45–75 ms) oscillations in the gamma band range (29–52 Hz) to the second of two tones presented with a brief gap of 70 ms when compared to children in a control group. This may be due to reduced synchronization in the Hebbian cell assemblies underlying phoneme representation (Heim, Keil, Choudhury, Thomas Friedman, & Benasich, 2013).

14.15 Reasons for Comorbidity of Auditory Processing Deficits and Language-related Impairments

There are several possible reasons (▸ Fig. 14.14) for APDs and language-related impairments to co-occur. Considering the heterogeneity of both disorders, the reasons are expected to vary for each individual, and more than one reason is possible in several cases. Some of these reasons are discussed below.

14.15.1 Shared Genetic Influences

Dichotic Listening Performance

Preliminary results suggest possible genetic influences on certain auditory processing tasks. Analyses of test correlations among 106 monozygotic (MZ) and 33 dizygotic (DZ) twin pairs has shown that dichotic listening ability is a highly heritable trait similar to height or insulin-dependent diabetes (Morell et al., 2007). Dichotic listening performance is poor in patients with mutations of the *PAX6* gene with associated reduction of interhemispheric fibers (Bamiou et al., 2004). Poor performance on dichotic tests has been reported in individuals with specific language impairments (Dlouha et al., 2007; Miller & Wagstaff, 2011) and dyslexia (Moncrieff & Black, 2008; Moncrief & Musiek, 2002; Simões & Schochat, 2010). Performance on dichotic listening performance can correctly classify 42% of the reading impaired samples, and if combined with other measures of executive functions, it can improve the classification accuracy to 90.74% (Asbjørnsen, Helland, Obrzut, & Boliek, 2003).

Musical Pitch Recognition and Speech Prosody Perception

Twin studies show that the variation in musical pitch recognition as measured by the Distorted Tunes Test, which requires listeners to judge whether simple popular melodies contain notes with incorrect pitch, is primarily related to highly heritable differences (Drayna, Manichaikul, de Lange, Snieder, & Spector, 2001). Congenital amusia, which is a deficit in processing musical pitch but not musical time, tends to be present in 39% of first-degree relatives, suggesting genetic transmission of the deficit (Peretz, Cummings, & Dubé, 2007). Deficits seen in amusics extend to deficits in speech processing. Individuals with amusia who speak a tonal language such as Mandarin show deficits in classifying prosody as appropriate or inappropriate during a speech comprehension task (Jiang et al., 2012). Independent studies of British and French Canadian amusics show that about 30% of amusics have difficulty discriminating a statement from a question on the basis of a final pitch fall or rise (Patel, Wong, Foxton, Loch, & Peretz, 2008). Compared with controls, amusics also show impaired performance in identifying and imitating statements and questions with embedded pitch direction differences in the final word (Liu, Patel, Fourcin, & Stewart, 2010). Approximately 30% of individuals with dyslexia may have difficulty in identifying pitch contours (Santurette et al., 2010).

Absolute Pitch Perception and Language Processing

At least one gene appears to promote the genesis of absolute pitch (the rare ability to label tones with their musical note names without using a reference) in individuals of European ancestry (Theusch, Basu, & Gitschier, 2009). There appears to be a close phenotypic and genetic relationship between absolute pitch and synesthesia with linkage on chromosomes 2 and 6q (Gregersen et al., 2013). Musicians with absolute pitch skills show significantly higher connectivity in the perisylvian language areas in the brain compared to relative pitch musicians and nonmusicians. The perisylvian areas are involved in higher-order auditory, working, and semantic memory processes (Jäncke, Langer, & Hänggi, 2012). Absolute pitch processors appear to be significantly quicker in identifying syllables from their first language, which suggests superior basic speech processing (Masataka, 2011).

Auditory Processing Deficits and Language Impairments

Auditory perceptual deficits are more likely in older language-impaired children with a positive family history of language/learning disorders than in those matched for language deficits but with a negative family history, suggesting a shared genetic component (Tallal, Townsend, Curtiss, & Wulfeck, 1991). The heritability of specific language impairments appears to depend on how the children are identified for inclusion in a study. Studies that include cases who have speech difficulties and who have been referred for intervention are more likely to show high heritability (Bishop & Hayiou-Thomas, 2008). Evidence of both speech and language deficits is more likely in children who have underlying APDs. The genetic connection is stronger between speech disorder and later reading, whereas language acquisition is prompted by both genetic and environmental factors (Hayiou-Thomas, 2008).

Generalist Genes

Many genes appear to be "generalists"; they have broad effects on development and can lead to several developmental phenotypes. Language is highly correlated genetically with general cognitive ability, reading skills, mathematics (Chow, Ho, Wong, Waye, & Bishop, 2013 Davis, Haworth, & Plomin, 2009) and writing (Olson et al., 2013). Twin studies show significant genetic correlations between language and reading (.44) disabilities with a higher correlation of .80 between general cognitive and language disabilities (Haworth et al., 2009). Disruption of a gene encoding a forkhead-domain transcription factor, forkhead box protein P2 (FOXP2), is related to a severe developmental disorder of verbal communication, including articulation, linguistic, and grammatical impairments. FOXP2 is expressed in the inferior olives, thalamus, cerebellum, basal ganglia, and cortical plate. It appears to be involved in the development of cortico-striatal and olivocerebellar circuits involved in motor control, which suggests that impairments in sequencing of movement and procedural learning may be central to the FOXP2-related speech and language disorder (Lai, Gerrelli, Monaco, Fisher, & Copp, 2003).

14.15.2 Defects in Shared Brain Regions

Acquisition of language, reading, and writing is augmented when auditory information is processed properly and is integrated with information across other relevant brain regions. The main cortical auditory areas are the temporal lobe and the sylvian fissure with insula. The sylvian or lateral fissure divides the frontal and parietal lobe from the temporal lobe and contains the transverse temporal or Heschl gyri involved in auditory processing. Interhemispheric connection is accomplished through the corpus callosum.

Corpus Callosum

Auditory areas of the corpus callosum (posterior midbody/isthmus) are shorter in individuals with dyslexia compared to age-matched controls (von Plessen et al., 2002). Individuals with perinatal corpus callosum damage show less accurate timber discrimination with slower reaction times during "same" or "different" judgment tasks at the age of 14 to 15 years. In addition, functional magnetic resonance imaging (fMRI) shows a deficit of activity in the right temporal lobe of the callosum-damaged group compared to an age-matched control group (Santhouse et al., 2002). Split-brain patients also have difficulty in verbally reporting intensity or frequency patterns (e.g., low-low-high) even though they can hum back the frequency patterns (Musiek, Pinheiro, & Wilson, 1980). Acallosal listeners are less accurate in localizing sounds occurring at midline and at other points in the auditory field than matched listeners (Poirier, Miljours, Lassonde, & Lepore, 1993). Right-handed patients with surgical sectioning of the corpus callosum have difficulty in repeating verbal stimuli presented to the left ear during dichotic listening tasks (Milner, Taylor, & Sperry, 1968; Musiek et al., 1989; Musiek & Wilson, 1979; Musiek et al., 1979). Left ear deficits are also apparent when patients with commissural section are presented with low-redundancy speech stimuli (Musiek et al., 1979). Children with callosal agenesis show deficits in phonemic discrimination (Temple & Ilsley, 1993). Other linguistic impairments are apparent in the presence of agenesis of the corpus callosum, including deficits in vocal prosody, phonological processing, syntax,

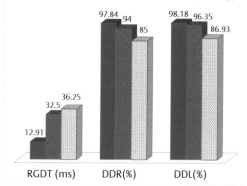

Fig. 14.15 Average random gap detection test (RGDT) and Dichotic Digits score in the Right (DDR) and Dichotic Digits score in the Left (DDL) ears in three groups of children (based on Boscariol et al., 2011).

pragmatics, restricted verbal expressions, and poor conversation skills (reviewed in Paul, 2011).

Perisylvian Cortex

Another example of a shared structure is the area surrounding the sylvian fissure known as the perisylvian cortex. The perisylvian cortex, along with the Wernicke area and the angular gyrus, integrates auditory and visual information important for language acquisition and literacy skills. If there are structural defects in these areas, auditory processing, speech, language, and reading can be impaired. An example of a structural anomaly is polymicrogyria, which is a developmental defect of the cortex characterized by several excessively small convolutions or gyri detectable using MRI. Children with polymicrogyria in the perisylvian cortex exhibit APDs (Fig. 14.15 Boscariol et al., 2010) and language-learning impairments (Boscariol et al., 2011). Children with diffuse polymicrogyria around the entire sylvian fissure may not speak at all or may show mixed phonologic and syntactic deficits. If the polymicrogyria are restricted only to the posterior aspects, the deficit may be restricted to phonologic programming (Guerreiro et al., 2002; de Vasconcelos Hage et al., 2006). Perisylvian polymicrogyria may be present in some cases with acquired aphasia associated with Landau–Kleffner syndrome (LKS) (Huppke, Kallenberg, & Gärtner, 2005). In familial polymicrogyria, children show developmental language disorders, whereas adults have the diagnoses of dyslexia showing co-occurrence of language and reading disorders in the presence of perisylvian polymicrogyria (Oliveira et al., 2008). Individuals with dyslexia also show neuronal ectopias and architectonic dysplasias mainly in the perisylvian region of the left hemisphere (Galaburda, Sherman, Rosen, Aboitiz, & Geschwind, 1985).

14.15.3 Shared Risk Factors

Prenatal Risk Factors

An example of a shared prenatal risk factor is maternal cocaine exposure during pregnancy. ABRs obtained from newborns with prenatal cocaine exposure show prolonged absolute (Tan-Laxa, Sison-Switala, Rintelman, & Ostrea, 2004) and interpeak latencies with greater prolongation of interpeak latencies with increased stimulus rates compared to nonexposed newborns (Cone-Wesson & Spingarn, 1993; Cone-Wesson & Wu, 1992; Lester et al., 2003; Salamy, Eldredge, Anderson, & Bull, 1990; Shih, Cone-Wesson, & Reddix, 1988). A reduced binaural interaction component is apparent in both the ABR and the auditory middle latency response in newborns with prenatal cocaine exposure compared to controls (Cone-Wesson, 2005). Infants with prenatal cocaine exposure show impaired auditory processing ability at the corrected gestational age of 38 to 39 weeks compared to age-matched controls during behavioral tasks (Potter, Zelazo, Stack, & Papageorgiou, 2000).

Prenatal cocaine exposure has a stable negative effect on receptive and expressive language skills at least during the first 6 years of life (Lewis et al., 2007). Greater prenatal cocaine exposure is related to more severe deficits in stable aptitudes for language skills (Bandstra, Vogel, Morrow, Xue, & Anthony, 2004). Subtle effects of prenatal cocaine exposure continue to appear for specific aspects of language, including syntax, semantics, and phonological processing, at the age of 10 years (Lewis et al., 2011).

Perinatal Risk Factors

An example of a shared perinatal risk factor is low birth weight. Up to 62% of infants with auditory neuropathy have low birth weight (Xoinis, Weirather, Mavoori, Shaha, & Iwamoto, 2007). Adolescents born with low birth weight show significantly poor left ear performance on dichotic tasks when they are asked to repeat the CV in the left ear first and then the one occurring in the right ear (Bless et al., 2013). Low birth weight is also a significant risk factor for the development of subsequent specific language impairments (Stanton-Chapman, Chapman, Bainbridge, & Scott, 2002).

Postnatal Risk Factors

An example of a shared postnatal risk factor is chronic otitis media. Infants with otitis media leading to degraded afferent signal transmission due to transient conductive hearing loss are at risk for developing central auditory impairment even after recovery of normal hearing (Whitton & Polley, 2011). Children with chronic otitis media in the right ear yield significantly poor scores on phonetic, phonological, and syntactic tasks compared to age-matched controls. In addition, their ABR power in the gamma frequency band (30 −60 Hz) is correlated significantly with phonetic scores, and the middle latency power in the same frequency band is correlated with both phonetic and phonologic scores (Uclés, Alonso, Aznar, & Lapresta, 2012).

14.15.4 Causal Connection

Children with hearing loss have difficulty in acquiring normal speech, language, and reading skills without intervention, and even a mild hearing impairment can interfere with educational and social development. Such findings show that normal auditory input is important for normal speech, language, and reading acquisition. Thus, another possible reason for the comorbidity of APDs and language-related impairments is a causal connection between the two. An underlying APD has the potential to lead to speech, language, and or reading problems, as shown in ▶ Fig. 14.16. The particular type of deficit need not be the same in all children with language-related problems. Deficits may occur in one or more types of processing (Amitay, Ahissar, & Nelken, 2002) discussed in this textbook.

In one study, performance on brief, rapidly presented, successive auditory processing and perceptual-cognitive tasks was assessed in infants with a family history of language impairments and those without such history. During the initial assessment at the age of 6 to 9 months, significant differences in mean thresholds of rapid auditory processing tasks were seen in the two groups of infants. Later testing revealed that threshold of rapid auditory processing at 7.5 months was the best predictor of emerging language at the age or 24 months. The same threshold when combined with being male

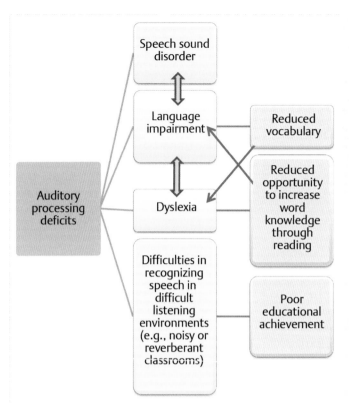

Fig. 14.16 Potential effects of auditory processing deficits.

predicted 39 to 41% of variance in language outcome at the age of 3 years. Thus, early deficits in rapid auditory processing abilities appear to precede and predict later language delays in some children (Benasich & Tallal, 2002).

The mismatch negativity (MMN) potentials of infants in response to bisyllabic words with different stress patterns suggest that infants are able to discriminate stress patterns in bisyllabic words (e.g., stress on the first syllable vs. stress on the second syllable) at the age of 5 months (Weber, Hahne, Friedrich, & Friederici, 2004). These MMN amplitudes can be used as a marker for later difficulties in speech production. When compared to matched controls, infants with very low production at the ages of 12 and 24 months display significantly reduced amplitudes of the MMN discrimination response to the trochaic stress (more stress on the first syllable) pattern in infancy, suggesting impaired prosodic processing of word stress during early development at the age of 5 months (Weber, Hahne, Friedrich, & Friederici, 2005).

It should be noted that not all children with hearing loss or APDs have language-related impairments. Some children can be expected to acquire normal speech and language skills due to the many contextual and situational redundancies available in language. This would be especially true in the presence of higher cognitive skills, including memory and abundant language stimulation at home in relatively quiet surroundings. Such children can be expected to rely more heavily on top-down processing strategies to both acquire and process spoken language in complex listening environments. However, their listening in complex environments can be enhanced through intervention, which may allow easier learning and better knowledge acquisition in educational environments.

14.16 Auditory Processing Evaluations in Children with Language Impairments

Audiologists should keep in mind that when language is impaired, children may not necessarily follow all test directions. It is important to keep the directions simple and to pay close attention to performance on practice test trials and the actual test trials. If responses suggest failure to understand instructions, the clinician needs to repeat the instructions and provide simpler practice test trials with associated visual cues. For example, for the random gap detection task, the child is required to indicate if he or she heard one or two sounds. The clinician can finger tap 1 or 2 sounds on a table in front of the child and ask the child to indicate the number of sounds heard. Once this task is mastered, the same activity can be repeated without visual cues before proceeding to the practice test trials of the actual test.

14.16.1 Use Simpler Tests

Some children with moderate to severe language impairments may have difficulty in mastering the concept of "same" or "different" judgments that are included in two forced-choice interval test paradigms (Fernell, Norrelgen, Bozkurt, Hellberg, & Löwing, 2002). Some children with language impairments have verbal working memory deficits (Leonard et al., 2007) and reduced memory scanning speeds (Sininger, Klatzky, & Kirchner, 1989). Performance on some tasks such as backward masking that involve visual and auditory senses or more than two forced-choice intervals can be compromised by nonverbal cognition or memory deficits. In such cases, the child is required not only to hear the signals, but to choose the correct interval based on visual images, such as three colored pictures requiring sensory mode shifts. These tasks require the child to hold the images of auditory stimuli in the short-term memory before providing a response. In one study involving the use of three forced-choice intervals, children with language impairments made a similar number of errors when the signal occurred during the first or the last (third) interval compared to children in the control group. However, more errors were apparent when the signal occurred during the second interval (Marler, Champlin, & Gillam, 2002), suggesting that the use of only two intervals could have minimized the influence of memory on test results.

Keep Response Requirements Simpler

Approximately 50% of children with language impairments also have dyslexia (McArthur, Hogben, Edwards, Heath, & Mengler, 2000), and some of these children may have associated visual processing deficits (Farmer & Klein, 1995). Thus, in testing auditory processing, requirements for processing visual stimuli displayed on computer screens (see an example in the previous paragraph), should be avoided. Also, asking children with dyslexia to choose a visual stimulus that matches the auditory stimulus may require more than just auditory processing as explained in the previous paragraph (e.g., greater cognitive effort involving memory and attention).

14.16.2 Minimize Boredom and Inattention

Each child should be monitored closely during both assessment and training for signs of inattention. Appropriate breaks should be provided as needed. Timely verbal reinforcements can significantly reduce boredom.

14.17 Training for Auditory Processing Deficits in Children with Language Impairments

In developing training for children, all comorbid conditions, such as ADHD and dyslexia, should be considered. For example, a child who has an APD and dyslexia may initially draw less benefit from auditory training that requires processing of visual stimuli, which is a requirement of many computer-driven programs. However, as the child becomes more confident about his or her auditory skills, visual components can be added to the training. Training designed to improve reading skills can improve language mastery related to technical vocabulary that is required in studying basic sciences. This, in turn, can improve educational achievements.

14.17.1 Improving the Efficiency of Speech/Language Therapy

Address the Underlying Deficit

It is important to address the underlying APD identified during the initial assessment using the strategies mentioned above and those described in Chapters 8 to 11. Depending on the particular deficit, part of the session can be devoted to addressing it until the child can perform like his or her peers. Addressing underlying APDs can result in improvement in phonological discrimination and language comprehension (Merzenich et al., 1996; Tallal et al., 1996), leading to improved efficiency of speech/language interventions. Engaging and adaptive auditory training designed to improve underlying temporal processing deficits can improve speech perception in children with language learning impairments (Nagarajan et al., 1998). Behavioral improvements in oral language and reading performance are accompanied by enhanced activation in relevant brain areas (Temple et al., 2003). In addition to improvement on standardized measures of language, computerized training designed to address underlying auditory deficits can improve neural mechanisms of selective auditory attention (Stevens, Fanning, Coch, Sanders, & Neville, 2008). When underlying APDs are addressed, even adults with aphasia who have specific sites of lesions show improvement (Dronkers et al., 1999). It is important to note that the training for addressing deficits should be based on the results of auditory processing evaluations. For example, if a child with language impairment does not have a temporal processing deficit, then training to improve temporal processing is unnecessary and is unlikely to lead to improvement in language skills.

14.17.2 Ensure Delivery of Ideal Sound Images

- For children with a weak ear as identified by ear deficits on dichotic tasks, the speech/language therapist should be on the side of the stronger ear. In group sessions, when possible, preferential seating arrangement should be offered in such a way that the stronger ear is facing the teacher. After the child has successfully completed ear strength balance or dichotic interaural intensity difference (DIID) training (see Chapter 10), this particular accommodation can be discontinued.
- For children with temporal processing deficits, use a slower speaking rate.
- Use a slightly louder stimulus delivery in quiet and low-reverberant surroundings. During individual (not group) therapy sessions in quiet environments with minimal reverberation, a slightly louder voice can deliver a distinct sound image to the child's ear with a better signal-to-noise ratio. For identification of monosyllabic words, children with learning problems need louder

levels compared to normal children (Elliott et al., 1979). Slightly louder delivery has already been integrated in some therapeutic approaches, such as the cycles approach (Hodson, 2007, 2011; Hodson & Paden, 1991).

- In relatively noisy environments such as classrooms, ensure a good signal-to-noise ratio to allow phonemic details to reach the child's ears with minimum degradation. Speech perception in noise is difficult for children with specific language impairments (Ziegler et al., 2011) and dyslexia (Boets et al., 2007; Dole, Hoen, & Meunier, 2012; Ziegler, Pech-Georgel, George, & Lorenzi, 2009). Phonological and phonemic awareness training is more effective when the signal-to-noise ratio is improved during training (Flexer, Biley, Hinkley, Harkema, & Holcomb, 2002). In noisy therapy rooms and classroom settings, personal FM devices can ensure good signal-to-noise ratio to the child's ears. In one randomized controlled study, 23 children with reading delays and ranging in from ages 6 to 11 years received a 6-week trial of personal FM systems. A significant improvement was noted in teachers' and children's ratings of classroom listening for difficult situations in the FM treatment group but not in the matched control group of 23 children (Purdy, Smart, Baily, & Sharma, 2009). In another study, after 1 year of use of an FM system, children with dyslexia showed improvement in their phonological awareness and reading skills, and their subcortical responses to sounds became less variable or more robust. A matched control group without FM devices did not show similar effects (Hornickel, Zecker, Bradlow, & Kraus, 2012).
- Use clear speech (see Chapter 8), which is produced by clear enunciations of all phonemes, deliberate pauses as appropriate to minimize slurring of words together, and stress on adjectives, verbs, and nouns (Picheny, Durlach, & Braida, 1985). When compared to conversational speech, clear speech is characterized by a slower speaking rate due to insertion of pauses between words and lengthening of durations of individual sounds. In conversational speech, when stops occur in the final position of a word, the associated bursts are often not released, whereas these are frequently released in clear speech. Vowels are frequently modified or reduced in conversational speech; in clear speech, vowels are modified to a lesser degree (Picheny, Durlach, & Braida, 1986). Elements in the 1000 to 3000 Hz range tend to

be louder in clear speech. In addition, low-frequency modulations have greater depth (Krause & Braida, 2004), which can make it easy to detect modulations. Clear speech is known to improve speech perception in noise in children with learning disabilities (Bradlow, Kraus, & Hayes, 2003).

Use Visual Aids

Use visual aids showing clear visual representations of speech, along with visual input, if possible. There are connections between auditory, visual, and articulatory areas that can be strengthened through auditory visual stimuli. For some patients, visual input may cause more confusion, but for others visual representations may improve speech/language processing or production. In one experiment, 13 patients with Broca aphasia were evaluated in three conditions: mimicking the speech of a talker whose mouth was visible on an iPod screen, mimicking a talker whose speech was only audible, and spontaneous speech (Fridriksson et al., 2012). When the mouth was visible, patients produced a greater variety of words when they could see the talker's mouth and hear the speech as compared to only hearing the speech or when speaking spontaneously. There was no difference when speaking spontaneously or when mimicking speech that could only be heard. This effect is most likely achieved through greater activation of brain areas involved in speech articulation. The authors of the study concluded that speech entrainment achieved through auditory-visual speech stimulation allows patients with Broca aphasia to double their speech output compared to spontaneous speech (Fridriksson et al., 2012).

14.18 Case Study

Consider the following patient, who was referred for a second opinion. The following is a summary of prior evaluations based on a file review of the patient, who was originally referred for an auditory processing and speech-language evaluation by the child's pediatrician. What types of recommendations can be made based on the file review?

14.18.1 Patient

The patient is a 9-year-old boy with supportive family.

14.18.2 Family History

The patient has no history of ADHD or hearing loss in the family.

14.18.3 Natal Risk Factors

The patient was delivered by emergency cesarean section. He was in the neonatal intensive care for 1 week due to transient tachypnea, or elevated respiratory rate.

14.18.4 Developmental History

All developmental milestones were within a normal range with the exception of speaking his first word, which was delayed until he was 3 years old.

14.18.5 Parent Concerns

The parents are concerned with poor academic progress, increasing frustration with schoolwork, and decreasing self-esteem due to academic struggles. The patient is beginning to notice he is different from his peers and is being teased for some of his struggles.

14.18.6 Current Academic Status

The patient is in an inclusive classroom and receives special education services in his regular classroom setting. He has completed third grade and will begin fourth grade in 1 month. Report cards indicate that the patient is behind grade level in all subject areas.

14.18.7 Teacher Concerns

Teachers report that the patient rushes through assignments and does not seek assistance when difficulties arise. He has difficulties following multiple-step directions and does not seem to process information.

14.18.8 Previous Evaluations

ADHD in the patient was ruled out through formal evaluation by a neuropediatrician. In 2006 the Differential Ability Scale Preschool Form indicated performance in the very low range, but the Developmental Activities Screening Inventory, second edition, suggested performance within normal limits. Results of other previous neuropsychological/educational assessments are shown in ▶ Table 14.3.

Table 14.3 Neuropsychological/Educational Assessment Results*

Area	Results

Intellectual abilities	Differential Abilities Scales, 2nd ed.
	• General cognition in the low average range
	Note from May 2010 based on Reynolds Intellectual Assessment
	• Low-average cognitive functioning
	  ○ Average nonverbal functioning
	  ○ Low-average verbal functioning

Academics	Wechsler Individual Achievement Test, 3rd ed. (WIAT III)
	• Basic reading and total reading:
	  ○ Average range
	• Written expression, mathematics, and math fluency:
	  ○ Below-average range
	Qualitative education assessment
	• Phonemic awareness, decoding, listening comprehension, word reading, oral fluency, and spelling:
	  ○ Relatively good performance
	• Expressive language, reading comprehension, written expression, and mathematics:
	  ○ Relatively weak areas
	• Across all academic areas:
	  ○ Sequencing difficulties as noted by struggles to organize information sequentially, solve problems in a specific order, and produce responses in an orderly fashion

Memory	Wide Range Assessment of Memory and Learning, 2nd ed. (WRAML-2):
	• General recognition memory and visual recognition:
	  ○ Superior range
	• Visual memory:
	  ○ High average
	• General memory, immediate verbal memory, attention/concentration, and verbal recognition:
	  ○ Average

Executive functioning abilities	Developmental Neuropsychological Assessment, 2nd ed. (NEPSY-II): • Executive functioning abilities well below expected level on some tasks, such as design fluency and comprehension of instructions to above expected level for word generation Behavior Rating Inventory of Executive Functioning (BRIEF) completed by the patient's mother and teacher: • Age appropriate with the possible exception of working memory
Overall adaptive function	Vineland Adaptive Behavior Scales: Parent/Caregiver Rating Report (VABS-II) completed by parents and teachers: • Adaptive behavior within the adequate range across all evaluated domains, including communication, daily living skills, and socialization

* Results from March 2011; only intellectual assessment results from May 2010.

14.18.9 Evaluation by Speech-Language Pathologists

A summary of all results from the various evaluations and recommendations is presented in ► Table 14.4. There is no indication of a formal evaluation of expressive language. The child reportedly discontinued therapy after 1 month of initiation of therapy.

14.18.10 Peripheral Hearing Assessment

Results of audiological evaluations are presented in ► Table 14.5. Findings show normal middle ear function, normal auditory sensitivity, and excellent speech recognition in quiet at most comfortable listening levels.

Table 14.4 Summary of Speech-Language Assessment, Services, and Recommendations

Age (years)	Description
2	Speech and language therapy initiated
3	Emergence of first word
7	Goldman–Fristoe Test of Articulation, 2nd ed. • Articulation: average range • Receptive language: average to below-average range • Expressive language: below-average to low range
Age 9	Word-Ordering Subtest of the Test of Language Development—Intermediate, 4th ed. Receptive language skills: below average, equivalent to 1-year younger children Peabody Picture Vocabulary Test, 4th ed. (PPVT-4) Receptive language skills: 27th percentile rank Behavioral observations: difficulty understanding multiple-step directions. Informal observation suggested that the patient appeared to have adequate expressive language skills but had difficulty finding the correct words when trying to explain more complex directions with reference to his video games. Test of Auditory Processing Skills, 3rd ed. (TAPS-3) 1. Phonologic Assessment Index: • Word discrimination • Phonological segmentation • Phonologic blending subtests ◦ Performance within developmentally normal range 2. Auditory Memory Index: • Number memory forward: below-normal performance • Number memory reversed: within normal range • Word memory: within normal range • Sentence memory subtests: below-normal performance 3. Auditory Cohesion Index: • Auditory comprehension: within normal limits • Auditory reasoning: below-normal limits; age-equivalent level of 5-years younger children. An example of an auditory reasoning task would be to tell the child, "When Jason fell out of the tree, he cried," then ask, "Why did Jason cry?" The correct response for this example would be "Jason got hurt when he fell," and an incorrect response would be "He fell out of the tree." 4. Optional auditory figure-ground subtest administered to test auditory attention: • Perfect scores for sets 1 and 2, indicating that attention was not a problematic factor in this assessment Recommendations: Language therapy was recommended to improve auditory reasoning, reading comprehension, and short-term memory.

14.18.11 Auditory Processing Evaluation

Objective Test Results

Acoustic Reflex Thresholds

Ipsilateral and contralateral thresholds were within normal limits in both ears, suggesting normally functioning connections between cochlear hair cells and auditory nerve fibers and normal low brainstem function.

Acoustic Reflex Threshold Decay

There was no significant decay in both ears, suggesting normal temporal maintenance of loud stimuli.

Behavioral Test Results

A summary of the conducted tests and administered screening measures is shown in ▶ Table 14.6 and ▶ Table 14.7. Performance on auditory closure, binaural interaction, and temporal resolution tasks is well within normal limits, showing normal skills

Table 14.5 Results of Peripheral Audiological Evaluation Conducted Prior to Auditory Processing Evaluation

Tests	Results
Otoscopy	Normal ear canals and tympanic membranes
Tympanometry	Suggested normal middle ear function
Acoustic reflex thresholds	Ipsilateral and contralateral thresholds within normal limits for 500, 1000, 2000, and 4000 Hz
Acoustic reflex decay	No decay noted at 500 or 1000 Hz ipsilaterally and contralaterally
Air conduction thresholds	Within normal limits, showing normal peripheral auditory sensitivity
Speech recognition thresholds	Within normal limits, confirming the results of air conduction thresholds
Speech recognition scores	Excellent recognition in quiet settings at most comfortable listening levels (100% in the right ear and 96% in the left ear)

Table 14.6 Percentage of correct scores on the Staggered Spondaic Word and SCAN-C Tests

Skill assessed	Test	Right Ear First Task		Left Ear First Task		Interpretation
		Right ear	Left ear	Right ear	Left ear	
Dichotic (binaural integration)	SSW test	70%	70%	80%	35%	Moderate impairment; Left ear deficit
		Significantly poor performance in LC, RC, RNC, and RLC conditions; significant ear and order effects; worst performance in the left ear competing condition.				
	Competing words (SCAN-C)	Right ear first task		Left ear first task		Left ear deficit
		Right ear	Left ear	Right ear	Left ear	
		60%	46.67%	100%	40%	
		Overall score: 25th percentile rank 2% of peers show the amount of right ear advantage in the left ear first task				
Dichotic (binaural separation)	Competing sentences (SCAN-C)	Right ear (ignore left ear)		Left ear (ignore right ear)		Left ear deficit
		100% correct		10% correct Normal cutoff is 74% at age 9 years (Bellis, 2003)		
		Overall score: 16th percentile rank				
Auditory closure	Filtered words (SCAN-C)	Right ear 70% correct		Left ear 85% correct		Normal
		25th percentile rank				
Speech perception in noise	AFG (SCAN-C)	Right ear 75% correct		Left ear 75% correct		Borderline normal

Abbreviation: AFG, auditory figure-ground; LC, left competing; RC, right competing; RNC, right non-competing; LNC, left non-competing; SSW, staggered spondaic word.

Table 14.7 Results of Binaural Interaction and Temporal Resolution Tests and Key Findings from Screening Questionnaires

Skill Assessed	Test	Score	Interpretation
Binaural interaction	Spondee masking level difference	11.5 (performance within normal limits of 5.5)	Normal
Temporal resolution	Random gap detection	Minimum gap detected: 5.2 ms Normal limits: 20 ms	Normal
Screening questionnaires			

Parental perception of listening performance at home	Children's Auditory Performance Scale	In noisy conditions:
		• Child unable to function
		  ○ When given complicated, multiple-step directions
		  ○ When not paying attention
		• Child has considerable or significant difficulty
		  ○ While listening to speech
			Poor performance in noisy conditions

	Children's Home Inventory for Listening Difficulties	Question from clinician: When the child is watching TV or playing with a noisy toy, walk into the room and talk to him or her without getting the child's attention. How difficult does it seem for your child to hear and understand the person? Response: The child misses all of the message.	

in these areas and no effect of any language deficits on auditory processing tests. Performance on a word recognition noise task appears to be in the borderline normal range, suggesting difficulties in noisy background. As shown in ▶ Fig. 14.17, a right ear advantage in the left ear first condition is apparent on the SSW and competing words tasks. It has been suggested that such differences in performance may occur due to confusion in determining the left and the right ear in children with language impairments (Richard, 2007). However, the SSW test does not rely on the child's making a decision about the left versus right ear. In the left ear first conditions, the noncompeting part of the spondee begins in the left ear. Thus, the child does not have to consciously think about the left or right ear. A right ear advantage is also apparent on the competing sentence task. More specifically, when the patient in this case study was asked to ignore the left ear, he was able to correctly repeat all 10 sentences presented in the right ear, but when he was

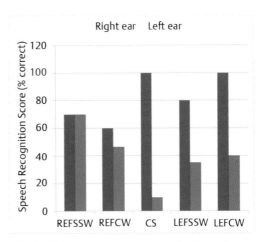

Fig. 14.17 Performance of a 9-year-old child on three dichotic tests. CW, competing words; CS, competing sentences; LEF, left ear first; REF, right ear first; SSW, staggered spondaic word test. The scores for the SSW are shown only for the competing conditions.

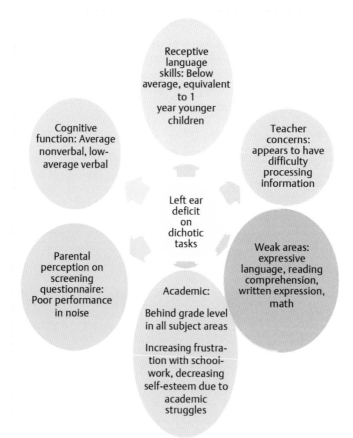

Fig. 14.18 Overall deficit pattern of a 9-year-old child with language impairment.

asked to ignore the right ear, he could correctly repeat only 1 of the 10 sentences presented to the left ear. In summary, a left ear weakness is apparent on three different dichotic tasks (SSW, competing words, and competing sentences). The left ear weakness can lead to difficulties in recognizing speech in noisy conditions, which are confirmed by the parental reports of the child's missing conversations in noisy conditions and the teachers' concerns about processing difficulties in the classroom. Most classrooms tend to be noisy, and some also tend to be reverberant. The child is expected to experience listening difficulties and academic struggles (▸ Fig. 14.18) due to the left ear weakness shown in ▸ Fig. 14.17.

14.18.12 Second Opinion/ Recommendations

1. Administration of the pitch pattern sequence test requesting for both nonverbal and verbal responses is recommended. The test will allow the assessment of auditory temporal sequence skills. Some children with language impairments have a deficiency in this area. As shown in ▸ Table 14.3, the child has sequencing difficulties as suggested by difficulties in organizing information sequentially, solving problems in a specific order, and producing responses in an orderly fashion. If a temporal pattern sequencing deficit is apparent, provide auditory training to improve function (see Chapter 9).

2. Address deficits shown on dichotic tasks (see Chapter 10).
   - Provide ear strength balance training with the following goals:
     - Improve left ear performance to at least 80% correct, during left ear first dichotic tasks.
     - Improve left and right ear performance to at least 80% correct, during the right ear first dichotic tasks.
     - Improve left ear performance to at least 80% correct during "ignore right ear" binaural separation tasks.

3. Provide speech perception in noise training to improve speech recognition performance to

within 1 SD of age-matched peers in background cafeteria-type or speech babble noise. The training should occur with the noise at the same location as speech and at a different location as the speech source (see Chapter 11).

4. Until all APDs are addressed, the child should be fitted with an FM device for classroom use and for use in resource rooms and speech-language therapy sessions. Teachers, special educators, parents, and the child should receive training in maintenance, monitoring, and accurate use of the FM device. Maintenance and use of the device should be written in the child's individualized education plan (IEP).

5. Six months after achievement of all auditory training goals, reassessments are recommended in the following areas:
   - General verbal cognition
   - Receptive and expressive language skills
   - Reading and writing skills
   - All academic areas

If deficits are still apparent, additional evaluations and follow-up remediation may be necessary, including continued use of the FM device.

6. Address the concerns related to teasing in collaboration with classroom teachers and any other professionals involved in the child's intervention.

14.19 Future Trends

It appears to be possible to correctly predict later speech and language development and reading skills based on speech evoked potentials obtained in the newborn period. Late evoked potentials in response to speech sounds (CV) recorded in neonates can predict performance on language tasks using the McCarthy Scale for Children's Abilities (McCarthy, 1972) at the age of 3 (Molfese & Molfese, 1985) and 5 years (Molfese & Molfese, 1997). In one study, 8-year-olds were classified into three groups of 17 with dyslexia, 7 poor readers, and 24 controls. Speech (/bi/ and /gi/) and nonspeech homologues of these sounds were used to elicit auditory event-related potentials (AERPs) when they were newborn infants. Six of the measures, including latencies and amplitudes recorded with various stimuli, were able to correctly classify all of the poor readers, 76.5% of the children with dyslexia and 79.2% of the children in the control group (Molfese, 2000). In another study, neonatal brain responses obtained with a different set of 9 CV speech stimuli composed of the consonants /b, d, g/ and the vowels /i, a, u/, were also able to predict

children's performance at the age of 8 years on the Wide Range Achievement Test 3 (WRAT-3; Wilkinson, 1993) of reading abilities (Molfese, Molfese, & Kelly, 2001).

Further refinement of such speech-evoked electrophysiological approaches using four or more measures (Molfese et al., 2001), use of modern imaging techniques, and consideration of family risk factor may allow correct prediction of speech and language delays and dyslexia in the future. For such children, intervention can begin early and capitalize on the maximum neural plasticity available during the critical periods of language development to either prevent or minimize the occurrence of future language-related disorders. Currently, ABRs are often recorded at birth to determine peripheral hearing sensitivity. These recordings can be expanded to use speech stimuli.

14.20 Review Questions

1. Discuss various components of language and review various categories of language impairments.
2. Discuss speech sound disorders and the potential impact of speech impairment in childhood.
3. Review the purposes of conducting speech and language assessments and various components of these assessments.
4. Provide three examples of interventions for language impairments and discuss the critical gaps in the evidence base for language intervention practices.
5. Provide three examples of interventions designed for speech sound disorders and discuss the need for research to improve the evidence base of intervention practices for speech sound disorders.
6. What are some possible difficulties in establishing best evidence for speech, language, and auditory processing deficits (APDs) using the medical model?
7. Discuss the various types of APDs that have been reported in children with language-related impairments using behavioral and objective measures.
8. Discuss potential reasons for comorbidity of language-related impairments and APDs.
9. What precautions should be taken in conducting auditory processing evaluations in children with language-related impairments?
10. How can the efficiency of speech-language interventions be improved in children with comorbid APDs?

References

[1] Ahissar, M., Protopapas, A., Reid, M., & Merzenich, M. M. (2000). Auditory processing parallels reading abilities in adults. Proceedings of the National Academy of Sciences of the United States of America, 97(12), 6832–6837.

[2] Ahmed, A., Parker, D., Adams, C., & Newton, V. (2006). Auditory temporal resolution in children with specific language impairment. Journal of Medical Speech-Language Pathology, 14, 79–96.

[3] American Psychiatric Association. (2013). Diagnostic and Statistical Manual of Mental Disorders (5th ed.). Arlington, VA: Author.

[4] American Speech-Language-Hearing Association (ASHA). (2004). Preferred practice patterns for the profession of speech-language pathology. Retrieved from www.asha.org/policy.

[5] Amitay, S., Ahissar, M., & Nelken, I. (2002). Auditory processing deficits in reading disabled adults. Journal of the Association for Research in Otolaryngology, 3(3), 302–320.

[6] Anthony, J., & Lonigan, C. (2004). The nature of phonological awareness: Converging evidence from four studies of preschool and early grade school children. Journal of Educational Psychology, 96, 43–55.

[7] Asbjørnsen, A. E., Helland, T., Obrzut, J. E., & Boliek, C. A. (2003). The role of dichotic listening performance and tasks of executive functions in reading impairment: A discriminant function analysis. Child Neuropsychology, 9(4), 277–288.

[8] Ayres, L. (1995). The efficacy of three training conditions on phonological awareness of kindergarten children and the longitudinal effect of each on later reading acquisition. Reading Research Quarterly, 30(4), 604–606.

[9] Baker, E., & McLeod, S. (2011). Evidence-based practice for children with speech sound disorders: 1. Narrative review. Language, Speech, and Hearing Services in Schools, 42(2), 102–139.

[10] Bamiou, D. E., Musiek, F. E., Sisodiya, S. M., et al. (2004). Deficient auditory interhemispheric transfer in patients with PAX6 mutations. Annals of Neurology, 56(4), 503–509.

[11] Bandstra, E. S., Vogel, A. L., Morrow, C. E., Xue, L., & Anthony, J. C. (2004). Severity of prenatal cocaine exposure and child language functioning through age seven years: A longitudinal latent growth curve analysis. Substance Use and Misuse, 39(1), 25–59.

[12] Basu, M., Krishnan, A., & Weber-Fox, C. (2010). Brainstem correlates of temporal auditory processing in children with specific language impairment. Developmental Science, 13 (1), 77–91.

[13] Benasich, A. A., & Tallal, P. (2002). Infant discrimination of rapid auditory cues predicts later language impairment. Behavioural Brain Research, 136(1), 31–49.

[14] Bishop, D. V. M., & Hayiou-Thomas, M. E. (2008). Heritability of specific language impairment depends on diagnostic criteria. Genes, Brain, and Behavior, 7(3), 365–372.

[15] Bishop, D. V. M., & McArthur, G. M. (2005). Individual differences in auditory processing in specific language impairment: A follow-up study using event-related potentials and behavioural thresholds. Cortex, 41(3), 327–341.

[16] Bless, J. J., Hugdahl, K., Westerhausen, R., et al. (2013). Cognitive control deficits in adolescents born with very low birth weight (≤1500 g): Evidence from dichotic listening. Scandinavian Journal of Psychology, 54(3), 179–187.

[17] Bloom, L. & Lahey, M. (1978). Language development and language disorders. New York: John Wiley & Sons.

[18] Boets, B., Wouters, J., van Wieringen, A., & Ghesquière, P. (2007). Auditory processing, speech perception and phonological ability in pre-school children at high-risk for dyslexia: A longitudinal study of the auditory temporal processing theory. Neuropsychologia, 45(8), 1608–1620.

[19] Boscariol, M., Garcia, V. L., Guimarães, C. A., et al. (2010). Auditory processing disorder in perisylvian syndrome. Brain and Development, 32(4), 299–304.

[20] Boscariol, M., Guimarães, C. A., Hage, S. R., et al. (2011). Auditory processing disorder in patients with language-learning impairment and correlation with malformation of cortical development. Brain and Development, 33(10), 824–831.

[21] Bradlow, A. R., Kraus, N., & Hayes, E. (2003). Speaking clearly for children with learning disabilities: Sentence perception in noise. Journal of Speech, Language, and Hearing Research, 46(1), 80–97.

[22] Camarata, S. M., & Nelson, K. E. (2006). Conversational recast intervention with preschool and older children. In R. McCauley & M. Fey (Eds.), Treatment of language disorders in children (pp. 237–264). Baltimore, MD: Paul Brookes.

[23] Carr, E. G., & Durand, V. M. (1985). Reducing behavior problems through functional communication training. Journal of Applied Behavioral Analysis, 18(2), 111–126.

[24] Chow, B. W., Ho, C. S., Wong, S. W., Waye, M. M., & Bishop, D. V. (2013). Generalist genes and cognitive abilities in Chinese twins. Developmental Science, 16(2), 260–268.

[25] Cirrin, F. M., & Gillam, R. B. (2008). Language intervention practices for school-age children with spoken language disorders: A systematic review. Language, Speech, and Hearing Services in Schools, 39(1), S110–S137.

[26] Clarke, E. M., & Adams, C. (2007). Binaural interaction in specific language impairment: An auditory evoked potential study. Developmental Medicine and Child Neurology, 49(4), 274–279.

[27] Cone-Wesson, B. (2005). Prenatal alcohol and cocaine exposure: Influences on cognition, speech, language, and hearing. Journal of Communication Disorders, 38(4), 279–302.

[28] Cone-Wesson, B., & Spingarn, A. (1993). Effects of maternal cocaine abuse on neonatal auditory brainstem responses. American Journal of Audiology, 2, 48–54.

[29] Cone-Wesson, B., & Wu, J. (1992). Audiologic findings in infants born to cocaine-abusing mothers. In L. M. Rosseti (Ed.), Developmental problems of drug exposed infants (pp. 25–35). San Diego, CA: Singular Publishing Group.

[30] Coplan, J., & Gleason, J. R. (1988). Unclear speech: Recognition and significance of unintelligible speech in preschool children. Pediatrics, 82(3, Pt. 2), 447–452.

[31] Davis, O. S. P., Haworth, C. M. A., & Plomin, R. (2009). Learning abilities and disabilities: Generalist genes in early adolescence. Cognitive Neuropsychiatry, 14(4-5), 312–331.

[32] deWeirdt, W. (1988). Speech perception and frequency discrimination in good and poor readers. Applied Psycholinguistics, 16, 163–183.

[33] Dodd, B. (1995). Differential diagnosis and treatment of children with speech disorders. London: Whurr.

[34] Dodd, B., & Bradford, A. (2000). A comparison of three therapy methods for children with different types of developmental phonological disorder. International Journal of Language and Communication Disorders, 35(2), 189–209.

[35] Dodd, B., Holm, A., Crosbie, S., & McCormick, P. (2005). Differential diagnosis of phonological disorder. In B. Dodd (Ed.), Differential diagnosis and treatment of children with speech disorders (pp. 44–70). London: Whurr.

[36] Dole, M., Hoen, M., & Meunier, F. (2012). Speech-in-noise perception deficit in adults with dyslexia: Effects of back-

ground type and listening configuration. Neuropsychologia, 50(7), 1543–1552.

[37] Dlouha, O., Novak, A., & Vokral, J. (2007). Central auditory processing disorder (CAPD) in children with specific language impairment (SLI): Central auditory tests. International Journal of Pediatric Otorhinolaryngology, 71(6), 903–907.

[38] Drayna, D., Manichaikul, A., de Lange, M., Snieder, H., & Spector, T. (2001). Genetic correlates of musical pitch recognition in humans. Science, 291(5510), 1969–1972.

[39] Dronkers, N. F., Husted, D. A., Deutsch, G., Tayler, M. K., Saunders, G., & Merzenich, M. M. (1999). Lesion site as a predictor of improvement after "Fast ForWord" treatment in adult aphasic patients. Brain and Language, 69, 450–452.

[40] Efron, R. (1963). Temporal perception, aphasia and déjà vu. Brain, 86, 403–424.

[41] Elliott, L. L., Connors, S., Kille, E., Levin, S., Ball, K., & Katz, D. (1979). Children's understanding of monosyllabic nouns in quiet and in noise. Journal of the Acoustical Society of America, 66(1), 12–21.

[42] Elliott, L. L., Hammer, M. A., & Scholl, M. E. (1989). Fine-grained auditory discrimination in normal children and children with language-learning problems. Journal of Speech and Hearing Research, 32(1), 112–119.

[43] Farmer, M. E., & Klein, R. M. (1995). The evidence for a temporal processing deficit linked to dyslexia: A review. Psychonomic Bulletin and Review, 2(4), 460–493.

[44] Fernell, E., Norrelgen, F., Bozkurt, I., Hellberg, G., & Löwing, K. (2002). Developmental profiles and auditory perception in 25 children attending special preschools for language-impaired children. Acta Paediatrica, 91(10), 1108–1115.

[45] Fey, M. E., & Finestack, L. H. (2009). Research and development in child language intervention: A 5-phase model. In R. G. Schwartz (Ed.), Handbook of child language disorders (pp. 513–529). New York: Psychology Press.

[46] Fey, M. E., Richard, G. J., Geffner, D., et al. (2011). Auditory processing disorder and auditory/language interventions: An evidence-based systematic review. Language, Speech, and Hearing Services in Schools, 42(3), 246–264.

[47] Flexer, C., Biley, K. K., Hinkley, A., Harkema, C., & Holcomb, J. (2002). Using sound-filed systems to teach phonemic awareness to pre-schoolers. Hearing Journal, 55(3), 38–44.

[48] Fortunato-Tavares, T., Rocha, C. N., Andrade, C. R., et al. (2009). Linguistic and auditory temporal processing in children with specific language impairment. Pro Fono, 21(4), 279–284.

[49] France, S. J., Rosner, B. S., Hansen, P. C., et al. (2002). Auditory frequency discrimination in adult developmental dyslexics. Perception and Psychophysics, 64(2), 169–179.

[50] Fridriksson, J., Hubbard, H. I., Hudspeth, S. G., et al. (2012). Speech entrainment enables patients with Broca's aphasia to produce fluent speech. Brain, 135(Pt. 12), 3815–3829.

[51] Galaburda, A. M., Sherman, G. F., Rosen, G. D., Aboitiz, F., & Geschwind, N. (1985). Developmental dyslexia: Four consecutive patients with cortical anomalies. Annals of Neurology, 18(2), 222–233.

[52] Gierut, J. A., Morrisette, M. L., Hughes, M. T., & Rowland, S. (1996). Phonological treatment efficacy and developmental norms. Language, Speech, and Hearing Services in Schools, 27, 215–230.

[53] Gillon, G. (2000). The efficacy of phonological awareness intervention for children with spoken language impairment. Language, Speech, and Hearing Services in Schools, 31, 126–141.

[54] Gillon, G. T. (2002). Follow-up study investigating the benefits of phonological awareness intervention for children

with spoken language impairment. International Journal of Language and Communication Disorders, 37(4), 381–400.

[55] Gopal, K. V., & Pierel, K. (1999). Binaural interaction component in children at risk for central auditory processing disorders. Scandinavian Audiology, 28(2), 77–84.

[56] Gregersen, P. K., Kowalsky, E., Lee, A., et al. (2013). Absolute pitch exhibits phenotypic and genetic overlap with synesthesia. Human Molecular Genetics, 22(10), 2097–2104.

[57] Guerreiro, M. M., Hage, S. R., Guimarães, C. A., et al. (2002). Developmental language disorder associated with polymicrogyria. Neurology, 59(2), 245–250.

[58] Hancock, T. B., & Kaiser, A. P. (2006). Enhanced milieu teaching. In R. McCauley & M. Fey (Eds.), Treatment of language disorders in children (pp. 203–233). Baltimore, MD: Paul Brookes.

[59] Haworth, C. M. A., Kovas, Y., Harlaar, N., et al. (2009). Generalist genes and learning disabilities: A multivariate genetic analysis of low performance in reading, mathematics, language and general cognitive ability in a sample of 8000 12-year-old twins. Journal of Child Psychology and Psychiatry, 50(10), 1318–1325.

[60] Hayiou-Thomas, M. E. (2008). Genetic and environmental influences on early speech, language and literacy development. Journal of Communication Disorders, 41(5), 397–408.

[61] Heath, S. M., Hogben, J. H., & Clark, C. D. (1999). Auditory temporal processing in disabled readers with and without oral language delay. Journal of Child Psychology and Psychiatry, 40(4), 637–647.

[62] Heim, S., Keil, A., Choudhury, N., Thomas Friedman, J., & Benasich, A. A. (2013). Early gamma oscillations during rapid auditory processing in children with a language-learning impairment: Changes in neural mass activity after training. Neuropsychologia, 51(5), 990–1001.

[63] Hickok, G., & Poeppel, D. (2007). The cortical organization of speech processing. Nature Reviews Neuroscience, 8(5), 393–402.

[64] Hodson, B. (2007). Evaluating and enhancing children's phonological systems: Research and theory to practice. Wichita, KS: Phonocomp.

[65] Hodson, B. W. (2011). Enhancing phonological patterns of young children with highly unintelligible speech. The ASHA Leader. retrieved from http://www.asha.org/Publications/leader/2011/110405/Enhancing-Phonological-Patterns-of-Young-Children-With-Highly-Unintelligible-Speech.htm

[66] Hodson, B., & Paden, E. (1991). Targeting intelligible speech: A phonological approach to remediation. Austin, TX: ProEd.

[67] Holm, A., Crosbie, S., & Dodd, B. (2007). Differentiating normal variability from inconsistency in children's speech: Normative data. International Journal of Language and Communication Disorders, 42(4), 467–486.

[68] Hornickel, J., Zecker, S. G., Bradlow, A. R., & Kraus, N. (2012). Assistive listening devices drive neuroplasticity in children with dyslexia. Proceedings of the National Academy of Sciences of the United States of America, 109(41), 16731–16736.

[69] Huppke, P., Kallenberg, K., & Gärtner, J. (2005). Perisylvian polymicrogyria in Landau-Kleffner syndrome. Neurology, 64(9), 1660.

[70] Jäncke, L., Langer, N., & Hänggi, J. (2012). Diminished whole-brain but enhanced peri-sylvian connectivity in absolute pitch musicians. Journal of Cognitive Neuroscience, 24(6), 1447–1461.

[71] Jiang, C., Hamm, J. P., Lim, V. K., Kirk, I. J., Chen, X., & Yang, Y. (2012). Amusia results in abnormal brain activity following

inappropriate intonation during speech comprehension. PLoS ONE, 7(7), e41411.

[72] Johnson, K. L., Nicol, T. G., Zecker, S. G., & Kraus, N. (2007). Auditory brainstem correlates of perceptual timing deficits. Journal of Cognitive Neuroscience, 19(3), 376–385.

[73] King, W. M., Lombardino, L. J., Crandell, C. C., & Leonard, C. M. (2003). Comorbid auditory processing disorder in developmental dyslexia. Ear and Hearing, 24(5), 448–456.

[74] Korkman, M., & Peltoman, A. K. (1993). Preventive treatment of dyslexia by a preschool training program for children with language impairments. Journal of Clinical and Child Psychology, 22, 277–287.

[75] Krause, J. C., & Braida, L. D. (2004). Acoustic properties of naturally produced clear speech at normal speaking rates. Journal of the Acoustical Society of America, 115(1), 362–378.

[76] Lai, C. S., Gerrelli, D., Monaco, A. P., Fisher, S. E., & Copp, A. J. (2003). FOXP2 expression during brain development coincides with adult sites of pathology in a severe speech and language disorder. Brain, 126(Pt. 11), 2455–2462.

[77] Lallier, M., Thierry, G., & Tainturier, M. J. (2013). On the importance of considering individual profiles when investigating the role of auditory sequential deficits in developmental dyslexia. Cognition, 126(1), 121–127.

[78] Lambert, J. M., Bloom, S. E., & Irvin, J. (2012). Trial-based functional analysis and functional communication training in an early childhood setting. Journal of Applied Behavior Analysis, 45(3), 579–584.

[79] Leonard, L. B. (1981). Facilitating linguistic skills in children with specific language impairment. Applied Psycholinguistics, 2, 89–118.

[80] Leonard, L. B. (1998). Children with specific language impairment. Cambridge, MA: MIT Press.

[81] Leonard, L. B., Ellis Weismer, S., Miller, C. A., Francis, D. J., Tomblin, J. B., & Kail, R. V. (2007). Speed of processing, working memory, and language impairment in children. Journal of Speech, Language, and Hearing Research, 50(2), 408–428.

[82] Leonard, L. B., Miller, C. A., & Finneran, D. A. (2008). Grammatical morpheme effects on sentence processing by schoolaged adolescents with specific language impairment. Language and Cognitive Processes, 24(3), 450–478.

[83] Lester, B. M., Lagasse, L., Seifer, R., et al. (2003). The Maternal Lifestyle Study (MLS): Effects of prenatal cocaine and/or opiate exposure on auditory brain response at one month. Journal of Pediatrics, 142(3), 279–285.

[84] Lewis, B. A., Kirchner, H. L., Short, E. J., et al. (2007). Prenatal cocaine and tobacco effects on children's language trajectories. Pediatrics, 120(1), e78–e85.

[85] Lewis, B. A., Minnes, S., Short, E. J., et al. (2011). The effects of prenatal cocaine on language development at 10 years of age. Neurotoxicology and Teratology, 33(1), 17–24.

[86] Liberman, A. M., Delattre, P. C., & Cooper, F. S. (1958). Some cues for distinction between voiced and voiceless stops in initial position. Language and Speech, 1, 153–167.

[87] Ling, D. (1976). Speech and the hearing-impaired child: Theory and practice. Washington, DC: Alexander Graham Bell Association for the Deaf.

[88] Liu, F., Patel, A. D., Fourcin, A., & Stewart, L. (2010). Intonation processing in congenital amusia: Discrimination, identification and imitation. Brain, 133(Pt. 6), 1682–1693.

[89] Lowe, A. D., & Campbell, R. A. (1965). Temporal discrimination in aphasoid and normal children. Journal of Speech and Hearing Research, 8(3), 313–314.

[90] Marler, J. A., Champlin, C. A., & Gillam, R. B. (2001). Backward and simultaneous masking measured in children with language-learning impairments who received computer-based training. American Journal of Speech-Language Pathology, 10, 258–268.

[91] Marler, J. A., Champlin, C. A., & Gillam, R. B. (2002). Auditory memory for backward masking signals in children with language impairment. Psychophysiology, 39(6), 767–780.

[92] Masataka, N. (2011). Enhancement of speech-relevant auditory acuity in absolute pitch possessors. Frontiers in Psychology, 2, 101.

[93] McAnally, K. I., & Stein, J. F. (1996). Auditory temporal coding in dyslexia. Proceedings of the Royal Society B: Biological Sciences, 263(1373), 961–965.

[94] McArthur, G. M., & Bishop, D. V. (2001). Auditory perceptual processing in people with reading and oral language impairments: Current issues and recommendations. Dyslexia, 7(3), 150–170.

[95] McArthur, G. M., & Hogben, J. H. (2001). Auditory backward recognition masking in children with a specific language impairment and children with a specific reading disability. Journal of the Acoustical Society of America, 109(3), 1092–1100.

[96] McArthur, G. M., Hogben, J. H., Edwards, V. T., Heath, S. M., & Mengler, E. D. (2000). On the "specifics" of specific reading disability and specific language impairment. Journal of Child Psychology and Psychiatry, 41(7), 869–874.

[97] McCormack, J., McLeod, S., McAllister, L., & Harrison, L. J. (2009). A systematic review of the association between childhood speech impairment and participation across the lifespan. International Journal of Speech-Language Pathology, 11(2), 155–170.

[98] McGivern, R. F., Berka, C., Languis, M. L., & Chapman, S. (1991). Detection of deficits in temporal pattern discrimination using the seashore rhythm test in young children with reading impairments. Journal of Learning Disabilities, 24(1), 58–62.

[99] Merzenich, M. M., Jenkins, W. M., Johnston, P., Schreiner, C., Miller, S. L., & Tallal, P. (1996). Temporal processing deficits of language-learning impaired children ameliorated by training. Science, 271(5245), 77–81.

[100] Miller, C. A., Leonard, L. B., & Finneran, D. (2008). Grammaticality judgements in adolescents with and without language impairment. International Journal of Language and Communication Disorders, 43(3), 346–360.

[101] Miller, C. A., & Wagstaff, D. A. (2011). Behavioral profiles associated with auditory processing disorder and specific language impairment. Journal of Communication Disorders, 44(6), 745–763.

[102] Milner, B., Taylor, L., & Sperry, R. W. (1968). Lateralized suppression of dichotically presented digits after commissural section in man. Science, 161(3837), 184–186.

[103] Molfese, D. L. (2000). Predicting dyslexia at 8 years of age using neonatal brain responses. Brain and Language, 72(3), 238–245.

[104] Molfese, D. L., & Molfese, V. J. (1985). Electrophysiological indices of auditory discrimination in newborn infants: The basis for predicting later language development. Infant Behavior and Development, 8, 197–211.

[105] Molfese, D. L., & Molfese, V. J. (1997). Discrimination of language skills at five years of age using event-related potentials recorded at birth. Developmental Neuropsychology, 13, 135–156.

[106] Molfese, D. L., Molfese, V. J., & Kelly, S. (2001). The use of brain electrophysiology techniques to study language: A basic guide for the beginning consumer of electrophysiology information. Learning Disability Quarterly, 24, 177–188.

[107] Moncrieff, D. W., & Black, J. R. (2008). Dichotic listening deficits in children with dyslexia. Dyslexia, 14(1), 54–75.

[108] Moncrieff, D. W., & Musiek, F. E. (2002). Interaural asymmetries revealed by dichotic listening tests in normal and dyslexic children. Journal of the American Academy of Audiology, 13(8), 428–437.

[109] Morell, R. J., Brewer, C. C., Ge, D., et al. (2007). A twin study of auditory processing indicates that dichotic listening ability is a strongly heritable trait. Human Genetics, 122(1), 103–111.

[110] Musiek, F. E., Kurdziel-Schwan, S., Kibbe, K. S., Gollegly, K. M., Baran, J. A., & Rintelmann, W. F. (1989). The dichotic rhyme task: Results in split-brain patients. Ear and Hearing, 10(1), 33–39.

[111] Musiek, F. E., Pinheiro, M. L., & Wilson, D. H. (1980). Auditory pattern perception in "'split brain'" patients. Archives of Otolaryngology, 106(10), 610–612.

[112] Musiek, F. E., & Wilson, D. H. (1979). SSW and dichotic digit results pre- and post-commissurotomy: A case report. Journal of Speech and Hearing Disorders, 44(4), 528–533.

[113] Musiek, F. E., Wilson, D. H., & Pinheiro, M. L. (1979). Audiological manifestations in "split brain" patients. Journal of the American Audiology Society, 5(1), 25–29.

[114] Nagarajan, S. S., Wang, X., Merzenich, M. M., et al. (1998). Speech modifications algorithms used for training language learning-impaired children. IEEE Transactions on Rehabilitation Engineering, 6(3), 257–268.

[115] Nelson, K.E. (1977). Facilitating children''s syntax acquisition. Developmental Psychology, 13, 101–107.

[116] Nickisch, A., & Massinger, C. (2009). Auditory processing in children with specific language impairments: Are there deficits in frequency discrimination, temporal auditory processing or general auditory processing? Folia Phoniatrica Logopaedica, 61(6), 323–328.

[117] O'Brien, B. A., Wolf, M., & Lovett, M. W. (2012). A taxometric investigation of developmental dyslexia subtypes. Dyslexia, 18(1), 16–39.

[118] Oliveira, E. P., Hage, S. R., Guimarães, C. A., et al. (2008). Characterization of language and reading skills in familial polymicrogyria. Brain and Development, 30(4), 254–260.

[119] Olson, R. K., Hulslander, J., Christopher, M., et al. (2013). Genetic and environmental influences on writing and their relations to language and reading. Annals of Dyslexia, 63(1), 25–43.

[120] Patel, A. D., Wong, M., Foxton, J. M., Loch, A., & Peretz, I. (2008). Speech intonation perception deficits in musical tone deafness. Music Perception, 25, 357–368.

[121] Paul, L. K. (2011). Developmental malformation of the corpus callosum: A review of typical callosal development and examples of developmental disorders with callosal involvement. Journal of Neurodevelopmental Disorders, 3(1), 3–27.

[122] Peretz, I., Cummings, S., & Dubé, M.-P. (2007). The genetics of congenital amusia (tone deafness): A family-aggregation study. American Journal of Human Genetics, 81(3), 582–588.

[123] Peterson, R. L., Pennington, B. F., & Olson, R. K. (2013). Subtypes of developmental dyslexia: Testing the predictions of the dual-route and connectionist frameworks. Cognition, 126(1), 20–38.

[124] Picheny, M. A., Durlach, N. I., & Braida, L. D. (1985). Speaking clearly for the hard of hearing: 1. Intelligibility differences between clear and conversational speech. Journal of Speech and Hearing Research, 28(1), 96–103.

[125] Picheny, M. A., Durlach, N. I., & Braida, L. D. (1986). Speaking clearly for the hard of hearing: 2. Acoustic characteristics of clear and conversational speech. Journal of Speech and Hearing Research, 29(4), 434–446.

[126] Poirier, P., Miljours, S., Lassonde, M., & Lepore, F. (1993). Sound localization in acallosal human listeners. Brain, 116 (Pt. 1), 53–69.

[127] Potter, S. M., Zelazo, P. R., Stack, D. M., & Papageorgiou, A. N. (2000). Adverse effects of fetal cocaine exposure on neonatal auditory information processing. Pediatrics, 105(3), E40.

[128] Purdy, S. C., Smart, J. L., Baily, M., & Sharma, M. (2009). Do children with reading delay benefit from the use of personal FM systems in the classroom? International Journal of Audiology, 48(12), 843–852.

[129] Richard, G. J. (2007). Cognitive-communicative and language factors associated with (central) auditory processing disorder: A speech-language pathology perspective. In G. D. Chermak & F. E. Musiek (Eds.), Handbook of (central) auditory processing disorder: Comprehensive intervention (Vol. 1, pp. 397–415). San Diego, CA: Plural Publishing.

[130] Robson, H., Grube, M., Lambon Ralph, M. A. L., Griffiths, T. D., & Sage, K. (2013). Fundamental deficits of auditory perception in Wernicke's aphasia. Cortex, 49(7), 1808–1822.

[131] Rocha-Muniz, C. N., Befi-Lopes, D. M., & Schochat, E. (2012). Investigation of auditory processing disorder and language impairment using the speech-evoked auditory brainstem response. Hearing Research, 294(1-2), 143–152.

[132] Rvachew, S., & Bernhardt, B. M. (2010). Clinical implications of dynamic systems theory for phonological development. American Journal of Speech-Language Pathology, 19(1), 34–50.

[133] Rvachew, S., & Nowak, M. (2001). The effect of target-selection strategy on phonological learning. Journal of Speech, Language, and Hearing Research, 44(3), 610–623.

[134] Salamy, A., Eldredge, L., Anderson, J., & Bull, D. (1990). Brainstem transmission time in infants exposed to cocaine in utero. Journal of Pediatrics, 117(4), 627–629.

[135] Santhouse, A. M., Ffytche, D. H., Howard, R. J., et al. (2002). The functional significance of perinatal corpus callosum damage: An fMRI study in young adults. Brain, 125(Pt. 8), 1782–1792.

[136] Santurette, S., Poelmans, H., Luts, H., Ghesquiére, P., Wouters, J., & Dau, T. (2010). Detection and identification of monaural and binaural pitch contours in dyslexic listeners. Journal of the Association for Research in Otolaryngology, 11(3), 515–524.

[137] Sharma, M., Purdy, S. C., & Kelly, A. S. (2009). Comorbidity of auditory processing, language, and reading disorders. Journal of Speech, Language, and Hearing Research, 52(3), 706–722.

[138] Shih, L., Cone-Wesson, B., & Reddix, B. (1988). Effects of maternal cocaine abuse on the neonatal auditory system. International Journal of Pediatric Otorhinolaryngology, 15(3), 245–251.

[139] Sices, L., Taylor, H. G., Freebairn, L., Hansen, A., & Lewis, B. (2007). Relationship between speech-sound disorders and early literacy skills in preschool-age children: Impact of comorbid language impairment. Journal of Developmental and Behavioral Pediatrics, 28(6), 438–447.

[140] Simões, M. B., & Schochat, E. (2010). (Central) auditory processing disorders in individuals with and without dyslexia. Pró Fono, 22(4), 521–524.

[141] Sininger, Y. S., Klatzky, R. L., & Kirchner, D. M. (1989). Memory scanning speed in language-disordered children. Journal of Speech and Hearing Research, 32(2), 289–297.

[142] Stanton-Chapman, T. L., Chapman, D. A., Bainbridge, N. L., & Scott, K. G. (2002). Identification of early risk factors for language impairment. Research in Developmental Disabilities, 23(6), 390–405.

[143] Stefanatos, G. A., Green, G. G., & Ratcliff, G. G. (1989). Neurophysiological evidence of auditory channel anomalies in developmental dysphasia. Archives of Neurology, 46(8), 871–875.

[144] Stevens, C., Fanning, J., Coch, D., Sanders, L., & Neville, H. (2008). Neural mechanisms of selective auditory attention are enhanced by computerized training: Electrophysiological evidence from language-impaired and typically developing children. Brain Research, 1205, 55–69.

[145] Stoel-Gammon, C., Stone-Goldman, J., & Glaspey, A. (2002). Pattern-based approaches to phonological therapy. Seminars in Speech and Language, 23(1), 3–14.

[146] Talcott, J. B., Witton, C., Hebb, G. S., et al. (2002). On the relationship between dynamic visual and auditory processing and literacy skills: Results from a large primary-school study. Dyslexia, 8(4), 204–225.

[147] Talcott, J. B., Witton, C., McLean, M. F., et al. (2000). Dynamic sensory sensitivity and children's word decoding skills. Proceedings of the National Academy of Sciences of the United States of America, 97(6), 2952–2957.

[148] Tallal, P., Miller, S. L., Bedi, G., et al. (1996). Language comprehension in language-learning impaired children improved with acoustically modified speech. Science, 271 (5245), 81–84.

[149] Tallal, P., & Newcombe, F. (1978). Impairment of auditory perception and language comprehension in dysphasia. Brain and Language, 5(1), 13–34.

[150] Tallal, P., & Piercy, M. (1973). Defects of non-verbal auditory perception in children with developmental aphasia. Nature, 241(5390), 468–469.

[151] Tallal, P., & Piercy, M. (1974). Developmental aphasia: Rate of auditory processing and selective impairment of consonant perception. Neuropsychologia, 12(1), 83–93.

[152] Tallal, P., Townsend, J., Curtiss, S., & Wulfeck, B. (1991). Phenotypic profiles of language-impaired children based on genetic/family history. Brain and Language, 41(1), 81–95.

[153] Tan-Laxa, M. A., Sison-Switala, C., Rintelman, W., & Ostrea, E. M., Jr. (2004). Abnormal auditory brainstem response among infants with prenatal cocaine exposure. Pediatrics, 113(2), 357–360.

[154] Tekieli Koay, M. E. (1992). Speech and speech disorders: Implications for central auditory processing. In J. Katz, N. Stecker, & D. Henderson (Eds.), Central auditory processing: A transdisciplinary view (pp. 169–176). St. Louis, MO: Mosby Year Book.

[155] Telkemeyer, S., Rossi, S., Koch, S. P., et al. (2009). Sensitivity of newborn auditory cortex to the temporal structure of sounds. Journal of Neurosciences, 29(47), 14726–14733.

[156] Temple, C. M., & Ilsley, J. (1993). Phonemic discrimination in callosal agenesis. Cortex, 29(2), 341–348.

[157] Temple, E., Deutsch, G. K., Poldrack, R. A., et al. (2003). Neural deficits in children with dyslexia ameliorated by behavioral remediation: Evidence from functional MRI. Proceedings of the National Academy of Sciences of the United States of America, 100(5), 2860–2865.

[158] Theusch, E., Basu, A., & Gitschier, J. (2009). Genome-wide study of families with absolute pitch reveals linkage to 8q24.21 and locus heterogeneity. American Journal of Human Genetics, 85(1), 112–119.

[159] Thompson, W. F., Marin, M. M., & Stewart, L. (2012). Reduced sensitivity to emotional prosody in congenital amusia rekindles the musical protolanguage hypothesis. Proceeding of the National Academy of Sciences of the United States of America, 109(46), 19027–19032.

[160] Uclés, P., Alonso, M. F., Aznar, E., & Lapresta, C. (2012). The importance of right otitis media in childhood language disorders. International Journal of Otolaryngology, Volume 2012, Article ID 818927, 10 pages.

[161] de Vasconcelos Hage, S. R., Cendes, F., Montenegro, M. A., Abramides, D. V., Guimarães, C. A., & Guerreiro, M. M. (2006). Specific language impairment: Linguistic and neurobiological aspects. Arquivos de Neuro-Psiquiatria, 64(2A), 173–180.

[162] Visto, J. C., Cranford, J. L., & Scudder, R. (1996). Dynamic temporal processing of nonspeech acoustic information by children with specific language impairment. Journal of Speech and Hearing Research, 39(3), 510–517.

[163] von Plessen, K., Lundervold, A., Duta, N., et al. (2002). Less developed corpus callosum in dyslexic subjects—a structural MRI study. Neuropsychologia, 40(7), 1035–1044.

[164] Watson, B. U. (1992). Auditory temporal acuity in normally achieving and learning-disabled college students. Journal of Speech and Hearing Research, 35(1), 148–156.

[165] Weber, C., Hahne, A., Friedrich, M., & Friederici, A. D. (2004). Discrimination of word stress in early infant perception: Electrophysiological evidence. Brain Research. Cognitive Brain Research, 18(2), 149–161.

[166] Weber, C., Hahne, A., Friedrich, M., & Friederici, A. D. (2005). Reduced stress pattern discrimination in 5-month-olds as a marker of risk for later language impairment: Neurophysiologial evidence. Brain Research, Cognitive Brain Research, 25 (1), 180–187.

[167] Weber-Fox, C., Leonard, L. B., Wray, A. H., & Tomblin, J. B. (2010). Electrophysiological correlates of rapid auditory and linguistic processing in adolescents with specific language impairment. Brain and Language, 115(3), 162–181.

[168] Weismer, S. E., & Robertson, S. (2006). Focused stimulation. In R. J. McCauley & M. Fey (Eds.), Treatment of language disorders in children (pp. 47–75). Baltimore, MD: Paul Brooks.

[169] Whitton, J. P., & Polley, D. B. (2011). Evaluating the perceptual and pathophysiological consequences of auditory deprivation in early postnatal life: A comparison of basic and clinical studies. Journal of the Association for Research in Otolaryngology, 12(5), 535–547.

[170] Wible, B., Nicol, T., & Kraus, N. (2002). Abnormal neural encoding of repeated speech stimuli in noise in children with learning problems. Clinical Neurophysiology, 113(4), 485–494.

[171] Wible, B., Nicol, T., & Kraus, N. (2004). Atypical brainstem representation of onset and formant structure of speech sounds in children with language-based learning problems. Biological Psychology, 67(3), 299–317.

[172] Wilkinson, G. S. (1993). The Wide Range Achievement Test: Manual. 3rd ed. Wilmington, DE: Wide Range.

[173] Wright, B. A., Lombardino, L. J., King, W. M., Puranik, C. S., Leonard, C. M., & Merzenich, M. M. (1997). Deficits in auditory temporal and spectral resolution in language-impaired children. Nature, 387(6629), 176–178.

[174] Xoinis, K., Weirather, Y., Mavoori, H., Shaha, S. H., & Iwamoto, L. M. (2007). Extremely low birth weight infants are at high risk for auditory neuropathy. Journal of Perinatology, 27(11), 718–723.

[175] Ziegler, J. C., Pech-Georgel, C., George, F., & Lorenzi, C. (2009). Speech-perception-in-noise deficits in dyslexia. Developmental Science, 12(5), 732–745.

[176] Ziegler, J. C., Pech-Georgel, C., George, F., & Lorenzi, C. (2011). Noise on, voicing off: Speech perception deficits in children with specific language impairment. Journal of Experimental Child Psychology, 110(3), 362–372.

Chapter 15

Auditory Neuropathy Spectrum Disorder Including Auditory Synaptopathy

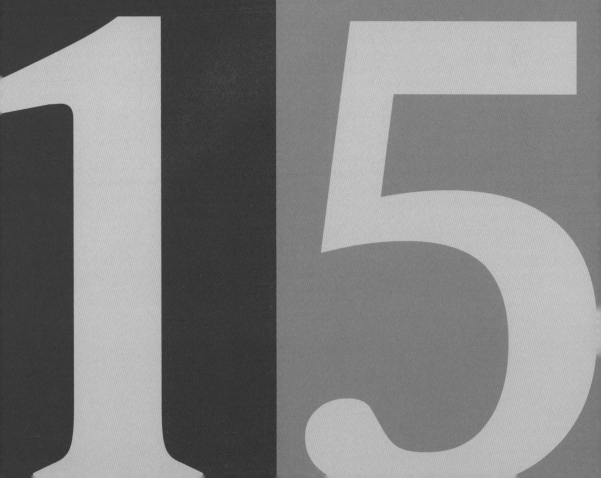

15 Auditory Neuropathy Spectrum Disorder Including Auditory Synaptopathy

Auditory neuropathy spectrum disorder (ANSD) is a type of auditory deficit characterized by an absent or abnormal auditory brainstem response (ABR) at relatively high stimulus rates possibly due to asynchronous neural firings in the presence of normal or nearly normal outer hair cell function, as reflected by the presence of otoacoustic emissions (OAEs) and/or a cochlear microphonic. The asynchronous neural firings lead to the absence of the auditory middle ear reflex. Many individuals with ANSD also show temporal auditory processing deficits (APDs). The use of the term *auditory neuropathy spectrum disorder* was recommended by a panel of experts who met in Como, Italy, at the Newborn Hearing Screening Conference in 2008 (Guidelines Development Conference, 2008). Other terms related to the disorder are *auditory dyssynchrony,* due to the lack of synchronous response of auditory neurons (Berlin, Hood, & Rose, 2001), and *auditory synaptopathy,* due to a deficit in the synapses between the inner hair cells and auditory neurons (Moser, Predoehl, & Starr, 2013).

15.1 Prevalence

Among children with sensorineural hearing loss, approximately 5% may have ANSD (Mittal et al., 2012); among those who are aided before the age of 3 years, the incidence appears to be 10% (Ching et al., 2013). Among children who have severe to profound hearing loss, a higher prevalence of 13 to 14% has been reported (Mittal et al., 2012; Sanyelbhaa Talaat, Kabel, Samy, & Elbadry, 2009). A similar incidence of 14% is estimated among individuals with severe to profound hearing loss. However, among all individuals with sensorineural hearing loss, the incidence is 1.2% (Penido & Isaac, 2013). The prevalence is 0.23% among infants and children who are at risk for hearing loss (Rance et al., 1999); among infants admitted to the neonatal intensive care unit (NICU), the rate of ANSD is 0.27% (Coenraad, Goedegebure, van Goudoever, & Hoeve, 2011) to 0.56% (Xoinis, Weirather, Mavoori, Shaha, & Iwamoto, 2007). Among babies admitted to the NICU who are referred after hearing screening, 8.7% appear to have ANSD (Coenraad et al., 2011). Among all babies referred after hearing screening, the prevalence is 19% (Maris, Venstermans, & Boudewyns, 2011). Among all newborns receiving hearing screening, the prevalence is estimated to be between 0.006 and 0.03% (Korver, van Zanten, Meuwese-Jongejeugd, van Straaten, & Oudesluys-Murphy, 2012).

15.2 Risk Factors

15.2.1 Environmental Risk Factors

Factors that increase the chance of ANSD include respiratory distress, meningitis, vancomycin administration (Coenraad et al., 2011), prematurity, hypoxia, kernicterus, severe neonatal jaundice (Saluja, Agarwal, Kler, & Amin, 2010), and extremely low birth weight (Xoinis et al., 2007). ANSD can also occur as a result of cryptococcal infection in adults with compromised immune systems (Celis-Aguilar, Macias-Valle, & Coutinho-De Toledo, 2012). Auditory neuropathy in adults can occur following exposure to noise (Furman, Kujawa, & Liberman, 2013) and ototoxins (Draper & Bamiou, 2009).

15.2.2 Genetic Factors

Syndromic, nonsyndromic, and mitochondrial genetic factors play a major role in ANSD. The inheritance patterns are autosomal dominant, autosomal recessive, X-linked, and mitochondrial. The inheritance pattern and genetic markers related to nonsyndromic ANSD, along with sites of pathology, are shown in ▶ Fig. 15.1 (Manchaiah, Zhao, Danesh, & Duprey, 2011). Gene mutations leading to congenital ANSD include *AUNA1*, or auditory neuropathy, dominant 1 (Kim et al., 2004), *PCDH9* (protocadherin 9; Grati et al., 2009), *OTOF* (otoferlin; Bae et al., 2013; Varga et al., 2003), *DIAPH3* (diaphanous-related formin 3; Bae et al., 2013; Schoen et al., 2010), *SLC26A4* (solute carrier family 26; Dahl et al., 2013), and *PJVK* (reported as *DFNB59*, deafness, autosomal recessive 59; Delmaghani et al., 2006). OTOF mutations may account for 3.2 to 7.3% of severe to profound recessive nonsyndromic hearing loss in Japan (Iwasa et al., 2013). Other mutations, such as those of the GJB2 (gap junction beta 2; Dahl et al., 2013; Santarelli et al., 2008), have been associated with ANSD.

Wang and colleagues (2005) conducted linkage analysis on a five-generation Chinese ANSD

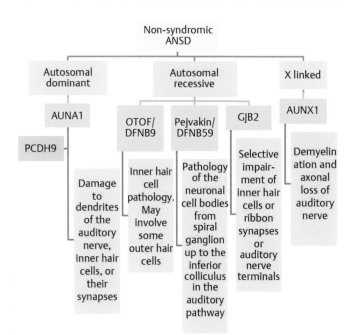

Fig. 15.1 Inheritance type and genetic markers related to nonsyndromic auditory neuropathy spectrum disorder (ANSD).

pedigree with 101 family members and discovered a region shared by 5 affected males and 4 female carriers located between markers DXS1220 and DXS8084 of the X chromosome (region Xq23–27.3). They named this locus auditory neuropathy X-linked recessive locus 1, or AUNX1. The affected members show a progressive hearing loss and decreased OAE amplitude. The ANSD in this family appears to be due to demyelination and axonal loss of the auditory nerve.

The various syndromes associated with ANSD are shown in ▶ Fig. 15.2 (Manchaiah et al., 2011). For example, ANSD has been noted in syndromes such as Friedreich ataxia (Rance, Corben, & Delatycki, 2012). Genes associated with syndromic ANSD include *pPM22, MPZ, NL-F, NDRG1, GJB1, OPA1, TMEM126A,* and *DDP,* along with mitochondrial DNA (mtDNA) and 12S ribosomal RNA (rRNA) (Wang et al; 2005 Manchaiah et al., 2011).

It is important to identify syndromes that are associated with ANSD given that rehabilitation strategies may differ based on other comorbid symptoms. For example, Leber's hereditary optic neuropathy is characterized by degeneration of retinal ganglion cells and their axons, which leads to loss of central vision in most patients. In the presence of ANSD in such patients (Ceranić & Luxon, 2004), rehabilitation strategies that rely on

vision to improve speech recognition may be ineffective. Other syndromes that include compromised vision are autosomal dominant optic atrophy (Kjer disease) (Haaksma-Schaafsma, van Dijk, & Dikkers, 2012), autosomal recessive optic atrophy (Meyer et al., 2010), Mohr-Tranebjaerg syndrome (Bahmad, Merchant, Nadol, & Tranebjaerg, 2007), and Refsum disease (Oysu, Aslan, Basaran, & Baserer, 2001). Syndromes such as Mohr-Tranebjaerg are associated with massive loss of spiral ganglion cells, along with loss of nearly all peripheral and central processes. Only 5 to 10% of the ganglion cells may survive (Merchant et al., 2001). Cochlear implantation in such patients is likely to be ineffective.

15.3 Sites of Pathology

Possible sites of lesion (▶ Fig. 15.3) are the cochlear inner hair cells, the synapse between the inner hair cells and the auditory nerve fibers coupled to the base of the hair cells, myelin and/or axonal impairment in the afferent auditory nerve fibers near the base of the hair cells (Moser et al., 2013; Starr, Picton, Sininger, Hood, & Berlin, 1996; Starr, Sininger, & Pratt, 2000), loss of spiral ganglion cells, impairment in the portion of the auditory nerve entering the cochlear nucleus, and impairments in

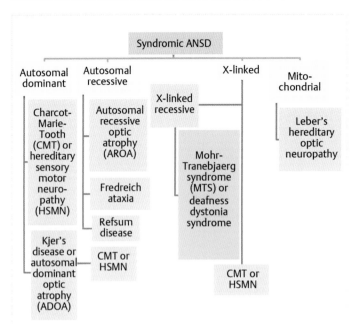

Fig. 15.2 Inheritance type and genetic markers of syndromic auditory neuropathy spectrum disorder (ANSD).

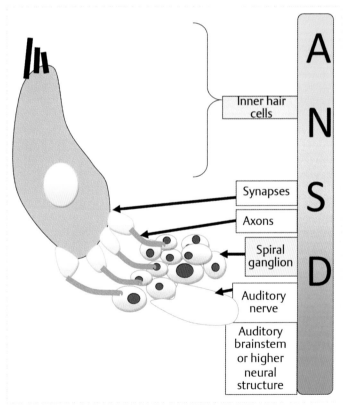

Fig. 15.3 Sites of pathology in auditory neuropathy spectrum disorder (ANSD).

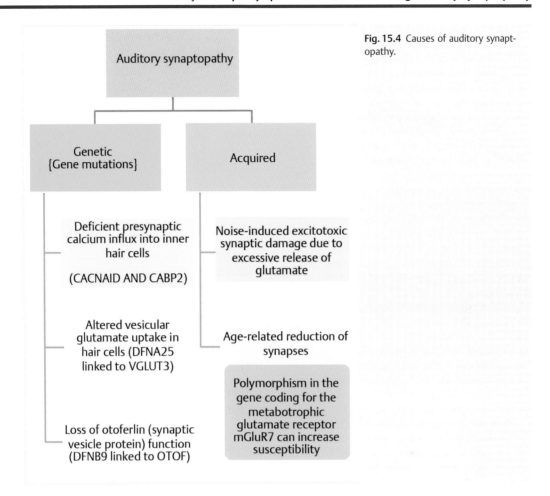

Fig. 15.4 Causes of auditory synaptopathy.

the higher neural structures, including the brainstem (Roche et al., 2010).

Selective loss of inner hair cells can occur in premature infants (Amatuzzi et al., 2001). Among seriously ill infants, as many as 27% of premature neonates may have selective inner hair cells loss, whereas only 3% of full-term babies show such pattern (Amutuzzi, Liberman, & Northrop, 2011). In some cases, the selective inner hair cell loss may be associated with intracochlear clots (Slack, Wright, Michaels, & Frohlich, 1986). These infants can be expected to fail ABR screenings during the neonatal period, especially when relatively high click rates (e.g., 37/s) are used during screenings (Amutuzzi et al., 2001). Because 95% of the afferent neural fibers are coupled to inner hair cells, selective loss of inner hair cells can lead to absence of the ABR.

The term *auditory synaptopathy* has been used when the site of dysfunction is located at the hair cell ribbon synapses. However, severe synaptopathy can lead to degeneration of nerve fibers, resulting in auditory neuropathy (Moser et al., 2013). Loss of presynaptic ribbons can reduce the reliability with which spikes are generated at stimulus onset, which can lead to dyssynchronous neural responses, resulting in the absence of the ABR. Presynaptic ANSD disrupting neurotransmitter release is associated with otoferlin mutations (Marlin et al., 2010). Otoferlin encoded by the *OTOF* gene is expressed in inner hair cells and is responsible for synaptic exocytosis at the auditory ribbon synapse (Roux et al., 2006). Possible causes of synaptopathy are shown in ▸ Fig. 15.4.

Some possible mechanisms for the lack of neural response may be decreased release of neurotransmitters leading to poor activation of dendrites (Santarelli et al., 2009), myelin and axonal impairment in the afferent nerve fibers (Moser et al., 2013; Starr et al., 1996, 2000), and mitochondrial dysfunction. Postsynaptic neuropathy that disrupts initiation of synchronous activity in nerve terminals is associated with OPA1 (optic atrophy type 1) mutations (Santarelli et al., 2011) and altered mitochondrial function (Huang, Santarelli, & Starr, 2009). Once initiated, conduction of the neural impulses can be affected along the auditory nerve in the presence of mutations, leading to hereditary motor and sensory neuropathies, such as Charcot–Marie–Tooth disease (Rance et al., 2012), or hereditary motor and sensory neuropathy (HMSN; Butinar et al., 1999) and Friedreich ataxia (Rance et al., 2008). In such disorders, both Schwann cells and axons can be affected, leading to slower nerve conduction and axonal degeneration (Butinar et al., 1999). Some children with Charcot–Marie–Tooth disease have demyelinating neuropathies (type 1), and others have pathologies affecting axons (type 2). Temporal processing and speech perception are affected in both types (Rance et al., 2012).

Syndromes such a Mohr–Tranebjaerg are characterized by 90 to 95% loss of cochlear neurons (Bahmad et al., 2007). Many children with cochlear nerve deficiency can yield findings that are characteristic of ANSD (Buchman et al., 2006). Comorbid conditions, including hypoplastic facial nerve, absent inferior vestibular nerve, absent horizontal or posterior semicircular canal, dilated superior semicircular canal, dilated vestibule, enlarged vestibular aqueduct (EVA), cystic cochlea, and a common cavity, have been noted in 56% of patients with cochlear nerve deficiency (Levi et al., 2013).

15.4 Behavioral Auditory Characteristics

15.4.1 Peripheral Auditory Sensitivity

Patients with ANSD can have either normal hearing (Rance, Corben, & Delatycki, 2012) or hearing loss (▶ Fig. 15.5). When hearing loss is present, the degree of hearing loss can vary from mild to profound, with about 55% having a moderate degree of hearing loss (Penido & Isaac, 2013). In individuals with near normal hearing, low-frequency (250 Hz) thresholds are generally elevated (Rance, Corben, & Delatycki, 2012). Some patients with ANSD can show wide variation in auditory sensitivity (Rance et al., 1999). In some patients, hearing loss is apparent only when the patients have fever. This is referred to as temperature-sensitive ANSD (Starr et al., 1998; Wang et al., 2010).

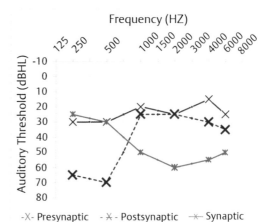

Fig. 15.5 Examples of left ear audiograms from patients with presynaptic, postsynaptic (based on Dimitrijevic et al., 2012), and synaptic (based on Moser, Predoehl, & Starr, 2013) sites of pathology.

15.4.2 Temporal Processing Deficits

Frequency Discrimination at Low Frequencies

Frequency discrimination is profoundly poor at frequencies below 4000 Hz in individuals with ANSD compared to matched peers. However, at higher frequencies above 4000 Hz, the discrimination tends to be similar to that apparent in matched controls (Zeng, Kong, Michalewski, & Starr, 2005). Such findings suggest that patients with ANSD may have difficulty in using temporal cues for low-frequency discrimination (Rance, McKay, & Grayden, 2004).

Temporal Integration

Individuals with ANSD have significantly more difficulty in detecting brief sounds lasting for 5 to 10 ms in duration compared to age-matched controls, resulting in a slightly elevated slope of the temporal integration function (Zeng et al., 2005).

Gap Detection

Gap detection thresholds of individuals with ANSD tend to be similar to that of age-matched controls (50 ms) at lower sensation levels of 5 to 10 dB, but at higher sensation levels of 40 to 50 dB, these individuals need larger gaps (15–20 ms) compared to age-matched controls (3 ms; Zeng et al., 2005).

Temporal Modulation Detection

Detection of rapid sinusoidal amplitude modulation appears to be poorer in children with Friedreich ataxia than for matched peers. Their mean amplitude modulation detection thresholds for a low-modulation frequency stimulus (e.g., 10 Hz) are similar to those found in matched peers (6.5 –6.9% modulation depth). However, when the modulation frequency is increased to 150 Hz, children with Friedreich ataxia need significantly larger modulation depths (34.7%) to detect amplitude changes compared to matched peers (11.6% modulation depth; Rance, Corben, & Delatycki, 2012). In another study, individuals with ANSD were found to have more difficulty in detecting both slow and fast temporal modulations compared to age-matched peers (Zeng et al., 2005). Both amplitude and frequency modulation detection thresholds (2 and 10 Hz modulation frequencies) are poorer in individuals with ANSD when compared to those in listeners with normal hearing, suggesting difficulty in extracting temporal envelope and fine structure cues. In addition, these thresholds are significantly correlated with speech recognition in noise (Narne, 2013).

Backward and Forward Masking

Individuals with ANSD show more backward and forward masking compared to age-matched controls. During forward masking, patients with ANSD continue to show significant masking effects even after a 100 ms separation between the signal and masker, whereas no masking is apparent in normal controls with 100 ms separation. During backward masking, a significant difference in masking is apparent between the two groups when the signal and masker are separated by 5 to 50 ms (Zeng et al., 2005).

Temporal Maintenance/Decay

Poor maintenance of neural responses to sounds or abnormal sound decay at 8000 Hz has been noted in patients with ANSD and disordered function of auditory nerve fibers. The decay is more pronounced in the presence of disordered function of hair cell ribbon synapses (temperature sensitive auditory neuropathy) and is also present at 250 Hz (Wynne et al., 2013).

In the presence of abnormal decay, ABRs for stimuli with relatively fast rates are expected to show deterioration with an increasing number of stimuli. For example, in a case with congenital fibrosis of the extraocular muscles type 1, a rapid decrease in amplitude and reproducibility of waves I and III was apparent after presentation of 2000 clicks at a rate of 19/s. Partial recovery occurred after a period of 5 minutes of silence, and complete recovery was apparent in a few more minutes. A suggested interpretation of these findings is that neuronal ionic pumps are unable to maintain homeostasis fast enough to cope with repetitive stimuli due to insufficient energy production by deficient mitochondria (Giraudet & Avan, 2012).

Localization Using Interaural Time Difference Cues

In normal-hearing individuals, the perception of the sound image changes from the center to the side of the head as the interaural time difference between the tones presented at the two ears is varied by changing the interaural phase difference from 0 to 90 degrees for a 500 Hz tone. In individuals with ANSD, the perception continues to remain at the center of the head, showing an inability to make use of the interaural time difference cues. However, they can use interaural level difference cues to correctly localize sounds (Zeng et al., 2005).

15.4.3 Binaural Beats

When a 500 Hz tone is presented to one ear and a 503 Hz tone to the other, normal-hearing individuals report the perception of beats. Individuals with ANSD report a fused sound image without any perception of beats, suggesting difficulty in perceiving the fast modulations inherent in the fused signal (Zeng et al., 2005).

15.4.4 Speech Perception in Noise

Some patients with ANSD have difficulty in recognizing speech that is more marked in noisy environments (Rance et al., 2007). Their performance in noise tends to be poorer compared to age-matched normal listeners and listeners with cochlear hearing loss (Zeng & Liu, 2006). One reason for this difficulty may arise from difficulty in making use of gaps in noise. The difficulty in using interaural time cues to separate speech and noise when the two sources are at different locations can also lead to poor speech recognition. There is a significant correlation between amplitude modulation detection and speech recognition in the presence

15.5 Objective Auditory Measures

15.5.1 Otoacoustic Emissions

OAEs are initially normal in the presence of ANSD. The amplitude of transient evoked OAEs (TEOAEs) may reduce significantly over time in about 21% of patients with ANSD, and emissions may disappear in approximately 2% of patients. Patients fitted with hearing aids may show more reduction in the TEOAE amplitudes compared to those who are not fitted with amplification (Sanyelbhaa Talaat, Khalil, Khafagy, Alkandari, & Zein, 2013).

15.5.2 Middle Ear Muscle Reflex

As previously mentioned, the acoustic reflex is absent or elevated above 95 or 100 dB hearing level (HL) in patients with ANSD in the presence of normal tympanometric findings and normal OAEs, suggesting normal middle ear function and normal outer hair cell function. Ipsilateral acoustic reflex testing at 1 and 2 kHz is recommended in those newborn hearing screening programs that rely only on OAEs. Infants with absent or elevated reflex thresholds in the presence of normal tympanograms and normal OAEs should be followed up with ABR (Berlin et al., 2005). Other investigators have recommended inclusion of the middle ear muscle reflex in screening programs of hearing loss (Bielecki, Horbulewicz, & Wolan, 2012).

15.5.3 Cochlear Microphonic

Displacement of the stereocilia toward the tallest row causes current flow into a hair cell (Flock, 1965), which is referred to as the mechanoelectrical transduction, the conversion of the mechanical vibrations into electrical energy. The cochlear microphonic (CM) is generated by these currents. Both outer and inner hair cells contribute to the CM, with greater contribution from the outer hair cells (Dallos & Cheatham, 1976).

The CM can be documented by recording responses for rarefaction and condensation clicks, then subtracting the rarefaction (R) response from the condensation (C) and dividing the result by 2 [(C − R)/2]. The response obtained using this procedure occurs within 1 ms. On average there is a time delay of about 0.6 ms from presentation of sound

due to the delay introduced by the tube of the insert earphone. In recording the CM, usually a recording is obtained while the insert earphone tubing is open and another recording is obtained after clamping the tube. If any responses appear after clamping the tube to block the stimulus presentation, they are considered artifacts. If there is no response after clamping the tube, then the CM recorded without clamping is judged to be a true response. In patients with ANSD, when OAEs are normal, the CM is normal, and the input–output function of the CM shows nonlinearity, suggesting normal outer hair cell function. In the absence of OAEs, the CM is reduced in amplitude, and the input–output function shows less nonlinearity (▶ Fig. 15.6), suggesting that the inner hair cells may be contributing to the CM (Shi et al., 2012). Other investigators have reported that the CM is often recordable in patients with ANSD in the absence of OAEs (Deltenre et al., 1999). This recordability can be attributed to contribution from intact inner hair cells to the CM or higher sensitivity of OAEs to the degree of outer hair cell loss.

15.5.4 Transtympanic Electrocochleography

Three patterns of cochlear potentials have been recorded using transtympanic electrocochleography

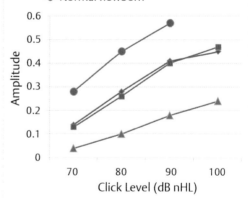

Fig. 15.6 Amplitude of the cochlear microphonic as a function of click levels across different groups. All of the mean values are based on the report of Shi et al. (2012) except for the newborn data, which are based on Young (2000).

in auditory neuropathy: presence of receptor summating potential (SP) without a neural compound action potential (CAP), which suggests presynaptic dysfunction of inner hair cells; presence of delayed later neural potentials (e.g., wave V) without a CAP, suggesting postsynaptic disorder of nerve terminals at the base of inner hair cells; and presence of both SP and CAP, suggesting postsynaptic disorder of the auditory nerve (Santarelli, Starr, Michalewski, & Arslan, 2008).

15.5.5 Auditory Brainstem Response

As mentioned previously, ABR is absent or is reduced in amplitude (Rance, Corben, & Delatycki, 2012) in the presence of ANSD. In the presence of some residual inner hair cells, the auditory nerve fibers contacting these inner hair cells may have reduced or insufficient spontaneous and evoked discharged rates (Salvi, Ding, Wang, & Jiang, 2000), which can lead to the absence or reduction of the surface recorded wave I and following components of the ABR. In some cases, the ABR may be absent initially but can be recorded later (Aldosari, Mabie, & Husain, 2003; Psarommatis et al., 2006) probably due to neuromaturation.

15.5.6 Auditory Steady-State Response

The auditory steady-state response (ASSR) is more often recordable in ANSD patients compared to the ABR. One report noted the absence of the ABR recorded with clicks at a rate of 19.9/s in 11 out of 13 patients with ANSD. The ASSR was recordable in 10 of the 13 patients across frequencies of 500 to 4000 Hz using modulation frequencies ranging from 77 to 103 Hz (Emara & Gabr, 2010). ASSR thresholds may allow estimation of behavioral thresholds in young children with ANSD (Attias, Buller, Rubel, & Raveh, 2006).

15.5.7 Cortical Potentials

Cortical potentials in children with ANSD can be modified by asking the children to pay active attention to the stimuli. In some cases, a response can be absent during passive recordings even in the presence of good speech perception skills (Alvarenga et al., 2012) but can appear when a child is actively attending to the stimuli (Michalewski, Starr, Nguyen, Kong, & Zeng, 2005). The P1 can be

recorded in approximately 70% of hearing aid users with ANSD (Sharma, Cardon, Henion, & Roland, 2011). Cortical evoked potentials may be useful in estimating auditory thresholds in infants with ANSD (He, Teagle, Roush, Grose, & Buchman, 2013).

One possible reason for the presence of auditory evoked cortical potentials in the absence of the ABR is central auditory system compensation for reduced input. The cortical neurons may increase their gain to compensate for reduced input from the auditory brainstem, leading to normal cortical evoked potentials (Salvi et al., 2000).

15.6 Intervention

The intervention strategies that can be used with infants with ANSD are shown in ▶ Fig. 15.7. Throughout intervention, guidance and support should be provided to parents to allow them to make well-informed decisions. In addition, the patients should receive ongoing monitoring of peripheral auditory sensitivity, OAEs, and ABRs.

15.6.1 Guidance and Support to Parents

The results of tests need to be explained to parents carefully, and the initial interventions strategies should be outlined. In the presence of severe to profound hearing loss, parents need to understand that a hearing aid will be tried initially and that it is useful to wait until the baby is at least 18 months old to allow for neuromaturation before considering cochlear implants. Throughout the intervention period, parents will need a supportive team. This is especially true when other comorbid deficits, such as vision problems, cognitive deficits, or cardiac abnormalities, are present. Audiologists should note that, without proper and repeated counseling and guidance related to the importance of hearing for adequate cognitive, speech and language, and social development, parents may give very low priority to the diagnosis of ANSD (Uus, Young, & Day, 2012). Because ANSD is an invisible disability, like other types of hearing loss, it can get easily ignored in the presence of other disabilities. To the best extent possible, the potential cause of the ANSD should be explored, not only for designing the intervention plan properly but also to allow parents to be knowledgeable about the cause. Generic referrals and counseling should be recommended as needed (Rawool, 2010a,b).

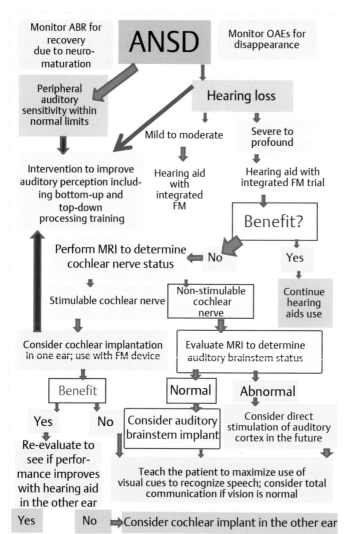

Fig. 15.7 Intervention techniques for auditory neuropathy spectrum disorder (ANSD).

15.6.2 Initial Intervention Strategies for Newborns

Newborns with reliable and stable audiograms showing moderate or more severe hearing loss should be fitted with hearing aids with integrated frequency modulation (FM) technology. For newborns with normal or near-normal hearing, use of FM devices is recommended in noisy situations. Initial approach for all newborns regardless of hearing sensitivity should include maximum auditory stimulation to stimulate synchronous responses, auditory training, and use of clear speech.

15.6.3 Personal Frequency Modulation Listening Devices

Children with ANSD who have normal or near-normal hearing may enjoy better speech perception in noise through the use of personal FM listening systems. In one study, 19 school-aged children with Friedreich ataxia and a cohort of matched control children were evaluated for their ability to understand speech in noise (Rance, Corben, & Delatycki, 2012). Consonant-nucleus-consonant (CNC) words were presented at 65 dB sound pressure levels (SPL) or comfortable listening levels in the presence of four-talker babble presented at the same levels to yield a signal-to-babble ratio of 0 dB. In this condition, mean phoneme scores for children with Friedreich ataxia was 22.3% (standard deviation [SD] 16), while that of children in the control groups was 55.9% (SD 5.6%), yielding a significant difference between the two groups. Use of personal FM devices improved the phoneme recognition performance of children with Friedreich ataxia to the level of their unaffected peers in noisy listening conditions designed to simulate average school classrooms (Rance, Corben, & Delatycki, 2012). Approximately 25% of patients with ANSD use FM devices with or without cochlear implants (Hood, Wilensky, Li, & Berlin, 2003).

15.6.4 Auditory Training

Individuals who show normal peripheral auditory sensitivity in the presence of ANSD may benefit from training geared toward improving temporal auditory processing skills, depending on the specific deficits identified during testing. In addition, some individuals who are fitted with hearing aids or cochlear implants and continue to experience difficulty in recognizing speech in noise could benefit from training to improve bottom-up and top-down processing, as discussed in Chapter 8. Neural plasticity has been demonstrated at subcortical levels. Improved brainstem responses to speech in noise associated with improved speech perception in noise have been recorded in young adults participating in auditory training (Song, Skoe, Banai, & Kraus, 2012). Auditory training can also improve auditory brainstem timing in children with autism spectrum disorders (Russo, Hornickel, Nicol, Zecker, & Kraus, 2010). Intervention strategies to improve speech perception in quiet and degraded conditions are discussed in Chapter 11, more specific training strategies for improving temporal processing are discussed in Chapter 9, and specific protocols for improving localization using interaural time cues are discussed in Chapter 10.

15.6.5 Clear Speech

Clear speech (see Chapter 8) is known to significantly improve the speech recognition performance of individuals with ANSD compared to conversational speech in quiet and noisy conditions. A significant advantage of clear speech over conversational speech has been documented in various listening conditions, as shown in ▶ Fig. 15.8. In patients with ANSD and cochlear implants, use of

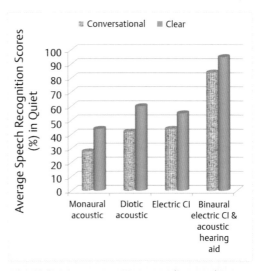

Fig. 15.8 Average recognition scores (% correct) in quiet for clear and conversational sentences across different conditions in listeners with auditory neuropathy spectrum disorder (ANSD) (based on Zeng & Liu, 2006). CI, cochlear implant.

clear speech can improve recognition in noise by approximately 20% (Zeng & Liu, 2006).

15.6.6 Modified Speech

Prolongation of rapidly changing acoustic speech elements and decreased speaking rate can improve speech perception in individuals with ANSD who have poor speech perception and have no auditory nerve deficiency. Hassan (2011) prolonged the formant transitions in consonants such as /ki-gi/and the pauses between consonant-vowel (CV) pairs. These modifications, especially the prolongation of consonant duration, improved phoneme discrimination in individuals with ANSD (Hassan, 2011). Adaptive training using such modified speech is known to improve the perception of average speech in individuals with temporal processing deficits (Tallal et al., 1996). Such a training approach may have the potential to improve speech perception in individuals with ANSD.

Because of the poor modulation detection thresholds shown by individuals with ANSD and the relationship of these thresholds to speech recognition in noise, envelope enhancement of the speech signal by enhancing the consonant portion and compressing the vowel portion has the potential to improve speech recognition (Apoux, Tribut, Debruille, & Lorenzi, 2004). Use of such schemes can improve speech recognition for many individuals with ANSD, although the degree of improvement can vary from only 8% to as much as 36%. Individuals who have very poor speech recognition for unprocessed speech show less improvement with this technique (Narne & Vaneja, 2012).

15.6.7 Hearing Aids

For individuals with mild to moderate hearing loss, hearing aids can compensate for the amplification normally provided by outer hair cells. In many individuals with normal OAEs, outer hair cells are assumed to be normal. However, in some cases, the OAEs disappear over time. Thus, hearing aids have been considered to be one option for compensating for hearing loss. Because of the presence of temporal processing deficits, linear amplification has been recommended because amplitude compression can reduce the amount of temporal modulations in aided signals (Zeng & Liu, 2006).

In some patients, some cochlear regions may have intact inner hair cells, and the selective inner hair cell loss in other regions is not complete, allowing the presence of residual inner hair cells. In addition, the supporting cells in the area and both inner and outer pillar cells may remain intact (Amutuzzi et al., 2011). The presence of neurotrophins in the supporting and pillar cells may allow continued survival of the remaining inner hair cells (Sobkowicz, August, & Slapnick, 2002). In such patients, at least partial benefit can be expected from hearing aids (Deltenre et al., 1999; Rance et al., 1999). Up to 50% of patients with auditory neuropathy show significant improvement with amplification (Rance, Cone-Wesson, Wunderlich, & Dowell, 2002). In one study, 8 out of 26 patients continued to use hearing aids with developmentally appropriate auditory progress, 4 of them achieved 60% or better open set recognition, and 2 hearing aid users achieved neuromaturation yielding normal ABRs at the age of 12 and 16 months. In addition, two of the patients continued to use a hearing aid in the nonimplanted ear because of the perceived benefit of using the aid in addition to cochlear implant (Pelosi et al., 2013). Another study demonstrated the added benefit of a hearing aid in the nonimplanted contralateral ear in addition to a cochlear implant compared to a cochlear implant alone (Runge, Jensen, Friedland, Litovsky, & Tarima, 2011). Some patients will continue to use hearing aids in the nonimplanted ear after perceiving little benefit from cochlear implants due to improved localization cues and better ability to

make use of visual cues for speech perception (Teagle et al., 2010).

Obligatory cortical evoked related potentials may offer a means of predicting the potential benefit from hearing aids, as the presence of such potentials with age-appropriate latency and morphology is correlated with significant open set speech perception abilities and the benefit from hearing aids (Rance et al., 2002). The P1 component of the long latency auditory evoked potential (LLAEP) in children with ANSD who are fitted with hearing aids suggests three possible outcomes: it could show normal latencies, delayed latencies, or abnormal or absent P1 response suggesting poor cortical maturation. Children who show abnormal cortical maturation or who do not benefit from hearing aids are expected to have a more severe form of neural dyssynchrony (Sharma et al., 2011).

15.6.8 Cochlear Implants

Generally, cochlear implants are considered as an option in the presence of severe to profound hearing loss. A trial period of hearing aids with integrated FM devices and auditory training is recommended before considering cochlear implants for newborns. The trial period should last for at least 18 months to allow for any spontaneous recovery from auditory neuropathy due to neuromaturation (Aldosari et al., 2003; Psarommatis et al., 2006; Raveh, Buller, Badrana, & Attias, 2007).

All children with ANSD are not expected to benefit optimally from cochlear implantation (Miyamoto, Kirk, Renshaw, & Hussain, 1999; Neary & Lightfoot, 2012; Rance & Barker, 2008, 2009). Approximately 27 to 38% of children with ANSD and cochlear implants can perform open set speech recognition tasks (Carvalho, Bevilacqua, Sameshima, & Costa Filho, 2011; Pelosi et al., 2013; Teagle et al., 2010). Among those who are able to perform open set speech recognition tasks, speech recognition scores can be less than 30% even after using the devices for 2 or more years. If not carefully selected for implantation, approximately 25% of children with ANSD may exhibit minimal benefit from cochlear implants (Gibson & Sanli, 2007; Teagle et al., 2010). This is especially true for individuals in whom the site of the lesion is in the auditory nerve, such as that seen in cochlear nerve deficiency (Teagle et al., 2010; Walton, Gibson, Sanli, & Prelog, 2008). A narrow or obliterated bony cochlear nerve canal on computed tomography (CT) scans and a deficient cochlear nerve on magnetic resonance imaging (MRI) are correlated with poor speech perception abilities after cochlear implants in children with ANSD. Such children also show no electrical stapedial reflex (ESR) during surgery and no electrical compound action potentials (ECAPs) following surgery. They also show minimal benefit from auditory verbal therapy (Jeong & Kim, 2013).

Although MRIs are more accurate in identifying cochlear nerves than CT scans, a very thin cochlear nerve may still be invisible during MRI (Song et al., 2011). Behavioral responses to environmental sounds or pure tones (Song et al., 2011) and ASSR testing may allow documentation of hearing at lower frequencies, suggesting the stimulability of the auditory nerve (Manolidis, Tonini, & Spitzer, 2006). Although the cochlear nerve may appear invisible or absent in radiologic images, innervation is still possible, and some children will benefit from cochlear implants (Warren, Wiggins, Pitt, Harnsberger, & Shelton, 2010). Electrodes designed especially to fit narrow diameters and intraoperative direct positioning of the electrode tips closer to the existing auditory nerve may improve outcomes in the presence of thinner cochlear nerves (Manolidis et al., 2006). A well-performed careful surgical approach (Chadha, James, Gordon, Blaser, & Papsin, 2009) and individualized rehabilitation program can improve success in such children (Arnlodner et al., 2004). Benefit from cochlear implantation may be possible with as few as 3500 neurons (Linthicum & Anderson, 1991). In some cases with demyelinating pathology located in the auditory nerve, cochlear implants can still provide some benefit (Postelmans & Stokroos, 2006). Even though hypoplasia of the cochlear nerve may lead to lower success than a normal nerve, some benefit is still possible following cochlear implantation (Zanetti et al., 2006). The success is most likely due to better synchrony of response firing through electrical stimulation provided by cochlear implants (Zeng & Liu, 2006).

Greater benefit from cochlear implants is expected when the site of the lesion is restricted to the inner hair cells or the synapses between the hair cells and the auditory nerve given that cochlear implants deliver a coded electrical current directly to the auditory nerve. In the presence of selective loss of inner hair cells, supporting cells in the area and both inner and outer pillar cells may be intact and normal. If the supporting and pillar cells generate sufficient neurotrophins for the maintenance of spiral ganglion cells (Stankovic

et al., 2004; Sugawara, Corfas, & Liberman, 2005), the patient can be expected to benefit from cochlear implants (Amutuzzi et al., 2011). Normal width of the bony cochlear nerve canal and the size of the cochlear nerve as detected by CT and MRI are reliable predictors of good speech perception after cochlear implants in children with ANSD (Jeong & Kim, 2013). Thus, preoperative MRI is recommended to rule out an absent or deficient auditory nerve, which can limit the benefit of cochlear implants (Adunka, Jewells, & Buchman, 2007). Good intraoperative ESR and good postoperative electrical compound action potentials suggest that the individual is likely to benefit from cochlear implants (Jeong & Kim, 2013; Teagle et al., 2010) due to good potential for electrical current-induced synchronous firing of auditory nerve fibers. Long-term outcomes suggest that 80% of patients with ANSD show 80% or higher open set speech recognition scores following cochlear implants (Breneman, Gifford, & Dejong, 2012).

The P1 component of the LLAEP is detectable in 85 to 100% of children with ANSD (excluding those with hypoplasia or agenesis of the auditory nerve or cochlear nerve deficiency) following cochlear implants. Shorter latencies of the P1 component are associated with better speech perception. Longer duration of sensory deprivation prior to cochlear implants is associated with longer P1 latencies, suggesting the need for early intervention (Alvarenga et al., 2012; Cardon & Sharma, 2013). Speech and language outcomes for cognitively and developmentally normal children with ANSD who are fitted with cochlear implants are similar to other children with cochlear implants without ANSD (Budenz et al., 2013).

Generally, high stimulation rates are used in cochlear implants to achieve better temporal sampling, stochastic-like firing in the auditory neurons, and wider dynamic range (Hong & Rubinstein, 2006). However, in the presence of slower neural conduction due to axonal loss or demyelination, individuals with ANSD may benefit more from low stimulation rates compared to high stimulation rates (Zeng et al., 2005). With an increase in the stimulation rates from 600 to 4800 pulses/s, the speech recognition performance in quiet and noise does not vary significantly with the exception of better vowel recognition in quiet at higher pulse rates (Shannon, Cruz, & Galvin, 2011). Thus, when patients with ANSD are implanted, it may be better to program the implants to provide slow stimulation rates.

15.6.9 Auditory Brainstem Implant

The cochlear nerve in some children with ANSD is absent. Such children derive either no or minimal benefit from cochlear implants. If other brain structures are normal, including the brainstem and higher centers, a child may be a candidate for a brainstem implant. As stated previously, MRI alone may not be sufficient in ruling out the presence of an auditory nerve for consideration of an auditory brainstem implant. A combination of MRI and preoperative behavioral responses to either pure tone or environmental sounds can be a better indicator of the presence or viability of cochlear nerves (Song et al., 2011). Some investigators have suggested a cochlear implant trial before considering an auditory brainstem implant because in many cases, the cochlear implant may provide a better outcome than the latter. An auditory brainstem implant should be considered only if there is an indication of an absent auditory nerve or severe hypoplasia of the nerve (Merkus et al., 2014), as speech perception outcomes with auditory brainstem implants may not always match the very high outcomes apparent in modern cochlear implants (Schwartz, Otto, Shannon, Hitselberger, & Brackmann, 2008). A shown in ▶ Fig. 15.9, children with auditory neuropathy can have other brain abnormalities, including prominent temporal horns, cerebrospinal fluid and/or ventricular abnormalities, brainstem/cerebellum abnormalities, white matter changes, cerebrum/midbrain abnormalities, demyelination, microcephaly, and a small optical nerve (Roche et al., 2010). Such abnormalities should be ruled out or carefully considered before recommending an auditory brainstem implant.

The auditory brainstem implant consists of a small paddle (8×3 mm), which includes an electrode array with 21 electrode contacts. It is placed on the cochlear nucleus, which is the first contact point within the auditory brainstem for auditory nerve fibers after exiting the cochlea. The cochlear nucleus has a tonotopic organization and different types of neurons, which are expected to be activated by the brainstem implant. In programming the implant processor, electrodes that elicit only nonauditory sensations, such as tingling on the same side of the body as the implant, are switched off and excluded from the implant program. The rate of major complications with auditory brainstem implant surgery is very low, and minor complications can be easily controlled and completely resolved over time (Colletti, Shannon, Carner, Veronese, & Colletti, 2010).

Patients with auditory brainstem implants can show excellent speech recognition even in adverse listening conditions consisting of only a 3 dB signal-to-noise ratio (Skarzyńsky, Behr, Lorens, Podskarbi-Fayette, & Kochanek, 2009). Open set speech recognition in patients with auditory brainstem implants and auditory nerve tumors can improve from 5% at first fitting to 37% after 12 months. Most individuals (84%) report satisfaction with their implant (Matthies et al., 2013). Auditory brainstem implants can allow telephone use in some adults with neurofibromatosis, indicating excellent speech recognition (Colletti, Shannon, & Colletti, 2012). In adults without tumors, open set speech recognition can vary from 10 to 100%, with an average score of 59%, although the performance in patients with neuropathy can be in the lower range (Colletti, Shannon, Carner, Veronese, & Colletti, 2009).

Approximately 80% of young children, including those with aplasia of the auditory nerve, show some benefit with reference to auditory and speech development within a period of 12 months following auditory brainstem implantation (Sennaroglu et al., 2009). In some children, auditory and speech development with auditory brainstem

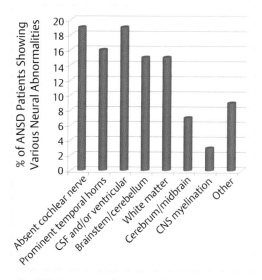

Fig. 15.9 Percentage of ANSD ears/patients showing abnormalities in various neural regions/structures (based on Roche et al., 2010). CNS, central nervous system; CSF, cerebrospinal fluid.

implants is similar to that apparent in age-matched peers with cochlear implants. Many children consistently use their devices and are aware of environmental sounds and produce simple words and sentences. Their auditory performance is significantly better with implantation and is associated with improvements in some cognitive measures (Colletti & Zoccante, 2008).

15.6.10 Use of Medications

Efficient high discharge rates of auditory neurons require healthy mitochondria with efficient ionic pumps for continuous energy production. Thus, auditory neuropathies due to mitochondrial defects may be vulnerable to neural degeneration. In the presence of mitochondrial dysfunction, a vicious cycle of impaired energy production by mitochondria may lead to free radical generation and increased oxidative stress. Thus, medications protecting against reactive oxygen species have been recommended to minimize neural death or degeneration from potential continuous overstimulation from cochlear implants and hearing aids (Giraudet & Avan, 2012). Neurotrophin gene therapy delivered via an injection in the lower basal turn of the scala media may also provide sustained protection of spiral ganglion neurons (Atkinson et al., 2012). Earlier intervention is necessary, as with increasing duration of deafness, neurotrophin therapy may be less effective in supporting the survival of spiral ganglion neurons (Wise et al., 2011).

15.7 Future Trends

The rehabilitation approach for newborns with ANSD is complicated, especially when they have severe to profound hearing loss. The possibility of neuromaturation may delay early cochlear implantation, leading to failure to effectively use early critical periods for speech and language development. In addition, the absence of the auditory nerve or other deficient neural structures may make cochlear or brainstem implants ineffective. One possible technology based on the radio-frequency or microwave auditory effect (chapter 10) that is likely to become available in the future will allow direct stimulation of the auditory cortex for speech and language development without any invasive surgeries that could compromise spontaneous recovery or neuromaturation.

As noted in chapter 10, U.S Patent No. 4,877,027 (1989) describes a device that is capable of inducing sounds in the head of a listener by radiating the head with microwaves in the range of 100 to 10,000 MHz that are modulated with a particular waveform. More specifically, high-frequency electromagnetic energy is projected through the head of the listener. The modulation of the electromagnetic energy allows creation of signals that are intelligible to humans regardless of their peripheral auditory sensitivity.

Another U.S. Patent No. 4,858,612 (1989) describes a method and apparatus for simulation of hearing by microwaves into the region of the auditory cortex. The device incorporates a microphone for picking up the sounds and converting them into electrical signals, which are analyzed and processed for generating several microwave signals at different frequencies. The multifrequency microwaves are then applied to the auditory cortical areas of the brain. By this method, sounds are perceived by the listener, which represent the original signal picked up by the microphone. The inventor notes that the hearing device simulates microwave radiation normally produced by the auditory cortex. The simulated brain waves are introduced into the region of the auditory cortex, which allows perception of the sound by the listener. The inventor claims that the hearing device can allow perception of sounds by individuals who have hearing loss due to damage to the ear or auditory nerve (Stocklin, 1989). The device was based on the hypothesis that the mammalian brain generates and uses electromagnetic waves as an integral part of the nervous system function (Stocklin & Stocklin, 1979).

A similar approach is described in "A Method for Encoding and Transmitting Speech by Means of the Radio Frequency Hearing Phenomenon" from the U.S. Air Force (1994) and is available from http://cryptome.org/rf-speech/rf-speech-02.pdf (Chapter 10). The researchers describe the possible uses of the apparatus for communication in environments such as space missions and hostage situations. This is most likely possible because the microwaves can be sent from a remote location, and the speech signal becomes perceptible only to the listener whose head is being radiated and remains inaudible to people surrounding the listener. More relevant to ANSD, the researchers note that, after appropriate transfer of the technology, this method will be able to improve communications for individuals who are otherwise deaf. As noted in chapter 10, more common term used for devices that send speech or voices directly to the auditory cortex is voice to skull (V2K) devices.

In commercializing such systems for use by individuals who have deficient neural structures, the projected microwave energy has to be carefully controlled to avoid damage to normal brain tissue (Brunkan, 1989). In addition, any other potential side effects, such as tinnitus and cataracts, need to be carefully controlled. Participants that could be ideal candidates for testing the efficacy of the technology are patients who have received cochlear implants with full-length electrodes in both ears. The inner hair cells in such cochleas are damaged during the surgery. A microwave hearing system could allow such patients to perceive music or speech during periods when both cochlear implants are inactive (e.g., while falling asleep). The perception of music and rhythmic humming after cochlear implantation even when the cochlear implant is inactive has been noted (Auffarth & Kropp, 2009). Up to 13% of patients report the perception of instrumental music and/or singing within their heads after cochlear implantation (Low, Tham, D'Souza, & Teng, 2013).

15.8 Review Questions

1. Discuss the audiometric result pattern apparent in the presence of auditory neuropathy spectrum disorder (ANSD). What are the different sites of pathologies in patients diagnosed with ANSD?
2. What are the risk factors for the occurrence of auditory neuropathy?
3. Why is it important to determine the possible cause of ANSD in each patient?
4. Review the auditory processing deficits apparent in patients with ANSD.
5. Review the results of objective measures used in the diagnosis of ANSD.
6. Discuss the initial intervention strategies for newborns diagnosed with ANSD.
7. Discuss the characteristics of patients with ANSD who may benefit from using hearing aids.
8. Under what circumstances and at what age should you consider cochlear implants for patients with ANSD? When can you expect optimal benefit from cochlear implants?
9. Under what circumstances should you consider auditory brainstem implants for patients with ANSD?
10. Discuss a potential future treatment option for patients with ANSD who have compromised auditory nerve and brainstem structures.

References

[1] Adunka, O. F., Jewells, V., & Buchman, C. A. (2007). Value of computed tomography in the evaluation of children with cochlear nerve deficiency. Otology and Neurotology, 28(5), 597–604.

[2] Aldosari, M., Mabie, A., & Husain, A. M. (2003). Delayed visual maturation associated with auditory neuropathy/dyssynchrony. Journal of Child Neurology, 18(5), 358–361.

[3] Alvarenga, K. F., Amorim, R. B., Agostinho-Pesse, R. S., Costa, O. A., Nascimento, L. T., & Bevilacqua, M. C. (2012). Speech perception and cortical auditory evoked potentials in cochlear implant users with auditory neuropathy spectrum disorders. International Journal of Pediatric Otorhinolaryngology, 76(9), 1332–1338.

[4] Amatuzzi, M., Liberman, M. C., & Northrop, C. (2011). Selective inner hair cell loss in prematurity: A temporal bone study of infants from a neonatal intensive care unit. Journal of the Association for Research in Otolaryngology, 12(5), 595–604.

[5] Amatuzzi, M. G., Northrop, C., Liberman, M. C., et al. (2001). Selective inner hair cell loss in premature infants and cochlea pathological patterns from neonatal intensive care unit autopsies. Archives of Otolaryngology–Head and Neck Surgery, 127(6), 629–636.

[6] Apoux, F., Tribut, N., Debruille, X., & Lorenzi, C. (2004). Identification of envelope-expanded sentences in normal-hearing and hearing-impaired listeners. Hearing Research, 189 (1-2), 13–24.

[7] Arnoldner, C., Baumgartner, W. D., Gstoettner, W., Egelierler, B., Czerny, C., Steiner, E., & Hamzavi, J. (2004). Audiological performance after cochlear implantation in children with inner ear malformations. International journal of pediatric otorhinolaryngology, 68(4), 457-467.

[8] Atkinson, P. J., Wise, A. K., Flynn, B. O., et al. (2012). Neurotrophin gene therapy for sustained neural preservation after deafness. PLoS ONE, 7(12), e5233.

[9] Attias, J., Buller, N., Rubel, Y., & Raveh, E. (2006). Multiple auditory steady-state responses in children and adults with normal hearing, sensorineural hearing loss, or auditory neuropathy. Annals of Otology, Rhinology, and Laryngology, 115 (4), 268–276.

[10] Auffarth, I. S., & Kropp, S. (2009). Musical hallucination in a patient after cochlear implantation. Journal of Neuropsychiatry and Clinical Neuroscience, 21(2), 230–231.

[11] Bae, S. H., Baek, J. I., Lee, J. D., et al. (2013). Genetic analysis of auditory neuropathy spectrum disorder in the Korean population. Gene, 522(1), 65–69.

[12] Bahmad, F., Jr., Merchant, S. N., Nadol, J. B., Jr., & Tranebjaerg, L. (2007). Otopathology in Mohr-Tranebjaerg syndrome. Laryngoscope, 117(7), 1202–1208.

[13] Berlin, C. I., Hood, L. J., Morlet, T., et al. (2005). Absent or elevated middle ear muscle reflexes in the presence of normal otoacoustic emissions: A universal finding in 136 cases of auditory neuropathy/dys-synchrony. Journal of the American Academy of Audiology, 16(8), 546–553.

[14] Berlin, C. I., Hood, L., & Rose, K. (2001). On renaming auditory neuropathy as auditory dyssynchrony. Audiology Today, 13, 15–17.

[15] Bielecki, I., Horbulewicz, A., & Wolan, T. (2012). Prevalence and risk factors for auditory neuropathy spectrum disorder in a screened newborn population at risk for hearing loss. International Journal of Pediatric Otorhinolaryngology, 76 (11), 1668–1670.

[16] Breneman, A. I., Gifford, R. H., & Dejong, M. D. (2012). Cochlear implantation in children with auditory neuropathy spectrum disorder: Long-term outcomes. Journal of the American Academy of Audiology, 23(1), 5–17.

[17] Brunkan, W. B. (1989). U.S. Patent No. 4,877,027. Washington, DC: U.S. Patent and Trademark Office.

[18] Buchman, C. A., Roush, P. A., Teagle, H. F., Brown, C. J., Zdanski, C. J., & Grose, J. H. (2006). Auditory neuropathy characteristics in children with cochlear nerve deficiency. Ear and Hearing, 227(4), 399–408.

[19] Budenz, C. L., Starr, K., Arndt, C., et al. (2013). Speech and language outcomes of cochlear implantation in children with isolated auditory neuropathy versus cochlear hearing loss. Otology and Neurotology, 34(9), 1615–1621.

[20] Butinar, D., Zidar, J., Leonardis, L., et al. (1999). Hereditary auditory, vestibular, motor, and sensory neuropathy in a Slovenian Roma (Gypsy) kindred. Annals of Neurology, 46 (1), 36–44.

[21] Cardon, G., & Sharma, A. (2013). Central auditory maturation and behavioral outcome in children with auditory neuropathy spectrum disorder who use cochlear implants. International Journal of Audiology, 52(9), 577–586.

[22] Carvalho, A. C., Bevilacqua, M. C., Sameshima, K., & Costa Filho, O. A. (2011). Auditory neuropathy/auditory dyssynchrony in children with cochlear implants. Brazilian Journal of Otorhinolaryngology, 77(4), 481–487.

[23] Celis-Aguilar, E., Macias-Valle, L., & Coutinho-De Toledo, H. (2012). Auditory neuropathy secondary to cryptococcal central nervous system infection in 2 immunocompromised patients. Otolaryngology–Head and Neck Surgery, 147(3), 597–598.

[24] Ceranić, B., & Luxon, L. M. (2004). Progressive auditory neuropathy in patients with Leber's hereditary optic neuropathy. Journal of Neurology, Neurosurgery, and Psychiatry, 75 (4), 626–630.

[25] Chadha, N. K., James, A. L., Gordon, K. A., Blaser, S., & Papsin, B. C. (2009). Bilateral cochlear implantation in children with anomalous cochleovestibular anatomy. Archives of Otolaryngology–Head and Neck Surgery, 135(9), 903–909.

[26] Ching, T. Y., Dillon, H., Marnane, V., et al. (2013). Outcomes of early- and late-identified children at 3 years of age: Findings from a prospective population-based study. Ear and Hearing, 34(5), 535–552.

[27] Coenraad, S., Goedegebure, A., van Goudoever, J. B., & Hoeve, L. J. (2011). Risk factors for auditory neuropathy spectrum disorder in NICU infants compared to normal-hearing NICU controls. Laryngoscope, 121(4), 852–85.

[28] Colletti, L., Shannon, R., & Colletti, V. (2012). Auditory brainstem implants for neurofibromatosis type 2. Current Opinion in Otolaryngology and Head and Neck Surgery, 20(5), 353–357.

[29] Colletti, L., & Zoccante, L. (2008). Nonverbal cognitive abilities and auditory performance in children fitted with auditory brainstem implants: Preliminary report. Laryngoscope, 118(8), 1443–1448.

[30] Colletti, V., Shannon, R., Carner, M., Veronese, S., & Colletti, L. (2009). Outcomes in nontumor adults fitted with the auditory brainstem implant: 10 years' experience. Otology and Neurotology, 30(5), 614–618.

[31] Colletti, V., Shannon, R. V., Carner, M., Veronese, S., & Colletti, L. (2010). Complications in auditory brainstem implant surgery in adults and children. Otology and Neurotology, 31 (4), 558–564.

[32] Dahl, H.-H. M., Ching, T. Y. C., Hutchison, W., Hou, S., Seeto, M., & Sjahalam-King, J. (2013). Etiology and audiological outcomes at 3 years for 364 children in Australia. PLoS ONE, 8(3), e59624.

[33] Dallos, P., & Cheatham, M. A. (1976). Production of cochlear potentials by inner and outer hair cells. Journal of the Acoustical Society of America, 60(2), 510–512.

[34] Delmaghani, S., del Castillo, F. J., Michel, V., et al. (2006). Mutations in the gene encoding pejvakin, a newly identified protein of the afferent auditory pathway, cause DFNB59 auditory neuropathy. Nature Genetics, 38(7), 770–778.

[35] Deltenre, P., Mansbach, A. L., Bozet, C., et al. (1999). Auditory neuropathy with preserved cochlear microphonics and secondary loss of otoacoustic emissions. Audiology, 38(4), 187–195.

[36] Draper, T. H., & Bamiou, D. E. (2009). Auditory neuropathy in a patient exposed to xylene: Case report. Journal of Laryngology and Otology, 123(4), 462–465.

[37] Emara, A. A., & Gabr, T. A. (2010). Auditory steady state response in auditory neuropathy. Journal of Laryngology and Otology, 124(9), 950–956.

[38] Flock, A. (1965). Transducing mechanisms in the lateral line canal organ receptors. Cold Spring Harbor Symposia on Quantitative Biology, 30, 133–145.

[39] Furman, A. C., Kujawa, S. G., & Liberman, M. C. (2013). Noise-induced cochlear neuropathy is selective for fibers with low spontaneous rates. Journal of Neurophysiology, 110(3), 577–586.

[40] Gibson, W. P., & Sanli, H. (2007). Auditory neuropathy: An update. Ear and Hearing, 28(2, Suppl.), 102S–106S.

[41] Giraudet, F., & Avan, P. (2012). Auditory neuropathies: Understanding their pathogenesis to illuminate intervention strategies. Current Opinion in Neurology, 25(1), 50–56.

[42] Grati, F. R., Lesperance, M. M., De Toffol, S., et al. (2009). Pure monosomy and pure trisomy of 13q21.2-31.1 consequent to a familial insertional translocation: Exclusion of PCDH9 as the responsible gene for autosomal dominant auditory neuropathy (AUNA1). American Journal of Medical Genetics Part A, 149A(5), 906–913.

[43] Guidelines Development Conference on the Identification and Management of Infants with Auditory Neuropathy. (2008). Auditory neuropathy spectrum disorder (ANSD) guidelines. Retrieved from www.thechildrenshospital.org/conditions/speech/danielscenter/ANSD-Guidelines.aspx. http://www.childrenscolorado.org/File%20Library/Conditions-Programs/ASL/ANSD-Monograph-Bill-Daniels-Center-for-Childrens-Hearing.pdf Retrieved on Nov 4, 2014.

[44] Haaksma-Schaafsma, S. C., van Dijk, P., & Dikkers, F. G. (2012). Auditory and optic neuropathy in Kjer's disease: Case report. Journal of Laryngoligy and Otology, 126(3), 309–312.

[45] Hassan, D. M. (2011). Perception of temporally modified speech in auditory neuropathy. International Journal of Audiology, 50(1), 41–49.

[46] He, S., Teagle, H. F., Roush, P., Grose, J. H., & Buchman, C. A. (2013). Objective hearing threshold estimation in children with auditory neuropathy spectrum disorder. Laryngoscope, 123(11), 2859–2861.

[47] Hong, R. S., & Rubinstein, J. T. (2006). Conditioning pulse trains in cochlear implants: Effects on loudness growth. Otology and Neurotology, 27(1), 50–56.

[48] Hood, L. J., Wilensky, D., Li, L., & Berlin, C. I. (2003). The role of FM technology in management of patients with auditory neuropathy/dys-synchrony. Proceedings of the International Conference ACCESS: Achieving Clear Communication. Employing Sound Solutions, 2003, 107–112. Retrieved December 2, 2013, from http://www.phonakpro.com/content/

dam/phonak/b2b/FM_eLibrary/ACCESS_Chapter_9_Linda_-Hood.pdf.

[49] Huang, T., Santarelli, R., & Starr, A. (2009). Mutation of OPA1 gene causes deafness by affecting function of auditory nerve terminals. Brain Research, 1300, 97–104.

[50] Iwasa, Y., Nishio, S. Y., Yoshimura, H., et al. (2013). OTOF mutation screening in Japanese severe to profound recessive hearing loss patients. BMC Medical Genetics, 14, 95.

[51] Jeong, S. W., & Kim, L. S. (2013). Auditory neuropathy spectrum disorder: Predictive value of radiologic studies and electrophysiologic tests on cochlear implant outcomes and its radiologic classification. Acta Otolaryngologica, 133(7), 714–721.

[52] Kim, T. B., Isaacson, B., Sivakumaran, T. A., Starr, A., Keats, B. J., & Lesperance, M. M. (2004). A gene responsible for autosomal dominant auditory neuropathy (AUNA1) maps to 13q14-21. Journal of Medical Genetics, 41(11), 872–87.

[53] Korver, A. M., van Zanten, G. A., Meuwese-Jongejeugd, A., van Straaten, H. L., & Oudesluys-Murphy, A. M. (2012). Auditory neuropathy in a low-risk population: A review of the literature. International Journal of Pediatric Otorhinolaryngology, 76(12), 1708–1711.

[54] Levi, J., Ames, J., Bacik, K., Drake, C., Morlet, T., & O'Reilly, R. C. (2013). Clinical characteristics of children with cochlear nerve dysplasias. Laryngoscope, 123(3), 752–756.

[55] Linthicum, F. H. Jr., & Anderson, W. (1991). Cochlear implantation of totally deaf ears: Histologic evaluation of candidacy. Acta Otolaryngologica, 111(2), 327–331.

[56] Low, W. K., Tham, C. A., D'Souza, V. D., & Teng, S. W. (2013). Musical ear syndrome in adult cochlear implant patients. Journal of Laryngology and Otology, 127(9), 854–858.

[57] Manchaiah, V. K., Zhao, F., Danesh, A. A., & Duprey, R. (2011). The genetic basis of auditory neuropathy spectrum disorder (ANSD). International Journal of Pediatric Otorhinolaryngology, 75(2), 151–158.

[58] Maris, M., Venstermans, C., & Boudewyns, A. N. (2011). Auditory neuropathy/dyssynchrony as a cause of failed neonatal hearing screening. International Journal of Pediatric Otorhinolaryngology, 75(7), 973–975.

[59] Marlin, S., Feldmann, D., Nguyen, Y., et al. (2010). Temperature-sensitive auditory neuropathy associated with an otoferlin mutation: Deafening fever! Biochemical and Biophysical Research Communications, 394(3), 737–742.

[60] Matthies, C., Brill, S., Kaga, K., et al. (2013). Auditory brainstem implantation improves speech recognition in neurofibromatosis type II patients. ORL Journal for Oto-Rhino-Laryngology and Its Related Specialties, 75(5), 282–295.

[61] Merchant, S. N., McKenna, M. J., Nadol, J. B., Jr., et al. (2001). Temporal bone histopathologic and genetic studies in Mohr-Tranebjaerg syndrome (DFN-1). Otology and Neurotology, 22(4), 506–511.

[62] Merkus, P., Di Lella, F.D, Di Trapani, GD, et al. (2014). Indications and contraindications of auditory brainstem implants: Systematic review and illustrative cases. European Archives of Otorhinolaryngology, 271(1), 3-13.

[63] Meyer, E., Michaelides, M., Tee, L. J., et al. (2010). Nonsense mutation in TMEM126A causing autosomal recessive optic atrophy and auditory neuropathy. Molecular Vision, 16, 650–664.

[64] Michalewski, H. J., Starr, A., Nguyen, T. T., Kong, Y. Y., & Zeng, F. G. (2005). Auditory temporal processes in normal-hearing individuals and in patients with auditory neuropathy. Clinical Neurophysiology, 116(3), 669–68.

[65] Mittal, R., Ramesh, A. V., Panwar, S. S., Nilkanthan, A., Nair, S., & Mehra, P. R. (2012). Auditory neuropathy spectrum disorder: Its prevalence and audiological characteristics in an Indian tertiary care hospital. International Journal of Pediatric Otorhinolaryngology, 76(9), 1351–1354.

[66] Miyamoto, R. T., Kirk, K. I., Renshaw, J., & Hussain, D. (1999). Cochlear implantation in auditory neuropathy. Laryngoscope, 109(2, Pt. 1), 181–185.

[67] Moser, T., Predoehl, F., & Starr, A. (2013). Review of hair cell synapse defects in sensorineural hearing impairment. Otology and Neurotology, 34(6), 995–1004.

[68] Narne, V. K. (2013). Temporal processing and speech perception in noise by listeners with auditory neuropathy. PLoS ONE, 8(2), e55995.

[69] Narne, V. K., & Vanaja, C. S. (2012). Speech identification with temporal and spectral modification in subjects with auditory neuropathy. ISRN Otolaryngology, Article ID 671247, 7 pages.

[70] Neary, W., & Lightfoot, G. (2012). Auditory neuropathy spectrum disorder: Examples of poor progress following cochlear implantation. Audiological Medicine, 10(3), 142–149.

[71] Oysu, C., Aslan, I., Basaran B., & Baserer, N. (2001). The site of the hearing loss in Refsum's disease. International Journal of Pediatric Otorhinolaryngology, 61(2), 129–134.

[72] Pelosi, S., Wanna, G., Hayes, C., et al. (2013). Cochlear implantation versus hearing amplification in patients with auditory neuropathy spectrum disorder. Otolaryngology–Head and Neck Surgery, 148(5), 815–821.

[73] Penido, R. C., & Isaac, M. L. (2013). Prevalence of auditory neuropathy spectrum disorder in an auditory health care service. Brazilian Journal of Otorhinolaryngology, 79(4), 429–433.

[74] Postelmans, J. T., & Stokroos, R. J. (2006). Cochlear implantation in a patient with deafness induced by Charcot-Marie-Tooth disease (hereditary motor and sensory neuropathies). Journal of Laryngology and Otology, 120(6), 508–510.

[75] Psarommatis, I., Riga, M., Douros, K., et al. (2006). Transient infantile auditory neuropathy and its clinical implications. International Journal of Pediatric Otorhinolaryngology, 70(9), 1629–1637.

[76] Rance, G., & Barker, E. J. (2008). Speech perception in children with auditory neuropathy/dyssynchrony managed with either hearing AIDS or cochlear implants. Otology and Neurotology, 29(2), 179–182.

[77] Rance, G., & Barker, E. J. (2009). Speech and language outcomes in children with auditory neuropathy/dys-synchrony managed with either cochlear implants or hearing aids. International Journal of Audiology, 48(6), 313–320.

[78] Rance, G., Barker, E., Mok, M., Dowell, R., Rincon, A., & Garratt, R. (2007). Speech perception in noise for children with auditory neuropathy/dys-synchrony type hearing loss. Ear and Hearing, 28(3), 351–360.

[79] Rance, G., Beer, D. E., Cone-Wesson, B., et al. (1999). Clinical findings for a group of infants and young children with auditory neuropathy. Ear and Hearing, 20(3), 238–252.

[80] Rance, G., Cone-Wesson, B., Wunderlich, J., & Dowell, R. (2002). Speech perception and cortical event related potentials in children with auditory neuropathy. Ear and Hearing, 23(3), 239–253.

[81] Rance, G., Corben, L., & Delatycki, M. (2012). Auditory processing deficits in children with Friedreich ataxia. Journal of Child Neurology, 27(9), 1197–1203.

[82] Rance, G., Fava, R., Baldock, H., et al. (2008). Speech perception ability in individuals with Friedreich ataxia. Brain, 131 (Pt. 8), 2002–2012.

[83] Rance, G., McKay, C., & Grayden, D. (2004). Perceptual characterization of children with auditory neuropathy. Ear and Hearing, 25(1), 34–46.

[84] Rance, G., Ryan, M. M., Carew, P., et al. (2012). Binaural speech processing in individuals with auditory neuropathy. Neuroscience, 226, 227–235.

[85] Raveh, E., Buller, N., Badrana, O., & Attias, J. (2007). Auditory neuropathy: Clinical characteristics and therapeutic approach. American Journal of Otolaryngology, 28(5), 302–308.

[86] Rawool, V. W. (2010a). Invisible hearing loss among multiple disabilities: Part 1. Ensuring auditory care. Hearing Review, 17(1), 18–21, 50.

[87] Rawool, V. W. (2010b). Invisible hearing loss among multiple disabilities: Part 2. The case of the missing hearing aids. Hearing Review, 17(2), 32–37.

[88] Roche, J. P., Huang, B. Y., Castillo, M., Bassim, M. K., Adunka, O. F., & Buchman, C. A. (2010). Imaging characteristics of children with auditory neuropathy spectrum disorder. Otology and Neurotology, 31(5), 780–788.

[89] Roux, I., Safieddine, S., Nouvian, R., et al. (2006). Otoferlin, defective in a human deafness form, is essential for exocytosis at the auditory ribbon synapse. Cell, 127(2), 277–289.

[90] Runge, C. L., Jensen, J., Friedland, D. R., Litovsky, R. Y., & Tarima, S. (2011). Aiding and occluding the contralateral ear in implanted children with auditory neuropathy spectrum disorder. Journal of the American Academy of Audiology, 22(9), 567–577.

[91] Russo, N. M., Hornickel, J., Nicol, T., Zecker, S., & Kraus, N. (2010). Biological changes in auditory function following training in children with autism spectrum disorders. Behavioral and Brain Functions, 6, 60.

[92] Saluja, S., Agarwal, A., Kler, N., & Amin, S. (2010). Auditory neuropathy spectrum disorder in late preterm and term infants with severe jaundice. International Journal of Pediatric Otorhinolaryngology, 74(11), 1292–1297.

[93] Salvi, R. J., Ding, D., Wang, J., & Jiang, H. Y. (2000). A review of the effects of selective inner hair cell lesions on distortion product otoacoustic emissions, cochlear function and auditory evoked potentials. Noise and Health, 2(6), 9–26.

[94] Santarelli, R., Cama, E., Scimemi, P., Dal Monte, E., Genovese, E., & Arslan, E. (2008). Audiological and electrocochleography findings in hearing-impaired children with connexin 26 mutations and otoacoustic emissions. European Archives of Otorhinolaryngology, 265(1), 43–51.

[95] Santarelli, R., Del Castillo, I., Rodríguez-Ballesteros, M., et al. (2009). Abnormal cochlear potentials from deaf patients with mutations in the otoferlin gene. Journal of the Association for Research in Otolaryngology, 10(4), 545–556.

[96] Santarelli, R., Starr, A., del Castillo, I., et al. (2011). Presynaptic and postsynaptic mechanisms underlying auditory neuropathy in patients with mutations in the OTOF or OPA1 gene. Audiological Medicine, 9, 59–66.

[97] Santarelli, R., Starr, A., Michalewski, H. J., & Arslan, E. (2008). Neural and receptor cochlear potentials obtained by transtympanic electrocochleography in auditory neuropathy. Clinical Neurophysiology, 119(5), 1028–1041.

[98] Sanyelbhaa Talaat, H., Kabel, A. H., Samy, H., & Elbadry, M. (2009). Prevalence of auditory neuropathy (AN) among infants and young children with severe to profound hearing loss. International Journal of Pediatric Otorhinolaryngology, 73(7), 937–939.

[99] Sanyelbhaa Talaat, H., Khalil, L. H., Khafagy, A. H., Alkandari, M. M., & Zein, A. M. (2013). Persistence of otoacoustic emissions in children with auditory neuropathy spectrum disorders. International Journal of Pediatric Otorhinolaryngology, 77(5), 703–706.

[100] Schoen, C. J., Emery, S. B., Thorne, M. C., et al. (2010). Increased activity of diaphanous homolog 3 (DIAPH3)/diapha-

nous causes hearing defects in humans with auditory neuropathy and in Drosophila. Proceedings of the National Academy of Sciences of the United States of America, 107 (30), 13396–13401.

[101] Schwartz, M. S., Otto, S. R., Shannon, R. V., Hitselberger, W. E., & Brackmann, D. E. (2008). Auditory brainstem implants. Neurotherapeutics, 5(1), 128–136.

[102] Sennaroglu, L., Ziyal, I., Atas, A., et al. (2009). Preliminary results of auditory brainstem implantation in prelingually deaf children with inner ear malformations including severe stenosis of the cochlear aperture and aplasia of the cochlear nerve. Otology and Neurotology, 30(6), 708–715.

[103] Shannon, R. V., Cruz, R. J., & Galvin, J. J., III. Effect of stimulation rate on cochlear implant users' phoneme, word and sentence recognition in quiet and in noise. Audiology and Neurootology, 16(2), 113–123.

[104] Sharma, A., Cardon, G., Henion, K., & Roland, P. (2011). Cortical maturation and behavioral outcomes in children with auditory neuropathy spectrum disorder. International Journal of Audiology, 50(2), 98–106.

[105] Shi, W., Ji, F., Lan, L., et al. (2012). Characteristics of cochlear microphonics in infants and young children with auditory neuropathy. Acta Otolaryngologica, 132(2), 188–196.

[106] Skarżyński, H., Behr, R., Lorens, A., Podskarbi-Fayette, R., & Kochanek, K. (2009). Bilateral electric stimulation from auditory brainstem implants in a patient with neurofibromatosis type 2. Medical Science Monitor, 15(6), CS100–CS104.

[107] Slack, R. W., Wright, A., Michaels, L., & Frohlich, S. A. (1986). Inner hair cell loss and intracochlear clot in the preterm infant. Clinical Otolaryngology and Allied Sciences, 11(6), 443–446.

[108] Sobkowicz, H. M., August, B. K., & Slapnick, S. M. (2002). Influence of neurotrophins on the synaptogenesis of inner hair cells in the deaf Bronx waltzer (bv) mouse organ of Corti in culture. International Journal of Developmental Neuroscience, 20(7), 537–554.

[109] Song, J. H., Skoe, E., Banai, K., & Kraus, N. (2012). Training to improve hearing speech in noise: Biological mechanisms. Cerebral Cortex, 22(5), 1180–1190.

[110] Song, M. H., Kim, S. C., Kim, J., Chang, J. W., Lee, W. S., & Choi, J. Y. (2011). The cochleovestibular nerve identified during auditory brainstem implantation in patients with narrow internal auditory canals: Can preoperative evaluation predict cochleovestibular nerve deficiency? Laryngoscope, 121 (8), 1773–1779.

[111] Stankovic, K., Rio, C., Xia, A., et al. (2004). Survival of adult spiral ganglion neurons requires erbB receptor signaling in the inner ear. Journal of Neuroscience, 24(40), 8651–8661.

[112] Starr, A., Picton, T. W., Sininger, Y., Hood, L. J., & Berlin, C. I. (1996). Auditory neuropathy. Brain, 119(Pt. 3), 741–753.

[113] Starr, A., Sininger, Y. S., & Pratt, H. (2000). The varieties of auditory neuropathy. Journal for Basic and Clinical Physiology and Pharmacology, 11(3), 215–230.

[114] Starr, A., Sininger, Y., Winter, M., Derebery, M. J., Oba, S., & Michalewski, H. J. (1998). Transient deafness due to temperature-sensitive auditory neuropathy. Ear and Hearing, 19(3), 169–179.

[115] Stocklin, P. L. (1989). U.S. Patent No. 4,858,612. Washington, DC: U.S. Patent and Trademark Office.

[116] Stocklin, P. L., & Stocklin, B. F. (1979). Possible microwave mechanisms of the mammalian nervous system. TIT Journal of Life Sciences, 9(1-2), 29–51.

[117] Sugawara, M., Corfas, G., & Liberman, M. C. (2005). Influence of supporting cells on neuronal degeneration after hair cell loss. Journal of the Association for Research in Otolaryngology, 6(2), 136–147.

[118] Tallal, P., Miller, S. L., Bedi, G., et al. (1996). Language comprehension in language-learning impaired children improved with acoustically modified speech. Science, 271 (5245), 81–84.

[119] Teagle, H. F., Roush, P. A., Woodard, J. S., et al. (2010). Cochlear implantation in children with auditory neuropathy spectrum disorder. Ear and Hearing, 31(3), 325–335.

[120] U. S. Air Force (1994). A method for encoding & transmitting speech by means of the radio frequency hearing phenomenon. Disclosure and record of invention, AF form 1279 to document inventions for consideration of patenting by the Air Force. 1994 Oct 27. Retrieved from http://cryptome.org/rf-speech/rf-speech-02.pdf

[121] Uus, K., Young, A., & Day, M. (2012). Auditory neuropathy spectrum disorder in the wider health context: Experiences of parents whose infants have been identified through newborn hearing screening programme. International Journal of Audiology, 51(3), 186–193.

[122] Varga, R., Kelley, P. M., Keats, B. J., et al. (2003). Non-syndromic recessive auditory neuropathy is the result of mutations in the otoferlin (OTOF) gene. Journal of Medical Genetics, 40(1), 45–50.

[123] Walton, J., Gibson, W. P., Sanli, H., & Prelog, K. (2008). Predicting cochlear implant outcomes in children with auditory neuropathy. Otology and Neurotology, 29(3), 302–309.

[124] Wang, D. Y., Wang, Y. C., Weil, D., et al. (2010). Screening mutations of OTOF gene in Chinese patients with auditory neuropathy, including a familial case of temperature-sensitive auditory neuropathy. BMC Medical Genetics, 11, 79–86.

[125] Wang, Q. J., Li, Q. Z., Rao, S. Q., et al. (2006). AUNX1, a novel locus responsible for X linked recessive auditory and peripheral neuropathy, maps to Xq23-27.3. Journal of Medical Genetics, 43(7), e33.

[126] Wang, Q., Li, R., Zhao, H., et al. (2005). Clinical and molecular characterization of a Chinese patient with auditory neuropathy associated with mitochondrial 12S rRNA T1095C mutation. American Journal of Medical Genetics Part A, 133A (1), 27–30.

[127] Warren, F. M., III, Wiggins, R. H., III, Pitt, C., Harnsberger, H. R., & Shelton, C. (2010). Apparent cochlear nerve aplasia: To implant or not to implant? Otology and Neurotology, 31(7), 1088–1094.

[128] Wise, A. K., Tu, T., Atkinson, P. J., et al. (2011). The effect of deafness duration on neurotrophin gene therapy for spiral ganglion neuron protection. Hearing Research, 278(1-2), 69–76.

[129] Wynne, D. P., Zeng, F. G., Bhatt, S., Michalewski, H. J., Dimitrijevic, A., & Starr, A. (2013). Loudness adaptation accompanying ribbon synapse and auditory nerve disorders. Brain, 136 (Pt. 5), 1626–1638.

[130] Xoinis, K., Weirather, Y., Mavoori, H., Shaha, S. H., & Iwamoto, L. M. (2007). Extremely low birth weight infants are at high risk for auditory neuropathy. Journal of Perinatology, 27(11), 718–723.

[131] Young, S. (2000). Cochlearmicrophonic and distortion product otoacoustic emissions in infants: A normative study. Unpublished master's thesis, University of Melbourne, Melbourne, Australia.

[132] Zanetti, D., Guida, M., Barezzani, M. G., et al. (2006). Favorable outcome of cochlear implant in VIIIth nerve deficiency. Otology and Neurotology, 27(6), 815–823.

[133] Zeng, F. G., Kong, Y. Y., Michalewski, H. J., & Starr, A. (2005). Perceptual consequences of disrupted auditory nerve activity. Journal of Neurophysiology, 93(6), 3050–3063.

[134] Zeng, F.-G., & Liu, S. (2006). Speech perception in individuals with auditory neuropathy. Journal of Speech, Language, and Hearing Research, 49(2), 367–380.

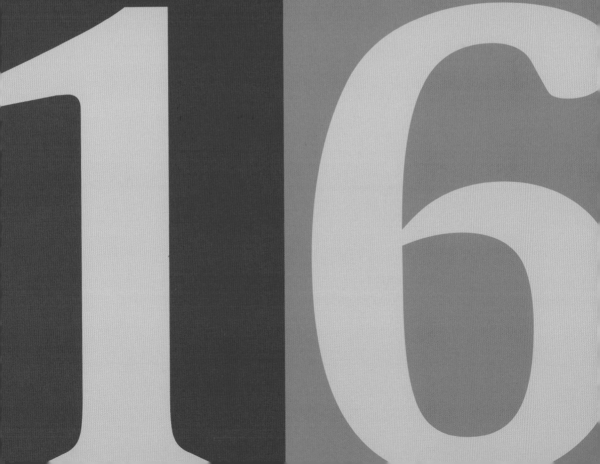

Chapter 16

Auditory Processing Deficits Due to Exposure to Ototoxins

16 Auditory Processing Deficits Due to Exposure to Ototoxins

Substances that can cause damage to the peripheral and central auditory systems are referred to as ototoxins (▶ Fig. 16.1). Exposure to various ototoxins can occur during work, recreation, and medical or other settings. Some ototoxins can cause central auditory deficits secondary to or in the absence of peripheral hearing loss. In assessing individuals with ototoxin exposures, the possibility of both peripheral and central auditory deficits should be considered using a comprehensive case history, audiometric results, and patient complaints.

WorkSafe Australia Guidelines (http://www.commerce.wa.gov.au/WorkSafe/Content/Safety_Topics/Noise/Further_information/Ototoxin.html) suggest that employees who are exposed to ototoxins and complain of hearing difficulties but have normal audiometric test results should be referred for evaluation of the central parts of the auditory system. Auditory processing deficits (APDs) can also be considered in cases where these deficits occur as a result of exposure to ototoxins in nonwork settings.

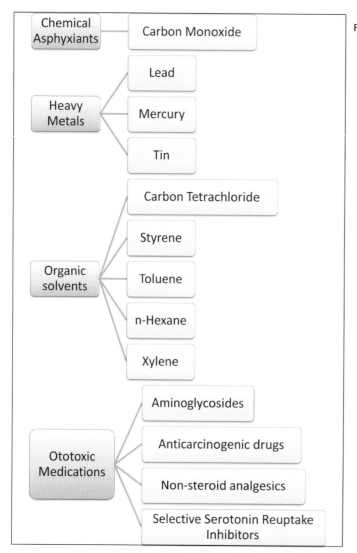

Fig. 16.1 Examples of ototoxins.

16.1 Ototoxins and Their Interactions with Noise

Employers should give specific attention to the interactive effects of work-related ototoxic substances and noise on workers' safety and health in conducting risk evaluations (European Union Directive 2003/10/EC/, 2003) and in providing workmen's compensation (WorkCover Australia, 2001). Ototoxins include asphyxiants (carbon monoxide), drugs (some chemotherapy agents, antibiotics, and aspirin and related medications), metals (arsenic, organic tin, mercury and derivatives, and manganese), and solvents (carbon disulfide, ethylbenzene, *n*-propylbenzene, toluene, *n*-hexane, styrene and methylstyrenes, trichloroethylene, and *p*-xylene) (European Agency for Safety and Health at Work, 2009). Ototoxic chemicals include hydrogen cyanide, diesel fuel, kerosene fuel, jet fuel, JP-8 fuel, organophosphate pesticides, and chemical warfare nerve agents (U.S. Army Center for Health Promotion and Preventative Medicine, USACHPPM, 2003). Ototoxins and noise can interact in worsening hearing loss, and the interactions can be synergistic or additive. Additive effects are predictable from the sum of the effects of exposure to noise or ototoxins alone. Synergistic effects are greater than those that can be predicted from the sum of the exposure to each of the agents.

16.2 Chemical Asphyxiants

Chemical asphyxiants, such as carbon monoxide, reduce oxygen delivery to tissues or oxygen use by tissues. The resultant oxidative stress leads to overproduction of unstable and reactive oxygen species (ROS) that can damage cochlear cells. Excessive glutamate release is apparent in the synapses under the inner hair cells from carbon monoxide ototoxicity (Kanthasamy, Borowitz, Pavlakovic, & Isom, 1994; Liu & Fechter, 1995), leading to auditory synaptopathy or auditory neuropathy spectrum disorder (see Chapter 15). Exacerbation of hearing loss beyond that caused by noise alone can occur at exposure levels of 200 parts per million (ppm) (Fechter, Chen, Rao, & Larabee, 2000; Rao & Fechter, 2000). Carbon monoxide poisoning after short-term exposure can cause sensorineural hearing loss with full or partial recovery (Razzaq, Dumbala, Shyam, & Moudgil, 2010; Shahbaz Hassan, Ray, & Wilson, 2003). Firefighters, foundry workers, miners, toll and tunnel workers, and vehicle mechanics have the potential to be exposed to excessive levels of carbon monoxide (Pouyatos & Fechter, 2007).

Carbon monoxide (asphyxiant) exposure can occur in homes from faulty stoves, water heaters, and furnaces. Razzaq and colleagues (2010) presented a case of sudden deafness in a man who had borrowed a friend's generator and used it in a closed space. Fortunately, in this case, at 3 months he reported full recovery of his hearing.

16.3 Heavy Metals

Some heavy metals have toxic effects on the body, including the auditory system. Ototoxic effects of such metals can occur in both occupational and nonoccupational settings. Some of the ototoxic metals are discussed below.

16.3.1 Lead

Lead is a natural bluish gray metal. Exposure to lead can occur from breathing workplace air or dust and consuming contaminated water or food. Lead is released in the environment through the burning of fossil fuels, mining, and the production of batteries, ammunition, metal products (solder and pipes), and x-ray shielding devices. Lead can damage kidneys and the reproductive system. It is also neuro- and ototoxic (Bleecker, Ford, Lindgren, Scheetz, & Tiburzi, 2003; Discalzi, Capellaro, Bottalo, Fabro, & Mocellini, 1992; Osman et al., 1999; Wu et al., 2000). Chronic low-level lead exposure as reflected in bone lead levels may increase the risk of age-related hearing loss (Park et al., 2010).

Lead exposure can also occur in nonwork settings. For example, lead is present in the Quikrete (Quikrete Companies Inc., Atlanta, GA) Color-PAK powder colorants, except for charcoal No. 1318, which can be used for coloring cement and concrete. Lead is also present in Mayco's (Hilliard, OH) Ceramic Clear Glaze (liquid), which is used for arts and crafts. Children can be exposed to lead by consuming lead-based paint chips or playing in polluted soil. Some pigments used in makeup and hair coloring contain lead. It is important to keep such products out of reach of children (Agency for Toxic Substances and Disease Registry [ATSDR], 2007).

Since August 2009, toys and children's products containing lead in excess of 300 parts per million (ppm) have been banned in the United States; this limit was subsequently lowered to 100 ppm in August 2011. The Consumer Safety Improvement Act of 2008 required the lead limit in toys to be less than 600 ppm within 180 days of the date of enactment of the act, less than 300 ppm after one year following the enactment of the act, and less than 100 ppm after three years following the enactment of the act unless such a lower limit was technologically not feasible for a product. (Consumer Product Safety Improvement Act, 2008). Some currently available children's toys and jewelry, however, may still contain high levels of lead. In 2011, two toys exceeded the 600 ppm limit including a toddler plastic book that could potentially be used by babies and toddlers as a teething instrument. A third toy exceeded the 100 ppm limit and the lead content in several other toys ranged from 74-100 ppm (Hossain & Rae, 2011). Parents need to be diligent when buying toys, especially when they are bought from small vendors with unknown manufacturers.

Blood lead levels greater than 7 µg/dL are significantly associated with hearing loss in adults in the 3 to 8 kHz range (Hwang, Chiang, Yen-Jean, & Wang, 2009). Lead exposure has been associated with anemia, and there is a relationship between blood hemoglobin levels and latencies of the auditory brainstem response (ABR). As the blood hemoglobin levels decrease, ABR latencies increase in children exposed to lead. Children with normal hearing but blood hemoglobin levels below 11 µg/dL show significantly prolonged latencies of waves I, II, III, IV, and V when compared to children with normal hemoglobin levels (Counter, Buchanan, & Ortega, 2012), which suggests central auditory deficits. Intellectual impairment can appear in children with blood lead concentrations below 10 µg/dL (Canfield et al., 2003).

16.3.2 Mercury (Methyl Mercury Chloride, Mercuric Sulfide)

Metallic mercury is a silvery odorless liquid (as seen in thermometers) that changes into a colorless, odorless gas after heating. Mercury salts (crystals) and inorganic mercury compounds are formed when mercury combines with other elements, such as chlorine, sulfur, and oxygen. Organic mercury compounds are formed when mercury combines with carbon. Exposure to mercury can occur from breathing air contaminated by mercury or from skin contact to mercury. Metallic mercury is used in the production of chlorine gas, caustic soda, thermometers, and mercury batteries. The U. S. Occupational Safety and Health Administration

(OSHA) limit for organic mercury is 0.1 mg for each cubic meter of workplace air (0.1 mg/m^3) and 0.05 mg/m^3 of metallic mercury vapor during 8-hour work shifts, assuming a 40-hour workweek.

High-level mercury exposure can damage the nervous system and kidneys, as well as a developing fetus. Mercury can more easily affect the brain in the methylmercury and metallic mercury vapor forms, increasing the risk of injury (ATSDR, 1999a). Mercury compounds, such as methyl mercury chloride and mercuric sulfide, are ototoxic in animals, and organic mercury can be toxic to the human auditory system (Chuu, Hsu, & Lin-Shiau, 2001; Musiek & Hanlon, 1999; Rice, 1998; Rice & Gilbert, 1992).

Exposure to mercury can also occur in nonwork settings. Mercury is present in all of the colors in the Quikrete Color-PAK (powder), except for charcoal No. 1318, which can be used for coloring cement or concrete. Mercury salts are used in some skin-lightening creams, antiseptic creams, and ointments.

Mercury vapor can be released from amalgam dental fillings; the vapor is inhaled, transferred to the blood, and gradually accumulated in the nervous and other systems (Berlin, 2003; Eggleston & Nylander, 1987). The amount of exposure to mercury vapor depends on the size and number of amalgam surfaces (Berlin, 2003; Clarkson, Magos, & Myers, 2003). A higher number of amalgam fillings is associated with poorer auditory thresholds at higher frequencies. The use of amalgam for dental fillings should be avoided as much as possible. In addition, during the removal of existing amalgam fillings at the end of their useful life, precautions such as high-volume air extraction can reduce mercury exposure to the patients, dentists, and dental assistants (Rothwell & Boyd, 2008).

In water, metallic mercury and mercury are metabolized by bacteria, leading to organic or methylmercury, which can build up in fish tissues. As an example, 50% of fish samples and 17% of hair samples collected from villagers close to a mercury processing plant in KwaZulu-Natal, South Africa, exceeded guidelines of the World Health Organization (WHO) possibly due to the disposal of mercury waste in the Mngceweni River, located near the plant (Papu-Zamxaka et al., 2010). The U. S. Environmental Protection Agency (EPA) limit is 2 parts of mercury per billion parts of drinking water (2 parts per billion, or 2 ppb), and the U.S. Food and Drug Administration (FDA) limit is 1 part of methylmercury per million parts of seafood (1 ppm).

Individuals who consume fish caught in a bay with high mercury content can suffer from severe neurologic defects, including hearing loss (Mizukoshi et al., 1989). Those who consume tuna fish regularly have higher levels of mercury in urine and blood than control subjects. In addition, their performance on temporal neurobehavioral tasks involving speed, such as color word reaction time, digit symbol reaction time, and finger-tapping speed, is significantly worse than control subjects (Carta et al., 2003).

Children who accidentally consumed bread made from seeds that were coated with mercury as a fungicide showed audiological impairment (Amin-Zaki, Majeed, Clarkson, & Greenwood, 1978). Andean children who were exposed to mercury vapor from gold-mining operations showed auditory brainstem abnormalities (Counter, 2003). Long-term methylmercury exposure appears to delay ABR latencies with incomplete recovery (Murata, Weihe, Budtz-Jørgensen, Jørgensen, & Grandjean, 2004), suggesting APDs.

16.3.3 Tin

An acute limbic-cerebellar syndrome including hearing loss has been reported in six industrial workers who had inhaled trimethyltin. The exposure occurred while the workers were cleaning a tank used in the manufacturing of dimethyltin (DMT). (Besser et al., 1987).

16.4 Organic Solvents

As suggested by the name, solvents are capable of dissolving one or more other substances. Organic solvents contain carbon in their molecular structure. Exposure to organic solvents can occur in various ways as alcohol, in paints and adhesives, and in heating (propane, kerosene) and automotive (diesel, gasoline) fuels. Workers are most frequently exposed to a mixture consisting mainly of xylene, toluene, and methyl ethyl ketone (MEK), or butanone. However. some workers, such as those in the glass-fiber-reinforced plastic industry are exposed to only styrene, and some, such as those in the rotogravure printing industry, are exposed to only toluene (Sliwińska-Kowalska et al., 2007).

Chronic exposure to solvents can lead to chronic solvent encephalopathy (CSE), which is characterized by mild to severe cognitive impairments, including attention deficits, reduced processing speed, and memory deficits (van Valen et al., 2012). Neuroradiological techniques have demonstrated dose-related neuropathology in patients with CSE that is correlated with performance on tasks involving attention and psychomotor speed (Visser et al, 2008). CSE can develop after 5 to 10 years of daily exposure near the occupational exposure limits (European Agency for Safety and Health at Work, 2009). In cases of very high exposures, CSE can occur in less than 5 years (van der Laan & Sainio, 2012). Workers older than 45 years are more likely to show symptoms of CSE (Keski-Säntti, Kaukiainen, Hyvärinen, & Sainio, 2010).

Toxic exposure to solvents can cause pulmonary edema, peripheral and central nervous system damage, cancer, and liver and kidney failure (Steyger, 2009). Solvent exposure increases the risk of high-frequency hearing loss (Rabinowitz et al., 2008). Exposure to jet fuel, which contains ototoxins such as *n*-hexane, *n*-heptane, toluene, and xylene, increases the adjusted odds of a permanent hearing loss when combined with noise exposure during the first 12 years of exposure. The adjusted odds of hearing loss increase by 70% with 3 years of exposure and by 140% with 12 years of exposure (Kaufman, LeMasters, Olsen, & Succop, 2005). However, under some circumstances, the hearing loss may be mostly noise-induced (Sliwińska-Kowalska et al., 2007).

Mild cortical atrophy (Keski-Säntti, Mäntylä, Lamminen, Hyvärinen, & Sainio, 2009) and a negative impact on dopamine-mediated frontostriatal circuits (Visser et al., 2008) have been reported in patients with CSE. Diffuse structural damage to subcortical cerebral white matter is apparent in some individuals exposed to toluene (Yücel, Takagi, Walterfang, & Lubman, 2008). Myelin, with its high lipid content, appears to be the target of solvents' lipophilic effects leading to neurotoxicity. Thus, the auditory nervous system can be compromised, including the acoustic middle ear muscle reflex. Although the major damage particularly during co-exposure to noise is to the cochlea, solvents may compromise the protective role played by the middle ear acoustic reflex, thus exposing the inner ear to higher noise levels (Campo, Maguin, & Lataye, 2007; Lataye, Maguin, & Campo, 2007; Maguin, Campo, & Parietti-Winkler, 2009). Solvent addicts who inhale glue or paint can suffer from auditory brainstem abnormalities or hearing loss (Ehyai & Freemon, 1983; Metrick & Brenner, 1982; Poulsen & Jensen, 1986), which can be expected to be prominent in the 4000 to 12,000 Hz frequency range. Solvent exposure can also cause poor performance on the dichotic digits test, suggesting central binaural deficits (Fuente et al., 2009). Individuals exposed to solvents report listening difficulties (Fuente, McPherson, & Hormazabal, 2013). Some of the ototoxic solvents are discussed below.

16.4.1 Carbon Tetrachloride

The commonly reported toxic effects of carbon tetrachloride in humans are on the liver, kidneys, and central nervous system (CNS). Carbon tetrachloride has been used in the past to make refrigerants and propellants for aerosol cans, as a solvent for oils, fats, lacquers, varnishes, rubber waxes, and resins, and as a grain fumigant and a dry-cleaning agent. Consumer and fumigant uses have been discontinued by the EPA. It is now used only in industrial settings. Besides industrial settings, exposure to carbon tetrachloride can occur from accidental releases in the air and from its disposal in landfills, where it may evaporate into the air or seep into drinking water sources. Indoor air may be contaminated by carbon tetrachloride due to building materials or products such as cleaning agents used in homes (ATSDR, 1994; U.S. EPA, 1987). Individuals who work with grains or viscose rayon have been exposed to carbon tetrachloride/carbon disulfide (80/20 fumigants), leading to auditory neuropathy in addition to optic neuropathy. Carbon disulfide can form several bonds with single ions of trace copper and zinc metals in the body leading to disruption of their metabolism which results in an increase in the copper and zinc levels in the CNS. Thus, one possible mechanism of carbon disulfide ototoxicity is similar to copper intoxication leading to extrapyramidal symptoms (Peters, Levine, Matthews, Sauter, & Chapman, 1986).

16.4.2 Styrene

Styrene is a colorless, oily liquid that evaporates easily. It has a sweetish aroma, but usually chemicals are added to it, which creates an unpleasant odor. It is absorbed through skin or airways and is metabolized mainly as mandelic acid and phenylglyoxal acid. It can cause damage to several organs, including mucosa, liver, kidneys, the respiratory system, and the CNS. According to the International Agency for Research on Cancer (IARC) (Vineis & Zeise, 2002), styrene has the potential to cause cancer in humans. Examples of industries that can expose workers to styrene are plastics, glass-fiber-reinforced plastics, synthetic rubber, insulators, and some agricultural products. Exposure to styrene can also occur from breathing air that is contaminated with styrene vapors from building materials, tobacco smoke, use of copying machines, and automobile exhaust. Other means of exposure are drinking or bathing in contaminated water and eating food packaged in polystyrene containers.

According to the EPA, lifetime daily exposure to 0.1 ppm styrene is expected to be safe. FDA regulations do not allow styrene concentration in bottled drinking water to exceed 0.1 ppm as cited in Agency for Toxic Substances and Disease Registry (ATSDR, 2007b). Occupational exposure limits for styrene are usually higher, with 12 ppm in Poland and up to 100 ppm in the United Kingdom (Hoet & Lison, 2008). OSHA (1997) also has a permissible exposure limit (PEL) of 100 ppm for an 8-hour workday, 40-hour workweek. Campo and Maguin (2007) proposed a limit of 30 ppm to protect hearing.

Workers who are exposed to both noise and styrene have significantly worse auditory thresholds between 2 and 6 kHz compared to those who are exposed to only noise (Morata et al., 2002). Workers who are exposed to a mixture of solvents with styrene as the main component and noise are more likely to have a hearing loss than workers who are exposed to only styrene or only noise (Sliwińska-Kowalska et al., 2003). A high-frequency hearing loss can occur even in workers who are exposed to both styrene and noise levels that are just within the permissible limits if the exposure occurs for 5 or more years (Morioka, Miyai, Yamamoto, & Miyashita, 2000).

16.4.3 Toluene

Toluene is a colorless liquid with a distinctive smell. Examples of industries/processes where workers can be exposed to toluene are leather tanning, printing, painting, and anywhere lacquers, dyes, and degreasing agents are used. Toluene can be absorbed through airways, skin, and the digestive track. It can damage the CNS and liver and irritate the respiratory tract. The PEL for toluene in air varies from 27 ppm in Poland to 200 ppm in the United States (Hoet & Lison, 2008).

The odds ratio estimates for hearing loss are 1.76 (95%, confidence interval [CI] 1.00–2.98) times greater for each gram of hippuric acid (the main toluene metabolite) per gram of creatinine in rotogravure printing workers who are exposed to an organic solvent mixture of toluene, ethyl acetate, and ethanol (Morata et al., 1997). Combined exposure to noise and toluene can be more damaging compared to exposure to either noise or toluene alone (Chang, Chen, Lien, & Sung, 2006; Morata, Dunn, Kretschmer, Lemasters, & Keith, 1993). Based on repeated monitoring of the German printing industry for 5 years, Schäper, Seeber, and van Thriel (2008) found no effect of toluene on auditory thresholds. The average exposure levels in this study for toluene in the printing area was 25.7 (± 20.1) ppm, and for the end-processing area it was 3.2 (± 3.1) ppm. Thus, average exposure levels of less than 50 ppm may not be toxic to human hearing. Stapedius reflex decay (Morata et al., 1993) and ABR abnormalities (Vrca, Karacić, Bozicević, & Malinar, 1996) have been noted in workers who are exposed to toluene.

16.4.4 *n*-Hexane

n-Hexane is a colorless volatile liquid with a disagreeable smell. A very high percentage of *n*-hexane can be absorbed by inhalation; it is then distributed to tissues and organs rich in lipids, such as the brain, peripheral nerves, liver, spleen, kidneys, and adrenal glands. Workers in the textile, furniture, printing, and shoe industries can be exposed to *n*-hexane along with other solvents, especially in the presence of poor air ventilation. Special glues used in the roofing and leather industries, quick-drying glues used in various hobbies, gasoline, and rubber cement contain *n*-hexane (ATSDR, 1999b). Solvents containing *n*-hexane are used to extract vegetable oils from crops such as soybeans. Chronic low-dose *n*-hexane exposure such as that apparent in industrial workers can cause axonal loss with sensory impairment. Subacute high-dose *n*-hexane exposure such as that apparent in glue sniffers is also neurotoxic and can cause swelling of axons with secondary demyelination, peripheral neuropathy, muscle wasting, and weakness (Huang, 2008; Kuwabara, Kai, Nagase, & Hattori, 1999).

Workers who receive a moderate exposure to *n*-hexane and toluene are more likely to have hearing loss compared to the nonexposed population. The risk of hearing loss is greater in workers who are exposed to noise in addition to these solvents (Sliwińska-Kowalska et al., 2005). The exposure to *n*-hexane can affect the auditory nervous system beyond the cochlea (Howd, Rebert, Dickinson, & Pryor, 1983) due to its neurotoxic effects. Auditory brainstem transmission time (wave I–V interpeak interval) is longer in patients with *n*-hexane neuropathies (Chang, 1987).

16.4.5 Xylene

Xylene is a colorless, aromatic volatile liquid that can take three forms, or isomers: *meta*-xylene, *ortho*-xylene, and *para*-xylene (*m*-, *o*-, and *p*-xylene). Xylene occurs naturally in petroleum and coal tar. Xylene exposure can occur through inhalation or skin contact. Workers in paint, biomedical laboratories, metal, furniture, and automobile garage industries can be exposed to xylene. The OSHA limit for xylene is 100 ppm for workplace air for 8-hour shifts (U. S. Department of Labor, Occupational Safety Health Administration, 1999), but other countries, such as Denmark, have a lower limit of 25 ppm (as cited in Johnson & Morata, 2010). The biological marker for xylene exposure is the detection of methylhippuric acid in urine. High exposure levels can cause dizziness and confusion.

Draper and Bamiou (2009) reported a patient with xylene exposure with no other risk factors who had normal otoacoustic emissions but absent ABR and acoustic reflexes, suggesting auditory neuropathy. His auditory complaints of difficulty hearing in complex surroundings and complex stimuli such as music began following xylene exposure. The prevalence of hearing loss among workers in a liquefied petroleum gas infusion factory was found to be as high as 56.8% (Chang & Chang, 2009) in the presence of relatively low noise doses. Medical laboratory workers exposed to a mixture of xylene isomers showed significantly prolonged absolute and interpeak ABR latencies, as well as poor performance on the pitch pattern sequence and dichotic digits tests, although the effect may be temporary (Fuente, McPherson, & Cardemil, 2013).

16.5 Ototoxic Medications

Several drugs can cause hearing loss (European Agency for Safety and Health at Work, 2009). Thus, noise-exposed workers who are on these medications can suffer additional hearing loss. Hearing loss due to ototoxic medications begins at higher frequencies, and with continuous ingestion, the loss can progress to lower frequencies. Ingestion of multiple ototoxic medications can lead to more severe damage to multiple structures in the cochlea.

16.5.1 Aminoglycosides

Aminoglycosides are narrow-spectrum antibiotics that can counteract aerobic gram-negative bacilli and are considered effective in treating severe infections such as septicemia. Aminoglycosides, including gentamicin, kanamycin, streptomycin, amikacin, tobramycin, and neomycin, can damage the cochlea, specifically the outer hair cells (Forge & Schacht, 2000; Govaerts et al., 1990; Hashino, Shero, & Salvi, 1997). They seem to invade the cochlea through the stria vascularis (Govaerts et al., 1990; Tran Ba Huy et al., 1983). Hearing loss occurs in about 20 to 30% of patients receiving aminoglycosides (Fausti et al., 1999; Fee, 1980; Lerner, Schmitt, & Seligsohn, & Matz, 1986; Moore, Smith, & Lietman, 1984).The dose and duration of treatment determine the presence and degree of hearing loss, but genetic predisposition can also be a factor.

Sequence analysis of the mitochondrial genome has implicated mutations at the 961, 1494, and 1555 loci in the 12S ribosomal RNA (rRNA) gene that can make individuals susceptible to aminoglycoside ototoxicity (Guan, Fischel-Ghodsian, & Attardi, 2000; Li et al., 2004; Wang et al., 2006; Zhao et al., 2004). For example, some individuals have a genetic predisposition to hearing loss due to aminoglycosides because of a substitution of guanosine at position 1555 in the mitochondrial rRNA by an adenosine (Prezant et al., 1993). As a preventive measure, a quick screening for the existence of this mutation is possible (Usami, Abe, Shinkawa, Inoue, & Yamaguchi, 1999). Approximately 10 to 20% of individuals with aminoglycoside-induced ototoxicity may show a mutation in the 12S rRNA gene (Fischel-Ghodsian, 1999).

Other factors that increase the risk of hearing loss are preexisting disorders of hearing, older age, use of other medications, including loop diuretics, and noise exposure. Auditory threshold shifts are worse when aminoglycoside exposure occurs along with or after noise exposure. Soldiers with blast and gunshot wounds often receive aminoglycosides during and after evacuation from war zones in noisy armored personnel carriers or aircrafts. Exposure to moderate or intense noise during combat injuries and medical evacuation and consequent aminoglycoside treatment can lead to noise-augmented aminoglycoside-induced hearing loss. In such cases, the possibility of hearing loss can be minimized by using non-ototoxic drugs or reducing the noise level (Li & Steyger, 2009) as much as possible. Another protective measure is to administer aspirin along with aminoglycosides, which can reduce the incidence of hearing loss by up to 75% (Sha, Qiu, & Schacht, 2006).

Aminoglycoside treatment is sometimes used in neonatal intensive care units (NICUs), where ventilators and other machines are producing noises. About 600,000 babies annually pass through NICUs in the United States, and many receive aminoglycosides for suspected bacterial sepsis for 2 days, or until a negative bacteriologic assay is reported (Escobar, 1999; Pillers, & Schleiss, 2005). A meta-analysis of studies published between 1991 and 2003 found that aminoglycoside toxicity based on auditory testing was 2.3% (10 of 436 cases) in children receiving one strong daily dose and 2.0% (8 of 406 cases) in children receiving multiple daily doses (Contopoulos-Ioannidis, Giotis, Baliatsa, & Ioannidis, 2004).

Some studies have reported alteration of ABRs of neonates who received aminoglycosides (Bernard, 1981). Although aminoglycosides are not associated with an increased risk of sensorineural hearing loss, they are associated with an increased risk of auditory neuropathy spectrum disorder (see Chapter 15) among NICU babies (Xoinis, Weirather, Mavoori, Shaha, & Iwamoto, 2007).

16.5.2 Anticarcinogenic Drugs

Cisplatin causes hearing loss in humans, with a marked loss of hair cells and spiral ganglions and damage to the stria vascularis (Helson, Okonkwo, Anton, & Cvitkovic, 1978; Kopelman, Budnick, Sessions, Kramer, & Wong, 1988; Macdonald, Harrison, Wake, Bliss, & Macdonald, 1994; Nagy et al., 1999). The reported incidence of cisplatin-induced hearing loss varies from 11 to 97% (Scheweitzer, 1993). Cisplatin-induced hearing loss is first apparent at frequencies above 8 kHz (Fausti et al., 1993), and it can progress after termination of treatment (Bertolini et al., 2004). The ototoxic effects of cisplatin can increase with co-exposure to aminoglycosides (Riggs, Brummett, Guitjens, & Matz, 1996), loop diuretics (Komune & Snow, 1981), and hazardous noise exposure (Gratton, Salvi, Kamen, & Saunders, 1990; Laurell, 1992). Potentiation of cisplatin ototoxicity by previous noise exposure has been reported in clinical cases (Bokemeyer et al., 1998).

Carboplatin, another anticarcinogenic drug, is less nephrotoxic than cisplatin. Carboplatin-induced oxidative injury has been reported in the inferior colliculus of male Wistar rats (Husain, Whitworth, Hazelrigg, & Rybak, 2003), suggesting central auditory deficits. If mannitol is used to disrupt the blood–brain barrier, carboplatin can successfully treat malignant brain tumors, but a high percentage of the patients can have hearing loss. The hearing loss can be prevented by administering sodium thiosulfate after closing of the blood –brain barrier (Neuwelt et al., 1998).

16.5.3 Nonsteroidal Analgesics and Antiinflammatory Drugs

High doses of salicylate (> 2.5 g/d) can cause a temporary threshold shift and/or tinnitus (Stypulkowski, 1990), but in some cases permanent hearing loss may occur (Jarvis, 1966; Kapur, 1965). According to the Drug Enforcement Agency of the U.S. Department of Justice, prescriptions for opiate-based drugs have skyrocketed in the past decade. Abuse of opiates can cause a temporary or permanent sensorineural hearing loss in some individuals. In some settings where illicit opium is easily available, such as in military deployments in areas such as Afghanistan, opiate and noise exposure can occur simultaneously. A combination of noise and opium exposure is also possible in recreational settings. Several case reports suggest that some individuals are susceptible to hearing loss from excessive consumption of opioids. (For a review, see Rawool & Dluhy, 2011.)

Rawool and Dluhy (2011) evaluated auditory sensitivity of individuals with a history of opiate abuse and/or occupational or nonoccupational noise exposure. Twenty-three men who reported opiate abuse served as participants in the study. Four of the individuals reported no history of noise exposure, 12 reported hobby-related noise exposure, and 7 reported occupational noise exposure, including 2 who also reported hobby-related noise exposure. Fifty percent (2/4) of the individuals without any noise exposure had a hearing loss confirming previous reports that some of the

population is vulnerable to the ototoxic effects of opiate abuse. Example of air conduction thresholds from a 33-year-old man with a history of opiate abuse is shown in ▶ Fig. 16.2. The percentage of the population with hearing loss increased with hobby-related (58%) and occupational (100%) noise exposure. Mixed multivariate analysis of variance (MANOVA) revealed a significant ear, frequency, and noise exposure interaction. The possibility that opiate abuse may interact with noise exposure in determining auditory thresholds needs to be considered in noise-exposed individuals who are addicted to opiates (Rawool & Dluhy, 2011).

Opioid receptors are present in the spiral ganglion and nerve fibers in the organ of Corti (Popper, Cristobal, & Wackym, 2004), suggesting the possibility of a neural hearing loss in addition to the sensory or cochlear site of lesion. Opioid receptors MOP-R, DOP-R, KOP-R, and NOP-R are widely distributed in the CNS and in peripheral sensory and autonomic nerves (Henricksen & Willoch, 2008). Heroin overdose has been associated with peripheral neuropathy (Dabby et al., 2006; Warner-Smith, Darke, & Day, 2002). Acute effects of opiates include decreased tone of peripheral blood vessels, which could disrupt blood flow to the cochlea and the brain. Niehaus and Meyer (1998) described a case of a 25-year-old heroin abuser who developed cerebral ischemic lesions. Cerebral magnetic resonance imaging (MRI) revealed bilateral border zone infarctions that were attributed to a heroin-associated vasculitis of the basal cerebral arteries.

MRI and new computational brain-mapping techniques suggest that chronic methamphetamine abuse may selectively damage the medial temporal lobe and the cingulate-limbic cortex leading to neuroadaptation, neurophil reduction, or cell death. Significant white matter hypertrophy may appear from reduced myelination and adaptive glial changes (Thompson et al., 2004). Such findings suggest the possibility of damage to the central auditory pathways and associated deficits.

In some cases, analgesics cause only a temporary hearing loss. The temporary or permanent status of the hearing loss may depend on the overall health of the individual and the degree and specific type of exposure. Abuse of hydrocodone with acetaminophen (Vicodin) may induce more permanent hearing loss compared to abuse of heroin, methadone, and amphetamines, which appear to induce a temporary hearing loss (Lopez, Ishiyama, & Ishiyama, 2012).

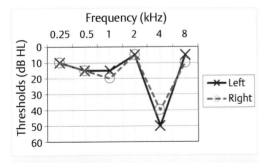

Fig. 16.2 Air conduction thresholds of a 33-year-old man with a history of opiate abuse. (based on Rawool & Dluhy, 2011).

16.5.4 Selective Serotonin Reuptake Inhibitors

Selective serotonin reuptake inhibitors (SSRIs), which are administered to chronically depressed individuals, can have negative effects on transient otoacoustic emissions, auditory processing skills, and evoked auditory responses. The enhancement of serotonin (5-HT) due to the intake of SSRIs may be a contributing factor (Gopal, Briley, Goodale, & Hendea, 2005).

16.6 Auditory Processing Deficits due to Ototoxins

The effects of various metals and solvents on vision, hearing, olfactory function, touch, and taste have been noted by various investigators. Different pathogenic mechanisms may be involved that act on sensory receptors, nerve fibers, and the CNS (Gobba, 2003). More specifically, processing of auditory stimuli can be poor in workers exposed to solvents (Laukli & Hansen, 1995; Morata et al., 1997; Niklasson et al., 1998; Odkvist, Arlinger,

Edling, Larsby, & Berholtz, 1987), even in the presence of auditory sensitivity within normal limits (Fuente & McPherson, 2007). Damage to the central auditory pathways is also possible following noise exposure. In cases where possibility to damage to the central auditory systems is suspected due to patient complaints or exposure to ototoxic substances, an auditory processing test battery is recommended. A matched control group of employees who are not exposed to solvents and/or noise should be included in evaluations. In evaluating individual patients, use of a normative data base established in each clinic is recommended.

16.7 Auditory Processing Test Battery

Further research will be useful in identifying the specific auditory processing skills that are affected due to exposure to ototoxins, including solvents and metals such as mercury. In the interim, a recommended battery for evaluating auditory processing skills in the context of occupational exposure to ototoxins is shown in ▶ Fig. 16.3. The

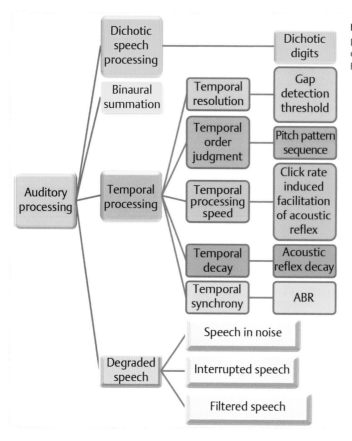

Fig. 16.3 Recommended auditory processing test battery for workers exposed to ototoxins (adapted from Rawool, 2012a).

test battery should be preceded by a complete audiological evaluation as described previously to document any peripheral hearing loss and word recognition difficulties in quiet and noise (Chapter 3). The inclusion of tests within the auditory processing test battery in ▶ Fig. 16.3 is based on the following considerations:

- Ease of administration and interpretation in clinical settings
- Evaluation of brainstem and cortical auditory pathways
- Evaluation of binaural (dichotic) and temporal auditory processing skills
- Minimal effect of hearing loss
- Minimal effect of linguistic competency. Individuals with poor linguistic competency (Chapters 3 and 4) may do poorly on tasks involving words or sentences, making it difficult to distinguish auditory processing from linguistic deficits. Degraded speech tasks should be avoided in the presence of questionable linguistic competency unless the tests are available in the native language of the person.
- Minimal effect of cognitive variables, including attention. Solvent-exposed workers may have some difficulty in modulating their attentional resources according to task demands, as apparent in similar P300 amplitudes for rare and oddball stimuli (Massioui et al., 1990). Vigilance decrement has also been noted during methylene chloride exposure (Winneke, 1982).
- Use of subjective and objective measures. Acute low-level exposure to organic solvents can result in prenarcotic states of depression of the CNS (Winneke, 1982). This can negatively affect the ability to perform behavioral tasks. Therefore, some objective measures are included in the test battery.
- Control of patient fatigue and learning effects. The recommended tests involve simple behavioral tasks or no response from patients. In addition, the fatigue effects can be controlled by interspersing objective measures among behavioral measures.

16.7.1 Temporal Resolution

Temporal resolution refers to the lowest limits of the auditory system to resolve time. One way to measure temporal resolution is to determine the gap detection thresholds (see Chapter 5). This is the minimum time gap that is necessary to detect the gap between two stimuli. Workers exposed to

solvents show poorer performance on the random gap detection test compared to nonexposed individuals (Fuente & McPherson, 2007; Fuente, McPherson, & Hickson, 2011; Fuente, McPherson, & Hormazabal, 2013).

16.7.2 Temporal Order Judgment

Temporal order judgment involves the accurate perception of the sequence of stimuli. Two or three stimuli differing in pitch (e.g., high, low, low) or duration (short, short, long) are presented with sufficient gaps between the stimuli. The patient's task is to accurately state or hum the sequence. Two tests are available for temporal order judgment: the pitch pattern sequence (PPS) and duration pattern sequence (see Chapter 5). Workers exposed to solvents show poor performance on the PPS tests (Fuente & McPherson, 2007; Fuente, McPherson, & Hickson, 2011, 2013). When age and hearing loss are used as covariates, styrene-exposed individuals show significantly poor performance on both pitch and duration pattern tests compared to nonexposed individuals (Zamyslowska-Szmytke, Fuente, Niebudek-Bogusz, & Sliwińska-Kowalska, 2009).

16.7.3 Temporal Processing Speed

The speed with which stimuli are processed over time can be referred to as the temporal processing speed. Progressive increase of reaction time/speed has been previously noted at toluene exposures of 300 ppm for 30 minutes (Winneke, 1982). Thus, it is important to assess auditory processing speed in workers exposed to solvents.

Acoustic reflex thresholds evoked with clicks presented at faster rates are lower than those elicited with clicks presented at slow rates (Rawool, 1995, 1996a). This improvement in thresholds is discussed in Chapter 5. Acoustic reflex thresholds obtained with a rate of 200 clicks/s (e.g., 80 dB peak equivalent sound pressure level [peSPL]) could be subtracted from those obtained at 50 clicks/s (e.g., 110 dB peSPL). The difference in the two thresholds (20 dB SPL) is the rate-induced facilitation (RIF) of the acoustic reflex. It appears that in the presence of reduced temporal processing speed, some of the clicks presented at higher rates are missed, leading to a smaller RIF. Thus, in the presence of a slower processing speed, the click RIF of acoustic reflex thresholds is reduced (Rawool, 1996b). The click RIF has not been evaluated on individuals with auditory processing difficulties but is more objective than other potential tests of temporal processing speed, such as recognition of time-compressed words, and is not influenced by linguistic or cognitive factors. Temporal processing speed can also be assessed by recording acoustic reflex latencies (see Chapter 5).

16.7.4 Temporal Response Maintenance (Decay)

Temporal response maintenance can be thought of as the ability of the auditory system to continue to evaluate high-level stimuli without fatigue. This ability can be determined using the acoustic reflex decay (Chapter 5). Workers who are exposed to solvents can show significant reflex decay, suggesting retrocochlear or brainstem pathology (Morata et al., 1997).

Although traditionally reflex decay has been measured over a fixed time frame (10 s), it can also be measured using a fixed number of stimuli, such as 1000 clicks (Rawool, 1996c). Furthermore, it can be measured at levels that approximate the exposure levels of workers to impulse types of noises. The elicited response patterns may identify workers who are more susceptible to noise or ototoxin exposure. When the reflex is recorded by presenting 1000 clicks at the rate of 50 or 100/s at 95 or 105 dB hearing level (HL), the reflex decays in about 5 to 10% of individuals, suggesting increased vulnerability to impulse noises. On the other hand, the reflex amplitude increases over time in about 5 to 10% of individuals, suggesting tough ears with lower risk of noise induced hearing loss. In the remaining subjects the amplitude either remains steady or fluctuates over time (see Chapter 5).

16.7.5 Temporal Synchrony

Temporal synchrony can be thought of as the ability of the auditory neurons to simultaneously fire in response to a broadband stimulus. The integrity of the click-evoked ABR relies heavily on the synchronous firings of several auditory neurons. Thus, ABR can be used as a measure of temporal synchrony. For this purpose, the ABR can be elicited using high-level stimuli, such as 70 and 80 dB normal hearing level (nHL), and absolute and interpeak latencies, amplitudes, and morphology of the waveforms can be analyzed. It is best to record two waveforms at each presentation level using rarefaction and condensation clicks because of differences in resulting waveform morphology across individuals (Rawool, 1998, 2007; Rawool & Zerlin, 1988). Relatively higher click repetition rates (e.g. 30 clicks/s) that can increase the sensitivity of the ABR (Rawool, 2007) without compromising the integrity of the waveforms are recommended for evoking the response.

Prolonged latencies and reduced amplitudes of the ABR have been noted in individuals exposed to solvents (Abbate, Giorgianni, Munaò, & Brecciaroli, 1993; Hirata, Ogawa, Okayama, & Goto, 1992; Kumar & Tandon, 1997; Nolfe, Palma, Guadagnino, Serra, & Serra, 1991; Vrca, Bozicević, Bozikov, Fuchs, & Malinar, 1997; Vrca et al., 1996). For example, workers exposed to *n*-hexane show prolonged I to V interpeak latencies (Chang, 1987; Huang & Chu, 1989). Prolonged interpeak I–III latencies have also been noted in some workers who are exposed to mercury and chlorinated hydrocarbons (Moshe et al., 2002). Some gas station attendants exposed to fuels for at least 3 years may show prolonged absolute and interpeak latencies and interaural asymmetries in the ABR (Quevedo, Tochetto, Siqueira, & Machado, 2012).

Individuals with blood concentration levels of lead greater than 50 µg/dL over the previous 3 years show longer I–V ABR interpeak latencies compared to age- and gender-matched nonexposed individuals (Discalzi et al., 1992). In addition, workers with the highest level of lead in blood show particularly longer I–V interpeak latencies. Workers exposed to mercury also show longer I–V interpeak latencies of the ABR compared to age-matched nonexposed individuals (Discalzi, Fabbro, Meliga, Mocellini, & Capellaro, 1993).

16.7.6 Binaural Interaction

Binaural interaction refers to the comparative evaluation and/or fusion of the stimuli presented simultaneously to the two ears at a central auditory level. For example, a stimulus can be presented slightly earlier in time to the right ear compared to that presented to the left ear. The stimulus is perceived as a single or fused image that is lateralized to the right side. The phenomenon of masking level difference (MLD) also involves binaural interaction (see Chapter 6). MLDs appear to be normal in workers exposed to solvents (Fuente, McPherson, & Hickson, 2011; Fuente, McPherson, Muñoz, & Pablo Espina, 2006), suggesting normal binaural interaction. If ABRs are recordable at low stimulus levels, binaural interaction may be investigated using ABRs (Rawool & Ballachanda, 1990) to confirm the findings obtained using behavioral measures.

16.7.7 Binaural Summation

Binaural summation can be measured objectively in the presence of acoustic reflex. The procedure is described in Chapter 6.

16.7.8 Dichotic Speech Processing

This type of processing involves simultaneous presentation of different stimuli to each ear. The listener is expected to repeat the stimuli presented to both ears either in a particular order for a directed listening task or without specification of any order for a free recall task. The percentage of correctly repeated stimuli is calculated (see Chapter 6).

Chronic solvent exposure can affect dichotic listening skills (Varney, Kubu, & Morrow, 1998). Although various stimuli, including consonant-vowels and words, can be used for testing dichotic processing skills, the best stimuli for testing in the context of hearing conservation probably are dichotic digits, which are least likely to be affected by hearing loss. Workers exposed to solvents perform poorly on the free recall dichotic digits task with simultaneous presentation of two digits to each ear (Fuente et al., 2011; Fuente & McPherson, 2007).

16.7.9 Modified Speech Tests

Modified speech tests (see Chapter 7) can show exaggerated deficits in those cases where worker compensation is being sought. In addition, workers whose primary language is not English may perform poorly on these tasks. Thus, such tasks should be administered to only carefully selected populations exposed to ototoxins.

Speech Perception in Noise

Workers exposed to ototoxins have more difficulty recognizing speech in noise when compared to nonexposed peers (Fuente, McPherson, & Hickson, 2013). Workers exposed to styrene need a larger speech-to-noise ratio to correctly recognize 40% of the speech signal in a background of noise compared to a control group (Johnson et al., 2006).

Filtered Speech

Workers exposed to a mixture of solvents have more difficulty recognizing filtered speech compared to age-matched nonexposed controls in the presence of normal peripheral sensitivity (Fuente, McPherson, & Hickson, 2011). The degree of abnormality in recognizing filtered speech can vary among workers exposed to industrial solvents (Laukli & Hansen, 1995).

Interrupted Speech

Many workers exposed to styrene show abnormally poor performance on an interrupted speech task (see Chapter 7) with 7 interruptions/s. Performance on interrupted speech tasks is correlated with recognition of speech in noise in workers exposed to styrene (Johnson et al., 2006). The sensitivity of interrupted speech to CNS lesions in workers exposed to industrial solvents has been noted by several investigators (Möller et al., 1989; Odkvist, Arlinger, Edling, Larsby, & Bergholtz, 1987; Odkvist et al., 1982).

16.8 Minimizing Ototoxin Exposure

Exploration of the use of less toxic compounds needs to continue in the future as a preventive measure. Other preventive measures are reduction to exposures by engineering controls to reduce environmental concentrations, improving general dilution ventilation or local exhaust ventilation, and reducing the PELs. For example, the PEL for noise can be reduced to an 8-hour time-weighted average (TWA) of 80 dB(A) from 90 dB(A) in the presence of simultaneous exposure to organic solvents (Campo & Maguin, 2007).

In designing workplaces, proper and quiet ventilation systems must be considered to reduce exposure to toxic fumes. When engineering controls are not technically feasible or are insufficient, face masks, protective clothing, and respirators should be provided to workers when necessary. To avoid skin contact with ototoxic chemicals, gloves should be worn, and in case of accidental skin contact, the involved body part (e.g., hands) should be washed or cleaned immediately. In general, good personal hygiene practices, including washing hands before eating and taking a shower before leaving the worksite, can reduce exposure.

16.9 Intervention Strategies

Both peripheral and central auditory deficits should be addressed in individuals exposed to ototoxins. If hearing aids are provided, they should be monitored at least annually along with auditory sensitivity. Assistive listening technology should be recommended as needed. Rehabilitation strategies to improve auditory perception should include both top-down and bottom-up processing deficits, as described in Chapter 8. In addition, deficit-specific training (see Chapters 9 to 11) should be provided based on the deficits apparent during the auditory processing test battery. Patients with CSE can also benefit from group sessions based on cognitive behavioral principles to address inadequate illness behaviors, along with cognitive strategy training sessions to compensate for residual memory problems (van Hout, Wekking, Berg, & Deelman, 2008).

16.10 Case Study

When a worker is seeking compensation, careful evaluation to ensure true responses on behavioral measures and inclusion of objective measures is necessary. Poor performance on behavioral measures can occur due to conscious malingering, eagerness to document experienced deficits, attentional issues, fatigue, and poor processing speed (van Valen et al., 2012). Cognitive malingering can occur in up to 45% of patients reporting exposure to occupational and environmental substances (Greve et al., 2006). Tests involving speech stimuli may be more vulnerable to exaggeration of deficits. In this particular case study, for the selected behavioral measures, the CD was paused after each stimulus group (e.g., after three tones in the pitch pattern sequence test) presentation to allow more time for the patient to respond to stimuli, as motor speed is often affected in patients with CSE (van Valen et al., 2012).

16.10.1 Reason for Self-Referral

Patient OE is 64 years old. He believes that he has suffered from hearing deficits due to work-related exposure to ototoxins and is interested in finding if his workers' compensation claim can be supported. He is specifically interested in receiving an evaluation of central processing skills.

A complete case history was obtained using the case history form presented in Rawool (2012b) and supplementing the form with additional probe questions based on the information noted in the case history.

16.10.2 Family History

The patient reports no family history of hearing loss. His father has a hearing loss due to work-related noise exposure. His mother has diabetes.

16.10.3 Medical History

Patient OE has been diagnosed with chronic beryllium disease (CBD) due to exposure to beryllium at the workplace. He also reports enlarged arteries on the left side of the heart, high blood pressure, abnormal cholesterol levels, arthritis, diabetes, and acid reflux. He has suffered from skin cancer, which was treated surgically. Other reported conditions are depression and anxiety.

Medications include Flovent (220 mg) and ProAir HFA (albuterol sulfate) inhalation aerosol for CBD since 2003, Cymbalta (duloxetine, 20 mg) for depression and anxiety, lorazepam (5 mg) for anxiety, Nexium (esomeprazole) for acid reflex, Crestor (rosuvastatin, 10 mg) for abnormal cholesterol levels, and Nasarel (flunisolide) for breathing difficulties. The patient reports no consumption of alcohol or any recreational drugs.

16.10.4 Hearing and Vestibular Symptoms History

Patient OE reports difficulty in hearing speech since 1981 or 1982. Family members at that time had to repeat what they were saying and would complain about the TV volume being too loud. He has also been experiencing tinnitus since the mid-1980s. The tinnitus is described as rapid clicking with almost no separation between the clicks.

He has experienced dizziness and balance issues since the 1980s and continues to experience sudden falls. He has been prescribed a cane to minimize falls. He reports during or after work he would often feel dizzy due to exposure to solvents, and sometimes the fume buildup in the workplace would be unbearable.

16.10.5 Ototoxin Exposure at Work

The patient was a chemical operator and was involved in field decontamination at a gaseous

Table 16.1 Work-related Exposure to Various Ototoxins*

Ototoxin in the Workplace	Period of Exposure	How Exposure Occurred
Trichloroethylene	Aug. 1974–Feb. 1980	Very high exposure levels during certain periods; exposure through skin contact and through breathing of fumes
Styrene	Aug. 1974–Feb. 1980	Patient operated incinerator for solvents, including styrene
Carbon tetrachloride	Aug. 1974–Feb. 1980	Patient operated incinerator for solvents, including carbon tetrachloride
Thorium	Aug. 1974–Feb. 1980	Patient operated incinerator for radioactive materials, including thorium
Carbon monoxide	Aug. 1974–Feb. 1980; some exposure in 1994–1999	Primarily from vehicles (trucks running inside buildings) where the patient was working or other pieces of equipment being operated inside the building
Diesel fuel	Aug. 1974–Feb. 1980	From forklifts inside buildings and diesel generators
Lead	Aug. 1974–Feb. 1980	Being around a lot of batteries in some of the process buildings and from cleaning batteries in battery room
Arsenic	Aug. 1974–Feb. 1980; July 1994–Dec. 2000	From trap changes and scrapping operations
Mercury	Aug. 1974–Feb. 1980	Patient operated incinerator for metals, including mercury; previous masks did not filter mercury
Pesticides and herbicides	Aug. 1974–Feb. 1980	During weed and grass control using Roundup weed killer; trifluralin pre-emergence herbicide may have been used outside the buildings, but huge ventilation fans often pulled fumes with a bad odor into building. Break rooms and other rooms in the building were sprayed for bugs using malathion often in the presence of workers.
PCB	Aug. 1974–Feb. 1980	Process buildings, electrical switchyards, lube oil X326 cleanup

* Information as reported by the patient while working as a chemical operator at a Gaseous Diffusion Plant.

diffusion plant. He was also exposed to dust during some parts of his work. Patient reports work-related exposure to various ototoxins, as shown in ▶ Table 16.1 and ▶ Fig. 16.4. Other factors in the workplace reported by the patient that could potentially increase the risk of hearing loss were intermittent exposure to excessive heat and whole-body vibrations due to vibrations of entire rooms (Boettcher, Henderson, Gratton, Danielson, & Byrne, 1987). The patient was also exposed to high levels of noise but wore hearing protection. The unprotected or protected noise levels are unknown.

16.10.6 Hearing Aid History

Patient was fitted with his first hearing aid in the left ear at age 40. Currently, he uses digital hearing aids in both ears on a regular basis but continues to report difficulty in understanding speech through hearing aids.

16.10.7 Current Audiological Evaluation

This evaluation consisted of peripheral and central auditory evaluation and was limited to

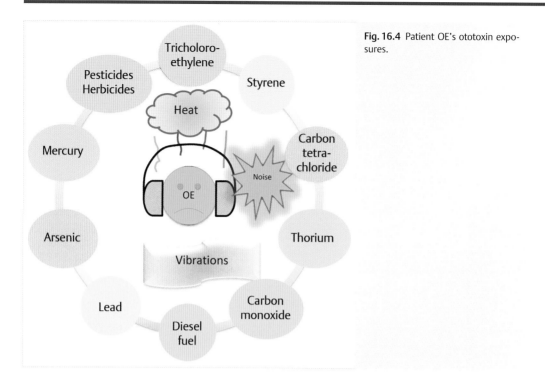

Fig. 16.4 Patient OE's ototoxin exposures.

approximately 3 hours due to time constraints. Only one session was used for the evaluation, as the patient lives a distance from the clinic. Objective tests were interspersed with subjective tests to control for fatigue effects during tests that required an active response from the patient. All testing was conducted using an audiometer, which is subjected to annual exhaustive calibrations and daily checks.

16.10.8 Peripheral Audiological Evaluation

Video-otoscopy

Otoscopic findings revealed intact tympanic membranes and some cerumen in both ears.

Acoustic Immittance Testing

Equivalent ear canal volumes were within normal limits bilaterally. Compensated static admittance was established within normal limits in both ears, suggesting normal mobility of the tympanic membrane/middle ear system. Ipsilateral and contralateral reflexes were elevated bilaterally at 500 Hz and 1000 Hz, suggesting mild dysfunction within the auditory reflex pathway.

Auditory Sensitivity

Testing was conducted using warble tones to allow clearer perception of the tones in the presence of tinnitus reported by the patient. Warble tone air and bone conduction results indicated mild to moderately severe sloping sensorineural hearing loss in both ears except at 500 Hz, where peripheral auditory sensitivity was within normal limits.

Speech Audiometry

Speech recognition thresholds (SRTs) were established at 25 dB HL in the right ear and 30 dB HL in the left ear. These results are consistent with the pure tone averages of 25 dB HL in the right ear and 30 dB HL in the left ear. Word recognition scores in quiet or noise were not established due to time constraints and to control for fatigue.

16.10.9 Auditory Processing Evaluation

Behavioral Measures

Stimuli for all subjective measures were presented through a CD coupled to the audiometer.

Dichotic Digits Task

For this test, a pair of digits was presented to each ear simultaneously, and the patient was asked to repeat all four digits in any order. The digits were presented at 40 dB SL (SRT of each ear). Initial practice with the task was provided with 25 pairs of digits. The patient's performance was 100% correct in the right ear and 88% correct in the left ear. These findings showed a right ear advantage. The results were within normal limits with a cutoff criterion of 80% correct for individuals with hearing loss.

Gap Detection Task

Gap detection ability was measured by presenting stimuli at comfortable listening levels with or without gaps between them. During the practice task, gaps were varied from 0 to 300 ms. During the test, stimuli were presented with gaps of the following duration: 0, 2, 5, 10, 15, 20, 25, 30, and 40 ms. Stimulus frequencies were 500, 1000, and 4000 Hz. The patient was asked to indicate if he heard one or two sounds after each presentation. The patient was able to detect gaps of 10 ms duration or lower in each ear for each of the test frequencies, suggesting good temporal resolution skills. Normal cutoff values are 20 ms.

Temporal Order Judgment

The patient was presented with a sequence of three tones to both ears at comfortable listening levels with sufficient intervals between them. The tonal sequence included tones of two different frequencies. The patient's task was to state the sequence correctly (e.g., high, low, low). Training was provided with 10 trials. Forty trials were used for the test. The patient was able to correctly judge the sequence in 70% of the trials. His 12/40 incorrect responses included six reversals (e.g., stimulus: high-low-high; response: low-high-low). Young adults with normal auditory sensitivity show performance of 78% correct or better on this task. The patient's performance was slightly below the normal range, suggesting a mild deficit in this area.

Objective Measures

Temporal Processing Speed

Processing speed was indirectly evaluated using reflex thresholds determined with various stimulus rates and evaluating the maximum improvement in thresholds with an increase in click rates from 50 to 300/s. In the left ipsilateral configuration, thresholds could not be established at the limits of the equipment (110 dB peSPL) for the slower click rates of 50 and 100/s. The reflex thresholds were established at 110 dB peSPL for the higher click rates of 150, 200, and 300/s, suggesting the possibility of 5 dB improvement in thresholds with an increase in click rates from 50 to 300/s. In the right ipsilateral configuration, the improvement in thresholds with an increase in click rates from 50 to 300/s was 5 dB, which is within normal limits. These findings suggested a processing speed within normal limits within the acoustic reflex pathway.

Temporal Decay or Maintenance

Temporal decay was measured by presenting stimuli 10 dB above the acoustic reflex threshold for a period of 10 seconds and recording the magnitude of the reflex over this period. More than 50% decrease in the magnitude suggests significant decay. The decay could not be determined for the left ipsilateral configuration at 500 and 1000 Hz and for the right ipsilateral configuration at 1000 Hz due to the limits of the equipment in presenting stimuli 10 dB above the reflex threshold. No decay was apparent in the right ipsilateral configuration at 500 Hz. Similarly, no decay was apparent in the right contralateral (stimulus to the right ear and probe in the left ear) and left contralateral (stimulus in the left ear and probe in the right ear) configurations at both 500 and 1000 Hz. Also, no decay was apparent using clicks in the left and right contralateral configurations. Overall, these findings suggested steady/normal processing of loud stimuli over a period of 10 seconds within the acoustic reflex pathway.

Binaural Summation

Binaural summation within the auditory brainstem was evaluated by comparing the reflex thresholds obtained with the contralateral steady and the contralateral pulsed configurations (see Chapter 6). In the contralateral pulsed configuration, the reflex-activating stimuli to one ear are alternated with the probe tone presented to the other ear. In the contralateral steady configuration, the reflex-activating stimuli to one ear and the probe tone to the other ear are presented

Table 16.2 Evaluation of Threshold Shifts Using Occupational Safety and Health Administration (1983) and National Institute for Occupational Safety and Health (1998) Criteria

Comparison Audiogram Dates	Is There Any OSHA (1983) Standard Threshold Shift?	Is there Any NIOSH (1998) Significant Threshold Shift?	Do Threshold Shifts Remain after Applications of OSHA (1983) Age Corrections?		Are There Any 15 dB or Greater Threshold Shifts at 8 kHz?
			OSHA standard threshold shift	NIOSH significant threshold shift	
1973 and 1981	None in both ears	15 dB at 6 kHz in the left ear; 20 dB at 4 kHz in the right ear	NA	With age corrections, shift in the right ear at 4 kHz remains significant	40 dB in the left ear; none in the right ear
1981 and 1994	16.66 dB standard threshold shift only in the left ear	20 and 25 dB shifts apparent at 3 and 4 kHz in the left ear; 15 dB shifts apparent at 3 and 4 kHz in the right ear	11.33 dB standard threshold shift in the left ear after age correction	After age corrections, shift at 4 kHz in the left ear remains significant	None in the left ear; 20 dB shift in the right ear
1994 and 2006	None in both ears	20 dB at 6 kHz in the left and right ears	NA	After applications of age corrections, no significant threshold shifts apparent during this period	15 dB at 8 kHz in the left and right ear, which is expected to be insignificant after age corrections
2006 and 2013	Only in the right ear; a shift of 15 dB	Not in the left ear; 20 and 15 dB at 2 and 3 kHz in the right ear	After age corrections, shift of 12.33 dB apparent in the right ear	After age corrections, shift at 2 kHz in the right ear remains significant	None in both ears

Abbreviation: NA, not applicable.

simultaneously, which leads to binaural summation. Thus, in normal individuals, the thresholds in the steady configuration are better (lower) by about 5 to 15 dB compared to those in the pulsed configuration. The click-evoked reflex threshold in the right contralateral pulsed configuration was 116 dB, and that in the contralateral steady configuration was 102 dB, showing a 14 dB improvement in threshold. In the left contralateral pulsed configuration, reflex threshold could not be obtained at the higher limit (120 dB) of the equipment, and that in the steady configuration was 115 dB, suggesting at least a 6 dB improvement in threshold in the steady configuration. These results indicate normal binaural summation, which suggests normal summative function within the auditory brainstem.

16.10.10 Case-study Conclusion

Variability in Previous Audiometric Results

Patient OE provided several previous audiograms for review. Previous audiological results show marked variation in thresholds for unknown reasons. Some possible reasons for the wide variations may be poor audiometric calibration, poor test environments, patient anxiety during testing, poor concentration due to a history of chronic solvent exposures, and a possible fluctuating component to the permanent hearing loss due to unstable cochlear dysfunction. The fluctuation in auditory sensitivity at 6 and 8 kHz could also result from variations in earphone placement.

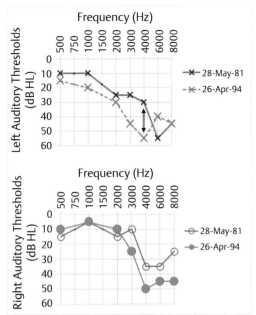

Fig. 16.6 Patient OE's left and right ear audiograms from 1981 and 1994. During 1981 and 1994, there was no exposure to workplace or nonwork ototoxins. Age-corrected significant threshold shift is shown by an arrow. After age correction, the threshold shift at 4 kHz in the left ear is 17 dB.

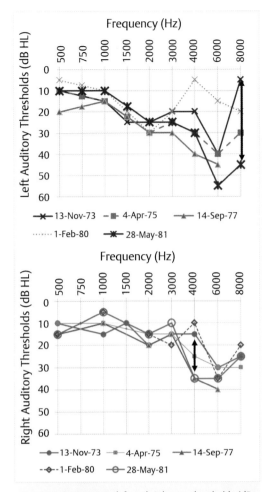

Fig. 16.5 Patient OE's left and right ear thresholds (dB hearing level [HL]) from 1973 to 1981. Arrows indicate marked threshold shifts.

Key Audiometric Findings

Findings since 1973 were compared and are summarized in ▶ Table 16.2.

1973 to 1981

Audiograms during this period were examined separately because maximum exposure to multiple ototoxins occurred at this time (▶ Table 16.1). The audiogram dated February 1, 1980, appears aberrant due to the appearance of significantly better thresholds at 4 and 6 kHz in the left ear and at 4 kHz in the right ear compared to the preemployment auditory sensitivity reading. The thresholds from this audiogram are shown in ▶ Fig. 16.5 but are excluded from the review. Comparison of the preemployment thresholds obtained on November 13, 1973, with those obtained on May 28, 1981, after termination of exposure to styrene, trichloroethylene, and other ototoxins including lead indicate an age-corrected significant threshold shift in the right ear at 4 kHz. In addition, a shift of 40 dB is apparent at 8 kHz in the left ear (▶ Fig. 16.5). Threshold shifts from some ototoxins such as lead and styrene have been reported at 8 kHz (Hwang et al., Sliwińska-Kowalska et al., 2003). The findings, along with the case history, suggest that work-related exposure to multiple ototoxins may have contributed to the hearing impairment.

1981 to 1994

Audiograms from 1981 and 1994 were compared to note any shifts occurring after cessation of exposure to workplace ototoxins. As shown in ▶ Fig. 16.6, an age-corrected significant threshold

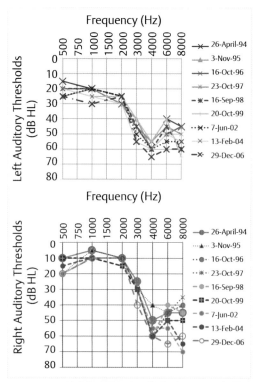

Fig. 16.7 Patient OE's left and right ear audiograms from 1994 to 2006.

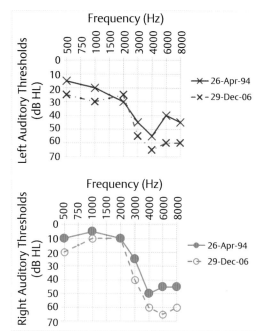

Fig. 16.8 Patient OE's left and right ear air conduction thresholds from 1994 and 2006.

shift is apparent at 4 kHz in the left ear. In addition, there is an age-corrected OSHA (1983) standard threshold shift in the left ear. Significant thresholds shifts have been reported after cessation of exposure to styrene at relatively high levels in rats (Campo, Lataye, Loquet, & Bonnet, 2001). The patient's hearing may have stabilized somewhere between the 1981 and 1994 tests, but other audiograms during this period were unavailable for this review.

1994 to 2006

During this period, the patient reported some exposures to arsenic and carbon monoxide. The audiograms from this period are shown in ▶ Fig. 16.7. The audiograms from 1994 and 2006 (▶ Fig. 16.8) reveal some worsening of auditory sensitivity. However, after accounting for potentially age-related worsening of hearing (OSHA, 1983), no significant threshold shifts are apparent.

2006 and 2013

Comparison of the 2006 audiogram to the current audiogram in 2013 shows a significant age-

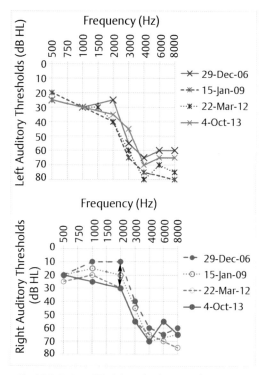

Fig. 16.9 Patient OE's left and right ear audiograms from 2006 to 2013. Age-corrected significant threshold shift is shown by an arrow.

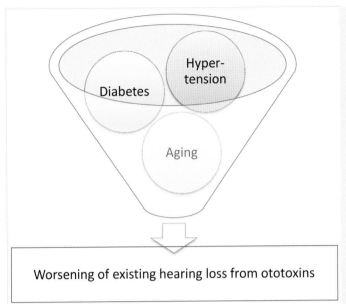

Fig. 16.10 Besides prior work-related exposure to ototoxins, risk factors for hearing loss for Patient OE during 2006 and 2013.

corrected threshold shift at 2 kHz and an OSHA (1983) standard threshold shift only in the right ear (▶ Fig. 16.9). Diabetes and hypertension since 2008 are additional risk factors for hearing loss during this period (▶ Fig. 16.10).

Current (2013) Peripheral Auditory Results

Current warble tone air and bone conduction results indicate mild to moderately severe sloping sensorineural hearing loss in both ears except at 500 Hz, where peripheral auditory sensitivity is within normal limits in the right ear. Compared to previous audiometric findings obtained on March 22, 2012, a significant improvement in auditory sensitivity was noted at 3 kHz in the left ear and at 6 kHz in the right ear. Speech recognition thresholds were consistent with pure tone averages in both ears. Tympanometric findings suggest normal middle ear function bilaterally. Acoustic reflex thresholds suggest mild dysfunction within the acoustic reflex pathways. Speech recognition scores in quiet and noise were not obtained due to time constraints. Also, test reliability of word recognition scores can be questioned unless the scores are near 90 to 100%, when the patient is seeking workers' compensation, as the task involves mere repetition of words. However, word recognition scores at 70 dB HL were 84% in the right ear and 80% in the left ear in 2012, suggesting a fair ability to recognize speech in quiet at loud or amplified levels.

Auditory Processing Results

Overall, the patient's performance was within normal limits on many of the tasks. There is mild deficit apparent on the temporal order judgment task, suggesting mild central auditory dysfunction. Acoustic reflex thresholds are present but elevated in both ipsilateral and contralateral configurations, suggesting mild dysfunction within the acoustic reflex pathways. Extensive time for the auditory system to recover following the last significant exposures in 1980 and consistent use of hearing aids may have reduced solvent-related APDs due to neural plasticity. It should also be noted that aging or any diabetic neuropathy may lead to or contribute to the mild APD (▶ Fig. 16.11).

16.10.11 Recommendations for the Patient

- Continued and consistent use of hearing aids is recommended to ensure consistent stimulation to the auditory system and to maximize neural plasticity.
- Finer adjustments to the patient's digital hearing aids to address specific complaints may improve speech intelligibility. The use of hearing aids should be supplemented with assistive listening technologies as needed.
- Auditory training involving both top-down and bottom-up processing (see Chapters 8 and 11) is recommended to improve speech recognition in

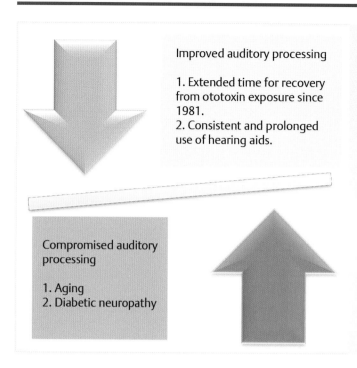

Fig. 16.11 Factors contributing to a mild auditory processing deficit in Patient OE.

Improved auditory processing

1. Extended time for recovery from ototoxin exposure since 1981.
2. Consistent and prolonged use of hearing aids.

Compromised auditory processing

1. Aging
2. Diabetic neuropathy

noise. Training to improve pitch pattern sequencing can also be beneficial (see Chapter 9).

- With reference to his tinnitus, the patient should note that tinnitus is a potential side effect of some of his medications, including lorazepam, Nexium, and ProAir HFA.
- With reference to dizziness and the prevention of falling, the patient should note that dizziness is a potential side effect of some of his current medications, including lorazepam, Nexium, and ProAir HFA.
- A comprehensive balance assessment and rehabilitation may improve balance and reduce the possibility of falls.
- Annual audiological and hearing aid reevaluations and are recommended.

16.11 Future Trends

Exposures to ototoxins such as solvents can lead to chronic solvent-induced encephalopathy resulting in disability and reduced work productivity. Regular multidisciplinary screenings of exposed populations may be cost-effective. Northern European countries have raised awareness of the condition through screening and other measures, such as lowering solvent exposures and offering protective measures to workers. As a result, cases with CSE have been decreasing in these countries (van der

Laan & Sainio, 2012). In the future, a similar effort will be implemented globally to reduce exposures to ototoxins.

A European consensus statement (van Valen et al., 2012) has been developed for facilitating prevention of CSE. The statement notes that there is no evidence of perceptual deficits in patients with CSE perhaps due to differences in vulnerability among workers and thus does not recommend any evaluation of peripheral or central auditory skills. Evaluation of the auditory system should be recommended in future revisions of any consensus statements and guidelines. Peripheral and central auditory assessments are especially important given the fact that peripheral and central APDs may have negative impact on the results of other neuropsychological tests used to diagnose CSE, including tests of verbal concept and reasoning. In addition, auditory deficits can lead to or exacerbate cognitive deficits as a result of sensory deprivation. Connections between APDs and working memory are discussed in Chapter 8, and the connection between slower processing and speech recognition is discussed in Chapter 17.

16.12 Review Questions

1. Under what circumstances are auditory processing evaluations recommended for workers exposed to ototoxins?

2. Review heavy metals that are ototoxic.

3. Review potentially ototoxic organic solvents.

4. What are the potential effects of aminoglycosides on the auditory system? Which populations are at greater risk for aminoglycoside-induced ototoxicity?

5. What are the potential effects of anticarcinogenic drugs on the auditory system?

6. What are the potential effects of opiate abuse on the auditory system?

7. What types of auditory processing deficits occur in some individuals exposed to ototoxins?

8. What should you consider in forming a auditory processing test battery for workers who are exposed to ototoxins?

9. Review the case study presented in this chapter. Given additional time, what other types of tests could you perform on Patient OE?

10. What are some future trends related to damage to the auditory system from exposure to ototoxins?

References

[1] Abbate, C., Giorgianni, C., Munaò, F., & Brecciaroli, R. (1993). Neurotoxicity induced by exposure to toluene: An electrophysiologic study. International Archives of Occupational and Environmental Health, 64(6), 389–392.

[2] Agency for Toxic Substances and Disease Registry (ATSDR). (1994). Toxicological profile for carbon tetrachloride (update). Atlanta, GA: Public Health Service, U.S. Department of Health and Human Services.

[3] Agency for Toxic Substances and Disease Registry (ATSDR). (1999a). Toxicological profile for mercury (CAS No. 7439–97-6). Atlanta, GA: Public Health Service, U.S. Department of Health and Human Services.

[4] Agency for Toxic Substances and Disease Registry (ATSDR). (1999b). Toxicological profile for n-hexane (CAS No. 110–54-3). Atlanta, GA: Public Health Service, U.S. Department of Health and Human Services.

[5] Agency for Toxic Substances and Disease Registry (ATSDR). (2007a). Toxicological profile for lead (update). Atlanta, GA: Public Health Service, U.S. Department of Health and Human Services.

[6] Agency for Toxic Substances and Disease Registry (ATSDR) (2007b). Styrene CAS # 100-42-5. Atlanta, GA: U.S. Department of Public Health and Human Services, Public Health Service. Retrieved from http://www.atsdr.cdc.gov/tfacts53.pdf

[7] Amin-Zaki, L., Majeed, M. A., Clarkson, T. W., & Greenwood, M. R. (1978). Methylmercury poisoning in Iraqi children: Clinical observations over two years. BMJ, 1(6113), 613–616.

[8] Berlin, M. (2003). Mercury in Dental Fillings: An Updated Risk Analysis in Environmental Medical Terms. Retrieved from http://www.sweden.gov.se/content/1/c6/01/76/11/fb660706.pdf.

[9] Bernard, P. A. (1981). Freedom from ototoxicity in aminoglycoside treated neonates: A mistaken notion. Laryngoscope, 91(12), 1985–1994.

[10] Bertolini, P., Lassalle, M., Mercier, G., et al. (2004). Platinum compound-related ototoxicity in children: Long-term follow-up reveals continuous worsening of hearing loss. Journal of Pediatric Hematology/Oncology, 26(10), 649–655.

[11] Besser, R., Krämer, G., Thümler, R., Bohl, J., Gutmann, L., & Hopf, H. C. (1987). Acute trimethyltin limbic-cerebellar syndrome. Neurology, 37(6), 945–950.

[12] Bleecker, M. L., Ford, D. P., Lindgren, K. N., Scheetz, K., & Tiburzi, M. J. (2003). Association of chronic and current measures of lead exposure with different components of brainstem auditory evoked potentials. Neurotoxicology, 24(4-5), 625–631.

[13] Boettcher, F. A., Henderson, D., Gratton, M. A., Danielson, R. W., & Byrne, C. D. (1987). Synergistic interactions of noise and other ototraumatic agents. Ear and Hearing, 8(4), 192–212.

[14] Bokemeyer, C., Berger, C. C., Hartmann, J. T., et al. (1998). Analysis of risk factors for cisplatin-induced ototoxicity in patients with testicular cancer. British Journal of Cancer, 77 (8), 1355–1362.

[15] Campo, P., Lataye, R., Loquet, G., & Bonnet, P. (2001). Styrene-induced hearing loss: A membrane insult. Hearing Research, 154(1-2), 170–180.

[16] Campo, P., & Maguin, K. (2007). Solvent-induced hearing loss: Mechanisms and prevention strategy. International Journal of Occupational Medicine and Environmental Health, 20(3), 265–270.

[17] Campo, P., Maguin, K., & Lataye, R. (2007). Effects of aromatic solvents on acoustic reflexes mediated by central auditory pathways. Toxicological Sciences, 99(2), 582–590.

[18] Canfield, R. L., Henderson, C. R., Jr., Cory-Slechta, D. A., Cox, C., Jusko, T. A., & Lanphear, B. P. (2003). Intellectual impairment in children with blood lead concentrations below 10 microg per deciliter. New England Journal of Medicine, 348 (16), 1517–1526.

[19] Carta, P., Flore, C., Alinovi, R., et al. (2003). Sub-clinical neurobehavioral abnormalities associated with low level of mercury exposure through fish consumption. Neurotoxicology, 24(4-5), 617–623.

[20] Chang, S. J., & Chang, C. K. (2009). Prevalence and risk factors of noise-induced hearing loss among liquefied petroleum gas (LPG) cylinder infusion workers in Taiwan. Industrial Health, 47(6), 603–610.

[21] Chang, S. J., Chen, C. J., Lien, C. H., & Sung, F. C. (2006). Hearing loss in workers exposed to toluene and noise. Environmental Health Perspectives, 114(8), 1283–1286.

[22] Chang, Y. C. (1987). Neurotoxic effects of n-hexane on the human central nervous system: Evoked potential abnormalities in n-hexane polyneuropathy. Journal of Neurology, Neurosurgery, and Psychiatry, 50(3), 269–274.

[23] Chuu, J. J., Hsu, C. J., & Lin-Shiau, S. Y. (2001). Abnormal auditory brainstem responses for mice treated with mercurial compounds: Involvement of excessive nitric oxide. Toxicology, 162(1), 11–22.

[24] Clarkson, T. W., Magos, L., & Myers, G. J. (2003). Human exposure to mercury: The three modern dilemmas. Journal of Trace Elements in Experimental Medicine, 16(4), 321–343.

[25] Consumer Product Safety Improvement Act of 2008. Pub. L. No. 110-314, Title 1, § 106, 122 Stat. 3033–3035 (2008).

[26] Contopoulos-Ioannidis, D. G., Giotis, N. D., Baliatsa, D. V., & Ioannidis, J. P. A. (2004). Extended-interval aminoglycoside administration for children: A meta-analysis. Pediatrics, 114 (1), e111–e118.

[27] Counter, S. A., Buchanan, L. H., & Ortega, F. (2012). Association of hemoglobin levels and brainstem auditory evoked responses in lead-exposed children. Clinical Biochemistry, 45(15), 1197–1201.

[28] Counter, S. A. (2003). Neurophysiological anomalies in brainstem responses of mercury-exposed children of Andean gold miners. Journal of Occupational and Environmental Medicine, 45(1), 87–95.

[29] Dabby, R., Djaldetti, R., Gilad, R., et al. (2006). Acute heroin-related neuropathy. Journal of the Peripheral Nervous System, 11(4), 304–309.

[30] Discalzi, G. L., Capellaro, F., Bottalo, L., Fabbro, D., & Mocellini, A. (1992). Auditory brainstem evoked potentials (BAEPs) in lead-exposed workers. Neurotoxicology, 13(1), 207–209.

[31] Discalzi, G., Fabbro, D., Meliga, F., Mocellini, A., & Capellaro, F. (1993). Effects of occupational exposure to mercury and lead on brainstem auditory evoked potentials. International Journal of Psychophysiology, 14(1), 21–25.

[32] Draper, T. H. J., & Bamiou, D. E. (2009). Auditory neuropathy in a patient exposed to xylene: Case report. Journal of Laryngology and Otology, 123(4), 462–465.

[33] Eggleston, D. W., & Nylander, M. (1987). Correlation of dental amalgam with mercury in brain tissue. Journal of Prosthetic Dentistry, 58(6), 704–707.

[34] Ehyai, A., & Freemon, F. R. (1983). Progressive optic neuropathy and sensorineural hearing loss due to chronic glue sniffing. Journal of Neurology, Neurosurgery, and Psychiatry, 46 (4), 349–351.

[35] Escobar, G. J. (1999). The neonatal "sepsis work-up": Personal reflections on the development of an evidence-based approach toward newborn infections in a managed care organization. Pediatrics, 103(1, Suppl. E), 360–373.

[36] European Agency for Safety and Health at Work. (2009). Combined Exposure to Noise and Ototoxic Substances: European Risk Observatory Literature Review. Luxembourg: Office for Official Publications of the European Communities.

[37] European Union (EU) Directive 2003/10/EC (2003). Directive 2003/10/EC of the European Parliament and of the Council of February 6th, 2003 on the minimum health and safety requirements regarding the exposure of workers on the risks arising from physical agents (noise). Seventeenth individual Directive within the meaning of Article 16(1) of Directive 89/391/EEC. Retrieved from: http://eur-lex.europa.eu/legal-content/EN/TXT/PDF/?uri=CELEX:32003L0010&from=EN

[38] Fausti, S. A., Henry, J. A., Helt, W. J., et al. (1999). An individualized, sensitive frequency range for early detection of ototoxicity. Ear and Hearing, 20(6), 497–505.

[39] Fausti, S. A., Henry, J. A., Schaffer, H. I., Olson, D. J., Frey, R. H., & Bagby, G. C., Jr. (1993). High-frequency monitoring for early detection of cisplatin ototoxicity. Archives of Otolaryngology–Head and Neck Surgery, 119(6), 661–666.

[40] Fechter, L. D., Chen, G. D., Rao, D., & Larabee, J. (2000). Predicting exposure conditions that facilitate the potentiation of noise-induced hearing loss by carbon monoxide. Toxicological Sciences, 58(2), 315–323.

[41] Fee, W. E., Jr. (1980). Aminoglycoside ototoxicity in the human. Laryngoscope, 90(10, Pt. 2, Suppl. 24), 1–19.

[42] Fischel-Ghodsian, N. (1999). Mitochondrial deafness mutations reviewed. Human Mutation, 13(4), 261–270.

[43] Forge, A., & Schacht, J. (2000). Aminoglycoside antibiotics. Audiology and Neurootology, 5(1), 3–22.

[44] Fuente, A., & McPherson, B. (2007). Central auditory processing effects induced by solvent exposure. International Journal of Occupational Medicine and Environmental Health, 20(3), 271–279.

[45] Fuente, A., McPherson, B., & Cardemil, F. (2013). Xylene-induced auditory dysfunction in humans. Ear and Hearing, 34 (5), 651–660.

[46] Fuente, A., McPherson, B., & Hickson, L. (2011). Central auditory dysfunction associated with exposure to a mixture of

[47] Fuente, A., McPherson, B.,& Hickson, L. (2013). Auditory dysfunction associated with solvent exposure. BMC Public Health, 13, 39.

[48] Fuente, A., McPherson, B., & Hormazabal, X. (2013). Self-reported hearing performance in workers exposed to solvents. Revista de Saúde Pública, 47(1), 86–93.

[49] Fuente, A., McPherson, B., Muñoz, V., & Pablo Espina, J. (2006). Assessment of central auditory processing in a group of workers exposed to solvents. Acta Otolaryngologica, 126 (11), 1188–1194.

[50] Fuente, A., Slade, M. D., Taylor, T., et al. (2009). Peripheral and central auditory dysfunction induced by occupational exposure to organic solvents. Journal of Occupational and Environmental Medicine, 51(10), 1202–1211.

[51] Gobba, F. (2003). Occupational exposure to chemicals and sensory organs: A neglected research field. Neurotoxicology, 24(4-5), 675–691.

[52] Gopal, K. V., Briley, K. A., Goodale, E. S., & Hendea, O. M. (2005). Selective serotonin reuptake inhibitors treatment effects on auditory measures in depressed female subjects. European Journal of Pharmacology, 520(1-3), 59–69.

[53] Govaerts, P. J., Claes, J., van de Heyning, P. H., Jorens, P. G., Marquet, J., & De Broe, M. E. (1990). Aminoglycoside-induced ototoxicity. Toxicology Letters, 52(3), 227–251.

[54] Gratton, M. A., Salvi, R. J., Kamen, B. A., & Saunders, S. S. (1990). Interaction of cisplatin and noise on the peripheral auditory system. Hearing Research, 50(1-2), 211–223.

[55] Greve, K. W., Bianchini, K. J., Black, F. W., et al. (2006). The prevalence of cognitive malingering in persons reporting exposure to occupational and environmental substances. Neurotoxicology, 27(6), 940–950.

[56] Guan, M. X., Fischel-Ghodsian, N., & Attardi, G. (2000). A biochemical basis for the inherited susceptibility to aminoglycoside ototoxicity. Human Molecular Genetics, 9(12), 1787–1793.

[57] Hashino, E., Shero, M., & Salvi, R. J. (1997). Lysosomal targeting and accumulation of aminoglycoside antibiotics in sensory hair cells. Brain Research, 777(1-2), 75–85.

[58] Helson, L., Okonkwo, E., Anton, L., & Cvitkovic, E. (1978). cis-Platinum ototoxicity. Clinical Toxicology, 13(4), 469–478.

[59] Henriksen, G., & Willoch, F. (2008). Imaging of opioid receptors in the central nervous system. Brain, 131(Pt. 5), 1171–1196.

[60] Hirata, M., Ogawa, Y., Okayama, A., & Goto, S. (1992). A cross-sectional study on the brainstem auditory evoked potential among workers exposed to carbon disulfide. International Archives of Occupational and Environmental Health, 64(5), 321–324.

[61] Hoet, P., & Lison, D. (2008). Ototoxicity of toluene and styrene: State of current knowledge. Critical Reviews in Toxicology, 38(2), 127–170.

[62] Hossain, N. & Rae, B. (2011) Trouble in Toyland, The 26th Annual Survey of Toy Safety. US PIRG Educational Fund, Washington.

[63] Howd, R. A., Rebert, C. S., Dickinson, J., & Pryor, G. T. (1983). A comparison of the rates of development of functional hexane neuropathy in weanling and young adult rats. Neurobehavioral Toxicology and Teratology, 5(1), 63–68.

[64] Huang, C.-C. (2008). Polyneuropathy induced by n-hexane intoxication in Taiwan. Acta Neurologica Taiwanica, 17(1), 3–10.

[65] Huang, C. C., & Chu, N. S. (1989). Evoked potentials in chronic n-hexane intoxication. Clinical Electroencephalography, 20(3), 162–168.

[66] Husain, K., Whitworth, C., Hazelrigg, S., & Rybak, L. (2003). Carboplatin-induced oxidative injury in rat inferior colliculus. International Journal of Toxicology, 22(5), 335–342.

[67] Hwang, Y. H., Chiang, H. Y., Yen-Jean, M. C., & Wang, J. D. (2009). The association between low levels of lead in blood and occupational noise-induced hearing loss in steel workers. Science of the Total Environment, 408(1), 43–49.

[68] Jarvis, J. F. (1966). A case of unilateral permanent deafness following acetylsalicylic acid. Journal of Laryngology and Otology, 80(3), 318–320.

[69] Johnson A.C. & Morata T.C. (2010). Occupational exposure to chemicals and hearing impairment. The Nordic Expert Group for Criteria Documentation of Health Risks from Chemicals. Nordic Expert Group. Gothenburg. Arbete och Hälsa, Vetenskaplig skriftserie, 44(4), 1– 177. Retrieved from https://gupea.ub.gu.se/bitstream/2077/23240/1/gupea_2077_23240_1.pdf

[70] Johnson, A. C., Morata, T. C., Lindblad, A. C., et al. (2006). Audiological findings in workers exposed to styrene alone or in concert with noise. Noise and Health, 8(30), 45–57.

[71] Kanthasamy, A. G., Borowitz, J. L., Pavlakovic, G., & Isom, G. E. (1994). Dopaminergic neurotoxicity of cyanide: Neurochemical, histological, and behavioral characterization. Toxicology and Applied Pharmacology, 126(1), 156–163.

[72] Kapur, Y. P. (1965). Ototoxicity of acetylsalicylic acid. Archives of Otolaryngology, 81, 134–138.

[73] Kaufman, L. R., LeMasters, G. K., Olsen, D. M., & Succop, P. (2005). Effects of concurrent noise and jet fuel exposure on hearing loss. Journal of Occupational and Environmental Medicine, 47(3), 212–218.

[74] Keski-Säntti, P., Kaukiainen, A., Hyvärinen, H. K., & Sainio, M. (2010). Occupational chronic solvent encephalopathy in Finland 1995-2007: Incidence and exposure. International Archives of Occupational and Environmental Health, 83(6), 703–712.

[75] Keski-Säntti, P., Mäntylä, R., Lamminen, A., Hyvärinen, H. K., & Sainio, M. (2009). Magnetic resonance imaging in occupational chronic solvent encephalopathy. International Archives of Occupational and Environmental Health, 82(5), 595–602.

[76] Komune, S., & Snow, J. B., Jr. (1981). Potentiating effects of cisplatin and ethacrynic acid in ototoxicity. Archives of Otolaryngology, 107(10), 594–597.

[77] Kopelman, J., Budnick, A. S., Sessions, R. B., Kramer, M. B., & Wong, G. Y. (1988). Ototoxicity of high-dose cisplatin by bolus administration in patients with advanced cancers and normal hearing. Laryngoscope, 98(8, Pt. 1), 858–864.

[78] Kumar, V., & Tandon, O. P. (1997). Neurotoxic effects of rubber factory environment: An auditory evoked potential study. Electromyography and Clinical Neurophysiology, 37 (8), 469–473.

[79] Kuwabara, S., Kai, M. R., Nagase, H., & Hattori, T. (1999). n-Hexane neuropathy caused by addictive inhalation: Clinical and electrophysiological features. European Neurology, 41 (3), 163–167.

[80] Lataye, R., Maguin, K., & Campo, P. (2007). Increase in cochlear microphonic potential after toluene administration. Hearing Research, 230(1-2), 34–42.

[81] Laukli, E., & Hansen, P. W. (1995). An audiometric test battery for the evaluation of occupational exposure to industrial solvents. Acta Otolaryngologica, 115(2), 162–164.

[82] Laurell, G. F. (1992). Combined effects of noise and cisplatin: Short- and long-term follow-up. Annals of Otology, Rhinology, and Laryngology, 101(12), 969–976.

[83] Lerner, S. A., Schmitt, B. A., Seligsohn, R., & Matz, G. J. (1986). Comparative study of ototoxicity and nephrotoxicity in patients randomly assigned to treatment with amikacin or gentamicin. American Journal of Medicine, 80(6B), 98–104.

[84] Li, H., & Steyger, P. S. (2009). Synergistic ototoxicity due to noise exposure and aminoglycoside antibiotics. Noise and Health, 11(42), 26–32.

[85] Li, R., Greinwald, J. H., Jr., Yang, L., Choo, D. I., Wenstrup, R. J., & Guan, M. X. (2004). Molecular analysis of the mitochondrial 12S rRNA and tRNASer(UCN) genes in paediatric subjects with non-syndromic hearing loss. Journal of Medical Genetics, 41(8), 615–620.

[86] Liu, Y., & Fechter, L. D. (1995). MK-801 protects against carbon monoxide-induced hearing loss. Toxicology and Applied Pharmacology, 132(2), 196–202.

[87] Lopez, I., Ishiyama, A., & Ishiyama, G. (2012). Sudden sensorineural hearing loss due to drug abuse. Seminars in Hearing, 33(3), 251–260.

[88] Macdonald, M. R., Harrison, R. V., Wake, M., Bliss, B., & Macdonald, R. E. (1994). Ototoxicity of carboplatin: Comparing animal and clinical models at the Hospital for Sick Children. Journal of Otolaryngology, 23(3), 151–159.

[89] Maguin, K., Campo, P., & Parietti-Winkler, C. (2009). Toluene can perturb the neuronal voltage-dependent Ca2 + channels involved in the middle-ear reflex. Toxicological Sciences, 107(2), 473–481.

[90] Massioui, F. E., Lille, F., Lesevre, N., Hazemann, P., Garnier, R., & Dally, S. (1990). Sensory and cognitive event related potentials in workers chronically exposed to solvents. Clinical Toxicology, 28(2), 203-219.

[91] Metrick, S. A., & Brenner, R. P. (1982). Abnormal brainstem auditory evoked potentials in chronic paint sniffers. Annals of Neurology, 12(6), 553–556.

[92] Mizukoshi, K., Watanabe, Y., Kobayashi, H., et al. (1989). Neurotological follow-up studies upon Minamata disease. Acta Otolaryngologica. Supplementum, 468, 353–357.

[93] Möller, C., Odkvist, L. M., Thell, J., et al. (1989). Otoneurological findings in psycho-organic syndrome caused by industrial solvent exposure. Acta Otolaryngologica, 107(1–2), 5–12.

[94] Moore, R. D., Smith, C. R., & Lietman, P. S. (1984). Risk factors for the development of auditory toxicity in patients receiving aminoglycosides. Journal of Infectious Diseases, 149(1), 23–30.

[95] Morata, T. C., Dunn, D. E., Kretschmer, L. W., Lemasters, G. K., & Keith, R. W. (1993). Effects of occupational exposure to organic solvents and noise on hearing. Scandinavian Journal of Work and Environmental Health, 19(4), 245–254.

[96] Morata, T. C., Fiorini, A. C., Fischer, F. M., et al. (1997). Toluene-induced hearing loss among rotogravure printing workers. Scandinavian Journal of Work and Environmental Health, 23(4), 289–298.

[97] Morata, T. C., Johnson, A. C., Nylen, P., et al. (2002). Audiometric findings in workers exposed to low levels of styrene and noise. Journal of Occupational and Environmental Medicine, 44(9), 806–814.

[98] Morioka, I., Miyai, N., Yamamoto, H., & Miyashita, K. (2000). Evaluation of combined effect of organic solvents and noise by the upper limit of hearing. Industrial Health, 38(2), 252–257.

[99] Moshe, S., Frenkel, A., Hager, M., Skulsky, M., Sulkis, J., & Himelfarbe, M. (2002). Effects of occupational exposure to mercury or chlorinated hydrocarbons on the auditory pathway. Noise and Health, 4(16), 71–77.

[100] Murata, K., Weihe, P., Budtz-Jørgensen, E., Jørgensen, P. J., & Grandjean, P. (2004). Delayed brainstem auditory evoked potential latencies in 14-year-old children exposed to methylmercury. Journal of Pediatrics, 144(2), 177–183.

453

[101] Musiek, F. E., & Hanlon, D. P. (1999). Neuroaudiological effects in a case of fatal dimethylmercury poisoning. Ear and Hearing, 20(3), 271–275.

[102] National Institute for Occupational Safety and Health (NIOSH). (1998). Criteria for a recommended standard: Occupational Noise Exposure–Revised Criteria 1998. Publication No. 98–126. Cincinnati, OH: Author.

[103] Nagy, J. L., Adelstein, D. J., Newman, C. W., Rybicki, L. A., Rice, T. W., & Lavertu, P. (1999). Cisplatin ototoxicity: The importance of baseline audiometry. American Journal of Clinical Oncology, 22(3), 305–308.

[104] Neuwelt, E. A., Brummett, R. E., Doolittle, N. D., et al. (1998). First evidence of otoprotection against carboplatin-induced hearing loss with a two-compartment system in patients with central nervous system malignancy using sodium thiosulfate. Journal of Pharmacology and Experimental Therapeutics, 286(1), 77–84.

[105] Niehaus, L., & Meyer, B. U. (1998). Bilateral borderzone brain infarctions in association with heroin abuse. Journal of the Neurological Sciences, 160(2), 180–182.

[106] Niklasson, M., Arlinger, S., Ledin, T., et al. (1998). Audiological disturbances caused by long-term exposure to industrial solvents: Relation to the diagnosis of toxic encephalopathy. Scandinavian Audiology, 27(3), 131–136.

[107] Nolfe, G., Palma, V., Guadagnino, M., Serra, L. L., & Serra, C. (1991). Evoked potentials in shoe-workers with minimal polyneuropathy. Electromyography and Clinical Neurophysiology, 31(3), 157–162.

[108] Occupational Safety and Health Administration (OSHA). (1983). 29 CFR 1910.95 OSHA. Occupational Noise Exposure; Hearing Conservation Amendment; Final Rule, effective 8 March 1983 (Fed. Reg. 48:9738–9785). Washington, DC: U.S. Department of Labor Publications.

[109] Occupational Safety and Health Administration. (1997). Occupational Safety and Health Standards. Regulations (Standards 29 CFR). 1910.1000 Table Z-2. [62 FR 42018, August 4, 1997]. Accessed June 4, 2011, from http://www.osha.gov.

[110] Occupational Safety and Health Administration (OSHA) (1983). 29 CFR 1910.95. Occupational Noise Exposure; Hearing Conservation Amendment; Final Rule, effective 8 March 1983. (Fed. Reg. 48: 9738-9785).

[111] Odkvist, L. M., Arlinger, S. D., Edling, C., Larsby, B., & Bergholtz, L. M. (1987). Audiological and vestibulo-oculomotor findings in workers exposed to solvents and jet fuel. Scandinavian Audiology, 16(2), 75–81.

[112] Odkvist, L. M., Bergholtz, L. M., Ahifeldt, H., Andersson, B., Edling, C., & Strand, E. (1982). Otoneurological and audiological findings in workers exposed to industrial solvents. Acta Otolaryngologica, 93(S386), 249–251.

[113] Osman, K., Pawlas, K., Schütz, A., Gazdzik, M., Sokal, J. A., & Vahter, M. (1999). Lead exposure and hearing effects in children in Katowice, Poland. Environmental Research, 80(1), 1–8.

[114] Papu-Zamxaka, V., Mathee, A., Harpham, T., et al. (2010). Elevated mercury exposure in communities living alongside the Inanda Dam, South Africa. Journal of Environmental Monitoring, 12(2), 472–477.

[115] Park, S. K., Elmarsafawy, S., Mukherjee, B., et al. (2010). Cumulative lead exposure and age-related hearing loss: The VA Normative Aging Study. Hearing Research, 269(1-2), 48–55.

[116] Peters, H. A., Levine, R. L., Matthews, C. G., Sauter, S., & Chapman, L. (1986). Synergistic neurotoxicity of carbon tetrachloride/carbon disulfide (80/20 fumigants) and other pesticides in grain storage workers. Acta Pharmacologica et Toxicologica (Copenhagen), 59(Suppl. 7), 535–546.

[117] Pillers, D.-A. M., & Schleiss, M. R. (2005). Gentamicin in the clinical setting. Volta Review, 105(3), 205–210.

[118] Popper, P., Cristobal, R., & Wackym, P. A. (2004). Expression and distribution of mu opioid receptors in the inner ear of the rat. Neuroscience, 129(1), 225–233.

[119] Poulsen, P., & Jensen, J. H. (1986). Brain-stem response audiometry and electronystagmographic findings in chronic toxic encephalopathy (chronic painter's syndrome). Journal of Laryngology and Otology, 100(2), 155–156.

[120] Pouyatos, B., & Fetcher, L. D. (2007). Chemicals and solvents affecting the auditory system. In K. C. M. Campbell (Ed.), Pharmacology and ototoxicity for audiologists (pp. 197–215). Clifton Park, NY: Thomson Delmar Learning.

[121] Prezant, T. R., Agapian, J. V., Bohlman, M. C., et al. (1993). Mitochondrial ribosomal RNA mutation associated with both antibiotic-induced and non-syndromic deafness. Nature Genetics, 4(3), 289–294.

[122] Quevedo, L. da S., Tochetto, T., Siqueira, M. A., & Machado, M. S. (2012). Auditory brainstem response in gas station attendants. Brazilian Journal of Otorhinolaryngology, 78(6), 63–68.

[123] Rabinowitz, P. M., Galusha, D., Slade, M. D., et al. (2008). Organic solvent exposure and hearing loss in a cohort of aluminium workers. Occupational and Environmental Medicine, 65(4), 230–235.

[124] Rao, D., & Fechter, L. D. (2000). Protective effects of phenyl-N-tert-butylnitrone on the potentiation of noise-induced hearing loss by carbon monoxide. Toxicology and Applied Pharmacology, 167(2), 125–131.

[125] Rawool, V. W. (1995). Ipsilateral acoustic reflex thresholds at varying click rates in humans. Scandinavian Audiology, 24(3), 199–205.

[126] Rawool, V. W. (1996a). Click-rate induced facilitation of the acoustic reflex using constant number of pulses. Audiology, 35(4), 171–179.

[127] Rawool, V. W. (1996b). Effect of aging on the click-rate induced facilitation of acoustic reflex thresholds. Journals of Gerontology Series A: Biological Sciences and Medical Sciences, 51(2), B124–B131.

[128] Rawool, V. W. (1996c). Acoustic reflex monitoring during the presentation of 1000 clicks at high repetition rates. Scandinavian Audiology, 25(4), 239–245.

[129] Rawool, V. W. (1998). Effects of click polarity on the auditory brainstem responses of older men. Audiology, 37(2), 100–108.

[130] Rawool, V. W. (2007). The aging auditory system: 1. Controversy and confusion on slower processing. Hearing Review, 14(7), 14–19.

[131] Rawool, V. W. (2012a). Comprehensive audiological, tinnitus, and auditory processing evaluations. In V. W. Rawool (Ed.), Hearing conservation: In occupational, recreational, educational, and home settings (pp. 106–135). New York: Thieme.

[132] Rawool, V. W. (2012b). Monitoring of auditory sensitivity and follow-up procedures. In V. W. Rawool (Ed.), Hearing conservation: In occupational, recreational, educational, and home settings (pp. 65–105). New York: Thieme.

[133] Rawool, V. W., & Ballachanda, B. B. (1990). Homo- and antiphasic stimulation in ABR. Scandinavian Audiology, 19(1), 9–15.

[134] Rawool, V., & Dluhy, C. (2011). Auditory sensitivity in opiate addicts with and without a history of noise exposure. Noise and Health, 13(54), 356–363.

[135] Rawool, V., & Zerlin, S. (1988). Phase-intensity effects on the ABR. Scandinavian Audiology, 17(2), 117–123.

[136] Razzaq, M., Dumbala, S., & Moudgil, S. S. (2010). Neurological picture: Sudden deafness due to carbon monoxide poi-

soning. Journal of Neurology, Neurosurgery, and Psychiatry, 81(6), 658.

[137] Rice, D. C. (1998). Age-related increase in auditory impairment in monkeys exposed in utero plus postnatally to methylmercury. Toxicological Sciences, 44(2), 191–196.

[138] Rice, D. C., & Gilbert, S. G. (1992). Exposure to methyl mercury from birth to adulthood impairs high-frequency hearing in monkeys. Toxicology and Applied Pharmacology, 115 (1), 6–10.

[139] Riggs, L. C., Brummett, R. E., Guitjens, S. K., & Matz, G. J. (1996). Ototoxicity resulting from combined administration of cisplatin and gentamicin. Laryngoscope, 106(4), 401–406.

[140] Rothwell, J. A., & Boyd, P. J. (2008). Amalgam dental fillings and hearing loss. International Journal of Audiology, 47(12), 770–776.

[141] Schäper, M., Seeber, A., & van Thriel, C. (2008). The effects of toluene plus noise on hearing thresholds: An evaluation based on repeated measurements in the German printing industry. International Journal of Occupational Medicine and Environmental Health, 21(3), 191–200.

[142] Schweitzer, V. G. (1993). Cisplatin-induced ototoxicity: The effect of pigmentation and inhibitory agents. Laryngoscope, 103(4, Pt. 2), 1–52.

[143] Sha, S.-H., Qiu, J.-H., & Schacht, J. (2006). Aspirin to prevent gentamicin-induced hearing loss. New England Journal of Medicine, 354(17), 1856–1857.

[144] Shahbaz Hassan, M., Ray, J., & Wilson, F. (2003). Carbon monoxide poisoning and sensorineural hearing loss. Journal of Laryngology and Otology, 117(2), 134–137.

[145] Sliwińska-Kowalska, M., Zamyslowska-Szmytke, E., Szymczak, W., et al. (2003). Ototoxic effects of occupational exposure to styrene and co-exposure to styrene and noise. Journal of Occupational and Environmental Medicine, 45(1), 15–24.

[146] Sliwińska-Kowalska, M., Zamyslowska-Szmytke, E., Szymczak, W., et al. (2005). Exacerbation of noise-induced hearing loss by co-exposure to workplace chemicals. Environmental Toxicology and Pharmacology, 19(3), 547–553.

[147] Sliwińska-Kowalska, M., Prasher, D., Rodrigues, C. A., et al. (2007). Ototoxicity of organic solvents: From scientific evidence to health policy. International Journal of Occupational Medicine and Environmental Health, 20(2), 215–222.

[148] Steyger, P. S. (2009). Potentiation of chemical ototoxicity by noise. Seminars in Hearing, 30(1), 38–46.

[149] Stypulkowski, P. H. (1990). Mechanisms of salicylate ototoxicity. Hearing Research, 46(1-2), 113–145.

[150] Thompson, P. M., Hayashi, K. M., Simon, S. L., et al. (2004). Structural abnormalities in the brains of human subjects who use methamphetamine. Journal of Neuroscience, 24 (26), 6028–6036.

[151] Tran Ba Huy, P., Meulemans, A., Wassef, M., Manuel, C., Sterkers, O., & Amiel, C. (1983). Gentamicin persistence in rat endolymph and perilymph after a two-day constant infusion. Antimicrobial Agents and Chemotherapy, 23(2), 344–346.

[152] U.S. Army Center for Health Promotion and Preventative Medicine (USACHPPM). (2003). Just the facts: Occupational ototoxins (ear poisons) and hearing loss (Pub. No. 51–002–0903). Aberdeen Proving Ground, MD: Author.

[153] U. S. Department of Labor, Occupational Safety & Health Administration (1999). Xylenes (o-, m-, p-isomers) Ethylbenzene, 1002. Retrieved from https://www.osha.gov/dts/sltc/methods/mdt/mdt1002/1002.html

[154] U.S. Environmental Protection Agency (EPA). (1987). Carbon tetrachloride health advisory. Washington, DC: Office of Drinking Water.

[155] Usami, S., Abe, S., Shinkawa, H., Inoue, Y., & Yamaguchi, T. (1999). Rapid mass screening method and counseling for the 1555A–G mitochondrial mutation. Journal of Human Genetics, 44(5), 304–307.

[156] van der Laan, G., & Sainio, M. (2012). Chronic solvent induced encephalopathy: A step forward. Neurotoxicology, 33 (4), 897–901.

[157] van Hout, M. S. E., Wekking, E. M., Berg, I. J., & Deelman, B. G. (2008). Psychosocial and cognitive rehabilitation of patients with solvent-induced chronic toxic encephalopathy: A randomised controlled study. Psychotherapy and Psychosomatics, 77(5), 289–297.

[158] van Valen, E., van Thriel, C., Akila, R., et al. (2012). Chronic solvent-induced encephalopathy: European consensus of neuropsychological characteristics, assessment, and guidelines for diagnostics. Neurotoxicology, 33(4), 710–726.

[159] Varney, N. R., Kubu, C. S., & Morrow, L. A. (1998). Dichotic listening performances of patients with chronic exposure to organic solvents. The Clinical Neuropsychologist, 12(1), 107–112.

[160] Vineis, P. & Zeise, L. (2002). Styrene-7, 8-oxide and Styrene. IARC Monograph 82, Retrieved from http://monographs.iarc.fr/ENG/Publications/techrep42/TR42-9.pdf

[161] Visser, I., Lavini, C., Booij, J., et al. (2008). Cerebral impairment in chronic solvent-induced encephalopathy. Annals of Neurology, 63(5), 572–580.

[162] Vrca, A., Bozicević, D., Bozikov, V., Fuchs, R., & Malinar, M. (1997). Brain stem evoked potentials and visual evoked potentials in relation to the length of occupational exposure to low levels of toluene. Acta Medica Croatica, 51(4-5), 215–219.

[163] Vrca, A., Karacić, V., Bozicević, D., Bozikov, V., & Malinar, M. (1996). Brainstem auditory evoked potentials in individuals exposed to long-term low concentrations of toluene. American Journal of Industrial Medicine, 30(1), 62–66.

[164] Wang, Q., Li, Q.-Z., Han, D., et al. (2006). Clinical and molecular analysis of a four-generation Chinese family with aminoglycoside-induced and nonsyndromic hearing loss associated with the mitochondrial 12S rRNA C1494 T mutation. Biochemical and Biophysical Research Communications, 340 (2), 583–588.

[165] Warner-Smith, M., Darke, S., & Day, C. (2002). Morbidity associated with non-fatal heroin overdose. Addiction, 97(8), 963–967.

[166] Winneke, G. (1982). Acute behavioral effects of exposure to some organic solvents: Psychophysiological aspects. Acta Neurologica Scandinavica. Supplementum, 92, 117–129.

[167] WorkCover Australia. (2001). WorkCover guides for the evaluation of permanent impairment. Sydney, Australia: Author.

[168] Wu, T. N., Shen, C. Y., Lai, J.S., et al. (2000). Effects of lead and noise exposures on hearing ability. Archives of Environmental Health, 55(2), 109–114.

[169] Xoinis, K., Weirather, Y., Mavoori, H., Shaha, S. H., & Iwamoto, L. M. (2007). Extremely low birth weight infants are at high risk for auditory neuropathy. Journal of Perinatology, 27(11), 718–723.

[170] Yücel, M., Takagi, M., Walterfang, M., & Lubman, D. I. (2008). Toluene misuse and long-term harms: A systematic review of the neuropsychological and neuroimaging literature. Neuroscience and Biobehavioral Reviews, 32(5), 910–926.

[171] Zamyslowska-Szmytke, E., Fuente, A., Niebudek-Bogusz, E., & Sliwińska-Kowalska, M. (2009). Temporal processing disorder associated with styrene exposure. Audiology and Neurootology, 14(5), 296–302.

[172] Zhao, H., Li, R., Wang, Q., et al. (2004). Maternally inherited aminoglycoside-induced and nonsyndromic deafness is associated with the novel C1494T mutation in the mitochondrial 12S rRNA gene in a large Chinese family. American Journal of Human Genetics, 74(1), 139–152.

Chapter 17

Age-related Deficits in Auditory Processing

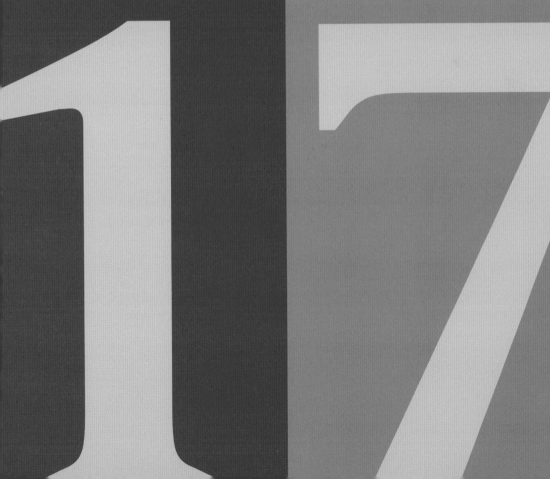

17 Age-related Deficits in Auditory Processing

Auditory processing skills can deteriorate with aging of the auditory system. Age-related changes in brain structure and function may contribute to poor sensory and cognitive function. Alternatively, cognitive declines may be a consequence of degraded auditory processing causing sensory deprivation. Thus, a complex interrelationship between speech recognition, cognitive performance, and slower processing can be expected. An in-depth understanding of this relationship can lead to more effective aural rehabilitation services to older individuals (Rawool, 2007a,b,c).

17.1 Aging within the Auditory Nervous System

Several studies have documented physiological changes within the aging auditory system that could lead to auditory processing deficits (APDs). Investigators have reported primary degeneration of the spiral ganglion (cell bodies of the auditory nerve fibers) or loss of fibers that can occur even in the absence of loss of sensory hair cells (Felder & Schrott-Fischer, 1995; Felix, Johnsson, Gleeson, & Pollak, 1990). ▶ Fig. 17.1 shows the loss of cochlear neurons with aging in individuals with normal counts of outer and inner hair cells. Approximately 100 neurons are lost per year of life. The neuronal loss may be related to a decrease in neurotrophin

expression in the organ of Corti with aging (Makary, Shin, Kujawa, Liberman, & Merchant, 2011).

Neuronal loss has been reported at other levels of the auditory system, including the cochlear nucleus, inferior colliculus, medial geniculate body, and temporal lobe (Brody, 1955; Hansen & Reske-Nielsen, 1965; Kirikae, Sato, & Shitara, 1964). Konigsmark and Murphy (1972) found a relation between age and a decrease in the volume of the cochlear nucleus that appeared to be associated with changes in axon size and degree of myelination. Degenerative changes in the myelin sheaths and axis cylinders have been reported by other investigators (Hansen & Reske-Nielsen, 1965). Other degenerative changes, such as cell size and cell shape irregularities and accumulation of lipofuscin pigments, have been observed in the cochlear nucleus, superior olivary nucleus, inferior colliculus, medial geniculate body, and inferior olive (Brody, 1976; Kirikae et al., 1964; Konigsmark & Murphy, 1972).

Based on functional magnetic resonance imaging (fMRI) studies, Peelle and colleagues (Peelle, McMillan, Moore, Grossman, & Wingfield, 2004) showed that sentences presented at a rapid rate recruit frontal brain regions such as the anterior cingulate and premotor cortex. These regions are also compromised in older individuals. Progressive loss of dendritic mass without obvious clinical symptoms has been reported especially in the frontal and temporal cortex with aging (Scheibel & Scheibel, 1975).

The above studies collectively suggest that compromised or slower neurotransmission in the neural auditory pathways is possible. Such slower processing can lead to poor auditory perception apparent in older individuals.

17.2 Behavioral Studies

17.2.1 Binaural Processing

Dichotic Digits

Older adults with normal peripheral sensitivity up to 4000 Hz have poorer scores than younger adults on the dichotic digits task in both free and directed recall conditions. In the directed recall condition, their performance tends to be worse in the left ear compared to that in the right ear, suggesting a corpus callosum deficit (Gootjes, Van Strien, & Bouma, 2004). Because of the poor performance in the left

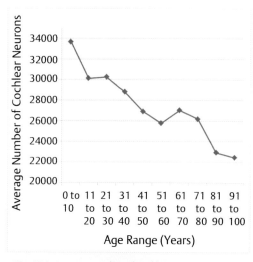

Fig. 17.1 Average number of cochlear neurons across different age groups (based on Makary et al., 2011).

ear, a larger right ear advantage is apparent in the 60- to 79-year-old group compared to younger adults (Strouse, Wilson, & Brush, 2000).

Binaural Sound Correlation

Individuals with normal hearing can reliably detect a break in the correlation (BIC) of sounds presented to two ears through headphones. However, younger adults can detect significantly shorter BICs than older adults. The age-related decline in the ability to detect a BIC is more obvious when the signal in one ear is delayed compared to the signal in the other ear. These deficits are expected to lead to difficulty in analyzing auditory scenes (Li, Huang, Wu, Qi, & Schneider, 2009). To detect a BIC, the central nervous system (CNS) needs to be efficient in comparing and contrasting the neural responses of the signals presented to the two ears. A loss of neural synchrony in the central auditory system may compromise this comparison, leading to difficulties in stream segregation (Wang, Wu, Li, & Schneider, 2011).

The ability to detect a BIC is better when the sounds are presented via loudspeakers placed on the right and left sides compared to when the sounds are presented through headphones. This improvement probably occurs due to additional spectral cues provided by interference between the sounds presented through the two loudspeakers. However, the advantage gained from listening through the loudspeakers compared to via the headphones is significantly less in older than younger adults (Qu et al., 2013).

17.2.2 Temporal Processing

Frequency Discrimination

The difference limens for 500 and 1000 Hz increase significantly with age (Clinard, Tremblay, & Krishnan, 2010). Age-related differences in frequency discrimination are largest at 500 Hz and decrease with an increase in frequency (He, Dubno, & Mills, 1998).

Gap Detection

McCroskey and Kasten (1980) varied the interstimulus interval between two tones and asked study participants to judge if they detected one tone (fusion) or two tones (flutter). The interval required for older participants to perceive two tones was longer. Other investigators have reported similar deterioration in gap detection due to aging (Gordon-Salant & Fitzgibbons, 1993; John, Hall, & Kriesman, 2012; Pichora-Fuller, Schneider, Benson, Hamstra, & Storzer, 2006; Schneider, Pichora-Fuller, Kowalchuk, & Lamb, 1994, 1998; Snell, 1997; Snell & Frisina, 2000; Strouse, Ashmead, Ohde, & Grantham, 1998). Older adults have significantly more difficulty in detecting 6 ms gaps than younger adults (Harris, Wilson, Eckert, & Dubno, 2012).

Duration Discrimination

The just noticeable difference (JND) in duration between a standard 1000 Hz tone of 40 ms and comparison tones of longer duration was evaluated in one study in the presence of maskers that were presented following the tonal stimulus with delays of 80, 240, and 720 ms (Phillips, Gordon-Salant, Fitzgibbons, & Yeni-Komshian, 1994). The JNDs for duration were significantly larger for older adults compared to younger adults in the 80 ms backward interference condition. These results show that when brief tones are followed closely by interfering stimuli, the duration discrimination performance of older adults is poorer when compared to younger adults, suggesting slower processing of durational characteristics of the signal in older listeners (Phillips et al., 1994). Although effects of age are more obvious in complex duration discrimination tasks, older adults also show significantly poor duration discrimination for simple tasks with the use of standard tones of 4000 Hz with a duration of 250 ms (Gordon-Salant & Fitzgibbons, 1999).

Gap Duration Discrimination

Older adults need larger durational differences in two gaps to detect differences in gap duration compared to younger adults even in the presence of normal hearing (Gordon-Salant & Fitzgibbons, 1999).

Temporal Modulation Detection

Frequency modulation detection is poorer in older than younger subjects, and age-related differences are greater at 500 Hz than at 4000 Hz (He, Mills, & Dubno, 2007). In one study, temporal modulation transfer functions (TMTFs) were measured at 75 dB sound pressure level (SPL) in 500 and 4000 Hz tonal carriers from young and older listeners with normal peripheral auditory sensitivity through 4000 Hz (He, Mills, Ahlstrom, & Dubno, 2008). Amplitude modulation detection thresholds for older adults became worse with increasing modulation frequency, indicating an age-related decline in temporal resolution for faster envelope fluctuations. Significant age-related differences were observed whenever amplitude modulation detection was dependent on temporal cues. These results suggest age-related deficit in synchronization of neural responses to both the carrier waveform (phase locking) and fluctuations in waveform envelope (envelope locking) (He et al., 2008).

Backward Masking

Some studies have shown an age-related decrease in temporal resolution using backward masking paradigms (Cobb, Jacobson, Newman, Kretschmer, & Donnelly, 1993). Older individuals also have difficulty in discriminating between phonemes varying in voice onset time (VOT; Strouse et al., 1998), which may be related to greater backward masking.

Temporal Order Thresholds

Older adults (55–70 years) require larger gaps between two tones (800 and 1200 Hz) to accurately judge the sequence of the tones compared to younger adults (20–35 years). The temporal order thresholds improve with practice. There is some variability in performance. Up to 13% of the older adults can accurately judge the sequence with a gap of 5.5 ms between the two tones; in comparison, 43% of the younger adults can accurately judge the sequence with the same gap (Fink, Churan, & Wittmann, 2005). A significant worsening of temporal order thresholds in adults older than 60 years has been noted for monaural 1 ms clicks presented in rapid succession (Szelag et al., 2011). Older adults with normal hearing need sequence component durations almost 3 times longer (95.6 ms) than younger adults (35.0 ms) to correctly judge the sequence of three tones differing in frequency around the frequency of 4000 Hz (Gordon-Salant & Fitzgibbons, 1999).

The above findings suggest that older individuals have difficulty processing rapidly changing information. Such changes in auditory temporal processing can make it difficult to perceive and understand rapid or degraded speech. Accurate perception of timing of successive auditory events is important for the perception of speech (de Boer & Dreschler, 1987).

17.2.3 Processing of Degraded Speech

Speech Perception in Noise

Older adults need significantly better signal-to-noise ratios than younger adults to yield equivalent speech recognition scores (SRSs), which suggests poor speech recognition in noise. When compared to the performance difference in the morning, the difference is larger in the evening, which is considered off-peak time for older adults (Veneman, Gordon-Salant, Matthews, & Dubno, 2013). Other studies have shown that older adults show significantly poorer performance on the Hearing in Noise Test (HINT) compared to younger adults when the noise is presented to the same ear as the speech signal (Mukari & Mamat, 2008).

When monosyllabic words are presented at a 0 dB signal-to-noise ratio, word recognition scores of older adults are significantly poor compared to those of younger adults with normal hearing (Krull, Humes, & Kidd, 2013). When the signal-to-noise ratio is 10 dB, and the words are presented at a 40 dB sensation level, individuals in the age range of 60 to 69 years show poor word recognition compared to younger individuals even in the presence of normal hearing and very good word recognition scores in quiet (Yilmaz, Sennaroğlu, Sennaroğlu, & Köse, 2007).

Interrupted Speech

When words are interrupted by digitally removing eight equal duration alternating segments and replacing the segments with silent periods to generate temporal glimpses of speech, the word recognition scores of older adults with normal hearing are significantly poorer than younger adults with normal hearing (Krull et al., 2013).

Older adults also perform significantly worse than younger adults when words are presented in the background of interrupted noise (Stuart & Phillips, 1996).

Filtered Speech

Older adults with normal hearing perform significantly worse than younger adults when spectral information in specific frequency bands is removed from words through filtering (Krull et al., 2013).

Reverberant Speech

Older adults with normal hearing show significantly poor recognition of speech with a reverberation time of 0.6 second compared to young adults. The presence of hearing loss can make the SRSs worse (Gordon-Salant & Fitzgibbons, 1999).

Time-Compressed Speech

Several investigators have reported age-related deterioration in recognizing time-compressed speech (Bergman et al., 1976; Gordon-Salant & Fitzgibbons, 1993, 1995, 1999, 2004; Konkle, Beasley, & Bess, 1977; Letowski & Poch, 1996; Schmitt & Carroll, 1985; Sticht & Gray, 1969; Stine, Wingfield, & Poon, 1986; Versfeld & Dreschler, 2002). Difficulty in recognizing rapid speech can be experienced by older individuals even in the presence of normal hearing.

Wingfield and colleagues (Wingfield, Poon, Lombardi, & Lowe, 1985) concluded that reductions in available processing time through the use of time-compressed speech had a disproportionate effect on the comprehension performance of the elderly study participants. They assumed that time compression has its effect more from removing normally available processing time than by degrading the speech signal itself. Gordon-Salant and Fitzgibbons (2001) suggested that older listeners have difficulty in recognizing fast speech due to trouble in processing the brief, limited acoustic cues for consonants that are inherent in rapid speech.

Overall, the above studies suggest that there is an age-related decline in the rate of information processing that makes it difficult for older listeners to understand rapid speech. Slower processing is probably at least in part related to slower neurotransmission speeds in the auditory pathways. The resulting communication difficulties, social isolation, and depression can contribute to an overall decrease in the quality of life of older individuals.

17.3 Objective Measures

The difficulties in rapid speech perception and temporal processing experienced by older individuals suggest slower processing within the aging auditory system. However, the age-related deficits in the tasks described above can also occur due to deficits in attention, memory, and/or cognition (Gordon-Salant, Yeni-Komshian, Fitzgibbons, &

Barrett, 2006; Moore, Peters, & Glasberg, 1992). Thus, whether or not slower processing occurs specifically within the aging auditory system can be questioned. However, objective measures that are not significantly affected by nonauditory factors, such as alertness level, attention, memory, and general intelligence, suggest that auditory processing is compromised or slower in the aging auditory pathway. Findings based on objective auditory measures are discussed below.

17.3.1 Age-related Transmission Delays (Slower Processing) in Evoked Potentials

Age-related transmission delays within the auditory pathways can be measured by using auditory evoked potentials. Birren and Fisher (1995) suggested that measurement of evoked potentials provides a window into the temporal nature of neural processing. More specifically, the latencies of evoked potentials can provide information on the time involved in processing the information as the information travels through the various segments of the auditory pathway. Evoked potentials allow description of the flow of information in a serial and hierarchical manner. Latencies of evoked potentials give an idea of the time required for processing the information by the auditory system following the onset of a stimulus. Interpeak latencies can provide information about the time required for processing from one generator (e.g., auditory nerve) to the next generator (e.g., superior olivary complex).

17.3.2 Auditory Brainstem Measures

Auditory Brainstem Response

Several studies have been conducted to evaluate the effect of age on latencies of the auditory brainstem response (ABR). Some investigators have reported a significant effect of age on latencies (Allison, Hume, Wood, & Goff, 1984; Allison, Wood, & Goff, 1983; Chu, 1985; Elberling & Parbo, 1987; Kelly-Ballweber & Dobie, 1984; Kjaer, 1980; Lenzi, Chiarelli, & Sambataro,, 1989; Maurizi, Altissimi, Otaviani, Paludetti, & Bambini, 1982; Robinson & Rudge, 1977; Rosenhall, Pedersen, & Dotevall, 1986; Rowe, 1978; Stürzebecher & Werbs, 1987), some investigators have reported a trend of age-related prolongation of latencies (Beagley & Sheldrake, 1978), some have reported a slight age effect (Jerger & Johnson, 1988; McClelland & McCrea, 1979; Otto & McCandless, 1982; Stockard, Stockard, & Sharbrough, 1978), and others have reported no effect of age on ABR latencies (Anias, Lima, & Kos, 2004; Ottaviani, Maurizi, D'Alatri, & Almadori, 1991). On the surface, the results appear to be controversial, as suggested by Boettcher (2002). One problem that is related to these results is that some investigators have not reported the statistical significance or non-significance of their findings (Burkard & Sims, 2001; Debruyne, 1986; Fujikawa & Weber, 1977).

After reviewing the ABR data from 11 different laboratories, Thornton (1987) suggested an interaction of age, gender, stimulus polarity, stimulus level, and stimulus rate. The use of all of these parameters varies in different age-related studies. In addition, the particular stimuli used in various studies include tone burst and clicks varying in duration from 0.1 to 0.5 ms. The selected age groups may also have an impact on the results. In some studies, the "younger" control groups include individuals up to the age of 51 years (Ottaviani et al., 1991).

Additional variation may be caused by monaural versus binaural stimulation and use or nonuse of contralateral noise. In the case of monaural stimuli, many investigators have not specified the ear of stimulation, and others reported using either the left or right ear depending on the auditory sensitivity. Soucek, Michaels, and Mason (1990) reported a prolongation of the III–V interpeak interval with age with stimulation of the right ear, but not the left ear. However, their results are confounded by the presence of hearing loss in older adults. Johannsen and Lehn (1984) found no ear effects, but they did not report the sample size; thus, it is difficult to ascertain whether the sample size was sufficient to reveal any ear effects.

Possible Interaction of Age with Stimulus Level and Polarity

Stimulus level is an obvious factor in determining ABR latencies and interacts with stimulus polarity (Rawool & Zerlin, 1988). Stimulus polarity itself has a significant effect on the ABR in the older population (Rawool, 1998), yet it has not been reported in some of the studies. Stimulus polarity can interact with intensity and can affect latencies, interpeak latencies, amplitude ratios, and waveform morphology (Rawool, 1998). The morphological changes in the wave IV–V complex (► Fig. 17.2)

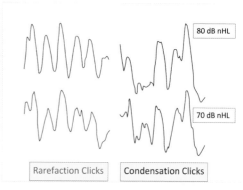

Fig. 17.2 Effect of click polarity and intensity on waveform morphology of the auditory brainstem response obtained from an older man (based on Rawool, 1998).

due to stimulus polarity (Rawool, 1998) can lead to contrary results, such as shortening and lengthening of interpeak or peak latency measures involving these two components, as reported by Johannsen and Lehn (1984).

Interaction of Age and Stimulus Rate

Another important factor that determines the effect of age on ABR latencies is the stimulus rate. Age effects tend to be more pronounced at higher click repetition rates (Debruyne, 1986; Fujikawa & Weber, 1977; Shanon, Gold, & Himelfarb, 1981). When very slow rates (e.g., 5.1/s) are used to elicit the ABR, no significant differences in latencies appear in the older and younger groups (Walton, Orland, & Burkard, 1999). This supports the notion that the aging auditory system may have difficulty in keeping up with stimuli occurring at faster rates.

Interaction of Age and Gender

Gender also has an impact on determining the age effect. For example, the age-related prolongation of latencies is more prominent in men (Allison et al., 1983, 1984; Elberling & Parbo, 1987; Kjaer, 1980; Patterson, Michalewski, Thompson, Bowman, & Litzelman, 1981; Stürzebecher & Werbs, 1987; von Wedel, 1979). When only men are included in the study, significant prolongation of latencies is reported with age (Maurizi et al., 1982) even in the presence of a small sample size (Kelly-Ballweber & Dobie, 1984). On the other hand, age effects seem to disappear when the sample size for each age group is small and the sample includes both men and women (Burkard & Sims, 2001) or when it includes only women (Harkins, 1981). Possible factors that may cause the age–gender interaction are difference in hormones and use or nonuse of estrogen by older women (Wharton & Church, 1990), more noise exposure in men causing subtle damage to outer hair cells, differences in head and brain size, and differences in whole-body temperature.

Interaction of Age and Hearing Loss

Another important factor that determines the age-related effect on ABR latencies is hearing loss. In the presence of sensory hearing loss, wave V latencies yielded with clicks are best predicted by hearing thresholds in the 4 to 8 kHz region (Marshall, 1983). Subjects with high-frequency hearing loss (4–8 kHz) show a greater wave I than wave V latency increase, which results in a reduced I–V interval (Coats, 1978; Elberling & Parbo, 1987; Keith & Greville, 1987). This is likely because wave I is predominantly generated from the more basal cochlear regions, whereas wave V comes from broader regions of the cochlea that include apical regions (Don & Eggermont, 1978). Age and high-frequency presbycusic hearing loss have opposite effects on the I–V interval; age prolongs it, whereas hearing loss shortens it (Elberling & Parbo, 1987).

Several studies have failed to match auditory sensitivity in the 4 and 8 kHz region in younger and older groups (Harkins, 1981; Martini, Comacchio, & Magnavita, 1991; Ottaviani et al., 1991). This may be the reason why some studies that have included participants with hearing loss have failed to find an age effect on the interpeak I–V latencies (Anias et al., 2004; Soucek & Mason, 1992). If the hearing loss dominates the interpeak wave I–V interval, then the interval may appear even shorter in older individuals (Martini et al., 1991; Oku & Hasegewa, 1997). In contrast, if the age effect dominates the I–V interval, then a longer interval may be seen in older individuals even in the presence of hearing loss (Rosenhall et al., 1986; von Wedel, 1979). When auditory sensitivity is normal, older individuals show longer wave V latencies when compared to younger adults (Hyde, 1985; Jerger & Hall, 1980).

In addition, gender interacts with hearing loss; men show more change in wave V latency with increasing hearing loss compared to women (Jerger & Johnson, 1988). The direction of the gender and hearing loss interaction for the I–V interval depends on how the data are plotted. When data are plotted as a function of auditory thresholds at 4 kHz, the interval seems to shorten with hearing loss in women, but not in men. When the data are plotted as a function of the average thresholds at 4 and 8 kHz, the I–V interval shortens more in men than in women (Jerger & Johnson, 1988).

Auditory Brainstem Response Results with Sufficient Control of Auditory Sensitivity

Investigators who have attempted to control for high-frequency hearing loss above 4 kHz have shown a significant effect of age on ABR latencies. Stürzebecher and Werbs (1987) included 69 women and 86 men in their study. The participants were divided into three age groups, and their pure tone average (PTA) at 2, 4, and 6 kHz was reported. The first group included individuals younger than 35 years, and their PTA was 7.3 dB. The second group included participants in the age range of 35 to 49 years and had a PTA of 10.6 dB. The third group included individuals above the age of 50 years, and their PTA was 12.8 dB. Significant differences between the first (under 35 years) and the third (over 50 years) group were found for latencies of waves III and V and interpeak latencies of I–V and III–V in males and for the wave V latency in females.

Elberling and Parbo (1987) obtained ABRs from 235 men and 249 women in the age range of 20 to 80 years. They used the averaged thresholds at 4 and 8 kHz as an index for the high-frequency hearing loss and conducted multiple regression analyses to evaluate the effect of age and hearing loss. They showed that, although hearing loss shortens the I–V interval, age increases both the I–V and I–III intervals.

Kelly-Ballweber and Dobie (1984) obtained ABRs from 12 young men (31–49 years) and 12 older men (64–76 years) in their study. The auditory sensitivity of the two groups was matched based on their PTA at 2, 4, and 8 kHz. For binaural as well as predicted binaural response based on monaural responses, wave V latency was significantly longer in older individuals.

Auditory Brainstem Responses Using Complex Stimuli

Walton and colleagues (1999) studied ABR recovery from forward masking using tone burst maskers and probes. Participants included two groups with normal hearing matched for auditory thresholds. The younger group included 10 adults in the range of 21 to 40 years. The older group included 10 adults in the range of 63 to 77 years. Probe tone bursts (1, 4, and 8 kHz) were presented at 40 dB above threshold, and the masker tone bursts (same frequency as the probe) were adjusted to a level that just eliminated the ABR to 40 dB sensation level (SL) probe when the probe onset occurred after masker offset. Forward masker intervals were 2, 4, 8, 16, 32, and 64 ms. Under forward masking conditions, wave V latency was prolonged for the shorter intervals and recovered to baseline latency by 64 ms. For the tone burst frequencies of 4 and 8 kHz, the mean latency shift was greater for the older group for forward masker intervals of 16 ms or less, but the shift was similar in the two groups for longer intervals. The prolonged recovery time from forward masking for older participants suggests deficient temporal processing for rapidly occurring stimuli.

Poth and colleagues (Poth, Boettcher, Mills, & Dubno, 2001) measured wave V of the ABR to two 50 ms broadband noise bursts separated by silent gaps varied in duration from 4, 8, 32, and 64 ms. The participants included eight younger and eight older adults with normal hearing. All adults had a measurable wave V response to the first noise burst. However, for the second noise burst, three of eight older adults did not have a measurable response with a gap duration of 4 and 8 ms, and one of the eight younger adults did not have a measurable response with a gap duration of 4 ms. These results suggest age-related deficits in resolving rapidly occurring stimuli at the level of the brainstem and show the individual variability in age-related deficits in temporal processing.

To summarize, when ABRs are elicited with fairly rapid stimuli, the latencies and interpeak latencies are prolonged with aging, suggesting slower processing in the aging auditory brainstem. There is some variability in this effect such that not all older systems demonstrate slowing, and men may show more slowing than women.

Frequency Following Response

A tool for detecting age-related desynchronization in the auditory brainstem is the frequency following response (FFR). The FFR reflects sustained phase-locked neural activity in the rostral brainstem (Krishnan, 2007). With advanced age, the tone–FFR phase coherence and FFR amplitudes for 1000 Hz and slightly lower frequencies are reduced significantly, suggesting reduction in the ability to sustain time-locked neural activity (Clinard et al., 2010).

When the FFR is elicited with the consonant-vowel (CV) /da/, the latencies of the sustained responses at the onset of vowel periodicity are delayed, and the amplitudes become smaller with increase in age. In addition, latencies of transient offset responses are prolonged. The degradation of the neural representation of the CV stimulus is related to the ability to encode simple tones (Clinard & Tremblay, 2013).

Binaural beats elicited by presenting tones of different frequencies (e.g., 390 and 430 Hz) simultaneously to the two ears can evoke the 40 Hz steady-state response. However, the response is recordable in fewer older participants compared to younger adults (Grose & Mamo, 2012).

Contralateral Suppression of Otoacoustic Emissions

Suppression of otoacoustic emissions (OAEs) is apparent when a noise is presented to the contralateral ear. The suppression allows measurement of the medial olivocochlear function, as described in Chapter 6. Older adults with normal hearing show reduced suppression of distortion product otoacoustic emissions (DPOAEs) compared to younger adults, which suggests an age-related deficit in the medial olivocochlear function (Kim, Frisina, & Frisina, 2002). The age-related reduction of suppression of DPOAEs is more evident in the frequency range of 3 to 8 kHz (Mukari & Mamat, 2008).

Acoustic Reflex

Elicitation of the acoustic reflex involves conduction of a relatively loud sound through the outer ear, the middle ear, and the cochlea. The neural impulses then travel through the auditory nerve to the cochlear nucleus and from the cochlear nucleus to the trapezoid bodies and/or to the superior olivary complexes (Borg, 1973; Rouiller, Capt, Dolivo, & De Ribaupierre, 1989). A message is then relayed to the stapedius motor neurons (Strutz, Münker, & Zöllner, 1988), which travels through the motor nerve fibers to the stapedius muscle. The contraction of the muscle changes the admittance characteristics of the middle ear. The related change in the middle ear admittance is recorded as the reflex. The acoustic reflex offers a unique opportunity to evaluate age-related changes involving efferent control of the auditory system.

Acoustic Reflex Latencies

Bosatra (1983) and Bosatra, Russolo, and Silverman (1984) reported a significant prolongation of acoustic reflex latency after the age of 60 years for 0.5, 1, and 2 kHz and broadband noise stimuli. These results suggest slower processing in the aging acoustic reflex pathway. Examples of acoustic reflex latency measures are provided in Chapter 5.

Rate-induced Facilitation of the Acoustic Reflex

Rawool (1996) showed that, at higher click rates, the acoustic reflex thresholds of older individuals are elevated, although at slower click rates, the reflex thresholds are similar to those obtained in younger study participants. These results suggest that the ability of the older auditory system to integrate stimuli presented at higher repetition rates is reduced. Some of the stimuli presented at fast rates are probably not registered by the aging auditory system due to slower processing.

Summary of Objective Measures of the Auditory Brainstem

The ABR, FFR, and acoustic reflex are not significantly affected by alertness, attention, and memory factors. The slowing apparent in these measures suggests that the aging auditory brainstem is slower in processing auditory stimuli. A great variability in age-related slowing can be expected so that some older individuals may show normal processing, whereas others may show very significant slowing. The variability may be related to gender and other factors, such as the overall health of the individual.

17.3.3 Auditory Thalamus and the Primary Auditory Cortex

The auditory middle latency response (AMLR, Chapter 4) can be used to document age-related transmission delays in the thalamus and the auditory cortex.

Analogous to the ABR studies reviewed in Rawool (2007a), the effect of aging on the AMLR appears to be controversial because of similar reasons. Studies that have included only female participants have failed to show significant prolongation of Pa latencies with aging (Azumi, Nakashima, & Takahashi, 1995; Chambers, 1992; Chambers & Griffith, 1991). Gender differences can be expected in the middle latency response, as age-related temporal lobe atrophy is more significant in elderly men than in women (Cowell et al., 1994). Gur and colleagues (1991) documented age-related changes in brain volume due to brain atrophy in normal subjects ranging in age from 18 to 80 years; sulcal atrophy was significantly more pronounced in older men than in women.

Some investigators have used stimulus rates that are probably too slow (5/s or lower) to accurately reveal age-related effects (Amenedo & Díaz, 1998; Paludetti, Maurizi, D'Alatri, & Galli, 1991). Others have failed to match the auditory sensitivity of the younger and older individuals in the higher frequency regions (Amenedo & Díaz, 1998; Lenzi et al., 1989; Martini, Maurizi, D'Alatri, & Galli, 1990; Woods & Clayworth, 1986). Nonetheless, a significant shift in Pa latencies reportedly occurs with age (Lenzi et al., 1989; Woods & Clayworth, 1986).

Kelly-Ballweber and Dobie (1984) carefully matched the auditory sensitivity of the younger and older participants and reported a significant prolongation of Pa latencies with age. In conclusion, when AMLRs are generated at relatively higher rates, and the auditory sensitivity is carefully matched, a significant prolongation of Pa latencies is apparent in older individuals. This suggests transmission delays within the aging thalamus and the primary temporal auditory cortex.

17.3.4 Temporal Lobe and Adjacent Parietal Lobe Areas

The auditory late response (ALR) can be used to evaluate age-related transmission delays in the temporal lobe and adjacent parietal lobe areas. The main components of the ALR and their characteristic latencies are P1 (50–80 ms), N1 (100–150 ms), P2 (150–200 ms), and N2 (180–250 ms). Based on existing evidence from scalp and intracranial recordings in listeners with normal hearing and temporal lobe lesions, Hall (1992) suggested that the generators for

ALR overlap and include the posterior portion of the superior temporal plane, lateral temporal lobe, and adjacent parietal lobe. Several investigators have reported latency increase in the ALR with advancing age (Goodin, Squires, Henderson, & Starr, 1978; Pfefferbaum, Ford, Roth, & Kopell, 1980), suggesting slower processing in the temporal lobe and related parietal lobe areas.

Late evoked potentials can be recorded in response to brief gaps that are inserted in a continuous broadband noise. The neurophysiological response to gap onset is marked by significantly longer latencies of the P2 component in older adults when compared to younger adults. In addition the amplitudes of N1, P2, and N2 components are significantly reduced in older adults compared to younger adults (Harris et al., 2012).

Cortical activity can be recorded by using MEG (Chapter 4). Such cortical responses can be evoked by changing the interaural phase of amplitude modulated tones. The responses are apparent for frequencies up to 1225 Hz in young adults but only up to 940 Hz in middle-aged adults and up to 760 Hz in older adults. The reduction in frequency range is significant in the older age group. In addition, the latencies of the P2 component in response to the change in interaural phase at 500 Hz are prolonged in the older age group compared to the younger age groups (Ross, Fujioka, Tremblay, & Picton, 2007). Similar effects of aging are apparent in auditory evoked potentials recorded using 63 surface electrodes. Such recordings show that the P2 peak latency in response to a sudden phase shift in the second harmonic of a harmonic complex is prolonged in middle-aged (48–57 years) adults compared to young (21–35 years) adults (Wambacq et al., 2009).

17.3.5 Multiple Cortical and Associated Sites

The P300 is recorded as a large positive voltage wave at approximately 300 ms in response to a rare oddball stimulus (Chapter 4). P300 generation involves multiple sites, including regions of the limbic system, particularly the hippocampus, mesencephalic reticular formation, medial thalamus, and prefrontal, frontal, centroparietal, and auditory cortices. Age-related increase in P300 latencies has been noted in previous investigations (Iragui, Kutas, Mitchiner, & Hillyard, 1993;

Polich, Howard, & Starr, 1985). For older adults in the age range of 60 to 74 years with auditory thresholds within 40 dB HL at 500, 1000, and 2000 Hz, the increase in P300 latency is estimated to be 2.85 ms/y (Cóser, Cóser, Pedroso, Rigon, & Cioqueta, 2010).

17.4 Relationship between Slower Processing in the Auditory Pathways and Speech Recognition

In this section, studies that suggest a relationship between slower processing or delayed neurotransmission and speech recognition will be reviewed. Such a relationship suggests the possibility that speech recognition deficits experienced by older individuals may be partially caused by neurotransmission delays in the auditory pathways.

17.4.1 Auditory Brainstem Response and Speech Recognition

Rawool (1989) examined the relationship between SRSs in noise and the ABR in participants with hearing loss in the age range of 40 to 60 years. Participants were selected based on fairly similar audiograms but different word recognition scores. A significant relationship was apparent between word recognition scores and latencies of waves I and II of the ABR. The latencies were prolonged in listeners with poor speech recognition (► Fig. 17.3).

In another study, older individuals (60–73 years) with average thresholds from 500 to 4000 Hz within 25 dB HL were evaluated using speech (/da/) evoked ABR in quiet and six-talker babble and the HINT. The participants were divided into two groups based on their HINT scores into high- and low-scoring groups and were matched for audiometric thresholds and intelligence. All ABR measures correlated with speech in noise perception. In addition, adults in the low-scoring group differed from the matched high-scoring group in terms of neural coding of speech. Individuals who scored poorly on HINT yielded ABRs in quiet with reduced neural representation of the fundamental frequency of the speech stimulus, along with reduced response magnitude, compared to the high-scoring group. The low-scoring group also showed greater disruption of ABRs in noise, suggesting greater

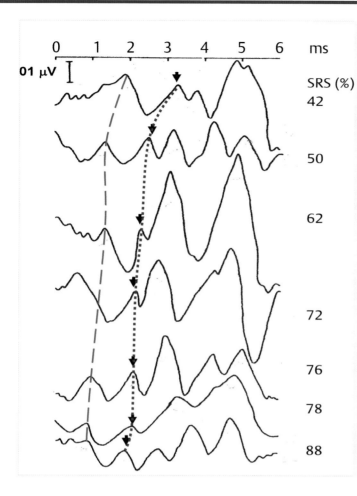

Fig. 17.3 Speech recognition scores (SRSs) of each older individual and the corresponding auditory brainstem response (ABR) waveform. The arrows indicate wave II of the ABR. Note that individuals with poorer SRSs have progressively poorer latencies. The individual with the highest SRS (88%) has the earliest latency for wave II. The green line shows prolongation of wave I latencies of the ABR with poorer SRS except for the participant with the SRS of 72%.

neural dyssynchrony (Anderson, Parbery-Clark, Yi, & Kraus, 2011).

17.4.2 Auditory Middle Latency Response and Speech Recognition

Paludetti and colleagues (1990) reported no relationship between speech understanding ability and AMLR in elderly people. However, the statistical bases for this conclusion were not provided, and the stimulus rate for eliciting the AMLR was too slow (5/s) to sufficiently stress the aging system.

Ali and Jerger (1992) studied the AMLR in two groups of older listeners, with 10 listeners in each group. Group A had speech understanding that was appropriate to the degree of hearing loss, whereas in group B it was disproportionately poor. The latency of Pa was significantly prolonged for participants in group B when compared to those in group A, even in the presence of somewhat better auditory sensitivity in group B than in group A. Thus, it appears that when AMLRs are elicited with relatively fast rates, prolongation of Pa latencies is associated with poorer speech recognition.

17.4.3 Auditory Late Response and Speech Recognition

Tremblay, Piskosz, and Souza (2003) recorded P1, N1, and P2 components of the ALR from younger and older adults. The ALRs were evoked by synthetic speech tokens representing 10 ms increments along a /ba/–/pa/ Voice Onset Time (VOT) continuum. The ability to discriminate the speech tokens was also assessed. Older adults had more difficulty discriminating 10 ms VOT contrasts than younger adults. In addition, the N1 and P2 latencies were prolonged in older participants. Thus, it appears that speech recognition deficits in older adults may be partially related to the neurotransmission delays reflected in the ALR.

17.4.4 P300 Response and Speech Recognition

Jerger and colleagues (Jerger, Alford, Lew, Rivera, & Chmiel, 1995) compared behavioral and electrophysiological responses to verbal and nonverbal dichotic listening tasks in younger and older adults. The results showed an increasing left ear deficit on verbal tasks and an increasing right ear deficit on nonverbal tasks due to age. The P300 latency measures similarly showed the effect of age with the use of both verbal and nonverbal stimuli.

17.4.5 Acoustic Reflex and Speech Recognition

Slower processing in the acoustic reflex pathways may be one of the reasons for the speech recognition difficulties experienced by older individuals, at least at higher presentation levels. The reflex attenuates only the low-frequency components of a complex sound and not the high-frequency components. Thus, it reduces the upward spread of masking of high-frequency sounds by low-frequency sounds (Borg & Counter, 1989). Mahoney, Vernon, and Meikle (1979) showed that speech recognition is better in the presence of a functioning reflex. Other investigators have similarly demonstrated the importance of acoustic reflex in speech recognition (Colletti, Fiorino, Verlato, & Carner, 1992).

In summary, several studies have demonstrated a correlation between speech measures and measures showing slower processing in the auditory and associated neural pathways.

17.5 Interrelationships among Slower Processing, Cognition, and Speech Recognition

17.5.1 Slower Signal/Neural Transmission Time Due to Age

Birren (1970) proposed that one of the most marked changes in old age is a general slowing of the rate of information processing. Continuous inputs of signals at fast rates are difficult for older people to process efficiently.

17.5.2 Physiological Changes in the Aging Central Nervous System

Using MRI, Sowell and colleagues (2003) found a significant decline in gray matter density with age. Birren, Woods, and Williams (1980) noted that reduction in synaptic density with age appears to come close to a reliably observed change that would slow the transmission of neurophysiological excitation. They suggested that this reduction could influence several key areas, such as the dentate gyrus of the hippocampus, which is associated with learning and memory. White matter lesion prevalence measured with MRI also appears to account for the age-related variance in individuals on tests of speed and executive ability (Rabbitt et al., 2007).

Another key set of nuclei that may be relevant is in the reticular system. The reduction in cells in the human locus ceruleus reported with age has potentially great significance for behavior. As part of the ascending reticular system, the locus ceruleus influences the level of excitation of the cerebellum, cerebrum, and limbic system. Such a nucleus could play a central role in the slowing of behavior with age (Birren et al., 1980).

Several other effects of aging can distress the CNS. The rate of cerebral blood flow diminishes with age, perhaps due to arteriosclerosis (Duara, London, & Rapoport, 1985). Conde and Streit (2006) found that the function of the microglia cells deteriorates with aging, and this may lead to neurodegeneration observed in the aging brain. Based on a review of the literature, Segovia, Porras, Del Arco, and Mora (2001) reported that the most significant and consistent finding in aging is the decrease in the density of glutamatergic N-methyl-d-aspartate (NMDA) receptors with age.

The suprachiasmatic nucleus (SCN) of the hypothalamus is considered to be a type of biological clock that governs circadian (hormonal rhythms, body core temperature, and sleep–wakefulness) time keeping. The age-related decrements in circadian cycles and the neuronal degeneration of the SCN suggest disturbance of the circadian pacemaker in the human brain with aging (Hofman & Swaab, 2006).

In summary, several changes have been reported in the aging central nervous system. Any of the above listed changes can lead to general slowing of behavior and/or lower cognition in aging.

17.5.3 Age-related Changes in Cognition

Generally speaking, the concept of cognition includes attention, memory, perceptual speed, response time, problem solving, and mental imagery. Decline of cognitive performance in older individuals has been reported in several investigations (Dore et al., 2007; Salthouse, 1985).

One way to examine the effect of aging on cognition is to consider two types of intelligence, crystallized and fluid. Crystallized intelligence can be thought of as the storage area of information that is learned and accumulated through the years, such as content knowledge and facts. In contrast, fluid intelligence refers to the ability to solve problems with novel applications of knowledge (Ackerman & Rolfhus, 1999). Typically, crystallized abilities tend to remain high and stable from young adulthood through old age, whereas fluid abilities plateau during the midlife years and decline around age 70 (Schaie, 2005). Thus, complex tasks that require taking in new information and analyzing it may become more difficult. The decline in fluid intelligence may be related to deficits that occur in memory, attention, and speed of processing with aging.

The process that allows us to temporarily store and manipulate information is referred to as working memory. Working memory declines with aging (Hedden & Gabrieli, 2004).

Difficulties in the allocation and maintenance of attention with aging have been reported (Broadbent & Heron, 1962; Rabbitt & Birren, 1967). Normal aging results in loss of attentional capacity (Berardi, Parasuraman, & Haxby, 2001; Greenwood, Parasuraman, & Alexander, 1997; Parasuraman & Giambra, 1991). Deficits are more obvious under circumstances of high attentional demands (Georgiou-Karistianis et al., 2007; Mouloua & Parasuraman, 1995; Parasuraman & Giambra, 1991; Parasuraman, Warm, & Dember, 1987). Depending on the difficulty of the response task, decreased attentional resources may contribute to poor performance on some auditory processing tasks (Szelag et al., 2011).

Aging reduces the speed with which incoming information is processed (Salthouse, 1996, 2000). Decreases in sensorimotor speed, perceptual speed, and reaction time speed with age have been reported (Earles & Salthouse, 1995). Reaction time, or the amount of time it takes to react to stimuli, varies with the complexity of the task and the expected response. When reaction time is used to study the "timeliness" in cognitive functions, older individuals appear to be on average slower than younger adults, regardless of the task or the experimental procedure (Baron & Cerella, 1993). When complex tasks are used for measuring gap detection, age-related deficits can be associated with deficits in processing speed and attention (Harris, Eckert, Ahlstrom, & Dubno, 2010).

17.5.4 Slower Processing, Lower Cognition, and Poor Speech Recognition

Slower processing due to deterioration in the CNS typically associated with aging could lead to a simultaneous decline in cognition and speech recognition abilities. For example, in Alzheimer's disease, impaired central auditory function is correlated with temporal lobe atrophy and cognition (Grimes, Grady, Foster, Sunderland, & Patronas, 1985). In addition, lower cognition can lead to poor speech recognition due to inefficient top-down processing of incoming speech stimuli. For example, an individual may have difficulty filling in missing elements using contextual cues. Poor speech recognition may lead to lower cognition due to deficient sensory input (▶ Fig. 17.4).

17.5.5 Slower Neural Processing and Cognition

Ertl and Schafer (1969) reported a significant correlation between intelligence quotient (IQ) and the visual evoked potential. The activity in the latency range from 11 to 136 ms was found to be greater in individuals with a higher IQ when compared to those with a lower IQ (Ertl, 1973; Ertl & Schafer, 1969).

Based on a carefully controlled study of healthy adults, Duffy and colleagues (Duffy, McAnulty, Jones, Als, & Albert, 1993) concluded that lower cognitive function is associated with longer evoked potential latencies, suggesting slower neural processing. The authors surmised that shorter evoked potential latencies associated with higher cognitive function may reflect better synaptic efficiency, which may be determined by the number of synapses, the ratio of excitatory to inhibitory synapses, and neuromodulatory influences.

Geisler and colleagues (Geisler, Morgan, Covington, & Murphy, 1999) examined the relationship between the P300 and slow wave components of the olfactory event-related potential (OERP) with neuropsychological performance in young and

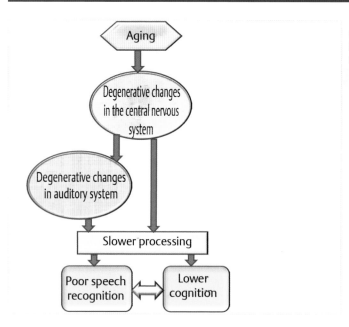

Fig. 17.4 The interrelationship between slower processing, speech recognition and cognition in aging.

elderly adults. Results showed that P3 latencies decline with age, and this decreased neuronal efficiency was associated with a reduction in neuropsychological performance indexed by the California Verbal Learning Test.

Jones and colleagues (1991) showed a similar correlation between cognitive flexibility and auditory evoked potentials. Collectively, these studies show a correlation between lower cognition and slower neural processing (as reflected in longer latencies of evoked potentials). Perhaps many of the benign effects of age on cognitive function can be accounted for by accumulations of latency prolongations across various stages of information processing.

17.5.6 Cognition and Speech Recognition

With reference to speech recognition, cognitive processing involves cortical function and is dependent on world knowledge, word dictionary saved in the memory, access to this memory, efficient retrieval, conceptual representation of the word, and use of situational or contextual cues to recognize the word. The extent to which previous experiences can be helpful in recognizing incoming stimuli is governed by complex cognitive processes, such as memory and recall of previously learned information (e.g., words and phrases) and problem solving, or being able to make use of the context to correctly recognize misunderstood words and fill in inaudible words.

A significant correlation between speech recognition ability for complex speech tasks and tests of cognitive capacity (digit span, arithmetic, block design, and verbal fluency) has been reported (Era, Jokela, Qvarnberg, & Heikkinen, 1986). Thomas and colleagues (1983) evaluated the relationship between speech recognition and cognition in 239 physically healthy, independent living elderly men and women with a mean age of 72 years. Participants were given the Speech Perception in Noise (SPIN) test, which consists of 50 short sentences spoken in a background of voice babble (multi-talker noise). Participants were asked to repeat the last monosyllabic word occurring at the end of each sentence. SPIN scores were correlated with the overall cognitive scores on the Jacobs cognitive screening examination, specifically the recall subsection of the cognitive screening examination, which tests the ability to recall four words after 3 minutes.

The ability to understand fast speech is partially dependent on the ability to quickly recall and recognize patterns (e.g., words) stored in the memory. As stated above, age-related deficits in memory can affect speech recognition (Thomas et al., 1983). van Rooij and Plomp (1990) reported that the speech recognition thresholds of older listeners can be partially predicted by reduced memory. Individuals with dementia show poor performance on several auditory processing tasks, including the dichotic digits and pitch pattern sequence tests (Gates, Anderson, Feeney, McCurry, & Larson, 2008).

Understanding fast speech requires rapid processing of continuous input without missing any elements, and memory for the earlier portions of the message must resist interference caused by the later parts of the message. In addition, if any elements are missed due to poor audibility or distortion, the missed elements must be manipulated to construct a cohesive picture of the message. Such manipulations are dependent on an efficient working memory, which is reduced with aging.

As discussed in Chapter 8, poor auditory perception can lead to poor working memory due to impaired verbal rehearsal. There is a significant correlation between working memory and speech recognition performance in noise (Desjardins & Doherty, 2013). Older listeners with hearing loss and poor working memory appear to be more susceptible to distortions caused by noise and by some types of hearing aid signal-processing schemes. When the speech signal is presented in the background of babble and is processed with frequency compression based on sinusoidal modeling, working memory accounts for 29.3% of the variability in understanding speech (Arehart, Souza, Baca, & Kates, 2013).

Slowing with age in the time it takes to look up a word and category in semantic memory has been reported (Petros, Zehr, & Chabot, 1983). van Rooij, Plomp, and Orlebeke (1989) concluded that the most important cognitive correlates of speech perception performance may be processing and sensorimotor speed. In a study involving 200 elderly subjects, Jerger, Jerger, and Pirozzolo (1991) demonstrated that the performance on the dichotic sentence identification (DSI) procedure, which requires the subject to identify two sentences presented simultaneously to each ear, is partially related to the speed of mental processing as measured by the Digit Symbol subtest of the revised Wechsler Adult Intelligence Scale (WAIS-R). A significant association between processing speed and speech recognition performance in noise has been reported for both younger and older listeners (Desjardins & Doherty, 2013). The critical signal-to-noise ratio needed to understand 50% of digit triplets in the background of a constant noise level increases with age and is related to a reduction in processing speed. Older adults with slower processing speed need a larger signal-to-noise ratio

compared to those with faster processing speed (Pronk et al., 2013).

It is necessary to sustain attention for accurate perception of rapid speech. It is also necessary to divide attention between continuous monitoring of the incoming stimuli and analyses and integration of the successive elements. Thus, age-related deficits in attention could have an effect on speech recognition.

It should be noted that some studies may fail to show any relationship between cognition and speech recognition if simple speech stimuli are used that are less demanding than those typically encountered in everyday natural communication environments (Sommers, 1997). Birren and Fisher (1995) suggested a hierarchical notion of the effects of slowing. The speed–knowledge continuum predicts that if the task involves primarily speed (e.g., fast speech), then age effects are expected to be large. If the task is primarily based on knowledge or crystallized intelligence, the age effects can be expected to be small (Birren & Fisher, 1995).

Decreased hearing due to aging may cause poor speech recognition, which in turn may impair abilities to receive or integrate environmental information correctly. A decrease in input and incorrect input of information could produce irreversible cognitive deficits similar to disuse atrophy. Sensory deprivation mechanisms have been used to explain the increased prevalence of paranoid psychosis in subjects with hearing loss (Berger & Zarit, 1978).

17.6 Intervention

Speech recognition deficits in older individuals appear to be interrelated to slower processing in the aging auditory system, general slowing in the central auditory system, and cognitive declines. Depending on the particular deficits present, the most effective aural rehabilitative efforts for older individuals should address the following aspects.

17.6.1 Amplification and Assistive Technology

Effective amplification and assistive listening devices can compensate for sensory deprivation caused by hearing loss and can deliver a clearly audible signal so that demands on available cognitive resources can be reduced. Improving audibility of high frequencies through amplification can also improve temporal processing in individuals with high-frequency hearing loss (Bacon & Gleitman, 1992; Bacon & Viemeister, 1985). In degraded listening conditions, the use of amplification should be supplemented with the use of assistive listening technology, including personal frequency modulation (FM) devices.

17.6.2 Auditory Training

Word recognition scores of older listeners can improve with training in background noise for the words used during training. The learning is generalized to unfamiliar speakers, and with brief refreshers the improved performance can be maintained over time (Burk & Humes, 2008). Training that begins with presentation of auditory stimuli at slower rates progressing to stimuli that are presented at faster rates may also be helpful. Auditory training has the potential for improving neural timing in the auditory brainstem (Russo, Nicol, Zecker, Hayes, & Kraus, 2005).

Practice in Listening to Rapid Speech

Blind adults frequently listen to prerecorded audiobooks or computerized audiotaped daily news at rapid playback rates. Such listening practice can average as much as 40 hours per week. As a result of such practice, older blind adults recognize time-compressed speech as well as younger adults, and their performance is significantly better than older sighted adults in quiet and noise. Thus, frequent practice in listening to speech at rapid rates may improve perception of rapid speech in sighted older adults (Gordon-Salant & Friedman, 2011).

17.6.3 Training to Improve Speed of Processing

Hertzog, Williams, and Walsh (1976) studied practice effects on the central perceptual processes and reported improvement in performance with practice. Response speed can also increase significantly with training in older individuals (Hoyer, Hoyer, Treat, & Baltes, 1978–1979). Individuals can improve their processing speed at home using readily available technology, such as a videotape-based speed-of-processing training protocol (Wadley et al., 2006). Training can also improve simultaneous processing of two tasks in older adults (Bherer et al., 2005).

17.6.4 Training to Improve Cognition

Mahncke and colleagues (2006) demonstrated an enhancement in cognitive function in older adults following intensive, plasticity-engaging training. Other studies have shown similar improvements in cognitive function in older adults with training (Ball et al., 2002; Günther, Schäfer, Holzner, & Kemmler, 2003). Strategies for improving attention and working memory are described in Chapter 8. Multimodal training can be used to improve cognitive function in healthy older adults and to slow the decline in individuals with dementia (Gates & Valenzuela, 2010).

17.6.5 Training for Simultaneous Improvement of Auditory and Cognitive Skills

Training that combines bottom-up auditory training exercises with top-down cognitive skills can improve neural timing, memory, speed of processing, and speech recognition in noise in older adults. The training decreases the temporal jitter in the speech-evoked ABR, yielding a less variable response (Anderson, White-Schwoch, Parbery-Clark, & Kraus, 2013).

17.6.6 Training in the Use of Contextual Cues

Older individuals can use contextual cues effectively to overcome the difficulty in recognizing fast speech (Wingfield et al., 1985). Thus, training in the use of contextual cues may be helpful for those individuals who are not using contextual cues effectively.

17.6.7 Adaptation of Healthy Habits

Earles and Salthouse (1995) demonstrated that the relationship between age and speed is partially mediated by health. Careful control of vascular risk factors can allow maintenance of healthy cognition (Duron & Hanon, 2008). It has been hypothesized that the maintenance of aerobic capacity through regular physical activity ensures an adequate delivery of oxygen to the nervous system and an attenuated deterioration in psychomotor performance. Exercise appears to be effective in reversing or at least slowing some age-related reduction in speed of cognitive processing (Rikli & Edwards, 1991).

Based on a review of literature, Dishman and colleagues (2006) concluded that voluntary physical activity and exercise training could favorably influence brain plasticity by facilitating neurogenerative, neuroadaptive, and neuroprotective processes. Thus, whenever possible, sedentary older individuals should be encouraged to engage in exercise with guidance and supervision as necessary.

17.7 Future Trends

In the future, assessment may become easier because of access to cheaper technology that will allow objective measures of APDs. Better training programs and techniques may also become available, as discussed in Chapter 8. Advances in digital technologies and research on the effectiveness of these technologies may lead to increasingly effective and sophisticated training systems incorporating a variety of auditory stimuli and interactive audiovisual displays (Pichora-Fuller & Levitt, 2012). Inclusion of three-dimensional visual displays and virtual listening environments may allow more effective simulation of real-life listening environments. In addition, future amplification devices are expected to implement more advanced speech-processing algorithms to allow easier recognition of speech in background noise (Healy, Yoho, Wang, & Wang, 2013).

17.8 Review Questions

1. Describe the physiological changes that have been noted in the neural auditory pathways of older individuals. Can age-related alterations in auditory neurons occur in the presence of intact inner and outer hair cells?
2. Describe the temporal processing deficits that have been noted in older adults.
3. Review age-related changes in the processing of modified/degraded speech signals.
4. Review age-related changes reflected in objective measures of the auditory brainstem.
5. Review age-related changes reflected in the auditory middle latency response.
6. Describe age-related changes reflected in the auditory late response and P300.
7. Review the relationship between objective measures of auditory processing and speech recognition.
8. Review age-related changes in cognition, including processing speed, working memory, and attention.
9. Discuss the relationship between cognition and speech recognition in older adults.
10. Describe a comprehensive approach for addressing age-related deficits in the processing of auditory stimuli.

References

[1] Ackerman, P. L., & Rolfhus, E. L. (1999). The locus of adult intelligence: Knowledge, abilities, and nonability traits. Psychology and Aging, 14(2), 314–330.

[2] Ali, A. A., & Jerger, J. (1992). Phase coherence of the middle-latency response in the elderly. Scandinavian Audiology, 21(3), 187–194.

[3] Allison, T., Hume, A. L., Wood, C. C., & Goff, W. R. (1984). Developmental and aging changes in somatosensory, auditory and visual evoked potentials. Electroencephalography and Clinical Neurophysiology, 58(1), 14–24.

[4] Allison, T., Wood, C. C., & Goff, W. R. (1983). Brain stem auditory, pattern-reversal visual, and short-latency somatosensory evoked potentials: Latencies in relation to age, sex, and brain and body size. Electroencephalography and Clinical Neurophysiology, 55(6), 619–636.

[5] Amenedo, E., & Díaz, F. (1998). Effects of aging on middle-latency auditory evoked potentials: A cross-sectional study. Biological Psychiatry, 43(3), 210–219.

[6] Anderson, S., Parbery-Clark, A., Yi, H. G., & Kraus, N. (2011). A neural basis of speech-in-noise perception in older adults. Ear and Hearing, 32(6), 750–757.

[7] Anderson, S., White-Schwoch, T., Parbery-Clark, A., & Kraus, N. (2013). Reversal of age-related neural timing delays with training. Proceedings of the National Academy of Sciences of the United States of America, 110(11), 4357–4362.

[8] Anias, C. R., Lima, M. A. M. T., & Kos, A. O. A. (2004). Evaluation of the influence of age in auditory brainstem response. Brazilian Journal of Otorhinolaryngology, 70, 84–89.

[9] Arehart, K. H., Souza, P., Baca, R., & Kates, J. M. (2013). Working memory, age, and hearing loss: Susceptibility to hearing aid distortion. Ear and Hearing, 34(3), 251–260.

[10] Azumi, T., Nakashima, K., & Takahashi, K. (1995). Aging effects on auditory middle latency responses. Electromyography and Clinical Neurophysiology, 35(7), 397–401.

[11] Bacon, S. P., & Gleitman, R. M. (1992). Modulation detection in subjects with relatively flat hearing losses. Journal of Speech and Hearing Research, 35(3), 642–653.

[12] Bacon, S. P., & Viemeister, N. F. (1985). Temporal modulation transfer functions in normal-hearing and hearing-impaired listeners. Audiology, 24(2), 117–134.

[13] Ball, K., Berch, D. B., Helmers, K. F., et al. Advanced Cognitive Training for Independent and Vital Elderly Study Group. (2002). Effects of cognitive training interventions with older adults: A randomized controlled trial. Journal of the American Medical Association, 288(18), 2271–2281.

[14] Baron, A., & Cerella, J. (1993). Laboratory tests of the disuse account of cognitive decline. In J. Cerella, W. Hoyer, J. Rybash, & M. Commons (Eds.), Adult information processing: Limits on loss (pp. 175-203). San Diego, CA: Academic Press.

[15] Beagley, H. A., & Sheldrake, J. B. (1978). Differences in brainstem response latency with age and sex. British Journal of Audiology, 12(3), 69–77.

[16] Berardi, A., Parasuraman, R., & Haxby, J. V. (2001). Overall vigilance and sustained attention decrements in healthy aging. Experimental Aging Research, 27(1), 19–39.

[17] Berger, K. S., & Zarit, S. H. (1978). Late-life paranoid states: Assessment and treatment. American Journal of Orthopsychiatry, 48(3), 528–537.

[18] Bergman, M., Blumenfeld, V. G., Cascardo, D., Dash, B., Levitt, H., & Margulies, M. K. (1976). Age-related decrement in hearing for speech: Sampling and longitudinal studies. Journal of Gerontology, 31(5), 533–538.

[19] Bherer, L., Kramer, A. F., Peterson, M. S., Colcombe, S., Erickson, K., & Becic, E. (2005). Training effects on dual-task performance: Are there age-related differences in plasticity of attentional control? Psychology and Aging, 20(4), 695–709.

[20] Birren, J. E. (1970). Toward an experimental psychology of aging. American Psychologist, 25(2), 124–135.

[21] Birren, J. E., & Fisher, L. M. (1995). Aging and speed of behavior: Possible consequences for psychological functioning. Annual Review of Psychology, 46, 329–353.

[22] Birren, J. E., Woods, A. M., & Williams, M. V. (1980). Behavioral slowing with age: Causes, organization and consequences. In L. W. Poon (Ed.), Aging in the 1980s: Psychological issues (pp. 293-308). Washington, DC: American Psychological Association.

[23] Boettcher, F. A. (2002). Presbyacusis and the auditory brainstem response. Journal of Speech, Language, and Hearing Research, 45(6), 1249–1261.

[24] Borg, E. (1973). On the neuronal organization of the acoustic middle ear reflex: A physiological and anatomical study. Brain Research, 49(1), 101–123.

[25] Bosatra, A. (1983). Reflex "delay" in sensorineural hearing-loss. Scandinavian Audiology. Supplement, 17, 40–42.

[26] Bosatra, A., Russolo, M., & Silverman, C. A. (1984). Acoustic reflex latency: State of the art. In S. Silman (Ed.), The acoustic reflex: Basic principles and clinical applications (pp. 301-328). Orlando, FL: Academic Press.

[27] Broadbent, D. E., & Heron, A. (1962). Effects of a subsidiary task on performance involving immediate memory by younger and older men. British Journal of Psychology, 53, 189–198.

[28] Brody, H. (1955). Organization of the cerebral cortex: 3. A study of aging in the human cerebral cortex. Journal of Comparative Neurology, 102(2), 511–516.

[29] Brody, H. (1976). An examination of cerebral cortex and brain stem aging. In R. D. Terry & S. Gershon (Eds.), Neurobiology of aging (pp. 171-181). New York: Raven Press.

[30] Burk, M. H., & Humes, L. E. (2008). Effects of long-term training on aided speech-recognition performance in noise in older adults. Journal of Speech, Language, and Hearing Research, 51(3), 759–771.

[31] Burkard, R. F., & Sims, D. (2001). The human auditory brainstem response to high click rates: Aging effects. American Journal of Audiology, 10(2), 53–61.

[32] Chambers, R. D. (1992). Differential age effects for components of the adult auditory middle latency response. Hearing Research, 58(2), 123–131.

[33] Chambers, R. D., & Griffiths, S. K. (1991). Effects of age on the adult auditory middle latency response. Hearing Research, 51(1), 1–10.

[34] Chu, N. S. (1985). Age-related latency changes in the brainstem auditory evoked potentials. Electroencephalography and Clinical Neurophysiology, 62(6), 431–436.

[35] Clinard, C. G., & Tremblay, K. L. (2013). Aging degrades the neural encoding of simple and complex sounds in the human brainstem. Journal of the American Academy of Audiology, 24(7), 590–599, quiz 643–644.

[36] Clinard, C. G., Tremblay, K. L., & Krishnan, A. R. (2010). Aging alters the perception and physiological representation of frequency: Evidence from human frequency-following response recordings. Hearing Research, 264(1-2), 48–55.

[37] Coats, A. C. (1978). Human auditory nerve action potentials and brain stem evoked responses. Archives of Otolaryngology, 104(12), 709–717.

[38] Cobb, F. E., Jacobson, G. P., Newman, C. W., Kretschmer, L. W., & Donnelly, K. A. (1993). Age-associated degeneration of backward masking task performance: Evidence of declining temporal resolution abilities in normal listeners. Audiology, 32(4), 260–271.

[39] Colletti, V., Fiorino, F. G., Verlato, G., & Carner, M. (1992). Acoustic reflex in frequency selectivity: Brain stem auditory evoked response and speech discrimination. In J. Katz, N. A. Stecker, & D. Henderson (Eds.), Central auditory processing: A transdisciplinary view (pp. 39-46). St. Louis, MO: Mosby Year Book.

[40] Conde, J. R., & Streit, W. J. (2006). Microglia in the aging brain. Journal of Neuropathology & Experimental Neurology, 65(3), 199-203.

[41] Cóser, M. J. S., Cóser, P. L., Pedroso, F. S., Rigon, R., & Cioqueta, E. (2010). P300 auditory evoked potential latency in elderly. Brazilian Journal of Otorhinolaryngology, 76(3), 287–293.

[42] Cowell, P. E., Turetsky, B. I., Gur, R. C., Grossman, R. I., Shtasel, D. L., & Gur, R. E. (1994). Sex differences in aging of the human frontal and temporal lobes. Journal of Neuroscience, 14(8), 4748–4755.

[43] de Boer, E., & Dreschler, W. A. (1987). Auditory psychophysics: Spectrotemporal representation of signals. Annual Review of Psychology, 38, 181–202.

[44] Debruyne, F. (1986). Influence of age and hearing loss on the latency shifts of the auditory brainstem response as a result of increased stimulus rate. Audiology, 25(2), 101–106.

[45] Desjardins, J. L., & Doherty, K. A. (2013). Age-related changes in listening effort for various types of masker noises. Ear and Hearing, 34(3), 261–272.

[46] Dishman, R. K., Berthoud, H.-R., Booth, F. W., et al. (2006). Neurobiology of exercise. Obesity (Silver Spring), 14(3), 345–356.

[47] Don, M., & Eggermont, J. J. (1978). Analysis of the click-evoked brainstem potentials in man using high-pass noise masking. Journal of the Acoustical Society of America, 63(4), 1084–1092.

[48] Dore, G. A., Elias, M. F., Robbins, M. A., Elias, P. K., & Brennan, S. L. (2007). Cognitive performance and age: norms from the Maine-Syracuse Study. Experimental aging research, 33(3), 205-271.

[49] Duara, R., London, E. D., & Rapoport, S. (1985). Changes in structure and energy metabolism of the aging brain. In C. E. Finch & E. L. Schneider (Eds.), Handbook of the biology of aging. New York (pp. 595-616): Van Nostrand Reinhold.

[50] Duffy, F. H., McAnulty, G. B., Jones, K., Als, H., & Albert, M. (1993). Brain electrical correlates of psychological measures: Strategies and problems. Brain Topography, 5(4), 399–412.

[51] Duron, E., & Hanon, O. (2008). Vascular risk factors, cognitive decline, and dementia. Vascular Health and Risk Management, 4(2), 363–381.

[52] Ertl, J. P. (1973). IQ evoked responses and Fourier analysis. Nature, 241, 209-210. Ertl, J. P., & Schafer, E. W. (1969). Brain response correlates of psychometric intelligence. Nature 223, 421 – 422.

[53] Earles, J. L., & Salthouse, T. A. (1995). Interrelations of age, health, and speed. Journals of Gerontology Series B: Psychological Sciences and Social Sciences, 50(1), 33–41.

[54] Elberling, C., & Parbo, J. (1987). Reference data for ABRs in retrocochlear diagnosis. Scandinavian Audiology, 16(1), 49–55.

[55] Era, P., Jokela, J., Qvarnberg, Y., & Heikkinen, E. (1986). Puretone thresholds, speech, understanding, and their correlates in samples of men of different ages. Audiology, 25(6), 338–352.

[56] Ertl, J. P., & Schafer, E. W. (1969). Brain response correlates of psychometric intelligence. Nature, 223(5204), 421–422.

[57] Felder, E., & Schrott-Fischer, A. (1995). Quantitative evaluation of myelinated nerve fibres and hair cells in cochleae of humans with age-related high-tone hearing loss. Hearing Research, 91(1-2), 19–32.

[58] Felix, H., Johnsson, L. G., Gleeson, M., & Pollak, A. (1990). Quantitative analysis of cochlear sensory cells and neuronal elements in man. Acta Otolaryngologica. Supplementum, 470, 71–79.

[59] Fink, M., Churan, J., & Wittmann, M. (2005). Assessment of auditory temporal-order thresholds: A comparison of different measurement procedures and the influences of age and gender. Restorative Neurology and Neuroscience, 23(5-6), 281–296.

[60] Fujikawa, S. M., & Weber, B. A. (1977). Effects of increased stimulus rate on brainstem electric response (BER) audiometry as a function of age. Journal of the American Audiology Society, 3(3), 147–150.

[61] Gates, G. A., Anderson, M. L., Feeney, M. P., McCurry, S. M., & Larson, E. B. (2008). Central auditory dysfunction in older persons with memory impairment or Alzheimer dementia. Archives of Otolaryngology–Head and Neck Surgery, 134(7), 771–777.

[62] Gates, N., & Valenzuela, M. (2010). Cognitive exercise and its role in cognitive function in older adults. Current Psychiatry Reports, 12(1), 20–27.

[63] Geisler, M. W., Morgan, C. D., Covington, J. W., & Murphy, C. (1999). Neuropsychological performance and cognitive olfactory event-related brain potentials in young and elderly adults. Journal of Clinical and Experimental Neuropsychology, 21(1), 108–126.

[64] Georgiou-Karistianis, N., Tang, J., Vardy, Y., et al. (2007). Progressive age-related changes in the attentional blink paradigm. Neuropsychology, Development, and Cognition. Section B, Aging, Neuropsychology, and Cognition, 14(3), 213–226.

[65] Goodin, D. S., Squires, K. C., Henderson, B. H., & Starr, A. (1978). Age-related variations in evoked potentials to auditory stimuli in normal human subjects. Electroencephalography and Clinical Neurophysiology, 44(4), 447–458.

[66] Gootjes, L., Van Strien, J. W., & Bouma, A. (2004). Age effects in identifying and localising dichotic stimuli: A corpus callosum deficit? Journal of Clinical Experimental Neuropsychology, 26(6), 826–837.

[67] Gordon-Salant, S., & Fitzgibbons, P. J. (1993). Temporal factors and speech recognition performance in young and elderly listeners. Journal of Speech and Hearing Research, 36(6), 1276–1285.

[68] Gordon-Salant, S., & Fitzgibbons, P. J. (1995). Recognition of multiply degraded speech by young and elderly listeners. Journal of Speech and Hearing Research, 38(5), 1150–1156.

[69] Gordon-Salant, S., & Fitzgibbons, P. J. (1999). Profile of auditory temporal processing in older listeners. Journal of Speech, Language, and Hearing Research, 42(2), 300–311.

[70] Gordon-Salant, S., & Fitzgibbons, P. J. (2001). Sources of age-related recognition difficulty for time-compressed speech. Journal of Speech, Language, and Hearing Research, 44(4), 709–719.

[71] Gordon-Salant, S., & Fitzgibbons, P. J. (2004). Effects of stimulus and noise rate variability on speech perception by younger and older adults. Journal of the Acoustical Society of America, 115(4), 1808–1817.

[72] Gordon-Salant, S., & Friedman, S. A. (2011). Recognition of rapid speech by blind and sighted older adults. Journal of Speech, Language, and Hearing Research, 54(2), 622–631.

[73] Gordon-Salant, S., Yeni-Komshian, G. H., Fitzgibbons, P. J., & Barrett, J. (2006). Age-related differences in identification and discrimination of temporal cues in speech segments. Journal of the Acoustical Society of America, 119(4), 2455–2466.

[74] Greenwood, P. M., Parasuraman, R., & Alexander, G. E. (1997). Controlling the focus of spatial attention during visual search: Effects of advanced aging and Alzheimer disease. Neuropsychology, 11(1), 3–12.

[75] Grimes, A. M., Grady, C. L., Foster, N. L., Sunderland, T., & Patronas, N. J. (1985). Central auditory function in Alzheimer's disease. Neurology, 35(3), 352–358.

[76] Grose, J. H., & Mamo, S. K. (2012). Electrophysiological measurement of binaural beats: Effects of primary tone frequency and observer age. Ear and Hearing, 33(2), 187–194.

[77] Günther, V. K., Schäfer, P., Holzner, B. J., & Kemmler, G. W. (2003). Long-term improvements in cognitive performance through computer-assisted cognitive training: A pilot study in a residential home for older people. Aging and Mental Health, 7(3), 200–206.

[78] Gur, R. C., Mozley, P. D., Resnick, S. M., et al. (1991). Gender differences in age effect on brain atrophy measured by magnetic resonance imaging. Proceedings of the National Academy of Sciences of the United States of America, 88(7), 2845–2849.

[79] Hall, J. W., III. (1992). Handbook of auditory evoked responses. Boston: Allyn & Bacon.

[80] Hansen, C. C., & Reske-Nielsen, E. (1965). Pathological studies in presbycusis: Cochlear and central findings in 12 aged patients. Archives of Otolaryngology, 82, 115–132.

[81] Harkins, S. W. (1981). Effects of age and interstimulus interval on the brainstem auditory evoked potential. International Journal of Neuroscience, 15(1-2), 107–118.

[82] Harris, K. C., Eckert, M. A., Ahlstrom, J. B., & Dubno, J. R. (2010). Age-related differences in gap detection: Effects of task difficulty and cognitive ability. Hearing Research, 264(1-2), 21–29.

[83] Harris, K. C., Wilson, S., Eckert, M. A., & Dubno, J. R. (2012). Human evoked cortical activity to silent gaps in noise: Effects of age, attention, and cortical processing speed. Ear and Hearing, 33(3), 330–339.

[84] He, N., Dubno, J. R., & Mills, J. H. (1998). Frequency and intensity discrimination measured in a maximum-likelihood procedure from young and aged normal-hearing subjects. Journal of the Acoustical Society of America, 103(1), 553–565.

[85] He, N. J., Mills, J. H., Ahlstrom, J. B., & Dubno, J. R. (2008). Age-related differences in the temporal modulation transfer function with pure-tone carriers. Journal of the Acoustical Society of America, 124(6), 3841–3849.

[86] He, N. J., Mills, J. H., & Dubno, J. R. (2007). Frequency modulation detection: Effects of age, psychophysical method, and modulation waveform. Journal of the Acoustical Society of America, 122(1), 467–477.

[87] Healy, E. W., Yoho, S. E., Wang, Y., & Wang, D. (2013). An algorithm to improve speech recognition in noise for hearing-

impaired listeners. Journal of the Acoustical Society of America, 134(4), 3029–3038.

[88] Hedden, T., & Gabrieli, J. D. E. (2004). Insights into the ageing mind: A view from cognitive neuroscience. Nature Reviews. Neuroscience, 5(2), 87–96.

[89] Hertzog, C. K., Williams, M. V., & Walsh, D. A. (1976). The effect of practice on age differences in central perceptual processing. Journal of Gerontology, 31(4), 428–433.

[90] Hofman, M. A., & Swaab, D. F. (2006). Living by the clock: The circadian pacemaker in older people. Ageing Research Reviews, 5(1), 33–51.

[91] Hoyer, F. W., Hoyer, W. J., Treat, N. J., & Baltes, P. B. (1978–1979). Training response speed in young and elderly women. International Journal of Aging and Human Developementent, 9(3), 247–253.

[92] Hyde, M. (1985). The effect of cochlear lesions on the ABR. In J. Jacobson (Ed.), The Auditory brainstem response (pp. 133-146). San Diego, CA: College Hill Press.

[93] Iragui, V. J., Kutas, M., Mitchiner, M. R., & Hillyard, S. A. (1993). Effects of aging on event-related brain potentials and reaction times in an auditory oddball task. Psychophysiology, 30(1), 10–22.

[94] Jerger, J., Alford, B., Lew, H., Rivera, V., & Chmiel, R. (1995). Dichotic listening, event-related potentials, and interhemispheric transfer in the elderly. Ear and Hearing, 16(5), 482–498.

[95] Jerger, J., & Hall, J. (1980). Effects of age and sex on auditory brainstem response. Archives of Otolaryngology, 106(7), 387–391.

[96] Jerger, J., Jerger, S., & Pirozzolo, F. (1991). Correlational analysis of speech audiometric scores, hearing loss, age, and cognitive abilities in the elderly. Ear and Hearing, 12(2), 103–109.

[97] Jerger, J., & Johnson, K. (1988). Interactions of age, gender, and sensorineural hearing loss on ABR latency. Ear and Hearing, 9(4), 168–176.

[98] Johannsen, H. S., & Lehn, T. (1984). The dependence of early acoustically evoked potentials on age. Archives of Otorhinolaryngology, 240(2), 153–158.

[99] John, A. B., Hall, J. W., III, & Kreisman, B. M. (2012). Effects of advancing age and hearing loss on gaps-in-noise test performance. American Journal of Audiology, 21(2), 242–250.

[100] Jones, K. J., Albert, M. S., Duffy, F. H., Hyde, M. R., Naeser, M., & Aldwin, C. (1991). Modeling age using cognitive, psychosocial and physiological variables: The Boston Normative Aging Study. Experimental Aging Research, 17(4), 227–242.

[101] Keith, W. J., & Greville, K. A. (1987). Effects of audiometric configuration on the auditory brain stem response. Ear and Hearing, 8(1), 49–55.

[102] Kelly-Ballweber, D., & Dobie, R. A. (1984). Binaural interaction measured behaviorally and electrophysiologically in young and old adults. Audiology, 23(2), 181–194.

[103] Kim, S., Frisina, D. R., & Frisina, R. D. (2002). Effects of age on contralateral suppression of distortion product otoacoustic emissions in human listeners with normal hearing. Audiology and Neurootology, 7(6), 348–357.

[104] Kirikae, I., Sato, T., & Shitara, T. (1964). A study of hearing in advanced age. Laryngoscope, 74, 205–220.

[105] Kjaer, M. (1980). Recognizability of brain stem auditory evoked potential components. Acta Neurologica Scandinavica, 62(1), 20–33.

[106] Konigsmark, B. W., & Murphy, E. A. (1972). Volume of the ventral cochlear nucleus in man: Its relationship to neuronal population and age. Journal of Neuropathology and Experimental Neurology, 31(2), 304–316.

[107] Konkle, D. F., Beasley, D. S., & Bess, F. H. (1977). Intelligibility of time-altered speech in relation to chronological aging. Journal of Speech and Hearing Research, 20(1), 108–115.

[108] Krishnan, A. (2007). Frequency-following response. In R. F. Burkard, J. J. Eggermont, & M. Don (Eds.), Auditory evoked potentials: Basic principles and clinical application (pp. 313-335). Baltimore, MD: Lippincott Williams & Wilkins.

[109] Krull, V., Humes, L. E., & Kidd, G. R. (2013). Reconstructing wholes from parts: Effects of modality, age, and hearing loss on word recognition. Ear and Hearing, 34(2), e14–e23.

[110] Lenzi, A., Chiarelli, G., & Sambataro, G. (1989). Comparative study of middle-latency responses and auditory brainstem responses in elderly subjects. Audiology, 28(3), 144–151.

[111] Letowski, T., & Poch, N. (1996). Comprehension of time-compressed speech: Effects of age and speech complexity. Journal of the American Academy of Audiology, 7(6), 447–457.

[112] Li, L., Huang, J., Wu, X., Qi, J. G., & Schneider, B. A. (2009). The effects of aging and interaural delay on the detection of a break in the interaural correlation between two sounds. Ear and Hearing, 30(2), 273–286.

[113] Mahncke, H. W., Connor, B. B., Appelman, J., et al. (2006). Memory enhancement in healthy older adults using a brain plasticity-based training program: A randomized, controlled study. Proceedings of the National Academy of Sciences of the United States of America, 103(33), 12523–12528.

[114] Mahoney, T., Vernon, J., & Meikle, M. (1979). Function of the acoustic reflex in discrimination of intense speech. Archives of Otolaryngology, 105(3), 119–123.

[115] Makary, C. A., Shin, J., Kujawa, S. G., Liberman, M. C., & Merchant, S. N. (2011). Age-related primary cochlear neuronal degeneration in human temporal bones. Journal of the Association for Research in Otolaryngology, 12(5), 711–717.

[116] Marshall, A. R. (1983). An investigation of the auditory brainstem response in subjects with high frequency cochlear hearing loss. Australian Journal of Audiology, 5(1), 11–18.

[117] Martini, A., Comacchio, F., & Magnavita, V. (1990). Auditory evoked responses (ABR, MLR, SVR) and brain mapping in the elderly. Acta Otolaryngologica (Supplementnum), 476, 97–103, discussion 104.

[118] Martini, A., Comacchio, F., & Magnavita, V. (1991). Auditory brainstem and middle latency evoked responses in the clinical evaluation of diabetes. Diabetic Medicine, 8(Spec. No.), S74–S77.

[119] Maurizi, M., Altissimi, G., Ottaviani, F., Paludetti, G., & Bambini, M. (1982). Auditory brainstem responses (ABR) in the aged. Scandinavian Audiology, 11(4), 213–221.

[120] McClelland, R. J., & McCrea, R. S. (1979). Intersubject variability of the auditory-evoked brain stem potentials. Audiology, 18(6), 462–471.

[121] McCroskey, R. L., & Kasten, R. N. (1980). Assessment of central auditory processing. In R. Rupp & K. Stockdell (Eds.), Speech protocols in audiology. New York: Grune & Stratton.

[122] Moore, B. C., Peters, R. W., & Glasberg, B. R. (1992). Detection of temporal gaps in sinusoids by elderly subjects with and without hearing loss. Journal of the Acoustical Society of America, 92(4, Pt. 1), 1923–1932.

[123] Mouloua, M., & Parasuraman, R. (1995). Aging and cognitive vigilance: Effects of spatial uncertainty and event rate. Experimental Aging Research, 21(1), 17–32.

[124] Mukari, S. Z.-M. S., & Mamat, W. H. W. (2008). Medial olivocochlear functioning and speech perception in noise in older adults. Audiology and Neurootology, 13(5), 328–334.

[125] Oku, T., & Hasegewa, M. (1997). The influence of aging on auditory brainstem response and electrocochleography in the elderly. ORL: Journal for Otorhinolaryngology and Related Specialties, 59(3), 141–146.

[126] Ottaviani, F., Maurizi, M., D'Alatri, L., & Almadori, G. (1990). Auditory brainstem responses in the aged. Acta Otolaryngologica (Supplementum), 476, 110–112, discussion 113.

[127] Otto, W. C., & McCandless, G. A. (1982). Aging and the auditory brain stem response. Audiology, 21(6), 466–473.

[128] Paludetti, G., Maurizi, M., D'Alatri, L., & Galli, J. (1990). Relationships between middle latency auditory responses (MLR) and speech discrimination tests in the elderly. Acta Otolaryngologica (Supplementum), 476, 105–109.

[129] Parasuraman, R., & Giambra, L. (1991). Skill development in vigilance: Effects of event rate and age. Psychology and Aging, 6(2), 155–169.

[130] Parasuraman, R., Warm, J. S., & Dember, W. N. (1987). Vigilance: Taxonomy and utility. In L. S. Mark, J. S.Warm, & R. L. Huston (Eds.), Ergonomics and human factors: Recent research (pp.11–32). New York: Springer-Verlag.

[131] Patterson, J. V., Michalewski, H. J., Thompson, L. W., Bowman, T. E., & Litzelman, D. K. (1981). Age and sex differences in the human auditory brainstem response. Journal of Gerontology, 36(4), 455–462.

[132] Peelle, J. E., McMillan, C., Moore, P., Grossman, M., & Wingfield, A. (2004). Dissociable patterns of brain activity during comprehension of rapid and syntactically complex speech: Evidence from fMRI. Brain and Language, 91(3), 315–325.

[133] Petros, T. V., Zehr, H. D., & Chabot, R. J. (1983). Adult age differences in accessing and retrieving information from long-term memory. Journal of Gerontology, 38(5), 589–592.

[134] Pfefferbaum, A., Ford, J. M., Roth, W. T., & Kopell, B. S. (1980). Age-related changes in auditory event-related potentials. Electroencephalography and Clinical Neurophysiology, 49(3–4), 266–276.

[135] Phillips, S. L., Gordon-Salant, S., Fitzgibbons, P. J., & Yeni-Komshian, G. H. (1994). Auditory duration discrimination in young and elderly listeners with normal hearing. Journal of the American Academy of Audiology, 5(3), 210–215.

[136] Pichora-Fuller, M. K., & Levitt, H. (2012). Speech comprehension training and auditory and cognitive processing in older adults. American Journal of Audiology, 21(2), 351–357.

[137] Pichora-Fuller, M. K., Schneider, B. A., Benson, N. J., Hamstra, S. J., & Storzer, E. (2006). Effect of age on detection of gaps in speech and nonspeech markers varying in duration and spectral symmetry. Journal of the Acoustical Society of America, 119(2), 1143–1155.

[138] Polich, J., Howard, L., & Starr, A. (1985). Effects of age on the P300 component of the event-related potential from auditory stimuli: Peak definition, variation, and measurement. Journal of Gerontology, 40(6), 721–726.

[139] Poth, E. A., Boettcher, F. A., Mills, J. H., & Dubno, J. R. (2001). Auditory brainstem responses in younger and older adults for broadband noises separated by a silent gap. Hearing and Research, 161(1-2), 81–86.

[140] Pronk, M., Deeg, D. J. H., Festen, J. M., et al. (2013). Decline in older persons' ability to recognize speech in noise: The influence of demographic, health-related, environmental, and cognitive factors. Ear and Hearing, 34(6), 722–732.

[141] Qu, T., Cao, S., Chen, X., et al. (2013). Aging effects on detection of spectral changes induced by a break in sound correlation. Ear and Hearing, 34(3), 280–287.

[142] Rabbitt, P., & Birren, J. E. (1967). Age and responses to sequences of repetitive and interruptive signals. Journal of Gerontology, 22(2), 143–150.

[143] Rabbitt, P., Scott, M., Lunn, M., et al. (2007). White matter lesions account for all age-related declines in speed but not in intelligence. Neuropsychology, 21(3), 363–370.

[144] Rawool, V. W. (1989). Speech recognition scores and ABR in cochlear impairment. Scandinavian Audiology, 18(2), 113–117.

[145] Rawool, V. W. (1996). Effect of aging on the click-rate induced facilitation of acoustic reflex thresholds. Journals of Gerontology. Series A, Biological Sciences and Medical Sciences, 51(2), B124–B131.

[146] Rawool, V. W. (1998). Effects of click polarity on the auditory brainstem responses of older men. Audiology, 37(2), 100–108.

[147] Rawool, V. W. (2007a). The aging auditory system: 1. Controversy and confusion on slower processing. Hearing Review, 14(7), 14–22.

[148] Rawool, V. W. (2007b). The aging auditory system: 2. Slower processing and speech recognition. Hearing Review, 14(8), 36, 38, 40, 42, 43.

[149] Rawool, V. W. (2007c). The aging auditory system: 3. Slower processing, cognition, and speech recognition. Hearing Review, 14(9), 38, 43, 44, 46, 48.

[150] Rawool, V. W., & Brouse, M. V. (2010). Effect of contralateral noise on the click-evoked human auditory middle latency response. Hearing Review, 17(6), 24–27, 50–53.

[151] Rawool, V., & Zerlin, S. (1988). Phase-intensity effects on the ABR. Scandinavian Audiology, 17(2), 117–123.

[152] Rikli, R. E., & Edwards, D. J. (1991). Effects of a three-year exercise program on motor function and cognitive processing speed in older women. Research Quarterly for Exercise and Sport, 62(1), 61–67.

[153] Robinson, K., & Rudge, P. (1977). Auditory evoked potentials in man: Psychopharmacology correlates of EPs. In J. E. Desmedt (Ed.), Progress in clinical neurophysiology (Vol. 2, 58–67). Basel, Switzerland: Karger.

[154] Rosenhall, U., Pedersen, K., & Dotevall, M. (1986). Effects of presbycusis and other types of hearing loss on auditory brainstem responses. Scandinavian Audiology, 15(4), 179–185.

[155] Ross, B., Fujioka, T., Tremblay, K. L., & Picton, T. W. (2007). Aging in binaural hearing begins in mid-life: Evidence from cortical auditory-evoked responses to changes in interaural phase. Journal of Neuroscience, 27(42), 11172–11178.

[156] Rouiller, E. M., Capt, M., Dolivo, M., & De Ribaupierre, F. (1989). Neuronal organization of the stapedius reflex pathways in the rat: A retrograde HRP and viral transneuronal tracing study. Brain Research, 476(1), 21–28.

[157] Rowe, M. J., III. (1978). Normal variability of the brain-stem auditory evoked response in young and old adult subjects. Electroencephalography and Clinical Neurophysiology, 44(4), 459–470.

[158] Russo, N. M., Nicol, T. G., Zecker, S. G., Hayes, E. A., & Kraus, N. (2005). Auditory training improves neural timing in the human brainstem. Behavioural Brain Research, 156(1), 95–103.

[159] Salthouse, T. A. (1985). A theory of cognitive aging. Amsterdam: North-Holland.

[160] Salthouse, T. A. (1996). The processing-speed theory of adult age differences in cognition. Psychological Review, 103(3), 403–428.

[161] Salthouse, T. A. (2000). Aging and measures of processing speed. Biological Psychology, 54(1-3), 35–54.

[162] Schaie, K. W. (2005). What can we learn from longitudinal studies of adult development? Research in Human Development, 2(3), 133–158.

[163] Scheibel, M. E., & Scheibel, A. B. (1975). Structural changes in the aging brain. In H. Brody, D. Harman, & J. M. Ordy (Eds.), Aging (Vol. 1, pp. 11–37). New York: Raven Press.

[164] Schmitt, J. F., & Carroll, M. R. (1985). Older listeners' ability to comprehend speaker-generated rate alteration of passages. Journal of Speech and Hearing Research, 28(2), 309–312.

[165] Schneider, B. A., Pichora-Fuller, M. K., Kowalchuk, D., & Lamb, M. (1994). Gap detection and the precedence effect in young and old adults. Journal of the Acoustical Society of America, 95(2), 980–991.

[166] Schneider, B., Speranza, F., & Pichora-Fuller, M. K. (1998). Age-related changes in temporal resolution: Envelope and intensity effects. Canadian Journal of Experimental Psychology, 52(4), 184–191.

[167] Segovia, G., Porras, A., Del Arco, A., & Mora, F. (2001). Glutamatergic neurotransmission in aging: A critical perspective. Mechanisms of Ageing and Development, 122(1), 1–29.

[168] Shanon, E., Gold, S., & Himelfarb, M. Z. (1981). Assessment of functional integrity of brain stem auditory pathways by stimulus stress. Audiology, 20(1), 65–71.

[169] Snell, K. B. (1997). Age-related changes in temporal gap detection. Journal of the Acoustical Society of America, 101(4), 2214–2220.

[170] Snell, K. B., & Frisina, D. R. (2000). Relationships among age-related differences in gap detection and word recognition. Journal of the Acoustical Society of America, 107(3), 1615–1626.

[171] Sommers, M. S. (1997). Speech perception in older adults: The importance of speech-specific cognitive abilities. Journal of the American Geriatric Society, 45(5), 633–637.

[172] Soucek, S., & Mason, S. M. (1992). Effects of adaptation on electrocochleography and auditory brain-stem responses in the elderly. Scandinavian Audiology, 21(3), 149–152.

[173] Soucek, S., Michaels, L., & Mason, S. M. (1990). Electrophysiology. In S. Soucek & L. Michaels (Eds.), Hearing loss in the elderly: Audiometric, electrophysiologic and histopathological aspects (pp. 47-83). London: Springer Verlag.

[174] Sowell, E. R., Peterson, B. S., Thompson, P. M., Welcome, S. E., Henkenius, A. L., & Toga, A. W. (2003). Mapping cortical change across the human life span. Nature Neuroscience, 6(3), 309–315.

[175] Sticht, T. G., & Gray, B. B. (1969). The intelligibility of time compressed words as a function of age and hearing loss. Journal of Speech and Hearing Research, 12(2), 443–448.

[176] Stine, E. L., Wingfield, A., & Poon, L. W. (1986). How much and how fast: Rapid processing of spoken language in later adulthood. Psychology and Aging, 1(4), 303–311.

[177] Stockard, J. J., Stockard, J. E., & Sharbrough, F. W. (1978). Nonpathologic factors influencing brainstem auditory evoked potentials. American Journal of EEG Technology, 18, 177–209.

[178] Strouse, A., Ashmead, D. H., Ohde, R. N., & Grantham, D. W. (1998). Temporal processing in the aging auditory system. Journal of the Acoustical Society of America, 104(4), 2385–2399.

[179] Strouse, A., Wilson, R. H., & Brush, N. (2000). Recognition of dichotic digits under pre-cued and post-cued response conditions in young and elderly listeners. British Journal of Audiology, 34(3), 141–151.

[180] Strutz, J., Münker, G., & Zöllner, C. (1988). The motor innervation of the tympanic muscles in the guinea pig. Archives of Otorhinolaryngology, 245(2), 108–111.

[181] Stuart, A., & Phillips, D. P. (1996). Word recognition in continuous and interrupted broadband noise by young normal-hearing, older normal-hearing, and presbyacusic listeners. Ear and Hearing, 17(6), 478–489.

[182] Stürzebecher, E., & Werbs, M. (1987). Effects of age and sex on auditory brain stem response: A new aspect. Scandinavian Audiology, 16(3), 153–157.

[183] Szelag, E., Szymaszek, A., Aksamit-Ramotowska, A., et al. (2011). Temporal processing as a base for language universals: Cross-linguistic comparisons on sequencing abilities with some implications for language therapy. Restorative Neurology and Neuroscience, 29(1), 35–45.

[184] Thomas, P. D., Hunt, W. C., Garry, P. J., Hood, R. B., Goodwin, J. M., & Goodwin, J. S. (1983). Hearing acuity in a healthy elderly population: Effects on emotional, cognitive, and social status. Journal of Gerontology, 38(3), 321–325.

[185] Thornton, A. R. D. (1987). Stimulus, recording and subject factors influencing ABR diagnostic criteria. British Journal of Audiology, 21(3), 183–189.

[186] Tremblay, K. L., Piskosz, M., & Souza, P. (2003). Effects of age and age-related hearing loss on the neural representation of speech cues. Clinical Neurophysiology, 114(7), 1332–1343.

[187] van Rooij, J. C., & Plomp, R. (1990). Auditive and cognitive factors in speech perception by elderly listeners: 2. Multivariate analyses. Journal of the Acoustical Society of America, 88(6), 2611–2624.

[188] van Rooij, J. C., Plomp, R., & Orlebeke, J. F. (1989). Auditive and cognitive factors in speech perception by elderly listeners:. 1. Development of test battery. Journal of the Acoustical Society of America, 86(4), 1294–1309.

[189] Veneman, C. E., Gordon-Salant, S., Matthews, L. J., & Dubno, J. R. (2013). Age and measurement time-of-day effects on speech recognition in noise. Ear and Hearing, 34(3), 288–299.

[190] Versfeld, N. J., & Dreschler, W. A. (2002). The relationship between the intelligibility of time-compressed speech and speech in noise in young and elderly listeners. Journal of the Acoustical Society of America, 111(1, Pt. 1), 401–408.

[191] von Wedel, H. (1979). Differences in brain stem response with age and sex. Scandinavian Audiology Supplement, 9, 205–209.

[192] Wadley, V. G., Benz, R. L., Ball, K. K., Roenker, D. L., Edwards, J. D., & Vance, D. E. (2006). Development and evaluation of home-based speed-of-processing training for older adults. Archives of Physical Medicine and Rehabilitation, 87(6), 757–763.

[193] Walton, J., Orlando, M., & Burkard, R. (1999). Auditory brainstem response forward-masking recovery functions in older humans with normal hearing. Hearing Research, 127(1-2), 86–94.

[194] Wambacq, I. J. A., Koehnke, J., Besing, J., Romei, L. L., Depierro, A., & Cooper, D. (2009). Processing interaural cues in sound segregation by young and middle-aged brains. Journal of the American Academy of Audiology, 20(7), 453–458.

[195] Wang, M., Wu, X., Li, L., & Schneider, B. A. (2011). The effects of age and interaural delay on detecting a change in interaural correlation: The role of temporal jitter. Hearing Research, 275(1-2), 139–149.

[196] Wharton, J. A., & Church, G. T. (1990). Influence of menopause on the auditory brainstem response. Audiology, 29(4), 196–201.

[197] Wingfield, A., Poon, L. W., Lombardi, L., & Lowe, D. (1985). Speed of processing in normal aging: Effects of speech rate, linguistic structure, and processing time. Journal of Gerontology, 40(5), 579–585.

[198] Woods, D. L., & Clayworth, C. C. (1986). Age-related changes in human middle latency auditory evoked potentials. Electroencephalography and Clinical Neurophysiology, 65(4), 297–303.

[199] Yilmaz, S. T., Sennaroğlu, G., Sennaroğlu, L., & Köse, S. K. (2007). Effect of age on speech recognition in noise and on contralateral transient evoked otoacoustic emission suppression. Journal of Laryngology and Otology, 121(11), 1029–1034.

Index